Current Techniques in
Operative Neurosurgery

Current Techniques in Operative Neurosurgery

edited by

Henry H. Schmidek, M.D., F.A.C.S.

Professor and Chairman,
Department of Neurosurgery
Hahnemann Medical College and Hospital
Philadelphia, Pennsylvania

and

William H. Sweet, M.D., D.Sc., F.A.C.S.

Professor of Surgery,
Harvard Medical School;
Chief of the Neurosurgical Service,
Massachusetts General Hospital
Boston, Massachusetts

GRUNE & STRATTON
A Subsidiary of Harcourt Brace Jovanovich, Publishers
New York San Francisco London

Library of Congress Cataloging in Publication Data

Hahnemann Symposium on Current Techniques in
Operative Neurosurgery, New York, 1976
Current techniques in operative neurosurgery.

Papers of a symposium was sponsored by
Hahnemann Medical College and Hospital of
Philadelphia.
Includes bibliographical references and index.
1. Nervous system—Surgery—Congresses.
I. Schmidek, Henry H. II. Sweet, William Herbert,
1910- III. Hahnemann Medical College and
Hospital of Philadelphia. III. Hahnemann Medical
College and Hospital of Philadelphia. IV. Title.
[DNLM: 1. Neurosurgery—Methods—Congresses.

WL368 H148c 1976]
RD593.H28 1976 617'.48 77-21649
ISBN 0-8089-1026-4

Grune & Stratton, Inc.
111 Fifth Avenue
New York, New York 10003

Distributed in the United Kingdom by
Academic Press, Inc. (London) Ltd.
24/28 Oval Road, London NW 1

Library of Congress Catalog Number 77-21649
International Standard Book Number 0-8089-1026-4

Printed in the United States of America

To our wives
and to Ian,
Alexandra, and
Jared.

CONTENTS

PREFACE

The increase in the diversity and complexity of neurosurgical procedures over the past decade dictates the need for a text dealing with these technical advances. This book is deliberately circumscribed to allow a detailed discussion of these procedures, their indications, and the intraoperative, preoperative, and postoperative management of the patient. Included are a spectrum of procedures ranging from those which are now standard but which deserve periodic review to those in which the clinical experience is inadequate but have a place in our armamentarium. Commissural myelotomy and longitudinal (Bishof's) myelotomy are examples of this latter category. We have major reservations about the place of the limited differential form of spinal posterior rhizotomy. Total trigeminal posterior rhizotomy carries with it a great likelihood of annoying denervation dysesthesias progressing all the way to a disabling anesthesia dolorosa. After total rhizotomy of one or more spinal posterior roots, such sensory sequelae are far less frequent. Moreover, idiopathic trigeminal neuralgia, the main indication for trigeminal denervation procedures, requires a much less thorough denervation for relief than is the case for the pain of disorders treated by spinal rhizotomy. Indeed the indications for even extensive total spinal rhizotomy are subjudice at present. However, the percutaneous operation is simpler than the open one and we agree that a few careful surgeons are appropriately attempting to determine what place it has, if any.

Special comments with respect to some of the chapters are in order. Re Chapters 6 and 17, on tumors of the glomus jugulare and the transbasal approach to tumors of the cranial base—a tour de force may be defined as a feat of endurance, skill or ingenuity. All three of these qualities are required to carry through to success, the major surgical tours de force described in these two chapters. An essential indication for doing such procedures is the likelihood that the neurosurgeons will be called on with some frequency to do such demanding operations. Indeed, even those who are already doing the tougher types of neurosurgery would perhaps do well to watch Dr. Robertson or Dr. Derome in action before undertaking their own first case of the type they describe.

By far the most controversial chapter for inclusion is the final one on "Posterior Lumbosacral Facet Coagulation." This is an accurate description of what is being attempted; however, the reservations regarding this operation are sufficiently vehement so that one of the editors has placed his comments in direct conjunction with the chapter.

The editors wish to thank our colleagues-coauthors for the major effort they have made in the preparation of their chapters and are hopeful that this book will be helpful to the neurosurgical fraternity. We would also like to thank Ms. Jane Krumrine and Mr. Robert Schaeffer of the Department of Continuing Education, Hahnemann Medical College and Hospital, Mrs. Audrey Simon of the Department of Neurosurgery, and Ms. Christine Russo, Medical Editor, for the editing and technical preparation of this book.

Henry H. Schmidek, M.D.
William H. Sweet, M.D., D.Sc.

August, 1977

CONTRIBUTORS

John E. Adams, M.D. *Guggenheim Professor, Department of Neurological Surgery, University of California Medical Center, San Francisco, California*

Ronald Brisman, M.D. *Associate in Neurological Surgery, New York Neurological Institute, Columbia-Presbyterian Medical Center; Columbia University, College of Physicians and Surgeons, New York, New York*

William A. Buchheit, M.D. *Professor and Chairman, Department of Neurosurgery, Temple University Hospital, Philadelphia, Pennsylvania*

Paul H. Chapman, M.D. *Assistant in Neurosurgery, Massachusetts General Hospital, Boston, Massachusetts*

Edwin W. Cocke, Jr., M.D. *Clinical Professor, Department of Otolaryngology and Maxillofacial Surgery, University of Tennessee Center for the Health Sciences, Memphis, Tennessee*

Louis W. Conway, M.D. *Department of Neurosurgery, Arnett Clinic and Hospital, Inc., Lafayette, Indiana*

Robert M. Crowell, M.D. *Assistant Visiting Neurosurgeon and Director, Microneurosurgical Laboratory, Neurosurgical Service, Massachusetts General Hospital and the Harvard Medical School, Boston, Massachusetts*

Charles W. Cummings, M.D. *Associate Professor, Department of Otolaryngology, State University Hospital, Upstate Medical Center, Syracuse, New York*

G. Debrun, M.D. *Department of Neuroradiology, University Hôpital, Henri Mondor, Creteil, France*

Patrick J. Derome, M.D. *Neurosurgeon, Hôpital Foch, St. Cloud, France*

Bernard E. Finneson, M.D. *Chief of Neurological Surgery, Crozer-Chester Medical Center; and Clinical Associate Professor, Department of Neurosurgery, Hahnemann Medical College and Hospital, Philadelphia, Pennsylvania*

Gale Gardner, M.D. *Assistant Professor, Department of Otolaryngology and Maxillofacial Surgery, University of Tennessee Center for the Health Sciences, Memphis, Tennessee*

J. Leonard Goldner, M.D. *Professor of Orthopaedic Surgery, Division of Orthopaedic Surgery, Duke University School of Medicine, Durham, North Carolina*

Robert R. Hansebout, M.D. *Associate Professor, Department of Neurology and Neurosurgery, McGill University; and Associate Neurosurgeon, Montreal Neurological Hospital and Institute, Montreal, Quebec, Canada*

Edgar M. Housepian, M.D. *Professor of Clinical Neurological Surgery, College of Physicians and Surgeons, Columbia University; and the New York Neurological Institute, Columbia-Presbyterian Medical Center, New York*

Yoshio Hosobuchi, M.D. *Associate Professor, Department of Neurological Surgery, University of California Medical Center, San Francisco, California*

Leslie P. Ivan, M.D. *Head, Division of Neurosurgery, Children's Hospital of Eastern Ontario, Ottawa, Ontario, Canada*

Craig H. Johnson, M.D. *Department of Neurosurgery, Temple University Hospital, Philadelphia, Pennsylvania*

Jonas Johnson, M.D. *Resident Otolaryngologist, State University Hospital, Upstate Medical Center, Syracuse, New York*

Edward R. Laws, Jr., M.D. *Assistant Professor, Department of Neurologic Surgery, Mayo Medical School, Mayo Clinic and Research Foundation, Rochester, Minnesota*

Robert D. Leffert, M.D. *Visiting Orthopaedic Surgeon and Chief, Department of Rehabilitation Medicine, Massachusetts General Hospital; and Assistant Professor, Department of Orthopaedic Surgery, Harvard Medical School, Boston, Massachusetts*

Paul M. Lin, M.D., M.Sc. *Clinical Associate Professor, Department of Neurological Surgery, Temple University Health Sciences Center, Philadelphia, Pennsylvania*

Robert Lippert, M.D. *Department of Neurological Surgery, University of California Medical Center, San Francisco, California*

Lester A. Mount, M.D. *Emeritus Professor of Clinical Neurological Surgery, College of Physicians and Surgeons, Columbia University; and The New York Neurological Institute, Columbia-Presbyterian Medical Center, New York*

Sean Mullan, M.D. *Professor and Chairman, Department of Neurosurgery, Pritzker School of Medicine, University of Chicago, Chicago, Illinois*

Ralph Rashbaum, M.D. *Division of Neurosurgery, University of Pennsylvania School of Medicine and Pennsylvania Hospital, Philadelphia, Pennsylvania*

Albert L. Rhoton, Jr., M.D. *Professor and Chief, Division of Neurological Surgery, University of Florida Health Center, Gainesville, Florida*

Howard A. Richter, M.D. *Chief, Department of Neurosurgery, Lankenau Hospital; and Clinical Assistant Professor, Department of Neurosurgery, Jefferson Medical College, Philadelphia, Pennsylvania*

James T. Robertson, M.D. *Professor and Chairman, Department of Neurosurgery, University of Tennessee Center for the Health Sciences, Memphis, Tennessee*

Robert A. Robinson, M.D. *Professor and Chairman, Department of Orthopaedic Surgery, The Johns Hopkins University School of Medicine; and Orthopaedic Surgeon-in-Charge, The Johns Hopkins Hospital, Baltimore, Maryland*

Bertram Selverstone, M.D. *Clinical Professor of Surgery (Neurosurgery), Brown University School of Medicine; and Director, Division of Neurosurgery, Miriam and Roger Williams Hospitals, Providence, Rhode Island*

Henry H. Schmidek, M.D. *Professor and Chairman, Department of Neurosurgery, Hahnemann Medical College and Hospital, Philadelphia, Pennsylvania*

Frederick A. Simeone, M.D. *Division of Neurosurgery, University of Pennsylvania School of Medicine; and Chief, Department of Neurosurgery, The Elliot Neurological Center of the Pennsylvania Hospital, Philadelphia, Pennsylvania*

Bennett M. Stein, M.D. *Professor and Chairman, Department of Neurosurgery, New England Medical Center, Boston, Massachusetts*

William H. Sweet, M.D., D.Sc. *Professor of Surgery, Harvard Medical School; and Chief, Neurosurgical Service, Massachusetts General Hospital, Boston, Massachusetts*

Edward Tarlov, M.D. *Assistant in Neurosurgery, Neurosurgical Service, Massachusetts General Hospital, Boston, Massachusetts*

John McLellan Tew, Jr., M.D. *Mayfield Neurological Institute, Cincinnati, Ohio*

Sumio Uematsu, M.D. *Assistant Professor, Department of Neurosurgery, The Johns Hopkins University School of Medicine, Baltimore, Maryland*

James R. Urbaniak, M.D. *Professor of Orthopaedic Surgery, Division of Orthopaedic Surgery, Duke University School of Medicine, Durham, North Carolina*

Kenneth E. Wood, M.D. *Senior Resident, Division of Orthopaedic Surgery, Duke University School of Medicine, Durham, North Carolina*

Nicholas T. Zervas, M.D. *Professor of Surgery (elect), Harvard Medical School; and Chief (elect), Neurosurgical Service, Massachusetts General Hospital, Boston, Massachusetts*

Current Techniques in
Operative Neurosurgery

CHAPTER 1
Direct Brain Revascularization

Robert M. Crowell

ISCHEMIC INFARCTION IS CAUSED by cerebrovascular occlusion with decreased blood flow. Surgical restoration of cerebral blood flow is, therefore, logical therapy to prevent ischemic stroke.

Cerebral revascularization by carotid endarterectomy can often benefit patients with extracranial occlusive disease.[1] Occlusive cerebrovascular disease, however, frequently affects intracranial arteries inaccessible to carotid endarterectomy.[2] Logical surgery for such cases is direct cerebral revascularization, including cerebral embolectomy and bypass procedures. These delicate procedures have become feasible only since the development of microneurosurgery.[3-5] Early results are tentative but promising, especially for superficial temporal-middle cerebral (STA-MCA) bypass. This report reviews procedures for direct cerebral revascularization; STA-MCA bypass is described in detail.

Procedures

Middle Cerebral Artery Embolectomy

Middle cerebral artery (MCA) embolectomy represents the most direct therapy for MCA embolic occlusion (Fig. 1-1).[6-8] Microsurgical methods may frequently restore MCA patency but rarely avert infarction. Reversible ischemia ripens to irreversible infarction faster than the surgeon opens the occlusion. At present MCA embolectomy cannot be recommended as standard therapy.

Long Grafts

For inaccessible internal carotid artery (ICA) lesions bypass grafting is a reasonable surgical approach (Fig. 1-2). To provide high flow, several authors have recommended interposition of free grafts between common carotid and cerebral vessels (ICA or MCA).[9-12] Early reports have indicated high flow (up to 300 ml/min), high morbidity and mortality (up to 30%), and low long-term patency (about 50%). A graft to a frontal branch of MCA may diminish complications.[12] In view of results to date, long grafting remains experimental.

Neurosurgical Service, Massachusetts General Hospital and Harvard Medical School, Boston, Massachusetts 02114

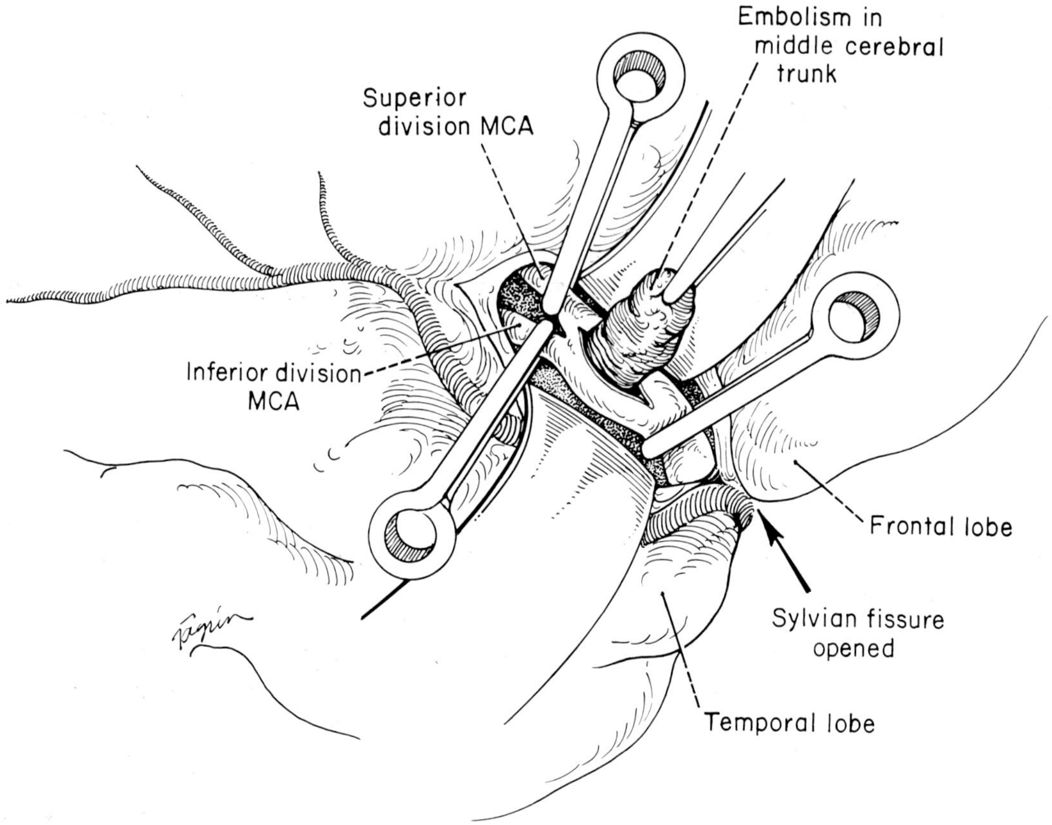

Fig. 1-1. Middle cerebral embolectomy. The right Sylvian fissure has been split to expose MCA. After Scoville clips are placed, the embolus is removed via microsurgical arterotomy. Finally MCA arterotomy is closed with microsuture technique.

Occipital-Posterior Inferior Cerebellar Artery (Occipital-PICA) Bypass

Recently this procedure (Fig. 1-3) has been used in a few cases for posterior circulation revascularization.[13-15] Technical feasibility and relative safety are established, but indications are unknown.

Superficial Temporal-Middle Cerebral Artery (STA-MCA) Bypass

STA-MCA bypass (Fig. 1-4) is presently the most promising form of direct cerebral revascularization, and the remainder of this report focuses on this procedure.

In 1967 Donaghy and Yasargil[3-4] first used microsurgical methods for STA-MCA bypass in man. Reichman[16] suggested several alterations in technique, including the use of two separate STA-MCA anastomoses, interrupted sutures tied down after all are placed, and bevelling of STA to promote flow back toward the MCA origin. Chater[2,17] recommended using the large angular branch of MCA to enhance flow and patency rates. Chater also advocated the use of a small Teflon cranioplastic button. Robertson[18] has proposed linear incision, instead of a flap, to accelerate surgery and preserve STA vasa vasorum. A short vein graft between STA and MCA has been proposed by Tew[19] to enhance flow.

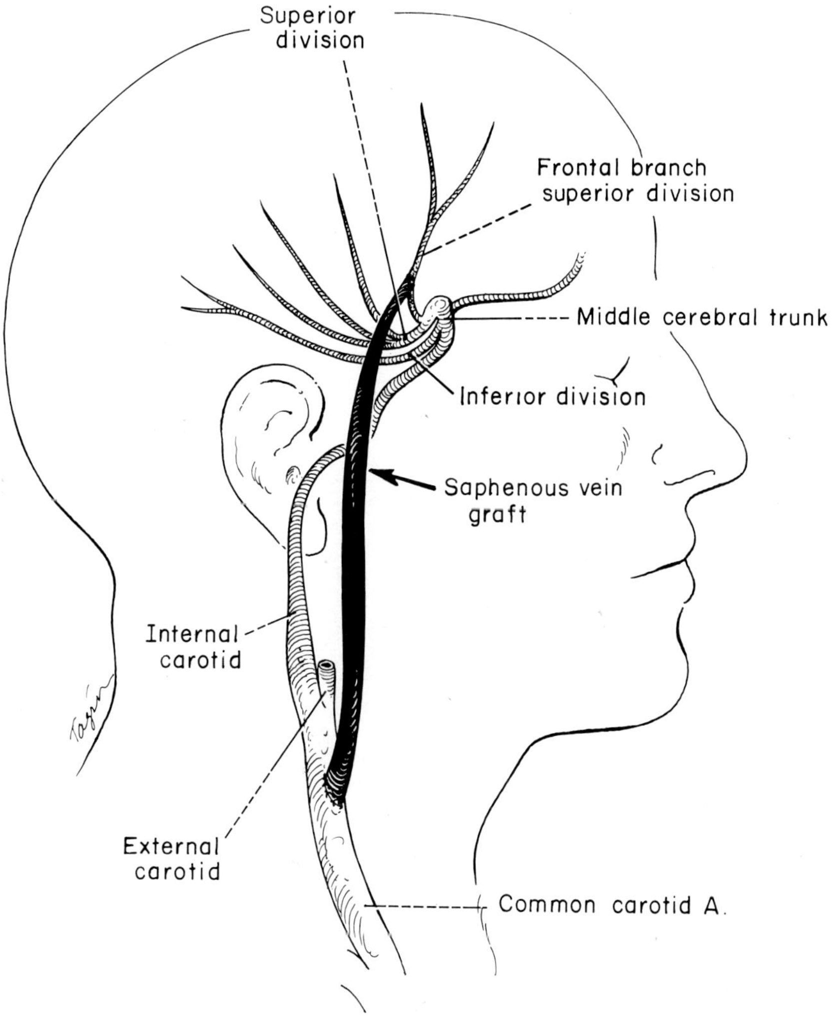

Fig. 1-2. Long graft. A free graft of saphenous vein (or radial artery) is interposed between common carotid and an MCA branch. Long grafts give high flow revascularization of the anterior circulation.

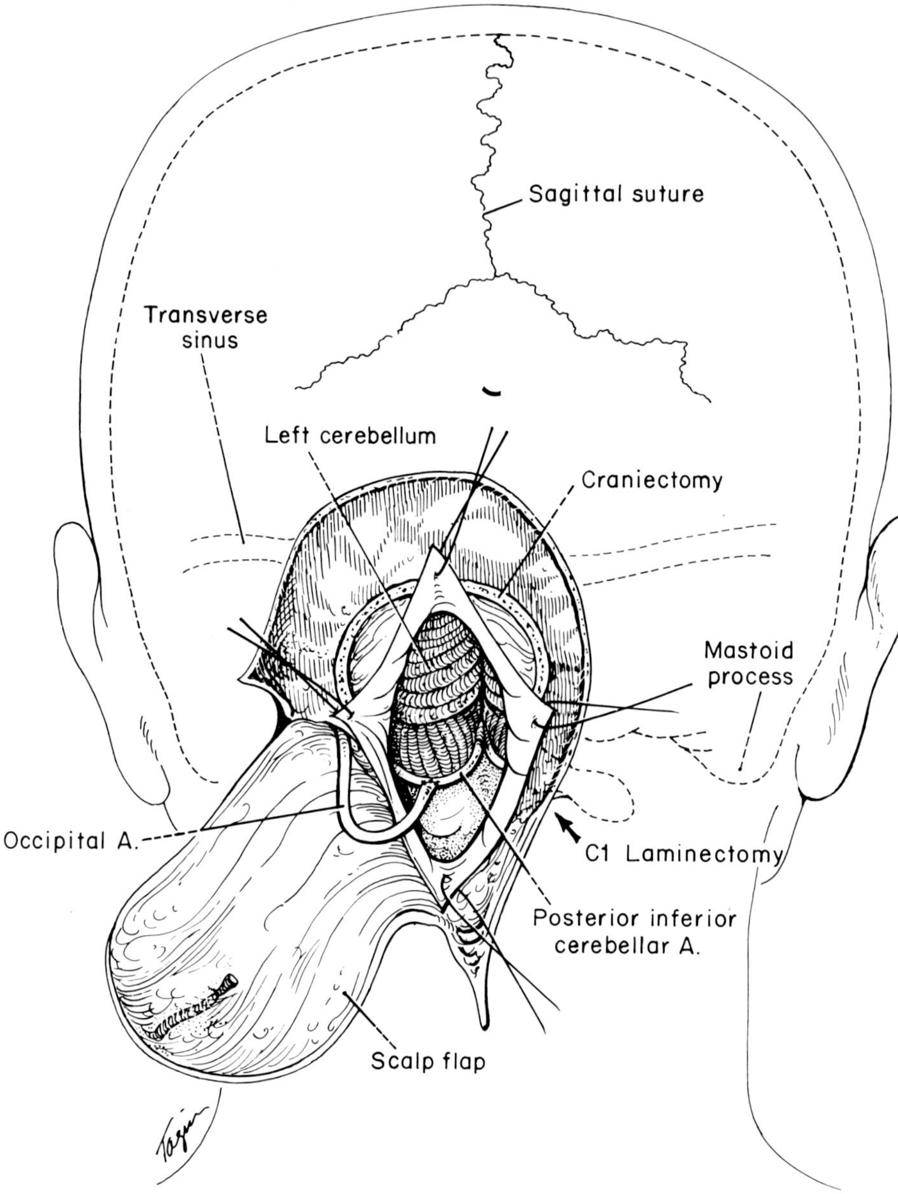

Fig. 1-3. Occipital-PICA graft. Suboccipital craniectomy and C1 laminectomy provide exposure of PICA caudal loop. Occipital artery anastomosis to PICA creates a new collateral to the posterior circulation.

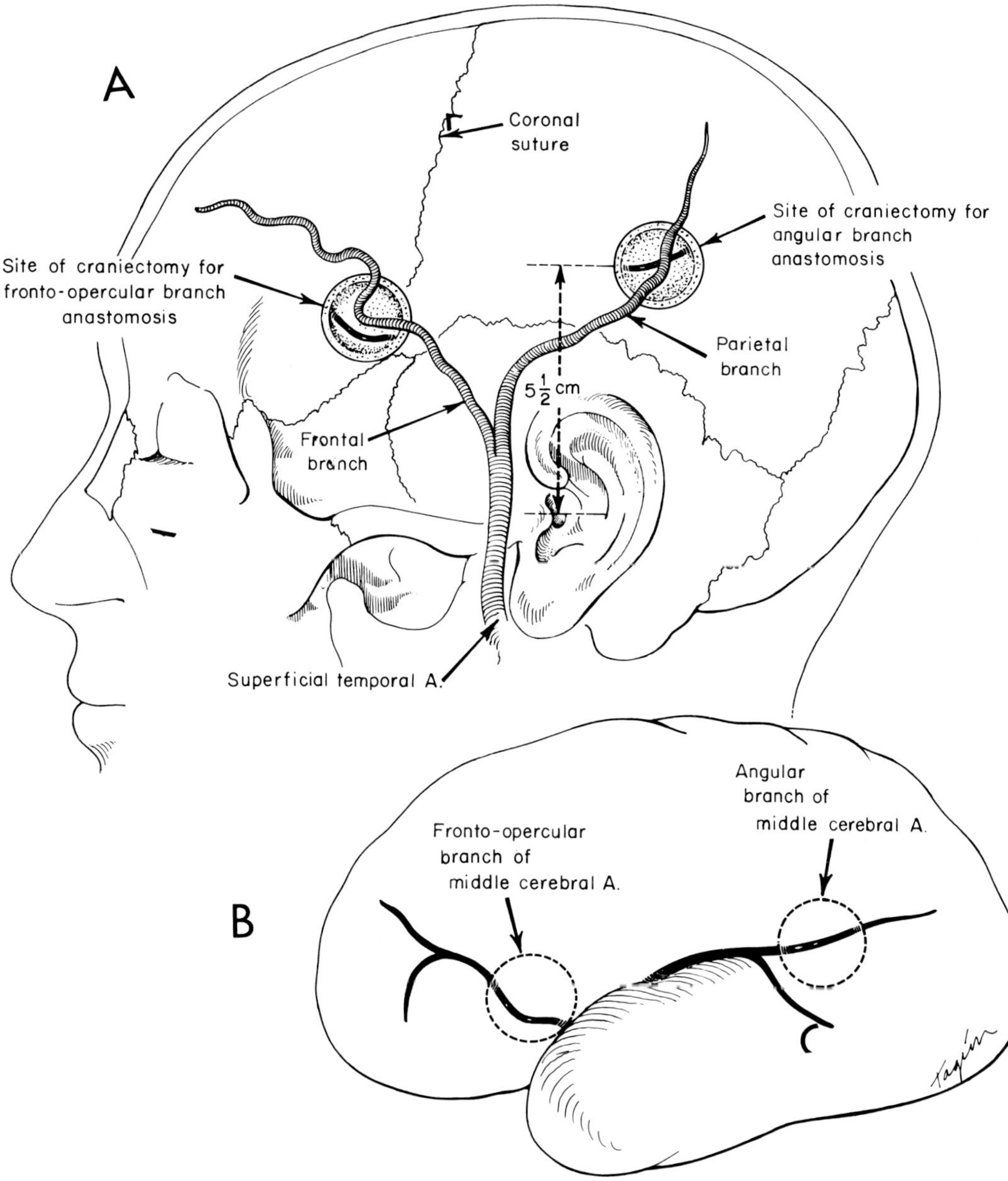

Fig. 1-4. Superficial temporal-middle cerebral artery bypass. **A.** Location of superficial temporal artery (STA) and branches. Craniectomy sites are indicated for exposure of MCA branches. **B.** Location of cortical branches of MCA used for bypass.

The therapeutic role of STA-MCA bypass has not been fully defined. However, in selected cases, STA-MCA bypass carries a low risk and appears to diminish the incidence of TIAs and infarctions.[2,4-5,16-17] Regional cerebral blood flow (rCBF) studies may assist in defining the indications for this procedure.[20-21]

Indications

In general this procedure is logical therapy for symptomatic cerebral ischemia inaccessible to carotid endarterectomy. Several tentative indications have been proposed:

1. *TIAs*. Bypass is probably best employed to prevent the evolution of TIAs into a frank stroke. Thus the best clinical indication is focal TIAs with paresis, paresthesiae, or dysphasia related to inaccessible ICA or MCA stenosis or occlusion.[2,4-5,16-17,20-22]
2. *Slow strokes*. Bypass may arrest or even reverse the gradual evolution (over days) of a stepwise ischemic stroke.[14,23]
3. *Planned occlusions*. Initial bypass grafting may provide needed cerebral collateral when carotid (or MCA) occlusion must be done for aneurysm.[4,24]
4. *Progressive dementia*. Multiple occlusions may rarely cause generalized hypoperfusion with dementia. STA-MCA grafting may reverse such syndromes.[25-26]
5. *Acute strokes*. Some evidence suggests emergency bypass may avert infarction,[27] but clinical data so far have not established a role for such surgery.[28]

Contraindications

Fixed deficits, even when moderate, are not improved through bypass grafting.[22] STA or MCA branches under 0.8 mm preclude useful bypass. When an embolic mechanism is likely, bypass probably will not help. Surgery is hazardous with extreme old age, severe cardiopulmonary disease, and uncontrolled diabetes and hypertension.

Preoperative Evaluation

Careful history taking is often crucial in establishing the indication for bypass (eg., TIAs). Physical examination should include careful palpation of STAs to help determine the suitability for bypass. Preoperative studies should include EKG, serum triglycerides, and serum cholesterol. In many cases cardiologic evaluation will be needed. Computed tomographic scanning identifies infarctions and unanticipated pathology (eg., tumors), which may preclude surgery. Transfemoral three-vessel angiography is essential to delineate cerebrovascular occlusions, collateral circulation, and potential bypass vessels. rCBF studies may be helpful in identifying candidates for surgery.[20-21]

Operative Technique

Yasargil and Donaghy[3,4] established the basic approach. Others have added modifications.[2,16-18]

Anesthesia

Atropine and Droperidol are given as premedication, and the patient's legs are wrapped prior to induction. General endotracheal anesthesia is used, usually halothane or a balanced technique (nitrous oxide, Innovar, and curare). Controlled ventilation is preferred. Precordial electrodes provide continuous EKG monitoring. A radial arterial line permits continuous blood pressure monitoring on a Tektronix portable oscilloscope. Infusions of colloid, dopamine, or nitroprusside maintain blood pressure in the normal range (for the individual patient) during induction and surgery. Arterial blood gases are sampled intermittently, and Pco_2 is maintained at 35 to 40 mmHg. Only in particularly long procedures is a Foley catheter inserted; for example, when the internal carotid artery is explored prior to STA-MCA grafting. Oxacillin is given prior to incision and for 48 hours after surgery; 2 g are administered intravenously every 6 hours.

Positioning

The patient lies supine, with the head turned away from the side to be operated. The operating table is flexed slightly so the head is above heart level. A small roll serves to elevate the shoulder on the side of surgery. The head rests on a doughnut. The operating table is tilted with the *side* adjustment to bring the temporal squama parallel to the floor. The side of the head is shaved to within 2 cm of the midline and well behind the ear when the angular branch of MCA is to be used.

Instruments

In addition to the usual craniotomy kit, several microsurgical instruments are essential. The Zeiss operating microscope No. 1 is preferred, with a 250-mm objective, 160-mm angled oculars, and 12.5× high-eyepoint eyepieces. The stereoscopic binocular observer tube is attached to the scope via a small beam splitter. (For a right-handed surgeon, the assistant is on the left to allow free access of the surgeon's dominant hand to the scrub nurse.) A No. 5 Dumont jeweler's forceps, adapted for bipolar coagulation, is required for precision hemostasis. A No. 5 Dumont jeweler's forceps and a 5-inch iris scissors serve well to prepare small arteries. Scoville clips (1 × 10 mm) are satisfactory for temporary occlusions. Miniature Gelpi retractors help to maintain exposure. A short blade-breaker holds a broken Gillette *Blue Blade*, which is used to incise the cortical vessel. Fine silastic tubing (0.025-inch outside diameter) serves as a stent during suturing. The anastomosis is performed with a 5-inch Barraquer curved needle holder and 10-0 monofilament nylon suture on a BV-6 needle (Ethicon).

Incision

Linear skin incisions permit (a) rapid STA preparation with preservation of vasa vasorum, and (b) satisfactory cortical exposure without large flaps and attendant edge necrosis. One or two incisions may be needed: one incision is always made over the larger STA branch (frontal or parietal) (Fig. 1-4). On the nondominant side, the angular MCA branch is exposed, either through an extension of the incision over frontal STA or through a separate incision when frontal STA is used. On the dominant side, a fronto-opercular MCA branch is exposed, either through the incision over frontal STA or through a separate incision when parietal STA is used.

The initial incision is made over the largest branch of STA. The course of this vessel is marked with a marking pen before induction of anesthesia (which often makes the vessel harder to palpate). Subcutaneous injection of local anesthetic is omitted. To avoid injury to the STA branch, the initial incision with a No. 15 blade is made only down to fat. Then surgeon and assistant elevate the scalp tissue with fine neurosurgical tissue forceps, and the plane superficial to STA is developed with Metzenbaum scissors. In this way a length of STA is exposed (Fig. 1-5).

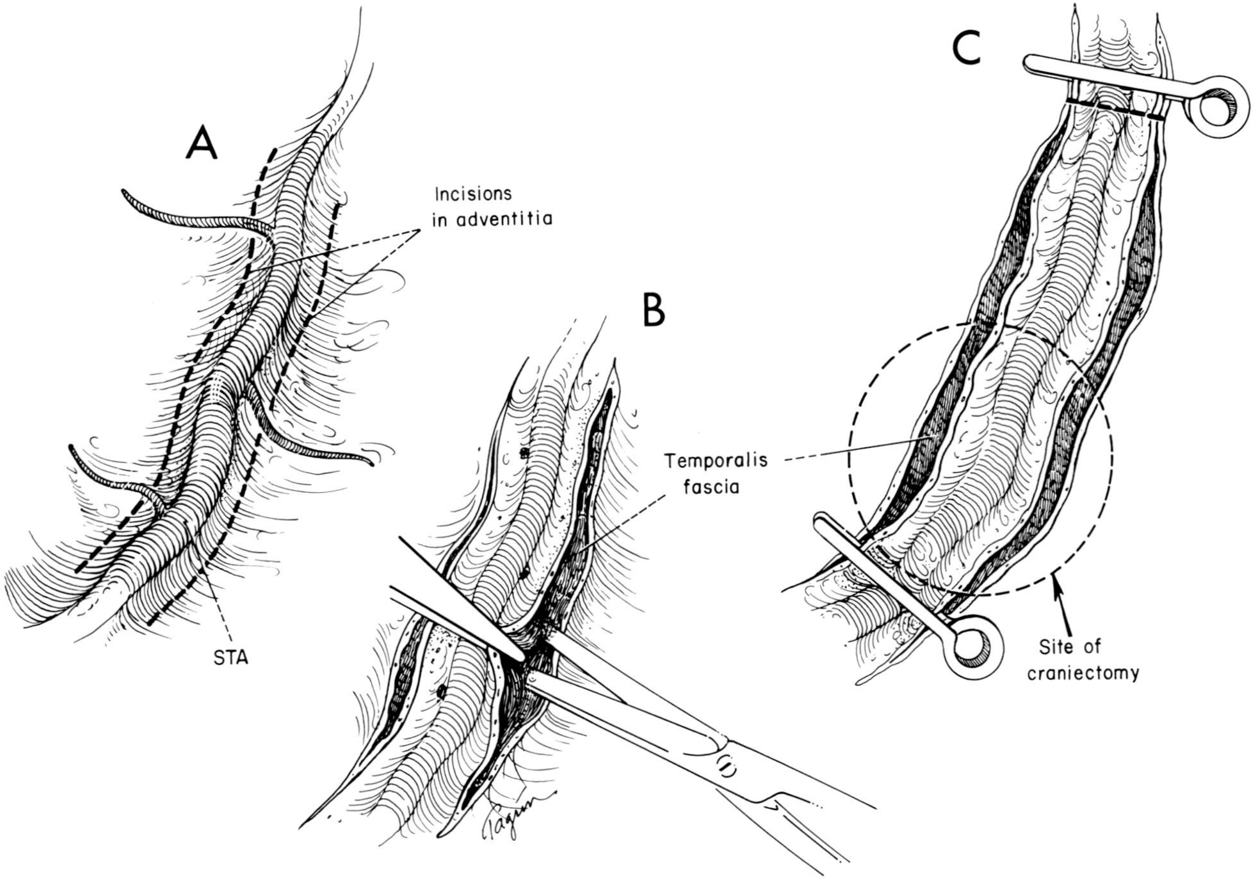

Fig. 1-5. STA-MCA bypass technique: STA preparation. **A.** Exposure. **B.** Undermining. **C.** Mobilization.

STA Preparation

Small flaps of scalp, about 1 cm wide, are elevated on each side of STA (Fig. 1-5). Miniature Gelpi retractors maintain exposure. Adventitia is incised, with a No. 15 blade, down to temporalis fascia, about 5 mm to each side of STA. Branches larger than 0.5 mm are divided between 4-0 silk ligatures. Other side branches and small bleeders are coagulated with a standard bipolar cautery. To facilitate these maneuvers, the surgeon uses the knife and a forceps, and the assistant uses a sucker and bipolar cautery. With a few spreading moves, the Metzenbaum scissors develop the plane between STA and temporalis fascia, thus completing isolation of the vessel. After isolation of the MCA branch segment (described below), the STA is further prepared. Satisfactory graft length is confirmed, and Scoville clips are applied at both ends. The distal end is cross-cut. A jeweler's forceps is used to dilate the STA tip. Flow against zero resistance is measured into a beaker. Heparinized saline is flushed into the STA through a No. 20 Medicut catheter, which is tied into the vessel with a 4-0 silk suture. This irrigation flushes out blood and helps to identify potential bleeders on the graft itself.

In some cases the STA segment must be brought from one incision to another. A tunnel is prepared by blunt dissection between galea and temporalis fascia. The STA tip is pulled through the tunnel by a terminal silk tie. Twists in STA are avoided.

MCA Preparation

Before surgery, the MCA branch for anastomosis is selected and its position marked on the scalp (Fig. 1-6). The angular branch is generally 5½ to 7 cm rostral to the external auditory canal. Fronto-opercular vessels can be used on the dominant hemisphere, just in

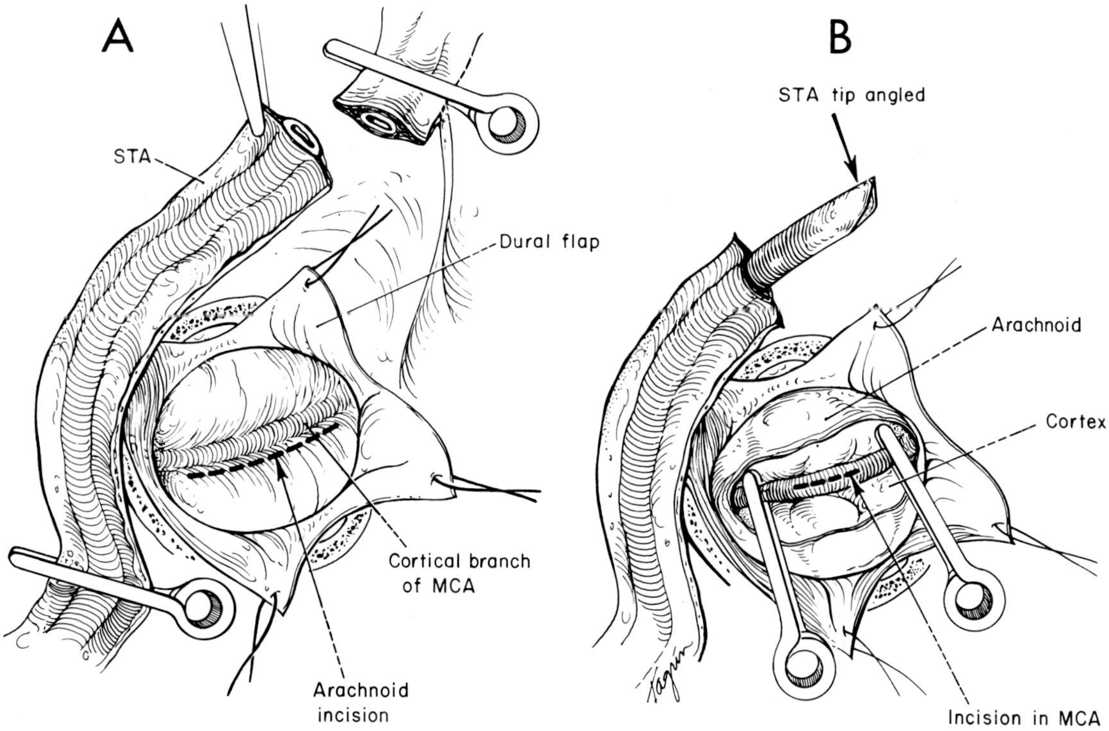

Fig. 1-6. STA-MCA bypass technique: MCA preparation. **A.** Craniectomy and dural opening expose MCA cortical branch. STA is routed to MCA. **B.** Arachnoid is opened, clips applied, and MCA arterotomy performed. STA tip has been freed of adventitia and tailored.

front of the coronal suture. An appropriate scalp incision, either that for STA exposure or a separate one, is made over the MCA branch to be used. Temporalis fascia and muscle are opened with cutting cautery. A burr hole is placed over the MCA branch. If meningeal arteries are encountered, their angiographic location vis-a-vis the MCA branch can direct further limited craniectomy for exposure. The dura is opened, and the craniectomy enlarged as needed to expose an adequate MCA branch. Bone edges are waxed, and dural to pericranial sutures are placed.

At 16× magnification, the arachnoid over MCA is cut with scissors. With the bipolar cautery set low (0-15), up to three small side branches may be coagulated, as needed, to prepare a 1-cm segment. (Generally one or two large side branches can be preserved by using temporary clips.) A strip of rubber dam is eased under the MCA to protect the cortex.

Tailoring of Vessels

The STA is cut at a length long enough to allow exposure of front and back suture lines (Figs. 1-6 and 1-7). The terminal 1 to 2 cm of adventitia is then excised. This maneuver, which permits enhanced exposure for suturing, is facilitated by the simultaneous use of three jeweler's forceps and a scissors at 16 to 25×. The STA tip is tailored to a curving bevel at 45° to the vessel's axis. The tip is dilated with a jeweler's forceps.

Final preparation of the MCA is achieved under 25× magnification, with the STA tip in full view. Scoville clips are placed on MCA, at least 8 mm apart. A short longitudinal

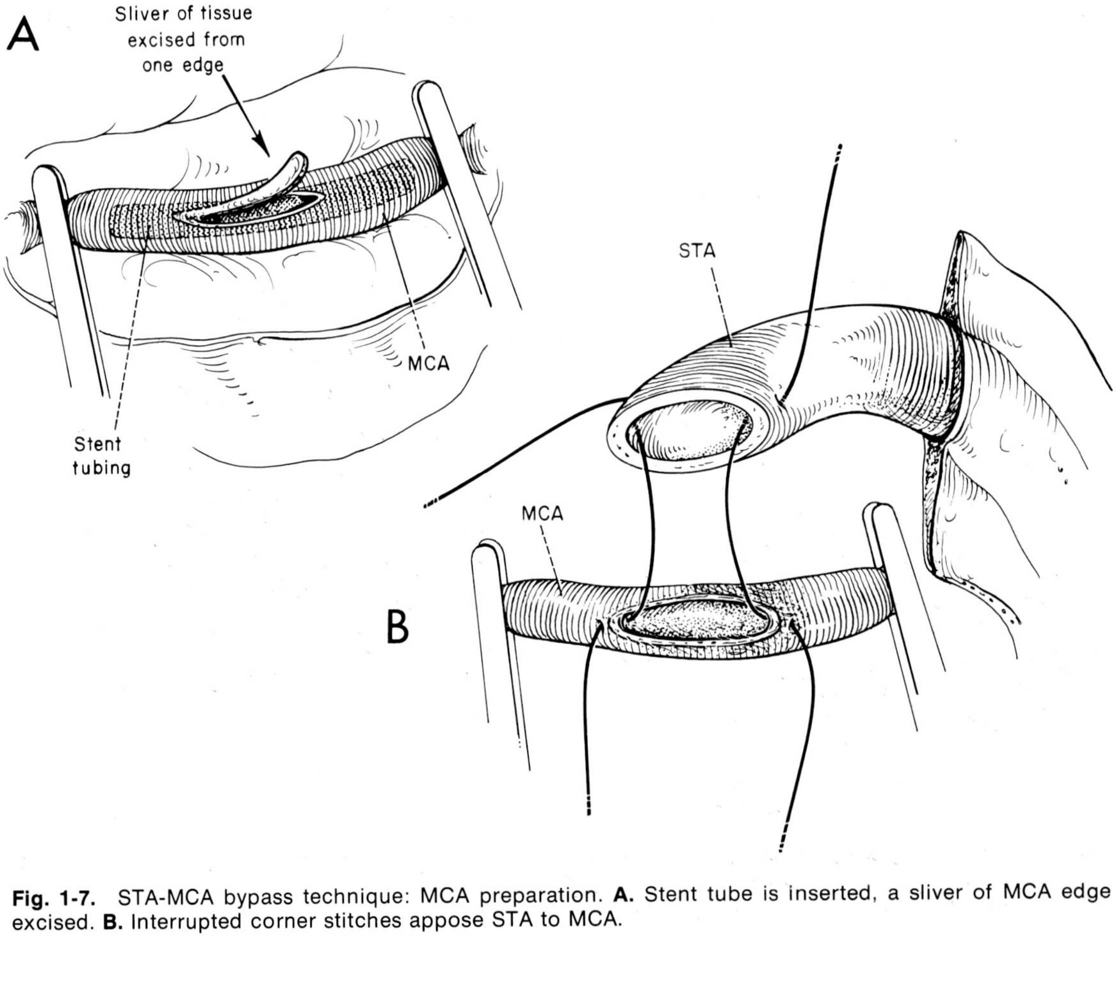

Fig. 1-7. STA-MCA bypass technique: MCA preparation. **A.** Stent tube is inserted, a sliver of MCA edge excised. **B.** Interrupted corner stitches appose STA to MCA.

arterotomy is made with a broken razor blade. With a single scissors cut, the arterotomy is lengthened to equal the maximal STA tip width. The vessel is irrigated with heparinized saline. A segment of silastic stent tubing, cut 2 mm longer than the arterotomy, is inserted into the vessel. A sliver of tissue is excised with scissors from the arterotomy edge.

Anastomosis

The STA is brought to the MCA opening, with bevel aiming back toward the origin of the MCA (Figs. 1-7 and 1-8). (Distal flow takes care of itself.) The Barraquer needle holder and jeweler's forceps are used to place 10-0 nylon sutures in each corner. These sutures are pulled through and tied down with jeweler's forceps. An additional 6 to 8 interrupted sutures are placed along the front wall. Tying down the sutures after all are placed provides maximum accuracy of placement. Bites are a bit larger on the STA side in order to promote overlap and intima-to-intima apposition. Sutures must accurately include STA atheroma, which may be quite thick in these patients. Sutures are placed slightly closer together near the corners, where leaks have a tendency to occur.

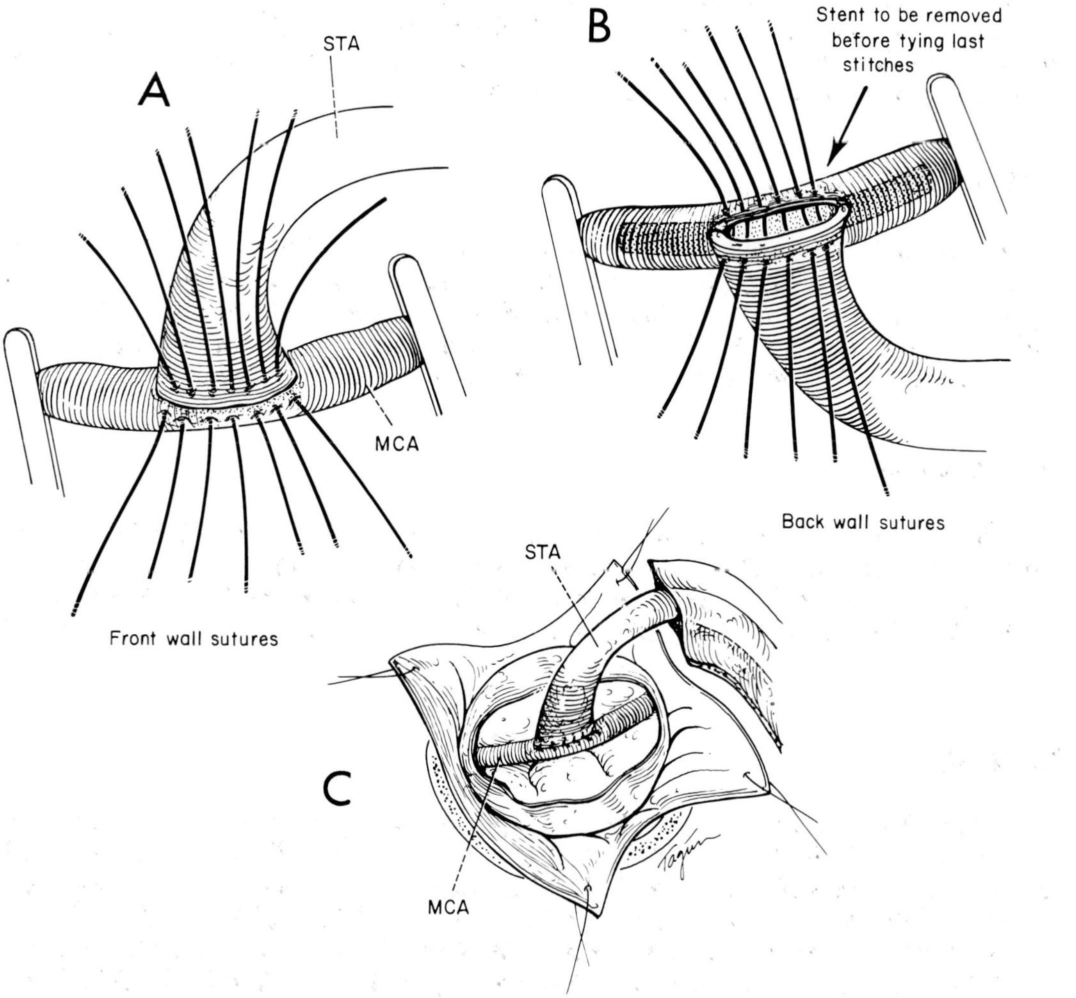

Fig. 1-8. STA-MCA bypass technique: anastomosis. **A.** Placement of interrupted sutures in front wall; sutures are tied after all are placed. **B.** Placement of back wall sutures; front wall suture line is inspected and stent removed before tying down last sutures.

After the STA is reflected aside to expose the back wall of the anastomosis, this suture line is completed. The front wall suture line is inspected from inside to confirm accurate suture placement. Then 6 to 8 interrupted sutures are used to close the back wall. Before the last two stitches are tied, the stent tube is gently removed, and the STA is opened briefly to expel clots and air.

The distal MCA clip is removed first, then the proximal MCA clip. Under 25× magnification, the suture line is inspected for leaks. A major pumper requires a stitch; suture line ooze will stop without suturing. The rubber dam is folded over the suture line, and a cottonoid provides pressure for 1 to 2 minutes. In some cases a strip of Gelfoam will be needed for hemostasis. Finally, the STA clip is removed to begin augmented cerebral flow. Graft flow may be measured with an electromagnetic flow probe and meter.

Closure

The dura is loosely approximated with interrupted 4-0 silk sutures. A Gelfoam pledget covers the dural exposure and surrounds the STA graft. After the graft is routed without kink or compression, the temporalis muscle is approximated with a few 3-0 silk sutures. The wound is irrigated with Bacitracin solution. The galea is closed with interrupted 3-0 silk and the skin with continuous 5-0 nylon. To preclude cerebrospinal fluid leakage, Steri-Strips are applied along the suture line. A small dressing is applied, together with a warning sign against pressure and a mark to indicate a palpable pulse.

Postoperative Management

For 24 to 48 hours, normal blood pressure is maintained with the aid of a radial arterial catheter, central venous catheter, and infusions of colloid, pressors, or nitroprusside. After 48 hours, when mobilization begins, blood pressure is controlled with oral agents. Aspirin (600 mg) and dipyridamole (50 mg) are given twice daily for 6 months to foster graft patency. Angiography is performed at 1 week to assess bypass patency.

Complications

Major reported complications are uncommon and include postoperative infarction (sometimes related to occlusion of graft or native collateral), intracerebral or extracerebral hematoma, meningitis, and cardiopulmonary sequelae of anesthesia.[2,4,16-17,20-22] Minor complications include transient focal deficits, seizures, wound infections, and scalp edge necrosis.

Discussion

Personal experience with 18 cases of STA-MCA bypass has been encouraging and parallel the results of others (Tables 1-1, 1-2, and 1-3).[2,4-5,16-17,20-22] Complications have been minor. Bypass has appeared to eliminate TIAs and prevent strokes: TIAs disappeared after surgery in 9 cases, and strokes never occurred in operated hemispheres (Table 1-2). (In one case with bilateral disease, infarction occurred contralateral to surgery in the second postoperative week.) One (perhaps two) slow strokes appeared to be improved. Bypass seemed helpful in preventing ischemia in one case in which ICA occlusion was done for a giant ICA aneurysm in the presence of poor native collateral supply. Acute strokes were not benefited, but the cases operated were not ideal.

Table 1-1. Case Material* (18 Grafts)

Presentations	No. of Cases	Angiogram	No. of Cases
TIAs	9	ICA occl	6
Acute stroke	4	ICA sten	3
Slow stroke	2	MCA occl	3
Dementia	1	Multiple	5
Other	2	Aneurysm	1

*Patients ranged in age from 39 to 64 years (avg = 58 years) and included 12 males and 4 females.

Table 1-2. Results

Flow	Angiograms	Clinical Outcome	
15-90 ml/min (av. 35)	1 occlusion	TIAs	0 (9 cases)
	16 open	Stroke	1 (opp side)
	1 ND	Better	2
		Worse	0
		No change	7

Table 1-3. Complications

	No. of Patients
Transient dysphasia	1
Transient paresis	1
Postoperative contralateral cerebral infarction	1
Seizures	1
Scalp edge necrosis	3
Scalp infection	1
Death	0

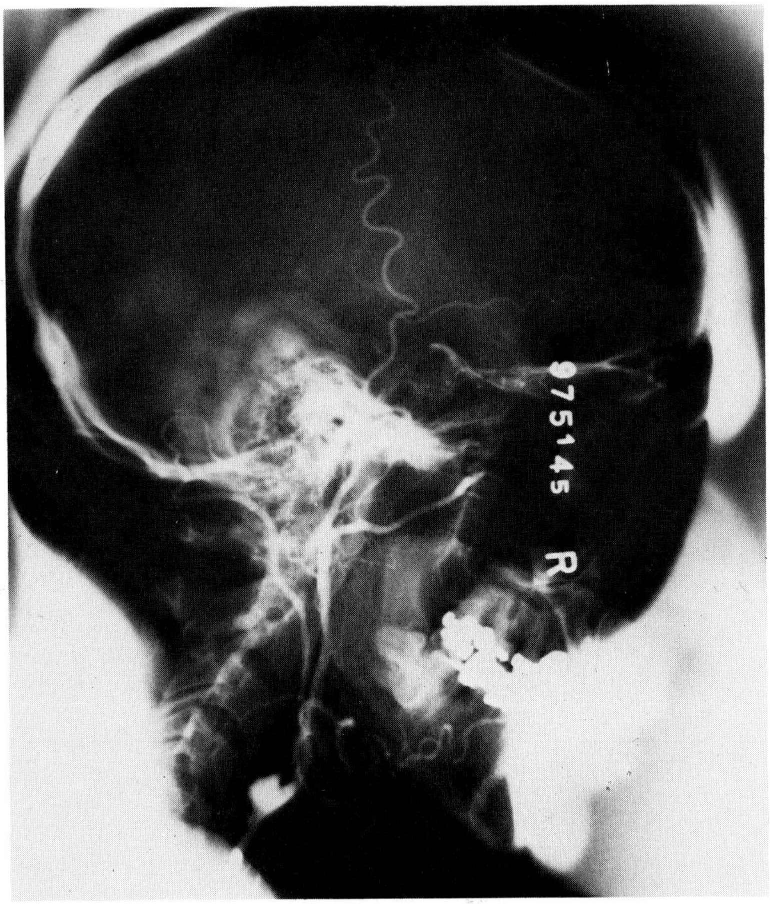

Fig. 1-9. *Case 1:* STA-MCA bypass eliminates TIAs. Right crotid angiogram shows ICA occlusion with poor reconstitution of intracranial ICA via ophthalmic artery. Patient has persistent TIAs.

Case reports serve to illustrate this experience:

Case 1. *(J.B.) In a man with ICA occlusion, STA-MCA bypass eliminates TIAs.* One year before admission, this 56-year-old man experienced the sudden onset of tingling and weakness in the left hand and forearm, which lasted about 30 minutes. On other occasions there was weakness in the left foot or tingling in the left side of the mouth. Similar spells recurred several times over a 9-month period. At another hospital angiography showed right ICA occlusion, and little backflow was obtained at carotid endarterectomy. Repeat angiography (Fig. 1-9) showed persistent right ICA occlusion with poor collateral to the right MCA from the right ophthalmic artery. After surgery, there were spells of tingling in the left cheek, two to three times per day, lasting for 3 to 5 minutes. Examination showed a blood pressure of 160/90 mmHg, slow speech, and denial of illness, together with mild weakness and sensory loss in the left arm and foot. A cardiology consultant recommended Dyazide to control hypertension and a diet to control hypercholesterolemia. A computed tomographic (CT) scan was unremarkable.

The right STA was anastomosed to the angular artery; flow at surgery was 30 ml/min. The postoperative course was smooth; power in the left limb improved subjectively and the spells of tingling disappeared. Arteriography showed filling of five branches of MCA through the STA graft (Fig. 1-9).

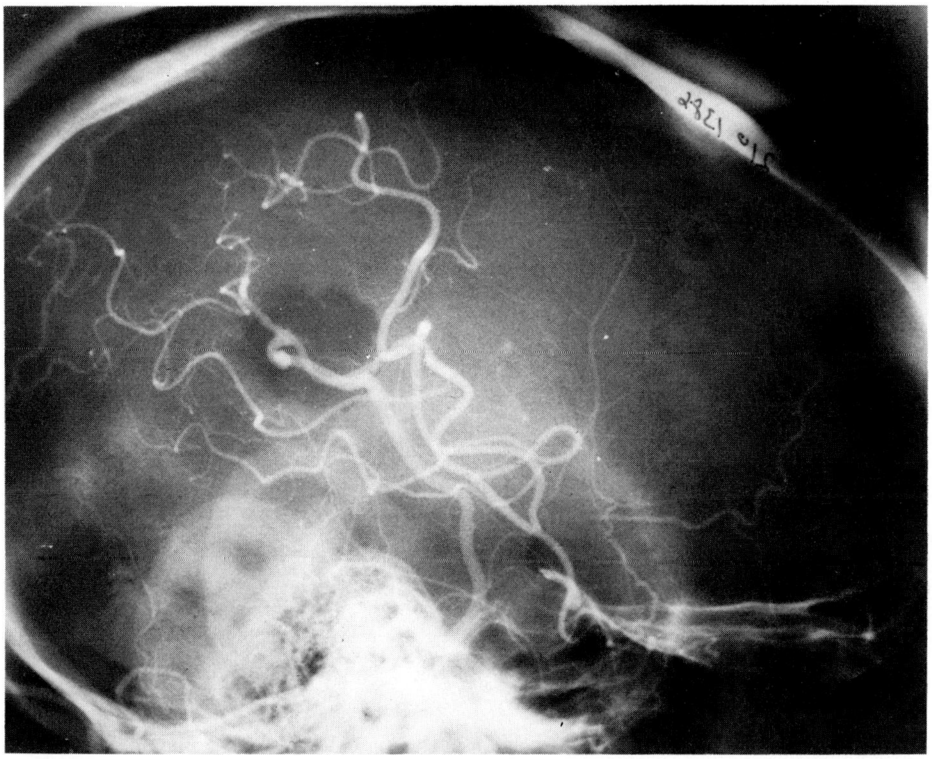

Fig. 1-9. (continued) Angiogram after STA-MCA bypass shows extensive MCA filling via graft. TIAs ceased.

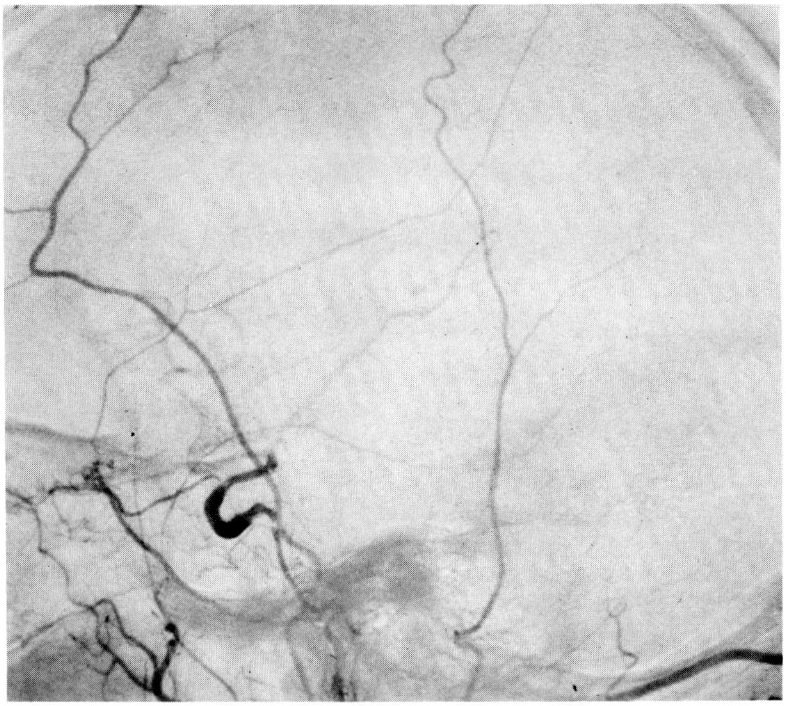

Fig. 1-10. *Case 2:* STA-MCA bypass arrests "slow stroke." Angiogram shows occluded left ICA with fair filling of intracranial ICA via ophthalmic artery. Patient presented with gradually progressive hemiparesis and dysphasia.

Case 2. *(A.H.) Bypass partially reverses a "slow" stroke.* A 62-year-old man who entered the hospital because he had spells of dysphasia and stepwise progressive weakness of the right hand and leg. A lone episode of mild hand weakness had led to angiography 3 months before; this study showed left internal carotid occlusion with poor collateral to the left MCA. He was treated with aspirin, dipyridamole, and Dyazide. During the 2 weeks preceding readmission, there were several episodes of temporary dysphasia and stepwise progressive right hemiparesis. On examination his blood pressure was 150/84 mmHg, power in the distal right arm was 5/10, with strength in the right leg 8/10. Repeat angiography was unchanged, except that dye passed retrograde in intracranial ICA down to the base (Fig. 1-10).

The cervical ICA was explored, but backflow could not be obtained. Therefore, STA was joined to a fronto-opercular branch of MCA; flow was 90 ml/min. Postoperative recuperation was smooth. Six weeks after surgery, there had been no spells, and power in the right hand was at least 8/10 while that in the leg was normal. An angiogram showed filling of five MCA branches through the graft (Fig. 1-10).

Future of Direct Cerebral Revascularization

STA-MCA bypass will probably prove to benefit patients with TIAs and inaccessible lesions. The procedure may also prove valuable for *slow* strokes, generalized hypoperfusion, and planned occlusions. Studies of regional cerebral blood flow and metabolism will likely help in the selection of candidates for surgery. Only critical controlled therapeutic trials can establish the validity of any of these indications.

Occipital-PICA bypass is clearly feasible; here, too, a controlled study of therapeutic efficacy will be required.

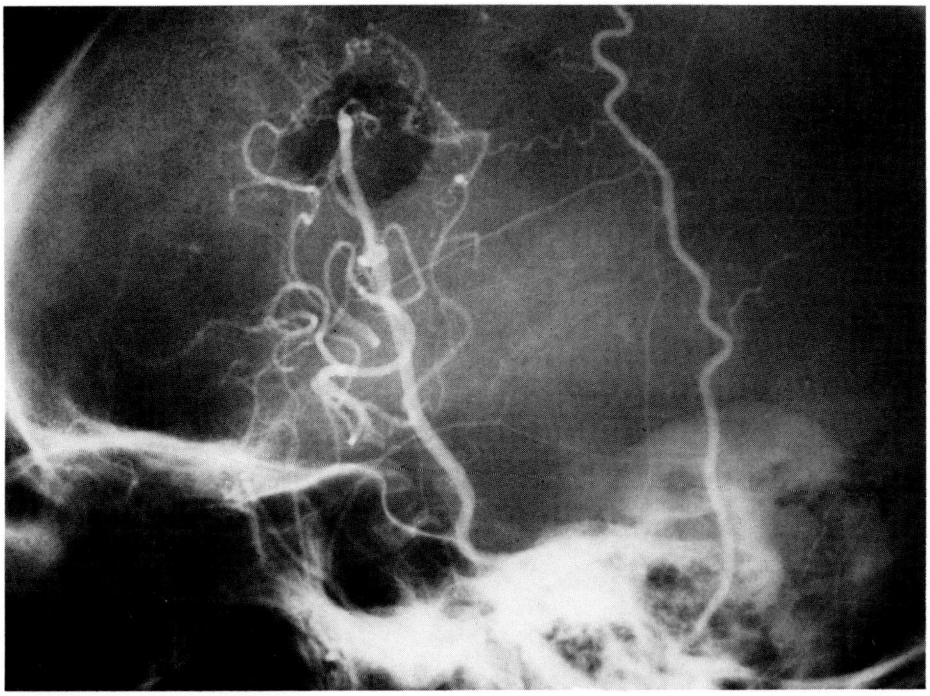

Fig. 1-10. (continued) Postoperative angiogram shows good filling of MCA via bypass. (ICA could not be opened in neck.) Virtually complete recovery after surgery.

Long grafting could become useful in preventive or emergency settings, if it can be hastened and its risk reduced. Nonsuture anastomosis, perhaps with adhesives, could go far to achieve speed, while the use of an MCA branch might lessen risks.[12]

Emergency direct cerebral revascularization awaits several developments: A test for tissue viability is needed to identify reversible cases; blood flow[29] or scanning studies[30] may permit such case selection. A method must be found to extend the period of reversibility until blood flow is restored; a number of methods under study hold promise (eg., barbiturates,[31] hypertension, etc.). Techniques for revascularization must be improved by decreasing the time of surgery and increasing the volume of flow; synthetic long grafts and tissue adhesives may some day provide rapid high-flow revascularization.

Acknowledgments

Drs. R.B. Morawetz and T.H. Jones assisted at bypass operations. Frank W. Marcoux ably carried out flow measurements. Mrs. Edith Tagrin did the superb line drawings. Ms. Mary Pat Kingsbury kindly prepared the manuscript. Dr. R.G. Ojemann provided constructive criticism. The research was supported in part by Teacher-Investigator Award NS11001, and grants NS10828 and NS13165 from the National Institute for Neurological and Communicative Disorders and Stroke.

REFERENCES

1. Ojemann RG, Crowell RM, Fisher CM, et al: Surgical treatment of extracranial carotid occlusive disease. *Clin Neurosurg 22*:214-263, 1975
2. Chater N, Mani J, Tonnemacher K: Superficial temporal artery bypass for cerebrovascular occlusive disease. *Cal Med 119*:9-13, 1973
3. *Micro-Vascular Surgery.* Edited by RMP Donaghy, MG Yasargil. Georg Thieme Verlag, Stuttgart, 1967
4. Yasargil MG: *Microsurgery Applied to Neurosurgery.* Georg Thieme Verlag, Stuttgart, 1968
5. Yasargil MG, Krayenbühl HA, Jacobson JH: Microneurosurgical arterial reconstruction. *Surgery 67*:221-233, 1970
6. Welch K: Excision of occlusive lesions of the middle cerebral artery. *J Neurosurg 13*:73-80, 1956
7. Chou SN: Embolectomy of middle cerebral artery. *J Neurosurg 20*:161-163, 1963
8. Garrido E, Stein BM: Middle cerebral artery embolectomy. Case Report. *J Neurosurg 44*:517-521, 1976
9. Woringer E, Kunlin J: Anastomose entre la carotide primitive et la carotide intra-cranienne on la Sylvienne par greffon selon la technique de la suture suspendue. *Neurochirurgie 9*:181-188, 1963
10. Lougheed W, Marshall BM, Hunter M, et al: Common carotid to intracranial internal carotid venous bypass graft. *J Neurosurg 34*:114-118, 1971
11. Neblett C: Presented at Microneurosurgery Symposium, Cincinnati, 1975
12. Epstein MH, Leibrock L, Long D: The anatomy of the so-called "middle cerebral trifurcation" and its potential for extracranial-intracranial bypass. Presented at the Congress of Neurological Surgeons, New Orleans, 1976
13. Ausman J: Presentation to Microneurosurgery Symposium, Cincinnati, 1975
14. Piepgras D, Sundt T: Presentation at Second International Symposium on Microneurosurgical Anastomoses for Cerebral Ischemia, Tegernsee, Germany, 1976
15. Khodadad G, Singh RS, Olinger CP: Prevention of the brain stem stroke by microvascular anastomosis in the vertebrobasilar system. in press, 1976.
16. Reichman OH, Davis DO, Roberts TS, et al: Anastomosis between STA and cortical branch of MCA for the treatment of occlusive cerebrovascular disease, *Reconstructive Surgery of Brain Arteries.* Edited by FT Marei. Akademiai Kiado, Budapest, 1974
17. Chater N: Surgical results and measurements of intraoperative flow in microneurosurgical anastomoses, *Microneurosurgical Anastomoses for Cerebral Ischemia.* Edited by G Austin. Charles C Thomas, Springfield, Illinois, 1976, pp 295-304
18. Robertson J: Personal communication, 1975
19. Tew JM: Reconstructive intracranial vascular surgery for prevention of stroke. *Clin Neurosurg 22*:264-280, 1974
20. Grazl O, Schmidek P, Spetzler R, et al: Clinical experience with extra-intracranial arterial anastomosis in 65 cases. *J Neurosurg 44*:313-324, 1976
21. Schmidek P, Gratzl O, Spetzler R, et al: Selection of patients for extra-intracranial bypass surgery based on rCBF measurements. *J Neurosurg 44*:303-312, 1976
22. Chater N, Popp J: Microsurgical vascular bypass for occlusive cerebrovascular disease: review of 100 cases. *Surg Neurol 6*:115-118, 1976
23. Weinstein P, Chater N: Presentation at Second International Symposium on Microneurosurgical Anastomoses for Cerebral Ischemia, Tegernsee, Germany, 1976
24. Peerless SJ: Role of cerebral revascularization after deliberate vessel occlusion during treatment of aneurysms or tumors. Presented to the Congress of Neurological Surgeons, New Orleans, 1976
25. Peerless SJ: Presented at First International Symposium on Microneurosurgical Anastomoses for Cerebral Ischemia, Loma Linda, California, 1973
26. Ferguson G: Presented at the Joint Symposium on Cerebrovascular Disease, Dallas, 1976
27. Crowell RM, Olsson Y: Effect of extracranial-intracranial vascular bypass graft on experimental acute stroke in dogs. *J Neurosurg 38*:26-31, 1973
28. Crowell RM: Superficial temporal-middle cerebral artery bypass graft for acute stroke. Presented at the Second International Symposium on Microneurosurgical Anastomoses for Cerebral Ischemia, Tegernsee, Germany, 1976
29. Morawetz RB, DeGirolami U, Ojemann RG, et al: Cerebral blood flow determined by hydrogen clearance during focal cerebral ischemia in waking monkeys. in press, 1976
30. Sokoloff L: The (14c)-deoxyglucose method for the quantitative determination of local cerebral glucose utilization, *Brain Blood Flow and Metabolism.* Edited by AM Harper. Churchill, Edinburgh, 1975
31. Smith AL, Hoff JT, Nielsen SL, et al: Barbiturate protection in acute focal cerebral ischemia. *Stroke 5*:1-7, 1974

CHAPTER 2

Treatment of Multiple and Asymptomatic Aneurysms

Lester A. Mount Ronald Brisman

THE TREATMENT OF MULTIPLE ANEURYSMS is in essence the treatment of asymptomatic aneurysms. All neurosurgeons agree that surgical treatment of symptomatic aneurysms is indicated, whenever possible. There is no unanimity of opinion regarding the treatment of an asymptomatic aneurysm. Representative of the diversity of opinion, covering the past 17 years, are the following: Poppen and Fager[1] in 1959, Pool and Potts[2] in 1965, Hamby[3] in 1959, Pouyanne and associates in 1970[4] and 1973[5], Moyes[6] in 1971, and Mount and Brisman in 1971[7] and 1973[8] advocated treatment of all intracranial aneurysms. Bjorkesten and Troupp[9] in 1960, McKissock and coworkers[10] in 1964, and Paterson and Bond[11] in 1973 did not think treatment of an unruptured aneurysm was indicated. Heiskanen and Marttila[12] suggested clipping the asymptomatic aneurysm if it could be reached through the same approach used to treat the symptomatic aneurysm, but they did not advise a second operation to clip it.

Incidence

In 1955 Bigelow[13] collected 2,737 patients with intracranial aneurysms, of which 10% were multiple. McKissock and associates[10], in 1964, reported an angiographic incidence of multiplicity in 14% of 1,686 cases and 28% in autopsy cases. In the Cooperative Study[14] 19% of 3,321 clinically diagnosed cases were multiple and in the autopsy series, 22%. Because of the high incidence of multiplicity, complete, four-vessel arteriography is required in any patient with an intracranial aneurysm.

Clinical Material

Between 1958 and 1976 there were 154 patients with multiple aneurysms, representing an incidence of 19%. Eighty-three percent were females. The average age for the group was the same as that for patients with single aneurysms; 59% occurred between the ages of 40 and 59. Blood pressure was elevated in 35%. Subarachnoid hemorrhage was the presenting symptom in 72%.

Department of Neurological Surgery, New York Neurological Institute, Columbia-Presbyterian Medical Center, College of Physicians and Surgeons, Columbia University, New York, New York 10032

Location of Aneurysms

One hundred fifty-four patients had 376 aneurysms, 253 of the internal carotid artery (30 of which were intracavernous), 69 of the middle cerebral, 31 of the anterior cerebral or anterior communicating arteries, and 23 of the posterior circulation (Table 2-1). In 96 patients the aneurysms were bilateral and in 58, unilateral. There were 90 patients with two aneurysms, 20 with three, 9 with four, and 2 with five. There were 62 patients with bilateral symmetric aneurysms, of which 56 involved the internal carotid (including seven intracavernous) and 9, the middle cerebral. One patient had bilateral symmetric aneurysms of both internal carotid arteries within the cavernous sinus and both middle cerebral arteries.

Table 2-1. Location of 376 Aneurysms in 154 Patients

Internal carotid	253
Middle cerebral	69
Anterior cerebral and anterior communicating	31
Posterior circulation	23

Results of Treatment

In the Cooperative Study the mortality rate was 70% in 252 patients who had multiple aneurysms and subarachnoid hemorrhage and were followed a maximum of 3 years.

Forty patients were treated nonsurgically and in 56 one aneurysm was treated surgically. Forty-four patients had both aneurysms treated by surgery, 9 had all three, 3 had all four, and 2 had all five (Table 2-2).

Table 2-2. Treatment

	No. of Patients
Nonsurgical	40
Surgical	
One aneurysm only	56
Both aneurysms	44
All three	9
All four	3
All five	2

Ninety-six patients did not have all their aneurysms treated, including 40 who had no surgical procedure at all. In this group there were good results in 54%, poor in 29%, and death occurred in 17%. (These results cannot be compared to those in surgically treated patients.) Of 50 patients with 137 aneurysms, all of which were treated surgically by intracranial clipping, muslin wrapping, plastic spraying, or extracranial carotid ligation, 91% had good results, 4.5% poor, and 4.5% died (Table 2-3). In the group of 37 patients with 89 aneurysms,

Table 2-3. Results of Surgical Treatment in 58 Patients Having 137 Aneurysms

Result	Percentage of Patients
Good	91
Poor	4.5
Died	4.5

Table 2-4. Intracranial Surgical Treatment of 37 Patients Having 89 Aneurysms

Result	Percentage of Patients
Good	94.6
Poor	2.7
Died	2.7

all of which were treated intracranially (61 operations), there were good results in 94.6%, poor in 2.7%, and death occurred in 2.7% (Table 2-4). In the 1 patient who died, both aneurysms were clipped at one operation. Today this patient would not be considered a satisfactory risk at the time he was operated upon. Twenty-four patients had elective craniotomies to treat 32 unruptured (multiple) aneurysms, with good results in 23 cases and no operative mortality (Table 2-5). The 1 patient with a poor result had an asymptomatic aneurysm of the middle cerebral artery at the origin of a large lenticulostriate artery. It was coated with Selverstone plastic material. This patient did well for 1 month and then developed sudden hemiparesis. Arteriography did not show the aneurysm or the lenticulostriate artery.

Table 2-5. Intracranial Surgical Treatment of 24 Patients Having 32 Unruptured Aneurysms

Result	No. of Patients
Good	23
Poor	1
Death	0

A severe neurologic deficit existed in 7% of the surgical patients and 15% of the nonsurgical patients at the time the decision was made as to whether to operate. Most of the patients treated conservatively were not operated upon because of the multiplicity of their aneurysms. This was thought, by some physicians, in the earlier part of the study (late 1950s), to contraindicate surgery. During this same period, some of the asymptomatic aneurysms were not treated surgically, as this was considered unnecessary by some doctors. However, the two groups are not comparable.

Discussion

The question is how to treat the asymptomatic aneurysm. In 1897 Gowers[15] wrote: "if there is an aneurysm, the prognosis is extremely grave for no one knows how near or how far may be the fatal rupture."

How near the fatal rupture may be is shown by a patient with a ruptured aneurysm of the left middle cerebral artery and a 3 mm unruptured one that arose from the right internal carotid artery. Her course was stormy, with persisting arteriospasm, but eventually the middle cerebral artery aneurysm was clipped. The patient slowly made an excellent recovery, but she was debilitated and apprehensive when she was sent home for further recuperation before her second operation. Two days later she was readmitted with fatal rupture of the 3 mm aneurysm of the right internal carotid artery, which was found at autopsy.

How far the fatal rupture may be is illustrated by a patient with two aneurysms, one at each internal carotid artery bifurcation, demonstrated by arteriography. The symptomatic one was clipped. Twenty-three years later the other aneurysm ruptured and the patient died.

The precarious nature of the unruptured aneurysm is demonstrated by autopsy examination, which in one case showed necrosis, phagocytosis, and hemorrhage in the wall of the aneurysm, indicating that it would soon have ruptured.

An existing aneurysm remains a permament threat to the patient as long as he lives. The natural history of the asymptomatic companion of a ruptured aneurysm indicates that there is continuing morbidity and mortality with each passing year. In this series of 158 patients, 99 from the literature and 59 of our own, the rate of subarachnoid hemorrhage was 10% and mortality was 4% in an average period of only 5 years (Table 2-6). The surgical results of the direct intracranial treatment of asymptomatic aneurysms were better. In 40 patients, 15 of Moyes and 24 of our own, there was no mortality and morbidity was 5%.

Table 2-6. Natural History of Unruptured Aneurysms

Source	No. of Patients at Risk	Time (yr)	No. Patients	
			SAH	Death
Heiskanen/Marttila	76	0.3-11	8	3
Mount/Brisman	59	0.1-10	4	1
Moyes	23	1.0-10	4	2
Total	158		16 (10%)	6 (4%)

SAH = Subarachnoid hemorrhage

The intracranial treatment of an unruptured aneurysm is like an anatomic dissection and, as shown above, is very safe when magnification is used (microscope, loops or both) and the operating team is skilled in aneurysm surgery. After treatment, the patient can resume his normal life style.

When should the asymptomatic aneuryms be treated? If it is in the same operative field, it should be treated at the same time as the symptomatic aneurysm. If a second operation is required, it should be done at the earliest feasible time. However, the timing as well as the decision to operate must be based on the patient's neurologic, mental, and medical status as well as the surgical accessibility of the aneurysm. Even the smallest aneurysms rupture; hence, the patient is in danger, regardless of the size of the aneurysm. The patient's physiologic age is more important than his chronologic age. Therefore, only his physiologic status is considered important.

It is recommended that all intracranial aneurysms be treated by surgery, preferably by direct intracranial methods, when there is a reasonable chance of success. An illustrative case is that of a patient who had five aneurysms, all of which were treated successfully. These were located on each internal carotid artery, one on the middle cerebral, one on the anterior communicating, and one at the apex of the basilar artery.

Summary

One hundred and fifty-four patients had a combined total of 376 aneurysms. Of 58 patients in whom 137 aneurysms were treated surgically, 91% had good results, 4.5% had poor results, and 4.5% died. In 37 patients who had all 89 of their aneurysms treated intracranially in 61 operations, the results were good in 94.6%, poor in 2.7%, and 2.7% died. Elective craniotomies to treat unruptured (multiple) aneurysms, in 24 patients produced good results in 23 and there was no mortality.

It is recommended that all multiple intracranial aneurysms be treated surgically, preferably by direct intracranial methods, when there is a reasonable chance of success.

REFERENCES

1. Poppen JL, Fager CA: Multiple intracranial aneurysms. *J Neurosurg 16*:581-589, 1959
2. Pool JL, Potts DG: *Aneurysms and Arteriovenous Anomalies of the Brain. Diagnosis and Treatment.* Harper and Row, New York, 1965, p 287
3. Hamby WB: Multiple intracranial aneurysms. *J Neurosurg 16*:558-563, 1959
4. Pouyanne H, Riemens V, Guerin J, et al: Les aneurysmes saculaires multiples du systeme carotidien. Indications et resultats de l'abord direct. *Neurochirurgie 16*:25-31, 1970
5. Pouyanne H, Banayan A, Guerin J, et al: Les aneurysmes sacculaires multiples du systeme carotidien supra clinoidien. Etude anatomoclinique et therapeutique. *Neurochirurgie 19: Suppl 1*, 1973
6. Moyes PD: Surgical treatment of multiple aneurysms and of incidentally discovered unruptured aneurysms. *J Neurosurg 35*:291-295, 1971
7. Mount LA, Brisman R: Treatment of multiple intracranial aneurysms. *J Neurosurg 35*:728-730, 1971
8. Mount LA, Brisman R: Treatment of multiple aneurysms—symptomatic and asymptomatic, *Clinical Neurosurgery*, vol. 21. Williams and Wilkins, Baltimore, 1974, pp 166-170
9. Bjorkesten G, Troupp H: Multiple intracranial arterial aneurysms. *Acta Chir Scand 118*:387-391, 1960
10. McKissock W, Richardson A, Walsh L, et al: Multiple intracranial aneurysms. *Lancet 1*:623-626, 1964
11. Paterson A, Bond MR: Treatment of multiple intracranial arterial aneurysms. *Lancet 1*:1302-1304, 1973
12. Heiskanen O, Marttila I: Risk of rupture of a second aneurysm in patients with multiple aneurysms. *J Neurosurg 32*:295-299, 1970
13. Bigelow NH: Multiple intracranial arterial aneurysms: an analysis of their significance. *Arch Neurol Psychiatry 73*:76-99, 1955
14. Sahs AL, Perret GE, Locksley HB, et al: Intracranial aneurysms and subarachnoid hemorrhage. A cooperative study. Lippincott, Philadelphia, 1969, p 50
15. Gowers WR: *A Manual of Diseases of the Nervous System,* vol. 2. Second edition. Blakiston, Philadelphia, 1897, p 538

CHAPTER 3

Techniques of Thrombosis of Carotid Cavernous Fistulae

John F. Mullan

THE SPONTANEOUS MORTALITY rate associated with carotid cavernous fistulae is low and results mainly from occasional nasal hemorrhage (3%). The incidence of neurologic deficit, in the form of hemiplegia or aphasia, is also low. Progressive ocular complications (70%), up to and including blindness, do occur.[1] Treatment therefore should be designed to prevent these ocular problems but should not invoke any measure traditionally prone to mortality, hemiplegia, or aphasia. Thus traditional treatment, which involves some form of occlusion of the carotid artery, is conceptionally undesirable and inadequate. Either the fistulous connection or the total venous sac must be shut off by a procedure that is virtually free from any risk of mortality, hemiplegia, or aphasia.

Detailed study of patients with fistulae has shown that each is different and that safe occlusion must be individually planned and may involve a variety of approaches and a variety of occlusive techniques.

The thrombogenic materials are:

1. Copper clad steel needles
2. Phosphor bronze wire (0.005 mm diameter)
3. Occlusive balloon
4. Conventional thrombogenic material (Gelfoam, oxidized cellulose, cotton).

It should be noted that an electric current is not advised in any instance.

Approaches to the carotid cavernous sinus are:

1. Anterior
2. Lateral
3. Posterior
4. Percutaneous transjugular

The types of fistulae that have been encountered are:

1. *Radiologically visible fistulous connection.* This is ideal and can be dealt with by stereotactic or direct insertion of copper-clad steel needles into the fistula, using the lateral approach.
2. *Fistula that drains exclusively anteriorly into the ophthalmic vein.* This group directs its

Department of Neurosurgery, Pritzker School of Medicine, University of Chicago, Chicago, Illinois 60637 entire force into the orbit and produces severe orbital problems. It is the simplest to deal with. By the anterior approach, the point of junction between the ophthalmic vein and the sinus is entered, and the sinus is packed with conventional thrombogenic material. In some of these in which there is very little cavernous sinus component and the artery opens almost directly into the ophthalmic vein, copper-needle insertion might be adequate.

3. *Fistula that drains exclusively posteriorly*. The posterior approach is a difficult one. Parkinson's triangle is devoid of nerves but the carotid artery lies in its depth, which is a problem for needle and wire insertion. We have used: (a) Direct insertion of wire or needles below and behind the third nerve, avoiding the artery by means of intraoperative angiography. (b) Direct insertion of thrombogenic material into the superior petrosal sinus and thence into the posterior cavenous sinus. The superior petrosal sinus is not always adequately developed. (c) Percutaneous retrograde insertion of an occlusive balloon via the jugular vein. The inferior petrosal sinus is not always adequately developed.
4. *Large fistula of long standing*. These are relatively simple to manage. Their specific problem is that the carotid cannot be visualized initially by intraoperative angiography. They are approached by the lateral route. Wire is first inserted intradurally into the safe anterior inferior corner. Alternatively the anterior inferior corner is packed by the anterior extradural approach. When this corner is occluded, the artery begins to show up on the arteriogram and further wire insertion can be carried out close to the artery, as indicated. These large fistulae may require 80 or more feet of wire.
5. *Smaller recent fistula draining in all directions*. These usually require a combination of several approaches. They may be difficult.
6. *Bilateral fistulae*. These are approached as unilateral fistulae, one at a time.
7. *Fistula with an intolerance to carotid compression*. It is believed that fistulae with this problem are not as dangerous as intact carotids with the same problem. However, since carotid cavernous fistulae carry little spontaneous mortality or hemispheric morbidity, it seems unjustifiable to ever take any risk of hemispheric insufficiency. Therefore, in bilateral instances in which the contralateral side was treated by carotid occlusion, and in unilateral cases intolerant to compression, all risk of carotid spasm must be avoided. Copper needles, which might cause carotid spasm if inserted flush with the artery, should either be avoided or inserted at a few millimeters distance from the artery, even if a small pouch persists.

Problems

Two have been encountered:

1. Occlusion of the posterior exit from the sinus, before the anterior exit is sealed, exacerbates orbital symptoms and demands immediate attention.
2. Occlusion of both anterior and posterior exits without obliteration of the middle results in a central aneurysm, with resulting temporary nerve paralysis. This too requires further treatment once the condition is recognized.

Therefore in planning the attack upon the fistula the sequence and extent of each thrombogenic measure should be carefully determined. In general it is desirable to complete unilateral occlusion in one stage, but staged occlusion is possible, either deliberately or if the initial procedure fails to achieve a complete result.

Technical Details

Superficial Temporal Artery Catheterization

Angiography is necessary for the lateral, posterior, and transjugular approaches but not for the anterior approach.

The essential components are: (a) use of intraluminal and perivascular papaverine, (b) clear delineation of the lumen so that the catheter is not misplaced in the wall, (c) secure anchoring of the catheter by pleated braids attached to the artery wall and surrounding deep tissues so that the catheter cannot possibly become displaced, and (d) continuous heparinized irrigation.

Use of a carotid needle or catheter for angiography is not recommended during a prolonged operative procedure. The superior thyroid artery is a better alternative.

Anterior Approach

Through a simple low temporal craniotomy the region of the foramen rotundum is located anteriorly in the extradural space. This guides the operator into the inferior orbital fissure. The bone between the superior and inferior orbital fissures is drilled out. The arterialized vein is seen running down from the roof of the orbit to the inferior fissure. Its presence at the point of entry into the sinus is confirmed by aspiration with a tuberculin syringe and fine needle. This point is entered by a fine scalpel and the sinus is gently packed by Gelfoam, oxidized cellulose, or cotton. These materials have different degrees of rigidity and are used in combination to secure gentle packing of the anterior sinus. The bulk depends upon the size of the cavernous distention. Care should be taken that the packing does not slide anteriorly into the vein instead of into the sinus (Figs. 3-1 and 3-2).

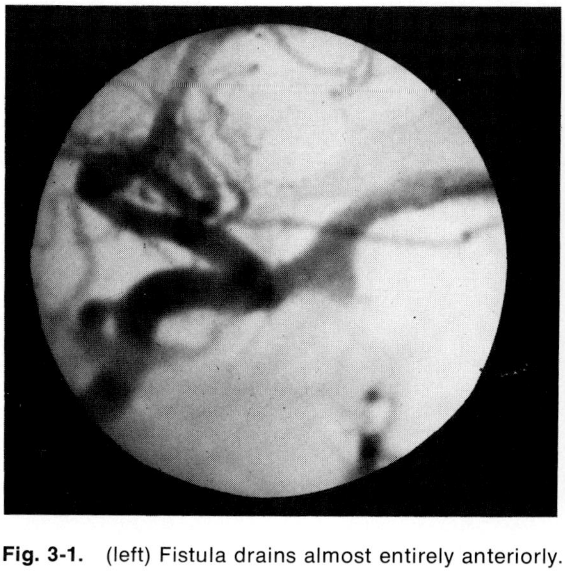

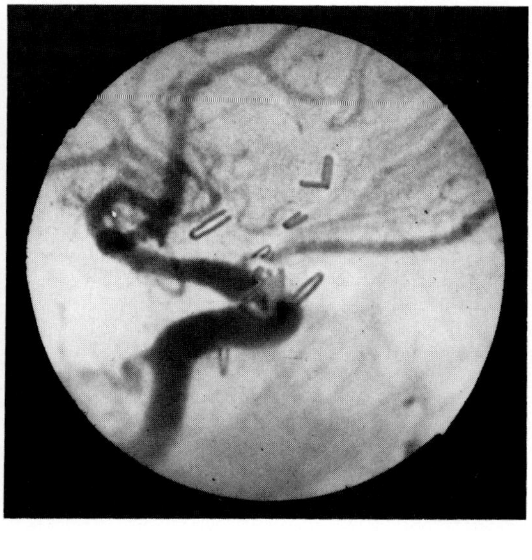

Fig. 3-1. (left) Fistula drains almost entirely anteriorly.

Fig. 3-2. (right) Fistula occluded by packing connection between ophthalmic vein and cavernous sinus.

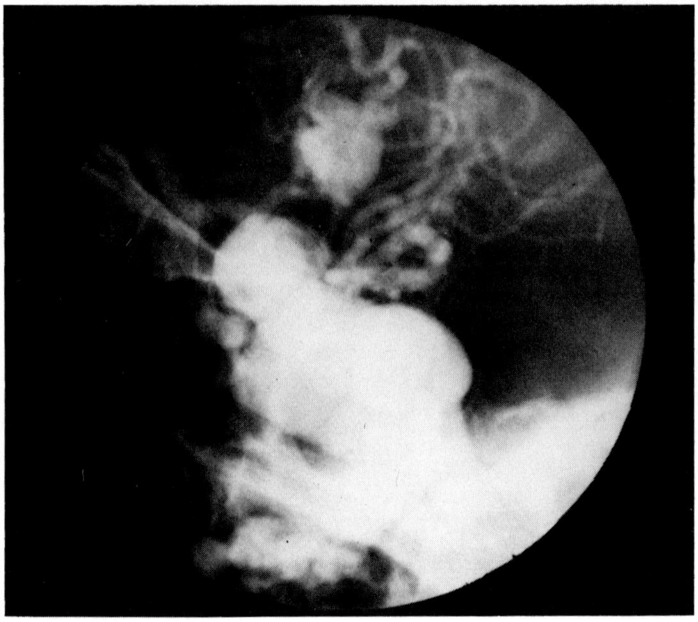

Fig. 3-3. Fistula of 6 years' duration with greatly distended sinus and distended middle cerebral veins. Carotid obscured by sinus.

Lateral Approach

Through the low temporal craniotomy, the dura is opened and the temporal lobe is elevated after lumbar drainage and mannitol. Radiologic markers are placed on the dura along the presumed path of the artery. Metal clips may be sewn to the dura or short steel needles of 0.01 mm diameter may be inserted at right angles into the dura. After angiography, phosphor bronze is inserted, by the method previously described,[2] through a point in the dura, which is radiologically free from artery. If the artery is not defined on the initial angiogram, wire is inserted anteroinferiorly (or the anteroinferior corner is packed by the anterior extradura approach, as already described). Wire insertion is completed when resistance prevents further entrance. Thrombosis may be completed at this point or may require further minutes, hours, days, or, in one instance, even 3 months. Usually it is complete within an hour (Figs. 3-3 and 3-4).

Posterior Approach

This also requires intraoperative angiography. It too is intradural. Wire or needles are inserted behind the radiographically outlined artery and below the visually identified third nerve. If conventional packing material is used, greater temporal retraction is necessary. The superior petrosal sinus is entered several millimeters behind its exit from the cavernous sinus and the material is packed forward in a gentle manner. This has resulted in a temporary sixth nerve palsy on one occasion.

Percutaneous Jugular Approach

A No. 5 Fogarty catheter has been used successfully. A No. 3 has proved to be flexible. The catheter enters the lateral sinus preferentially. Appropriate manipulation usually guides it into the inferior petrosal sinus but this attempt has not always been successful (Fig. 3-5).

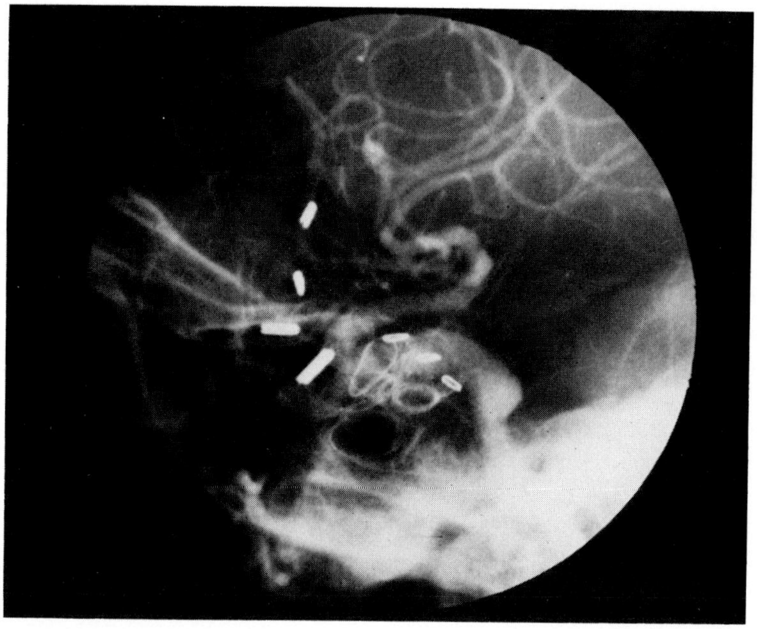

Fig. 3-4. Cavernous sinus occluded by wire inserted first into the anterior inferior corner. Three posterior clips are dural markers.

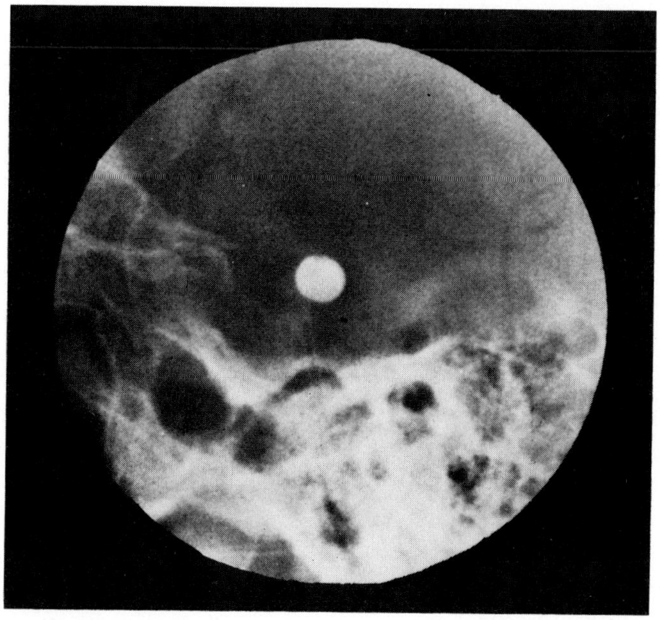

Fig. 3-5. Percutaneous transjugular, transinferior petrosal sinus insertion of balloon catheter. This is applicable to some fistulae from the region of the meningohypophyseal artery.

Combined Approach

In most instances more than one approach is necessary for each individual fistula.

Results

In a previous study 7 cases were reported and the techniques of stereotactic insertion of copper needles and craniotomy insertion of thrombogenic wire were described.[2] One temporary sixth nerve palsy was encountered. We have since treated 17 further patients. There was one temporary sixth nerve palsy. In another recent patient the fistula was temporarily converted into an aneurysm. A partial ophthalmoplegia became complete and has again been resolved. There was no mortality and no sign of insufficiency of hemispheric blood flow in any patient.

REFERENCES

1. Hamby, WG: *Carotid Cavernous Fistula.* Charles C Thomas, Springfield, Illinois, 1966
2. Mullan S: Experiences with surgical thrombosis of intracranial berry aneurysms and carotid cavernous fistulas. *J Neurosurg 41*:657-670, 1974

CHAPTER 4

Coating of Intracranial Aneurysms with Nontoxic Adherent Plastics

Bertram Selverstone

Prevention of subarachnoid hemorrhage after an initial ictus is the usual purpose of operations for intracranial aneurysms. Indirect procedures, such as ligation of a carotid or anterior cerebral artery, although technically simple, cannot be relied upon to provide permanent protection against rebleeding nor are they without hazard of cerebral infarction immediately, or of vascular insufficiency in later years.

Until intraluminal catheter techniques become generally applicable, direct exposure and treatment of the aneurysm, usually by a clip or ligature, is generally agreed to be the method of choice. However, a clip on the neck of the aneurysm may exclude from the circulation significant branches arising from the sac, especially in anterior communicating and middle cerebral aneurysms. A clip may not satisfactorily occlude a sessile aneurysm, or it may seriously deform and compromise the parent vessel. Even in an aneurysm with a well-formed neck, there is frequently a significant length of aneurysmal wall between a properly placed clip and the parent artery. Not uncommonly, this segment and its ostium may be the site of an atheromatous plaque, further compromising the defective segment of vessel wall, which is exposed to arterial pressure. Another unfortunate problem is the fact that even a well-designed, well-chosen, and well-placed clip may be dislodged from its site postoperatively, presumably as a result of arterial pulsation, with immediate or subsequent fatal hemorrhage.

Coating an aneurysm may serve several purposes. It may be used to (a) reinforce the wall of the aneurysm without employing clips or ligatures; (b) reinforce that portion of an aneurysm that cannot safely be excluded from the circulation by clipping; and (c) lock in place a clip, whether well or precariously placed, which cures an aneurysm but may be dislodged postoperatively. Coating is particularly applicable when significant cerebral arteries traverse or emerge from the aneurysmal sac. Also, the formation of a propagating intraluminal thrombus or an embolus at the site of intimal crushing may be prevented by eliminating clips or ligatures.

The use of muscle, gauze, or other material to wrap an aneurysm is a qualitatively different process from the use of adherent plastics to reinforce an aneurysm. These techniques cannot be expected to provide an immediate blood-tight seal and their efficacy

Department of Surgery (Neurosurgery) Brown University and Division of Neurosurgery, Miriam and Roger Williams Hospitals, Providence, Rhode Island

depends upon the provocation of a reactive fibrosis. Protection during the high-risk period following an initial hemorrhage is incomplete at best.

The selection of coating as a method of treating an aneurysm may be made either before or during operation, as the configuration of the lesion and its associated vessels becomes apparent. However, the author believes that the coating procedure should be available in all cases, since even with the use of clips, it offers significant additional protection. The decision to be made at operation therefore is whether the aneurysm is to be treated by coating alone, or by clipping and coating. In about 5% of cases in which coating alone has been planned, leakage or frank hemorrhage occurs from the sac during dissection, requiring the use of one or two clips before coating.

Preoperative Considerations

Diagnosis and treatment of patients in whom aneurysms are to be coated does not differ significantly from accepted methods employed for other techniques. The patient who is conscious is placed on complete bed rest, given epsilon aminocaproic acid, 5 g as a loading dose and 35 g daily by slow intravenous drip. Prophylactic anticonvulsants, sedatives, and tranquilizers are used (usually Dilantin, phenobarbital, and Librium). Hypotensive agents are administered after consultation with an internist, if arterial pressure is elevated. A stool softener is given.

Within 1 to 2 days, complete angiography is done by the femorocerebral route, with appropriate oblique and magnified views, as necessary, to provide as accurate a picture as possible of the configuration of the sac and of any small vessels emerging from or in intimate relation to the sac.

If the patient is unconscious and fails to improve rapidly, or has lateralizing or localizing signs suggesting the presence of an intracerebral clot complicating subarachnoid hemorrhage, a CAT scan without contrast enhancement will quickly determine whether a clot is actually present or whether some other cause—frequently vascular spasm—is responsible for the patient's clinical state. If a clot is present, angiography is required to define the aneurysm and permit evacuation of all or part of the clot, with or without treating the aneurysm. If no clot is shown by the CAT scan, angiography can be delayed until the patient's condition is suitable for operation. In either case these patients may benefit from generous doses of glucocorticoids (dexamethasone 8 to 16 mg every 6 hours intravenously). This medication should be tapered as soon as possible, since it may inhibit protective fibrosis about the aneurysm. It is recommended on the day preceding operation. When the condition of the patient is stable, angiography should be done as in the more favorable cases.

It is abundantly clear that the state of consciousness at the time of operation is the crucial factor in the patient's ability to recover satisfactorily from major aneurysm surgery. Operation should therefore be delayed until the patient is alert and oriented, using hypotensive and antifibrinolytic medication as noted above. If a clot is not present and the patient fails to return to a measurable state of consciousness, either persistent cephalus may be present. There are real hazards to operation in the presence of spasm, but if communicating hydrocephalus is present, the operation can be done, followed by ventriculoperitoneal shunt. Shunting should not precede treatment of the aneurysm lest it lead to a change in the position of the brain, which could provoke further bleeding from the aneurysm. The presence of communicating hydrocephalus may be recognized in the CAT scan by ventricular dilatation with accompanying dilatation of the cisterna ambiens. If there is persistent arterial spasm, a further delay, followed by further angiography when there is clinical evidence of significant improvement, may be the best course.

Operation

Controlled respiration is used with hyperventilation to decrease the volume of the brain. (The skill of the anesthetist in intubating the trachea with minimal irritation is of obvious importance.) A Foley catheter is placed in the bladder and mannitol, 20%, is given intravenously, beginning with the induction of anesthesia. The usual dose is 2.0 g/kg of body weight, to be given over a period of 40 to 60 minutes. Two lumbar puncture needles, No. 18 or 17, are placed for cerebrospinal fluid drainage, which is not begun until the dura has been opened. In no instance has bleeding occurred after cerebrospinal fluid drainage, even though as much as 200 ml or more has been withdrawn on occasion. In two instances, both anterior communicating aneurysms, bleeding has been found immediately upon opening the dura. In each case the dura was closed with a pericranial graft to allow for postoperative edema, the bone flap stored in a freezer, and the scalp closed. One of these patients survived the hemorrhage and was operated on successfully several weeks later, with replacement of the bone flap subsequently. The second patient never fully regained consciousness after this, her third hemorrhage and ultimately expired.

The patient's position on the table is lateral, with the right side up, for right-sided and midline aneurysms. The head is placed in the lateral position for internal carotid, middle cerebral, and basilar aneurysms and at 45° for anterior communicating and anterior cerebral aneurysms. Pin fixation was formerly used but has subsequently proved to be unnecessary.

The table is tilted to bring the head above the level of the cardiac atrium. A small frontotemporal free bone flap is turned, and a bony subtemporal decompression made down to the base. An essentially similar flap is used for internal carotid, middle cerebral, and basilar aneurysms, extending the flap somewhat anteriorly for anterior communicating aneurysms. Elevation of the head, hyperventilation, mannitol, and cerebrospinal fluid drainage are all relied upon to obtain access to the lesion, essentially without retraction. Scoville brain retractors are used over Telfa strips, exerting the most minimal traction to simply displace and maintain the position of the frontal and temporal lobes. Exertion of any force on the retractors is to be avoided at all cost.

Internal Carotid Aneurysms at Posterior Communicating Origin

In these aneurysms the bleeding point is usually near the distal point of the fundus. Bleeding has usually ceased, either because of adhesion to the medial surface of the temporal lobe, if the sac is supratentorial, or because the adhesion to the oculomotor nerve and adjacent arachnoid and dura if the sac is infratentorial. The exact configuration of the aneurysm can usually be predicted, both clinically (oculomotor nerve signs are more common in infratentorial aneurysms) and angiographically, but such predictions are not always certain. In cases of doubt, therefore, it is important to expose the aneurysm primarily by displacing the frontal rather than the temporal lobe, with additional maneuvers decided upon after the precise configuration of the sac has been determined. In this, as in other aneurysms, the use of induced hypotension with sodium nitroprusside may be useful during dissection of the sac.

As soon as the optic nerve has been exposed just medial to the anterior clinoid process, the overlying arachnoid is opened and the adjoining internal carotid artery is followed posteriorly to the origin of the aneurysm. If the arachnoid becomes adherent as one progresses posteriorly, the vessel is followed external to the arachnoid until it becomes free again. Arachnoid is never torn from the vessel during this part of the dissection lest the site of the adhesion, which has stopped the bleeding, be disturbed.

If the aneurysmal sac is seen to extend below the tentorium, exposure is obtained readily by coagulating and dividing bridging veins from the temporal tip and anteromedial surface to the cavernous, sphenoparietal, and superior petrosal sinuses. With the withdrawal of cerebrospinal fluid from below and the use of mannitol and hyperventilation, it is easy to gently assist the spontaneous recession of the temporal tip posteriorly in order to bring the proximal part of the aneurysm easily into view; there is no need to expose the tip or distal part of the fundus of the aneurysm.

If the sac is supratentorial and adherent to the temporal lobe, gentle displacement of the frontal lobe will bring the proximal part of the aneurysm into view without displacing the temporal lobe. The amount of neck (if any) and sac which should be exposed will depend on the configuration of the aneurysm, but adhesions to the temporal pia-arachnoid need not be disturbed.

Aneurysms of the internal carotid-posterior communicating junction may be classified as follows:

1. Flask-shaped with a neck long enough to be clipped.
2. Globular, ellipsoidal, or irregular, with an extremely short neck.
3. Sessile, with the sac at least as wide as the base.
4. Dome-shaped, with the base of the sac its widest point. Some of these are considered to be large infundibula of the posterior communicating origin.

Each of these four types may be supra- or subtentorial and each may possess, at its origin from the parent vessel, an atherosclerotic plaque.

In dealing with these aneurysms the coating technique, if available during the operative procedure, provides considerable flexibility. In the author's opinion this technique should be available in every case, whether or not the aneurysm is considered suitable for clipping, in order to anchor the clip in place, if for no other reason. There do appear to be however, adequate additional reasons for use of a nontoxic coating technique, with or without clips, in all cases.

Aneurysms with Narrow Neck. If the neck of the aneurysm is narrow and does not contain atheroma, a suitable Heifetz, Mayfield, Yarsargil, or other spring clip may be placed on it, with or without clearing the arachnoid from its surface. The neck should be inspected under magnification before and while the clip is being placed, using either the microscope or a suitable, concentrically lighted binocular loupe, providing from 3 to 6 diameters of magnification. Even in favorable cases, careful inspection of the clip after it is placed will usually reveal a significant length of aneurysmal neck between the clip and the parent vessel. Coating with adherent plastics will prevent the development of additional aneurysmal dilatation of this proximal part of the neck over the ensuing months or years. The coating should include the parent vessel, for a length of approximately 1.0 cm, the neck of the aneurysm, and the clip itself, which should be coated to prevent post-operative dislodgment. If an atherosclerotic plaque is present at the origin of the neck, the clip may be placed at a more distal point along the neck, or even on the fundus of the sac, the proximal portion of the sac and neck coated, and the clip locked in position with adherent plastic.

Globular, Ellipsoidal, or Irregular Aneurysm. With a large sac and a neck too short to be clipped safely, these aneurysms may sometimes by ligated with reasonable safety; a Sundt clip with gelatin foam or Avitene should be available in case the ligature cuts through the neck. Here again, coating will protect against new sac formation in the proximal part of the neck of the aneurysm. If the neck appears to be unusually fragile, either in this or the preceding type of aneurysm with a well-formed neck, the first step in the coating (polyvinyl-polyvinylidene chloride copolymer) may be applied with an artist's airbrush to strengthen the neck before applying the clip (v.i). It is sometimes safer to apply a long clip across the sac and to coat the parent vessel, short neck, proximal sac, and clip. If the sac is too wide for this maneuver to be practicable, an aneurysm adherent to the temporal lobe may usually be safely dissected free by opening the pia-arachnoid, which is sealing the site of bleeding. The aneurysm may then be coated as a whole, without clipping.

If bleeding occurs during dissection of this or other type of internal carotid aneurysms, the bleeding point is picked up in the sucker and a clip applied. The clip applied should be adequate to control bleeding, with no thought of cure. The aneurysm is then dealt with as if bleeding had not occurred. Temporary carotid occlusion using a Mayfield or Heifetz clip may help to control bleeding. The maximum time required to control hemorrhage in such circumstances has so far been 1 minute and 50 seconds. For this reason moderate hypothermia (28° to 30°C) is no longer used routinely but is now reserved for situations in which the need for temporary occlusion seems unusually likely.

If a long clip across a subtentorial sac is contemplated and found impracticable, and if the bleeding point is sealed as it often is by adhesion to the oculomotor nerve, the sac and nerve may be coated together. Substantial recovery of oculomotor nerve paresis may still occur. This technique has appeared to the author to be safer than dissection of the nerve from the sac in circumstances in which a long clip cannot be placed safely across the sac.

Sessile Internal Carotid Aneurysm. This type of aneurysm usually can be clipped at some convenient point on the sac, chosen for ease of exposure or circumferential dissection, without disturbing the site of bleeding. If this maneuver is not practicable, because of the danger of deformation of the parent vessel, or simply because of the large size of the collapsed sac, the aneurysm may be dissected free as in the previous type, and coated without clipping. It should be noted that in order to clip a sac 10 mm in diameter, a clip with jaws at least 16 mm in length must be used.

At this point it should be mentioned that when an aneurysm can be fully dissected with reasonable safety, coating alone should be considered, since the application of a clip, which may crush or abrade the endothelium of the aneurysm may increase the liklihood of the formation of a postoperative thrombus or embolus. If the coating material is nontoxic and nonpermeating, one would expect the likelihood of this catastrophic complication of aneurysm surgery to be lessened.

Dome-Shaped or Infundibular Aneurysm. These aneurysms often cannot be clipped without serious deformation of the internal carotid artery. If a clip is placed, its situation is likely to be most precarious and should be avoided if possible. The point of bleeding has often been sealed by arachnoid alone, which can be carefully circumcised under magnification and left in place. The aneurysm can then be coated without the use of clips. If bleeding occurs during dissection, a wide, square-ended Mayfield clip may be applied end-first to the bleeding point, again without attempting to cure the aneurysm. No matter how precariously the clip may have been placed, coating will anchor it in position and reinforce the remainder of the sac along with the adjacent portion of the artery. Treatment of an aneurysm of this type without coating is both hazardous and unreliable.

Internal Carotid Aneurysms at the Bifurcation

Aneurysms in this location are among the most hazardous to treat because there is danger of disturbing vessels entering the anterior perforated space from the proximal part of the middle cerebral artery and from adjacent portions of the anterior cerebral and internal carotid arteries. Dense adhesions are frequently present between the proximal part of the aneurysm, both neck and fundus, and the adjacent surfaces of the middle and anterior cerebral arteries. Further, the origins of one or both vessels are frequently compromised by the origin of the aneurysm, and placement of a clip may compromise the lumen of the middle cerebral, anterior cerebral, or both arteries. Treatment of these aneurysms by coating minimizes dissection of perforators and may make it unnecessary to separate the neck of the aneurysm from its adherence to major vessels.

Thus a simplified technique may be employed to treat bifurcation aneurysms when coating is used. Angiograms are studied with care in order to predict the site of the adhesion, which is usually between the bleeding site and the frontal or temporal cortex, usually the former. Elevation of the head, mannitol, hyperventilation, and cerebrospinal fluid drainage should permit gentle separation of frontal and temporal lobes with minimal retraction. The carotid bifurcation and aneurysm are exposed; no attempt is made to dissect the neck away from major arteries on either side. The aneurysm is followed to the most proximal point of its cortical adhesion. Just proximal to this point, the pia is entered and a few cubic millimeters of cortex sucked away, just enough to permit circumcision of the adherent area of pia or pia-arachnoid, which remains attached to the sac.

The aneurysm, adjacent origins of the middle and anterior cerebral arteries, and the distal 6 or 8 mm of the internal carotid artery are then coated, displacing these structures only minimally from their original positions.

Bleeding, during dissection to expose these aneurysms, may be catastrophic. In some cases moderate hypothermia should be considered because it may become necessary to clip temporarily the internal carotid and both major branches. However, with bleeding, it is preferable simply to pick up the bleeding point in the sucker and to place a clip, no matter how close to the margin of the leak or how precariously it is placed, in order to provide hemostasis for 4 to 5 minutes. It is immediately anchored to the sac by coating and the aneurysm and vessels coated as described above.

Aneurysms of the Middle Cerebral Artery

Coating middle cerebral artery aneurysms has transformed treatment of these lesions from a nightmare to what has often been a relaxed and uncomplicated procedure.[2] Most of these aneurysms arise from the trifurcation of the middle cerebral artery at about the limen insulae. A few do occur proximal to this point on the main trunk of the vessel. These latter are sessile usually, and in intimate relation to the perforating vessels to the caudate and lenticular nuclei and to the internal capsule. They are exposed by gently opening the arachnoid over the proximal portion of the sylvian fissure, and are coated in much the same manner as are aneurysms of the carotid bifurcation. These are dangerous lesions in which dissection should be kept to a minimum. Many cannot be clipped without compromising important perforating vessels. Coating with adherent plastics has made treatment of these aneurysms relatively safe. Mortality is low and there is much less danger of hemiparesis and hemiplegia than was formerly the case.

The more common trifurcation aneurysms may be exposed in a similar fashion. However, the author prefers to expose them by removing a plug of superior and middle temporal convolution, about 1.5 cm in diameter, centered approximately 2.0 cm behind the temporal tip. The main trunk of the vessel, as seen through the pia, leads into the aneurysm. Adhesions at the bleeding site are protected by approaching the lesion in this manner. The site of adherence can usually be identified easily as a dark area adherent to the overlying pia.

Under 3 to 6 power magnification, numerous vessels are seen winding about the sac; one or more major branches may emerge from the sac. These vessels may be dissected from the sac, a tedious process that presumably carries some risk of thrombosis as well as hemorrhage. Coating makes it unnecessary to clip the sac and thus obviates the need to dissect the vessels in relation to it. The pial adhesion to the sac is circumcised without disturbing it, and the nonadherent portion of pia-arachnoid is removed from the sac and from its feeding and emerging vessels. The aneurysm and adjacent vessels are then coated.

As with other aneurysms, if bleeding occurs, a clip is applied to close the bleeding point;

it is anchored in place when the aneurysm is coated. In two instances the bleeding point was controlled with smooth Cushing forceps while the coating was applied. The forceps were gently removed just before the outer coat polymerized completely.

Anterior Communicating Aneurysms

Exposure and treatment of these aneurysms is among the most hazardous of neurosurgical undertakings. Dissection of the sac may produce spasm and bleeding from important small perforating vessels to the hypothalamus. Excessive manipulaton or application of clips may be followed by thrombosis or embolism in an anterior cerebral artery. Not uncommonly, a clip intended to occlude the sac will compromise the origin of one or both anterior cerebral arteries. When clips are relied upon for necessary hemostasis alone, and coating is used as the primary modality, these hazards may be lessened.

Ordinarily the operation is done from the right side, unless the anterior cerebral artery is essentially a left azygos vessel. Relying upon the reduction of brain volume by the patient's position, hyperventilation, mannitol, and cerebrospinal fluid drainage, the internal carotid bifurcation is exposed. A small resection of the inferomedial part of the orbital cortex is made, and the proximal part of the anterior cerebral artery on the side of the craniotomy is exposed through the cortex. The overlying pia-arachnoid is left intact. Depending upon the configuration of the aneurysm, a decision is then made as to whether the left anterior cerebral artery should also be exposed. If so, the region of the aneurysm is avoided until, through a similar cortical resection, the opposite anterior cerebral artery is brought into view. Cortical tissue is gently sucked away, using a very fine sucker, and the perforating long and short branches of the anterior cerebral arteries are carefully preserved. The overlying arachnoid is left intact and the base of the aneurysm slowly approached by following one or both anterior cerebral arteries medially.

Meanwhile, the angiographic films are carefully and continuously reviewed during dissection in order to determine quite precisely the relationship of the aneurysm to the anterior cerebral arteries and to adjacent structures. As with other aneurysms, adhesion to free arachnoid or to pia or pia-arachnoid has usually been responsible for controlling the original bleeding. The point of hemorrhage is usually in the distal part of the sac. The adhesion may be to one or the other frontal lobe, either its inferior or its interhemispheric surface, to the optic chiasm, or tract, or to the lamina terminalis.

As the base and fundus of the aneurysm come into view, estimates of the position of its apex are continuously revised and every effort made to avoid this region. Dissection is continued by sucking small increments of cortex, keeping the pia or pia-arachnoid intact. Even if most of the aneurysm is clearly seen through the pia-arachnoid, the subarachnoid space is avoided as long as possible. A small secondary bulge or teat, or an area of dark discoloration is watched for, carefully avoided, and its overlying arachnoid cut around and preserved. Arachnoid or pia-arachnoid should be removed from the sac only if it is nonadherent. Adherent areas should be circumcised and preserved with the sac. If the sac appears unduly fragile as it is being dissected, it may be reinforced from time to time by spraying with the first coat, the polyvinyl-polyvinylidene chloride copolymer, which polymerizes immediately when dried with a stream of gas from the airbrush. Although aneurysms that point anteriorly or laterally are, of course, easier to expose than those that point posteriorly, less than 10% of anterior communicating aneurysms should bleed during dissection. If bleeding does occur, a circumstance especially likely if the sac must be dissected from the optic nerve, chiasm, or tract, the bleeding point is immediately picked up in the tip of the sucker and a Heifetz or Mayfield clip of suitable size and shape is applied. Hemostasis alone is sought in this maneuver and no attempt is made to cure the aneurysm; working too far proximally on the sac may deform or occlude the origin of an anterior cerebral artery.

The author has always held in readiness a Mayfield or Heifetz clip so that it can be temporarily placed on an internal carotid or anterior cerebral artery, but it has usually been possible to control bleeding without proximal clipping.

As dissection of the sac proceeds, it is important to be aware, at all times, of the position of the proximal and distal trunks of both anterior cerebral arteries. If this is done, a decision may safely be made during dissection to place a clip directly across the sac without exposing the site of the original hemorrhage. Placing such a clip across the distal part of the sac minimizes manipulation and dissection of the base of the aneurysm and of the anterior cerebral arteries in this region, which is rich in important perforating vessels. The clip, sac, and parent vessels are then coated. If, however, the sac can be dissected free without disturbing adherent pia-arachnoid, it should be coated without clipping, thus avoiding damage to its endothelial lining and consequent possible thrombosis or embolism.

Other Aneurysms

Aneurysms at the bifurcation of the anterior cerebral into the pericallosal and callosomarginal arteries are readily exposed along the falx through a small right frontal parasagittal flap. These aneurysms may be coated with or without clipping.

The author has treated only five aneurysms of the posterior circulation by coating. As in all cases of bifurcation aneurysms, the fundus of a basilar bifurcation aneurysm may be clipped and the lesion coated in order to avoid dissection through the posterior perforated space to clip its neck. Sessile aneurysms, especially those of the basilar trunk, may also be particularly suitable for coating. In one vertebral artery aneurysm it was not possible to occlude its neck without shutting off the posterior inferior cerebellar artery. A clip was therefore placed across the fundus, just proximal to the site of the original hemorrhage, and the clip, aneurysm, and adjacent vertebral artery coated.

Coating of Intracranial Aneurysms

Reinforcement of aneurysms with plastics was first reported in 1956 by Dutton,[3] who used methyl methacrylate to provide an investment about the lesion. Selverstone and associates[2,4-9] reported the use of adherent plastics for this purpose in 1958 and subsequently. This basic technique is still employed, with a number of modifications that have reduced the time of polymerization from about 45 minutes to from 3 to 5 minutes.

Other authors subsequently employed a number of agents,[10,11] but none provides an adherent coating without chemical bonding to tissue. Such a reaction must inevitably produce a zone of necrosis whenever the agent comes in contact with adventitia.[12] It may be assumed that a dead space ultimately will be present between the adhesive and the adventitia of the aneurysm.

The technique we employ makes use of an initial coat of an artificial latex that is well tolerated by tissue and when polymerized in situ by evaporation of its water base is intimately adherent by physical coaptation rather than by chemical bonding. This microdispersion of polyvinyl-polyvinylidene chloride copolymer is sprayed through a simple artist's airbrush onto the moist surface of the aneurysm and its associated vessels.

Helium is used to drive the airbrush, since this gas warms rather than cools with expansion, and is thus unlikely to provoke spasm in the feeding vessel. The supply of latex is then shut off, leaving a thin, virtually invisible coating of adherent plastic.

This initial coat provides relatively little strength in itself, but it does provide a dry surface, adherent to the aneurysm, to which a second coat, a mixture of two-component epoxy resins, is applied. The second coat polymerizes in 3 to 5 minutes with an increase in temperature of only 2° to 5°C, providing a strong, resilient coating for the aneurysm.

Technique of Coating

1. The aneurysm is exposed along with its parent vessels. Adherent vessels need not be dissected from the sac. Pia and arachnoid, which are adherent to the sac and usually constitute the fragile seal of the site of hemorrhage, are left in place.
2. If clips or ligatures have been placed, they are not disturbed.
3. Insofar as possible, adjacent structures are removed from contact with the sac.
4. If cerebrospinal fluid collects near the sac, a narrow cottonoid strip and sucker are used to keep the field as dry as possible.
5. Minute oozing from adventitial vessels is controlled by means of thrombin, 3% hydrogen peroxide, or Avitene.
6. If spasm of feeding vessels is present, it has always been possible to correct it by the application of absorbent cotton saturated with 3% papavarine solution, which may require as long as 10 to 15 minutes to be effective.
7. Moistened gelatin foam is placed over adjacent structures to mask them from the coating process. No ill effects have been observed however when masking has been incomplete.
8. A stream of helium is then directed to the aneurysm and feeding vessels through the artist's airbrush, with the valve from the "color bottle" closed.
9. As soon as obvious surface moisture has evaporated, the valve is opened to disperse the dilute artificial latex in a fine mist about the lesion.
10. If the aneurysm cannot be turned so that all surfaces face the stream, the mist that floats in the air within the craniotomy opening will nevertheless be deposited on all free surfaces.
11. The valve is then closed and the stream of helium again directed on the aneurysm and feeding vessels. The faintly milky, thin layer of latex dries to a transparent invisible coat.
12. The coating process is repeated three or four times, the entire process requiring about 5 minutes.
13. The two syringes containing the two components of the epoxy resin coating, in stoichiometric amounts, are mixed in the barrel of a small plastic syringe, stirred vigorously, and extruded through a plastic cannula to coat the aneurysm, a small segment of its parent vessels, and clips, if they have been used.
14. The undersurface of the aneurysm may, if necessary, be coated by extruding some of the resin on a thin piece of dry gelatin foam. This is slid into place beneath the aneurysm and brought up against its undersurface. Additional resin is added from above, until the coating is continuous. The gelatin foam is allowed to remain in place.
15. Alternatively, if desired, a single layer of medium-mesh cotton gauze may be used to contain the epoxy coat, wrapping it loosely around the sac.
16. The moist gelatin foam strips used as a protective mask initially may now be removed.
17. Hardness of the resin is checked by palpation with a small dissector. When polymerized, the resin is firm but somewhat resilient.
18. The procedure is completed in routine fashion.

Postoperative Care and Complications

There are no special features in the postoperative care of these patients. If hypothermia has been employed, temperature is allowed to rise to normal levels in 36 to 48 hours. A soft rubber catheter is left in the subarachnoid space near the aneurysm, draining into a rubber glove outside the dressing. Fifty to 100 ml of gradually clearing pink fluid usually drains within the first 36 to 48 hours, and the catheter is then removed.

Dexamethasone has been continued postoperatively in the same dose as that administered during the immediate preoperative period; it is gradually withdrawn within 6 to 8 days. Dilantin, 250 mg, is given intravenously immediately after operation and thereafter the dose is increased to 300 mg daily by mouth. It is continued for 2 years in most instances, and the dose is controlled by occasional determinations of blood levels, which are kept in the low therapeutic range unless a seizure occurs.

There have been no instances in which significant signs of meningeal irritation have occurred in patients whose aneurysms have been coated by the technique described, nor has there been any indication of unusual postoperative fever.

Rebleeding after an aneurysm has been fully coated has not been documented. In one patient in whom an anterior communicating aneurysm extended through the lamina terminalis into the third ventricle, where it was adherent to the diencephalon, the fundus of the aneurysm was not fully coated. Rebleeding occurred in this patient postoperatively, necessitating reoperation 3 months later. During reoperation, the sac was fully freed, withdrawn from the third ventricle, and coated. This patient has no abnormal sensory or motor findings but is functioning at a significantly reduced intellectual level.

The entire series of approximately 200 aneurysms that have been coated by this technique is now being reviewed. A brief assessment of the last 25 cases included 16 internal carotid, 6 anterior communicating, and 3 middle cerebral artery aneurysms. All of these patients are alive. One additional patient in whom the aneurysm could not be operated upon has expired. All treated patients have resumed their former occupations, except 2, mentioned earlier, who had anterior communicating aneurysms with a history of multiple hemorrhages. These patients have not as yet regained normal mental status and may never do so.

One patient was demented following two subarachnoid hemorrhages. His aneurysm was operated upon, with some misgivings because of his mental status. He subsequently proved to have communicating hydrocephalus and has returned to his normal business activities following ventriculoperitoneal shunt.

REFERENCES

1. Aitken RI, Drake CG: A technique of anesthesia with induced hypotension with subsequent correction of intracranial aneurysm, *Clinical Neurology*, vol 21. Williams and Wilkins, Baltimore, 1974, pp 107-113
2. Selverstone B: Aneurysms at middle cerebral "trifurcation"; treatment with adherent plastics. *J Neurosurg 19*:884-888, 1962
3. Dutton JEM: Intracranial aneurysm. A new method of surgical treatment. *Br Med J 2*:585-586, 1956
4. Selverstone B, Ronis N: Coating and reinforcement of intracranial aneurysms with synthetic resins. *Bull Tufts N Engl Med Center 4*:8-12, 1958
5. Selverstone B: Vascular reinforcement with adherent plastics. *N Engl Vasc Soc Proc 19*:37, 1960-1961
6. Selverstone B: Reinforcement of intracranial aneurysms with adherent plastics. Proceedings of the British Society of Neurology and Surgery. *J Neurol Neurosurg Psychiatr 24*:92, 1961
7. Selverstone B: Treatment of intracranial aneurysms with adherent plastics. Proceedings of the Boston Society of Psychiatry and Neurology. *N Engl J Med 265*:100, 1961
8. Selverstone B, Dehghan R, Ronis N, et al: Adherent synthetic resins in exerimental surgery. *Arch Surg 84*:80-84, 1962
9. Selverstone B: Treatment of intracranial aneurysm with adherent plastics, *Clinical Neurosurgery*, vol 9. Williams and Wilkins, Baltimore, 1963, pp 201-213
10. Sugar O, Tsuchiya G: Plastic coating of intracranial aneurysms with "EDH-adhesive." *J Neurosurg 21*:114-117, 1964
11. Chou S-N, Ortiz-Suarez HJ, Brown WE: Technique and material for coating aneurysms, *Clinical Neurosurgery*, vol 21. Williams and Wilkins, Baltimore, 1974, pp 182-193
12. Sachs E, Jr, Erbinger A, Margolis G, et al: Fatality from ruptured intracranial aneurysm after coating with methyl-2-cyanoacrylate. *J Neurosurg 24*:889-891n 1966

CHAPTER 5

Treatment of Certain Intracerebral Vascular Lesions with Releasable Balloon Catheter

G. Debrun

THE BEST AVAILABLE TREATMENT for a cavernous carotid fistula is to release an inflated balloon into the cavernous sinus to occlude the fistula and preserve carotid blood flow, a procedure first carried out by Serbinenko.[1] Our own technique, in which an inflatable, detached balloon is used, has been described,[2-7] but a more detailed presentation may be useful.

Technique

Making the Latex Sleeve

Stainless steel moulds are made in different shapes and sizes; mould diameter varies between 0.2 and 1.0 mm. The mould is dipped in pure latex, then placed in an oven and treated with steam at 100°C for 30 minutes. The sleeves are then slipped off the mould and small, latex, finger-shaped sleeves (Figs. 5-1 and 5-2A and B) are obtained.

Making the Balloon

To make the balloon, the sleeve is pulled over catheter A (Fig. 5-2C), and tied onto it with a thin elastic thread cut from a latex glove (Fig. 5-3). The thread is wound around catheter A five times (Figs. 5-4, 5-5, and 5-6A). On the last loop three simple knots are made and the two ends of the thread cut close to the knot with scissors. It may be easier to do this under a magnifying glass. That part of the sleeve under the knot is then cut off (Figs. 5-6B and 5-7).

Department of Neuroradiology, University Hospital Henri Mondor, 94010 Cretail, France

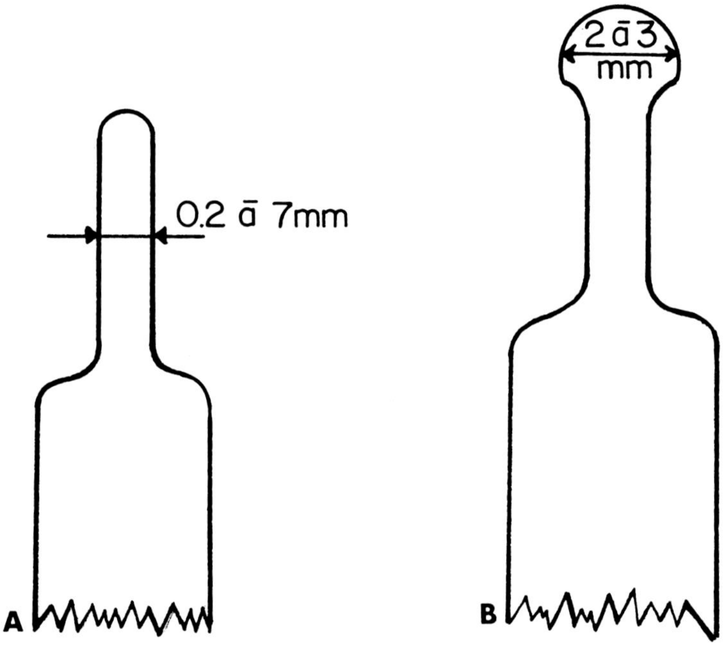

Fig. 5-1. Different shapes of stainless steel moulds.

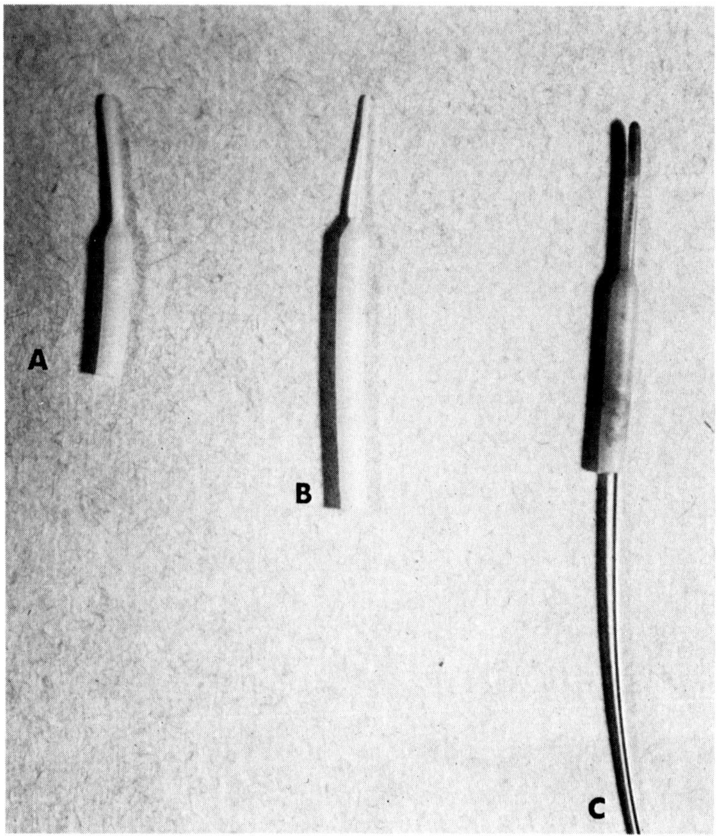

Fig. 5-2. A and B. Two different shapes of latex sleeves. **C.** Catheter A enters a sleeve.

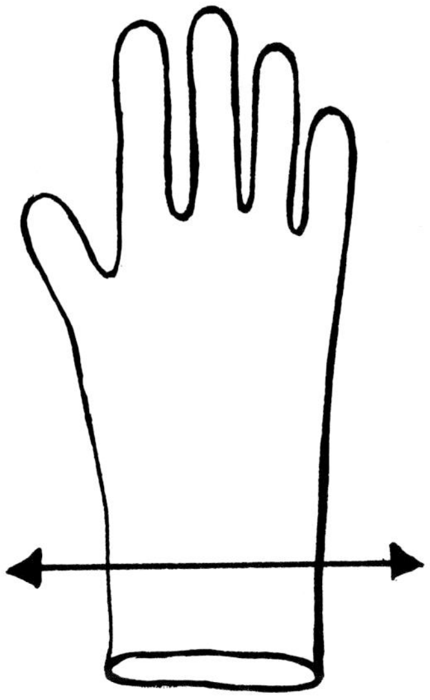
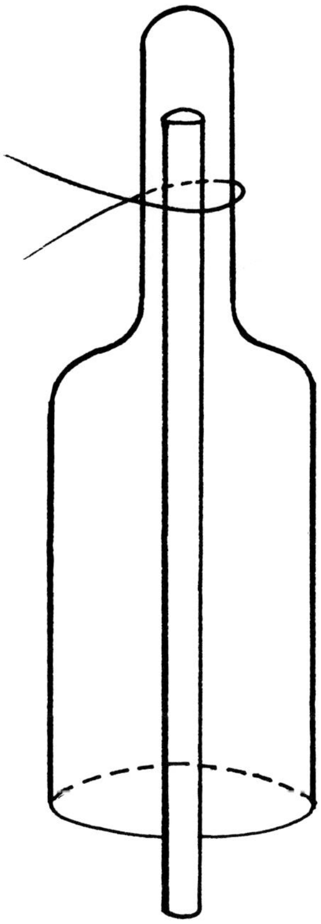
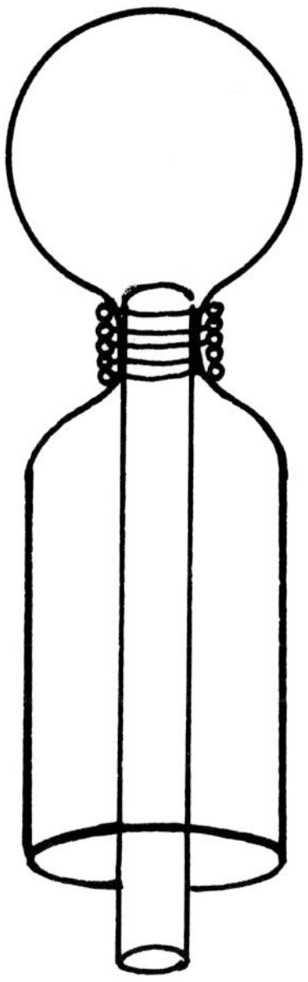

Fig. 5-3. (left) The elastic thread is cut off from a latex glove, as shown by the arrow.

Fig. 5-4. (middle)

Fig. 5-5. (right)

Releasing the Balloon

The balloon is released by a second coaxial catheter B, which is slipped over catheter A to push the balloon off (Figs. 5-6C and 5-8). The balloon aperture is immediately closed by the elasticity of the rubber thread.

This balloon may be released, filled with iodinated contrast medium without leaking immediately, but it progressively (2 to 4 weeks) deflates because the contrast medium passes out through the latex membrane of the balloon. For this reason, it must be replaced with a polymerizing mixture so that the balloon will retain its dimensions permanently.

Introducing Catheters A and B into the Internal Carotid Artery

Both the inner catheter A and the outer catheter B are introduced into the internal carotid with an introducer C, inserted by the Seldinger technique. The internal diameter (ID) of the introducer is 1.8 mm, which is wide enough to allow catheters A and B, as well as continuous isotonic glucose infusions or iodinated contrast medium for preoperative angiographic control, to be passed. We therefore use a lambda-shaped (λ) pipe attached to the rear end of the introducer C (Fig. 5-9). Catheters A and B are passed through the straight part of

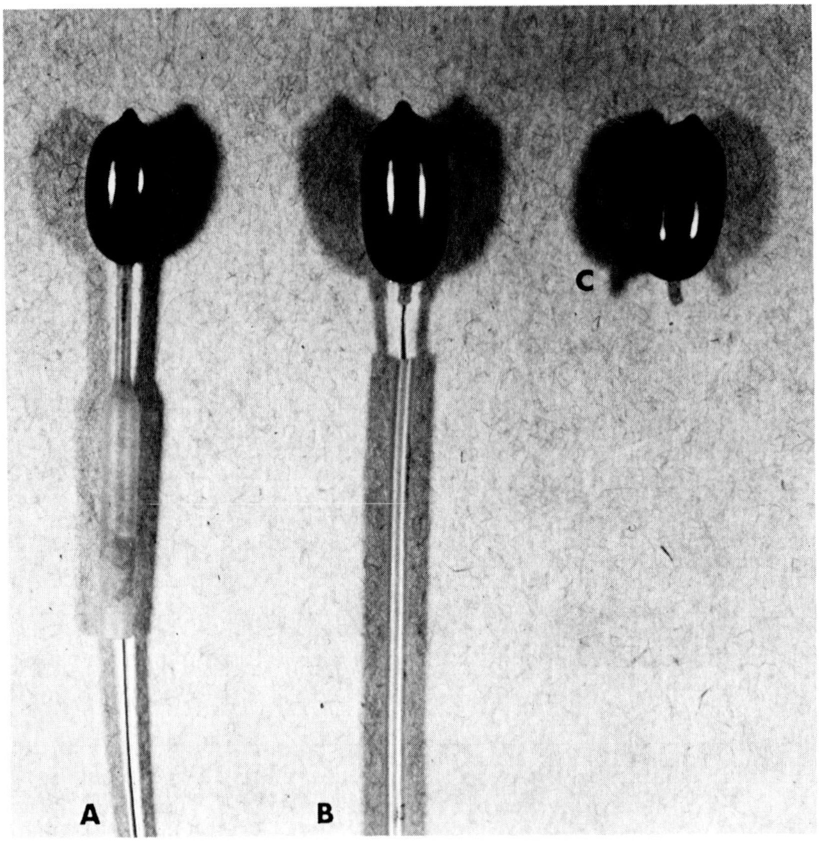

Fig. 5-6. **A.** The sleeve has been ligated over catheter A. **B.** The proximal part of the sleeve has been cut off. Both the ligature and coaxial catheter B are visible. **C.** The same balloon after it has been released.

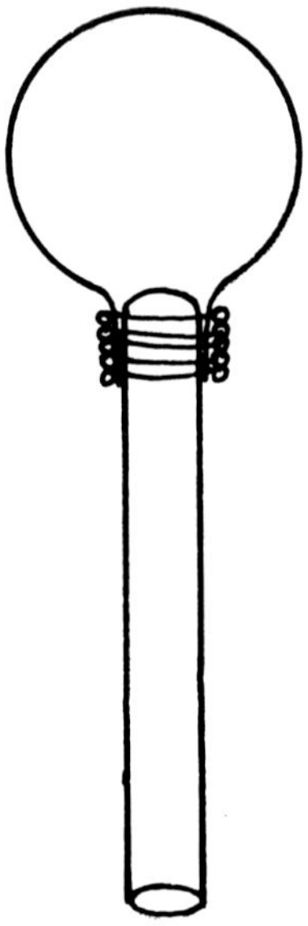

Fig. 5-7.

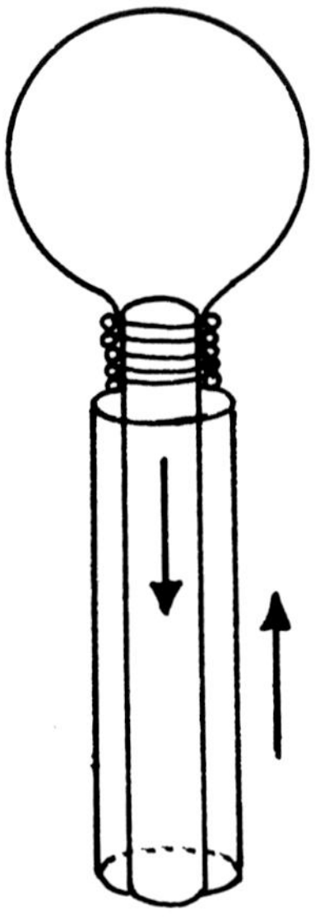

Fig. 5-8.

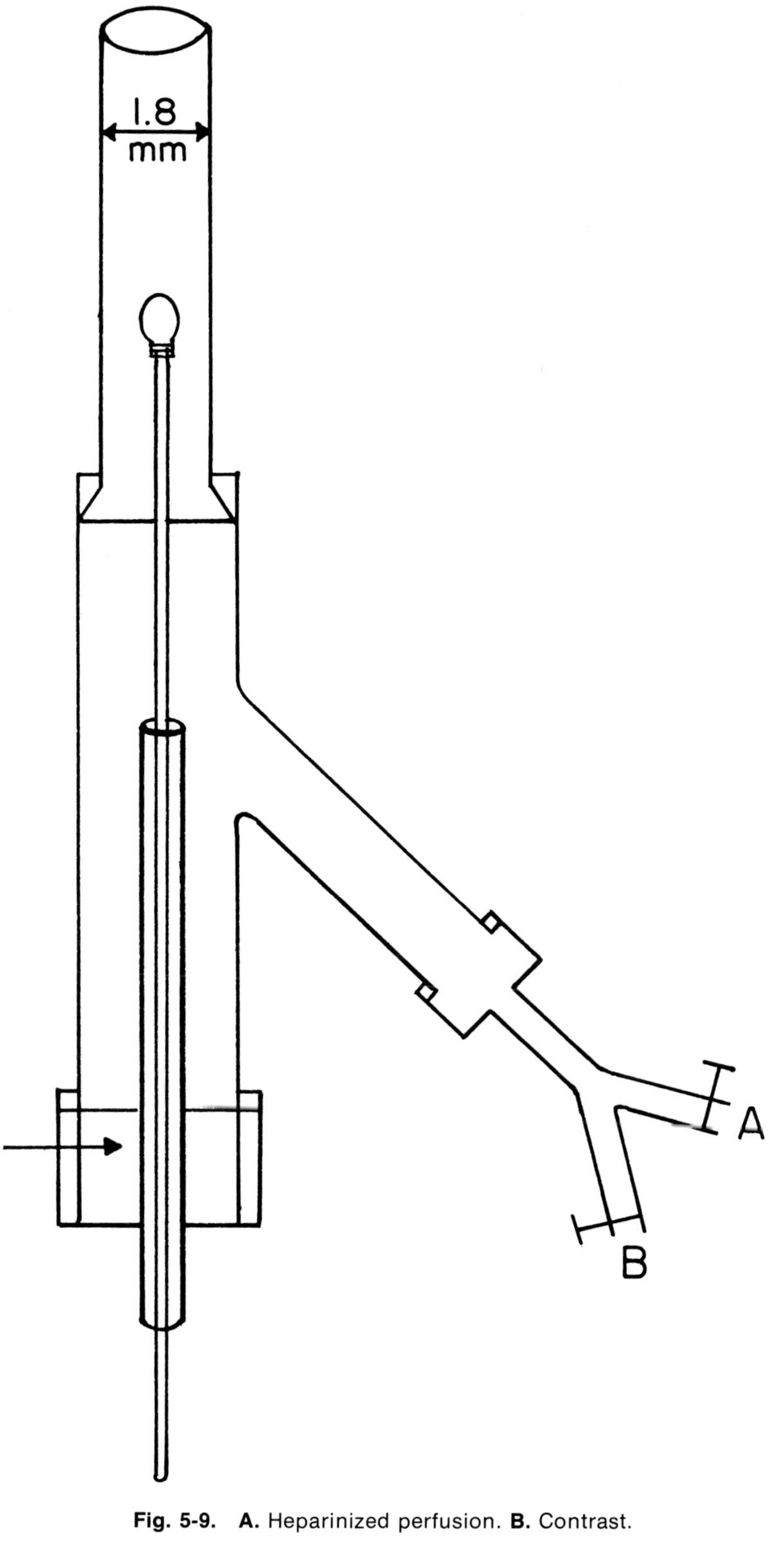

Fig. 5-9. **A.** Heparinized perfusion. **B.** Contrast.

the λ-shaped tube. Blood loss along the coaxial catheter B is prevented by a seal made of cotton soaked in heparinized jelly.

The balloon can be made visible by injecting iodinated contrast medium, when it is passed beyond introducer C. To see the balloon while it is in the introducer, a silver clip can be placed inside it before catheter A is placed in the sleeve. The clip is directed into the end of the sleeve, which is tied over it with a polyethylene thread.* When the balloon has left introducer C and been inflated with 0.05 ml of contrast medium, carotid blood flow and the thrust applied to catheter A are enough to drive the balloon into the carotid sinus.

Experimental Studies

In a series of experiments, carotid jugular fistulas were created in dogs. A week later the common carotid artery was punctured as far as possible below the fistula and an introducer placed in the artery. Carotid arteriography (Fig. 5-10A) shows the fistula. The carotid artery is not opacified above the level of the fistula because of the shunt. The balloon catheter is introduced through the introducer, guided under fluoroscopy, through the fistula into the jugular vein (Fig. 5-10B), and the balloon inflated until it occludes the fistula. Carotid arteriography confirms that the fistula remains occluded and that carotid blood flow is preserved. The balloon is released and further arteriography performed (Fig. 5-10C) to ensure that the balloon remains inflated in good position, the fistula is occluded, and carotid blood flow is preserved. The carotid artery above the level of the fistula is now opacified.

We have also created carotid aneurysms in dogs experimentally (Fig. 5-11), using a portion of vein implanted on the cervical carotid artery. One week later the carotid artery was studied arteriographically (Fig. 5-11A) by means of a carotid introducer. If there is no evidence of spontaneous thrombosis of the aneurysm, the balloon catheter is introduced under fluoroscopy into the aneurysm and the balloon inflated with iodinated contrast medium until its volume equals that of the aneurysm (Fig. 5-11B). Maintenance of carotid blood flow is checked arteriographically before the balloon is released, because if it is overinflated, it may obstruct the carotid. The balloon is then released (Fig. 5-11C) and a final arteriograph confirms that carotid blood flow is preserved. Three weeks later, the balloon is still opacified and carotid blood flow is normal (Fig. 5-11D).

Indications

The ease with which the balloon is drawn into an arteriovenous shunt by the flow contrasts with the difficulty encountered when the balloon is inserted into an aneurysmal cavity. For this reason the best indications for this technique are post-traumatic carotid cavernous and the infrequent vertebrovertebral fistulas. Definitive clinical cure without impairing internal carotid flow can be achieved sufficiently often and easily to make use of a Fogarty catheter less satisfactory for these types of lesions. The goal of treatment is to place the balloon in the cavernous sinus on the venous side of the fistula and to inflate the balloon until the fistula is no longer visible on control angiograms and carotid blood flow is preserved.

Spontaneous nontraumatic carotid cavernous fistulas are a different pathologic entity and are not indications for the balloon technique. Generally, several small feeding vessels

Catheter A: BD 7608, 0.25mm ID. 0.51mm OD; Biotrol, France, 1 rue du Foin 75140, Paris, Cedex 3 No. 1 has an ID of 0.3mm and an OD of 0.7mm; Teflon BD 6426 has an ID of 0.38mm and an OD of 0.69mm.

Catheter B: Ingenor-Surgimed, catheter 15 slips over BD 7608 and BD Teflon 6426, which must be straightened until it will enter Surgimed 15. Ingenor-Surgimed 14 slips over Biotol 1.

Surgimed 7666, ID 0.8mm, OD 2.4mm

Ethicon 1724

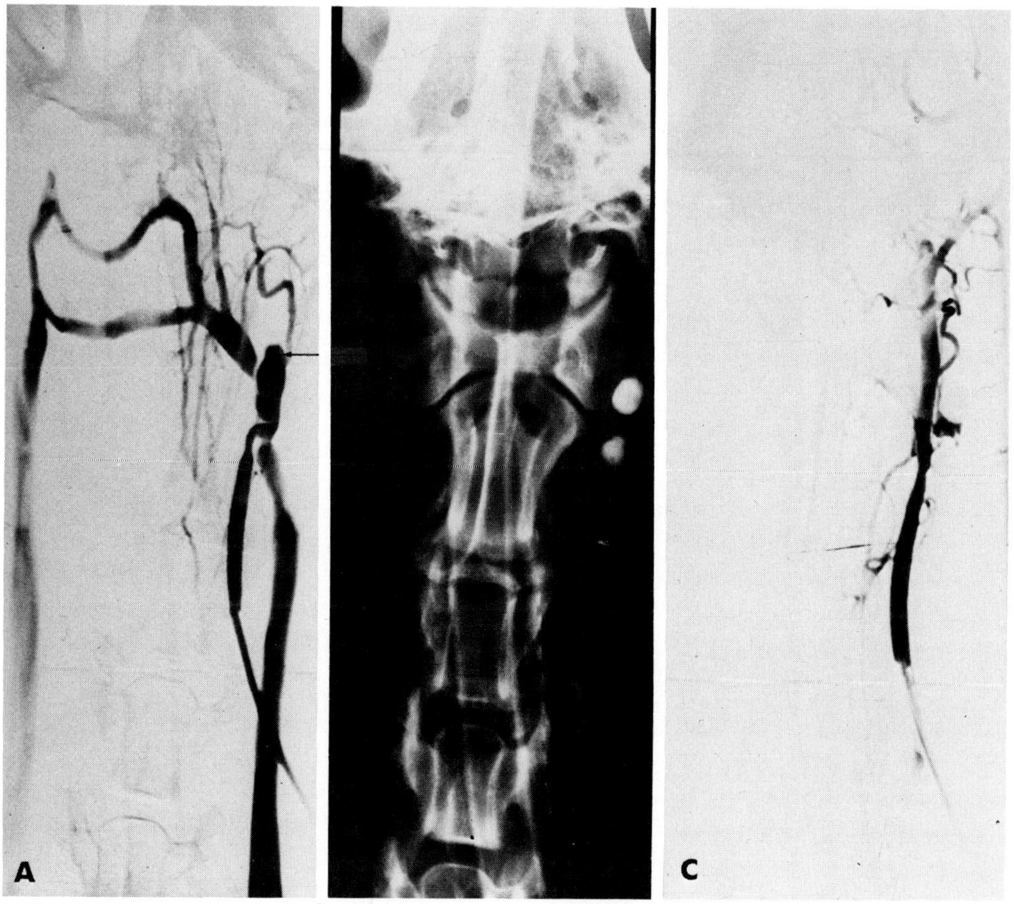

Fig. 5-10. Experimental carotid jugular fistula in a dog. **A.** The jugular vein has been ligated above the fistula. (arrow) The distal part of the carotid artery is not opacified because of the shunt. **B.** The highest balloon has been released in the jugular vein; the lowest balloon is still attached to the catheter. **C.** Control arteriography after the second balloon has been released. The fistula is occluded. The distal part of the carotid artery is now opacified.

arise from the internal carotid artery in the cavernous sinus, in addition to many feeding vessels from branches of the external carotid. The feeding vessels from the external carotid artery must be embolized. Weeks later the ophthalmologic signs will have disappeared and in some cases internal carotid arteriography may show that the feeding vessels from this branch have also disappeared.

For this reason the internal carotid artery of these patients must not be occluded surgically too soon.

Inoperable cerebral angiomas, with a small number of large feeding arteries, are good indications for this technique. Catheterization of the feeding artery with a double-lumen balloon catheter is preferable to proximal obstruction of the feeding vessels. The balloon, when inflated, occludes the artery and silicone is injected, which polymerizes, occluding the bed of the angioma. This technique must be repeated for each feeding vessel, and has been used to treat only one angioma. Although the clinical result was very good partial opacification of the angioma was still apparent at angiography. It is too early to say whether or not this technique will produce good results in the future, but it should not be forgotten.

Surgery remains the best treatment for *aneurysms*, because it is very difficult and hazardous to try to enter the neck of an aneurysm with the balloon catheter. However,

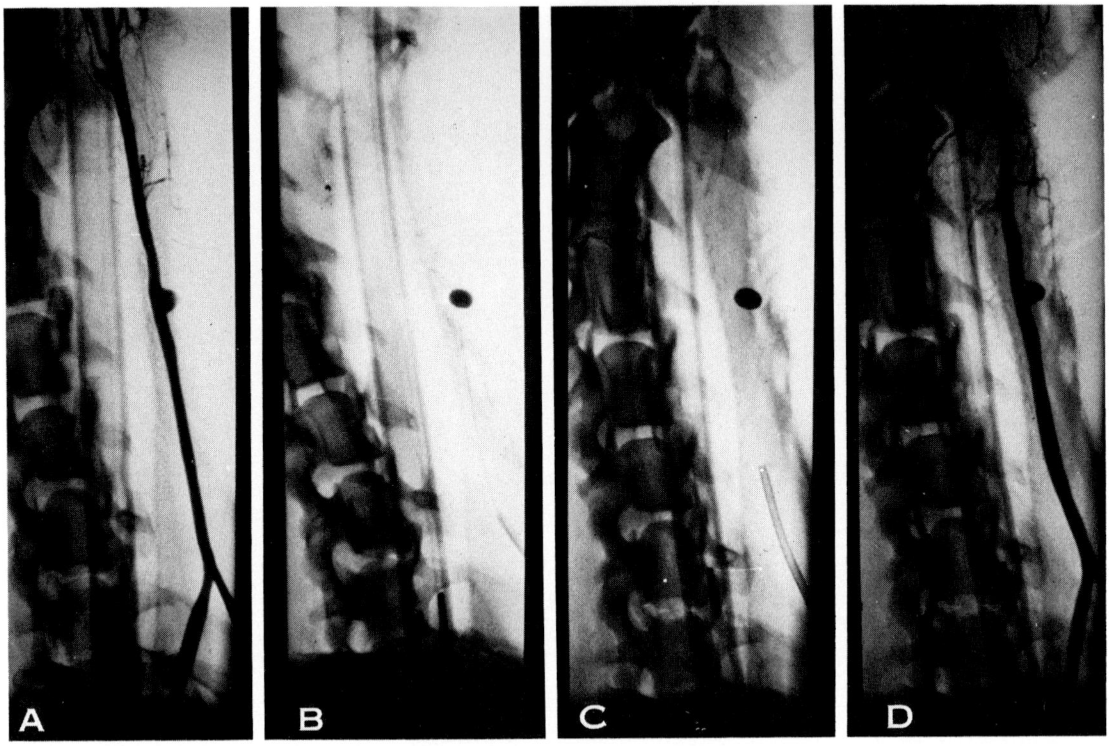

Fig. 5-11. Experimental carotid aneurysm in a dog. **A.** Aneurysm before treatment. **B.** Balloon inflated in the aneurysmal cavity; catheter still visible. **C.** Balloon has been released; carotid blood flow is preserved. **D.** Three weeks later the balloon is still opacified; the carotid artery is normal.

infraclinoid aneurysms of the carotid siphon, and certain basilar aneurysms cannot be operated upon and in these cases the balloon technique should be considered. All complications have been encountered during attempts to enter an aneurysmal cavity, never when treating an arteriovenous malformation. It is useless and indeed dangerous to try to enter an aneurysm with the balloon if there is spasm. There was one death from rupture of the aneurysmal sac.

In conclusion, the balloon technique must be considered excellent for the treatment of all post-traumatic carotid cavernous fistulas, but is only rarely indicated in certain nonsurgical aneurysms or brain angiomas.

Treatment of a Post-Traumatic Carotid Cavernous Fistula

The first step in the treatment of a post-traumatic carotid cavernous fistula using a detachable balloon inflated with polymerizing substance, is a thorough study of the location of the fistula by subtracted serial angiographic films, at least three films per second. Blood flow through the shunt is generally so rapid that the exact level of the fistula cannot be seen. However, vertebral angiography with compression of the feeding carotid artery in the neck will, in most cases, opacify the carotid siphon by retrograde flow and the level of the shunt can be seen (Fig. 5-12A and B). The contralateral carotid artery is always injected, with compression of the feeding carotid, to determine if the blood supply to the cerebral hemisphere, on the side of the fistula, can be insured by anastomosis via the circle of Willis in case it becomes necessary to cut off carotid flow on the side of the fistula.

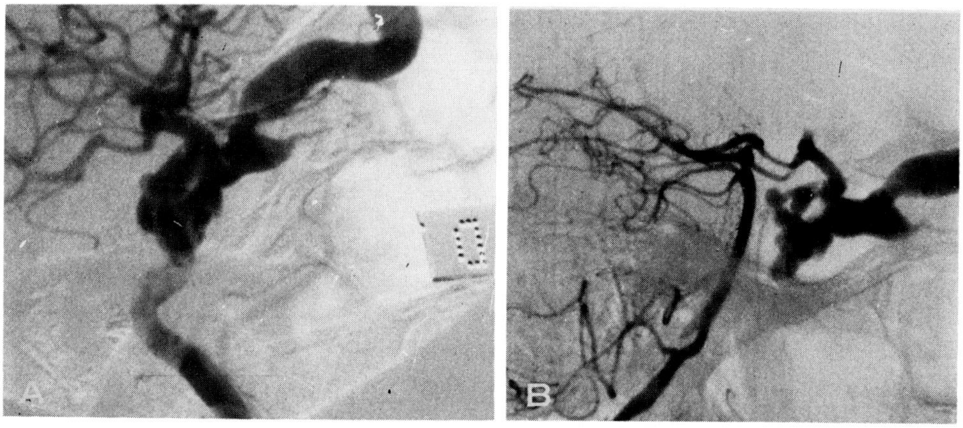

Fig. 5-12. **A.** Right carotid-cavernous fistula, right carotid arteriography. The exact level of the fistula cannot be seen. **B.** Same fistula. Vertebral arteriography with compression of the right carotid. The fistula is clearly seen on the anterior curve of the carotid siphon.

After introducer C has been placed in the internal carotid, balloon catheter A and coaxial catheter B are introduced into the carotid artery. At first, only balloon catheter A is removed. The balloon is inflated with 0.05 ml of iodinated contrast medium and its progress is followed under lateral fluoroscopy. It is difficult to follow the balloon through dense petrous bone and television subtraction with video-recording would help. As soon as the balloon has progressed beyond the petrous portion of the carotid canal, it once again can be seen quite easily. When it reaches the carotid siphon, it tends to be drawn upwards by the flux through the fistula, and a slight flutter or a directional change indicates that it has entered the cavernous sinus. In the last case treated, it was possible to push the balloon into the orbit through the superior ophthalmic vein.

When the balloon does not enter the cavernous sinus rapidly, it should be kept in the neighborhood of the supposed position of the fistula; small to-and-fro motions should be applied to the catheter as balloon volume is varied. If these measures are not successful, the balloon must be replaced with a smaller one.

When the balloon is inside the cavernous sinus, it must be inflated until the fistula is occluded, ie., with about 0.20 ml of iodinated contrast medium. The tap is closed. Preservation of carotid blood flow as well as closure of the fistula are confirmed by AP and lateral serial angiograms (the injection of contrast is carried out through the introducer C (Fig. 5-9B). Any abnormality, such as leakage of contrast into the cavernous sinus or irregularity in carotid blood flow, implies that the amount of contrast in the balloon should be modified until perfect conditions are obtained. In a few cases all the above procedures may fail, probably because the aperture of the fistula is too small or is directed in such a way that the balloon cannot enter it (Fig. 5-13). In this case the balloon should be released in the carotid artery, opposite the neck of the fistula, plugging the carotid artery.

Final Release of the Balloon

Once its final position has been achieved, the balloon is deflated and the iodine contrast it contained is carefully measured. Part of the contrast remaining in catheter A cannot be removed. This volume (0.05 to 0.07 ml) must be known, since it will be reintroduced into the balloon when the polymerizing substance is injected. The substance we use, which is still in a trial stage, is a fluid silicone oil, mixed, just prior to use, with a catalyst. The viscosity of this substance increases after 1 minute, and it must be rapidly sucked into an insulin syringe (1.0

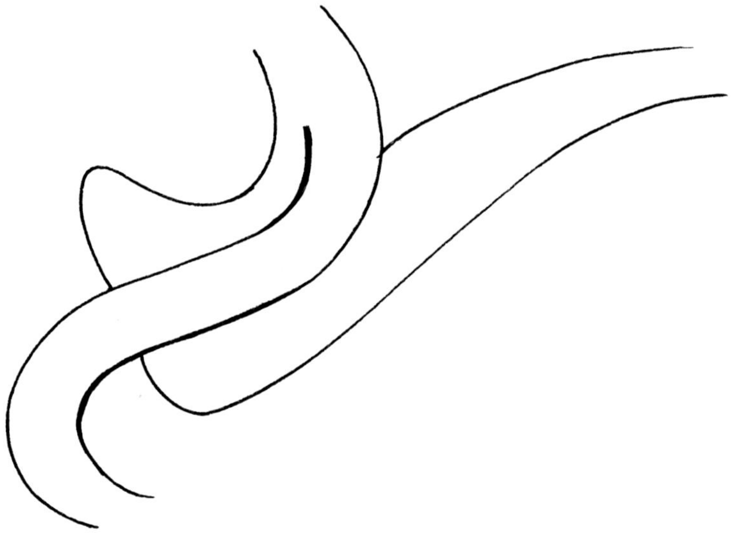

Fig. 5-13. Carotid cavernous fistula due to dissection of the internal carotid artery; the fistulous aperture is so located that it makes the balloon introduction into it impossible.

ml with 100 graduations) and the proper volume injected immediately. We have tried to opacify the silicone with a small amount of tantalum powder, but the powder increases the viscosity of the silicone and can obstruct catheter A before the end of the injection. Therefore this approach has not been pursued further.

Since the density of the iodine contrast medium is higher than that of the silicone, a layering effect will be seen in the inflated balloon.

Once the silicone has been injected, the tap of catheter A is closed. After a 10-minute waiting period, it is released. Then, coaxial catheter B is brought to the base of the balloon. A certain resistance is felt, indicating that the catheter has reached the balloon. At this point traction is exerted on the inner catheter A, while the outer catheter B is kept firmly in place, and release of the balloon can be felt distinctly. This step is controlled radioscopically and the balloon must not move at the time it is released. Both catheters A and B are then withdrawn from introducer C and a new arteriogram, AP and lateral, taken as a check.

The ateriogram must show:

1. The balloon is in the cavernous sinus, outside the carotid artery.
2. The contrast medium used for the arteriogram is not leaking into the cavernous sinus.
3. Carotid blood flow is normal.

Results

Ten patients with carotid cavernous fistulas have been treated (Table 5-1). The first patients were treated with balloons inflated with iodine contrast only (6 of 10 patients). This is a simpler technique but we have found that the volume of the balloon decreased gradually during the weeks following treatment. Of course this decrease in volume cannot occur when silicone is used. In two cases, after the balloon deflated, the fistula was definitely occluded but in place of the balloon there was a false aneurysm of the carotid siphon in the cavernous sinus. These two patients were treated with a second balloon inflated with silicone.

In one case the aperture of the fistula took the form of a very small, short canal between the internal carotid and the cavernous sinus. It was very difficult to enter this canal, but we succeeded in doing so by using a small balloon that could not be inflated with more than 0.05

Table 5-1. Summary of Cases of Carotid Cavernous Fistulas Treated by the Balloon Technique

Patients Treated	Balloon Inflated With Contrast and Released	Balloon Inflated With Silicone and Released	Carotid Blood Flow Preserved
SEM	+	−	+
LAC	+	−	−
FRA	+	−	−
TRI	+	−	+
FUS	+	−	+
LAC	+	−	−
GUI	−	+	+
DRA	−	+	−
BIR	−	+	+
CRO	−	+	+

ml of contrast. As catheter A contains 0.05 ml of contrast, which cannot be aspirated, it was impossible, in this case, to use silicone because it would have reached but not entered the balloon after 0.05 ml of contrast was reintroduced into it. Thus there are certain limitations to the technique when silicone is used.

Carotid blood flow was preserved in 6 of the 10 cases, one of which is illustrated in Figure 5-14. In the remaining 4 cases, the fistula could not be entered in 3 and the balloon was

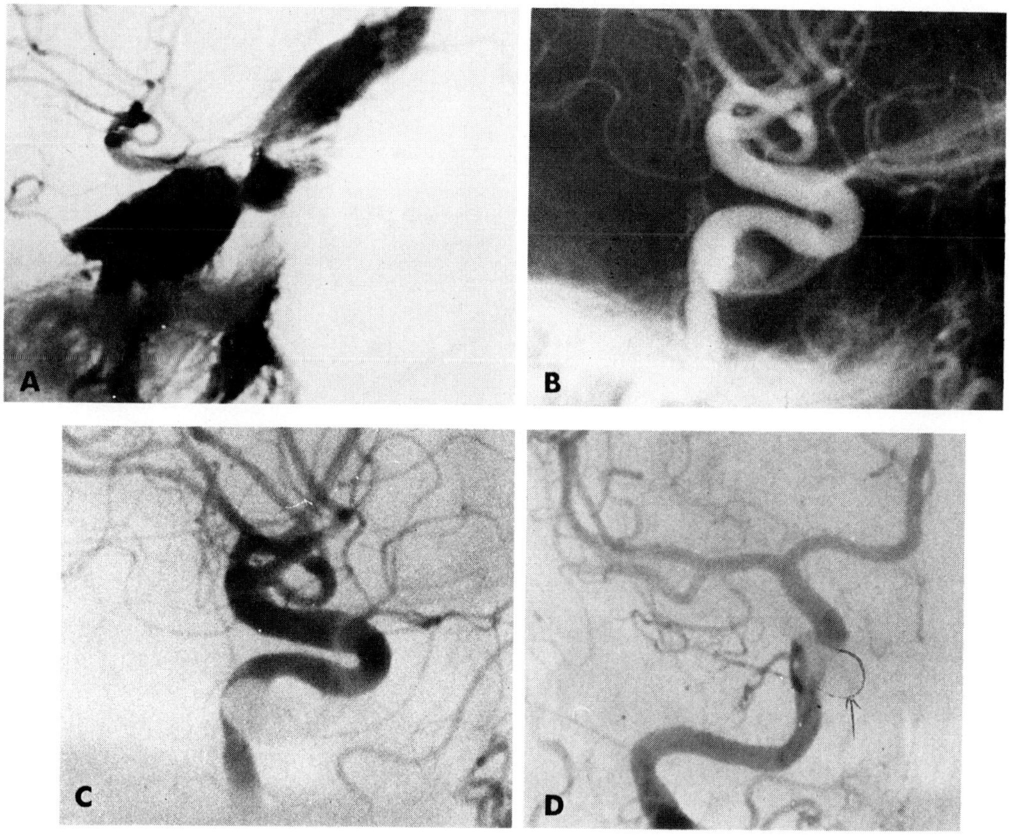

Fig. 5-14. **A.** Right post-traumatic carotid-cavernous fistula. **B.** Control arteriography. The fistula is occluded by a balloon inflated with silicone and released in the cavernous sinus. Level of iodinated contrast is visible. Carotid blood flow is preserved. **C.** Lateral view. **D.** The Balloon is seen in the cavernous sinus, on the left side of the carotid siphon.

released in the carotid siphon close to the fistula. In the last case, the internal carotid was occluded at the time of systematic angiographic control, 2 months after the procedure. These 10 patients now have a normal eye on the side of the fistula; they no longer have the previously audible subjective bruit, and none has had any complication. No oculomotor palsies nor trigeminal pain occurred despite the fact that a balloon was inflated in the cavernous sinus. Control angiograms were taken in all patients 2 months after the procedure, which confirmed the disappearance of the fistula. The 4 patients in whom the internal carotid was occluded were investigated by contralateral carotid and vertebral angiography (Table 5-2).

Table 5-2. Summary of Cases of Aneurysm of Cavernous Portion of Carotid Sinus Treated with the Balloon Technique

	Patients			
Treatment	SCE	OUL	GUI	AMR
Balloon inflated with contrast	+	+	−	−
Balloon inflated with silicone	−	−	+	+
Carotid blood flow reserved	+	+	+	+

We have treated 2 patients with arteriovenous malformations of the vertebrobasilar territory (Table 5-3). One had a vertebrovertebral fistula at C1-C2 level (Fig. 5-15A and B) with complaints of disturbance of deep sensation in the left lower leg and a right cervical murmur. In this patient the introducer was placed in the right vertebral artery by the femoral approach, and a balloon, inflated with iodinated contrast medium, was released in the fistula. Eight days later (Fig. 5-14C), the balloon was still visible, the fistula was occluded, and vertebral blood flow was preserved. This patient is in perfect health 12 months later and the cervical bruit has disappeared.

Table 5-3. Vertebrovertebral Fistulas Treated by the Balloon Technique

	Patients	
Treatment	LAP	BAB
Balloon inflated with contrast	+	+
Balloon inflated with silicone	−	−
Vertebral flow preserved	+	−

The second patient had a dural angioma supplied by many vessels arising from both the internal and external carotid arteries and the left vertebral artery. A balloon, inflated with contrast medium, was released at the origin of this latter feeding vessel, with a good immediate result but an angiographic control done elsewhere showed that the left vertebral artery was occluded.

We have treated 4 aneurysms of the cavernous portion of the internal carotid artery. In 2 cases the balloon was inflated with iodinated contrast medium and in 2 with silicone. The carotid blood flow was always preserved (Fig. 5-16 shows one of these cases).

Complications

Two important complications occurred during attempts to treat aneurysms. As stated above, one patient had an aneurysm of the end of the internal carotid, judged inoperable; he was comatose (grade IV). The internal carotid blood flow was very slow and there was spasm close to the neck of the aneurysm.

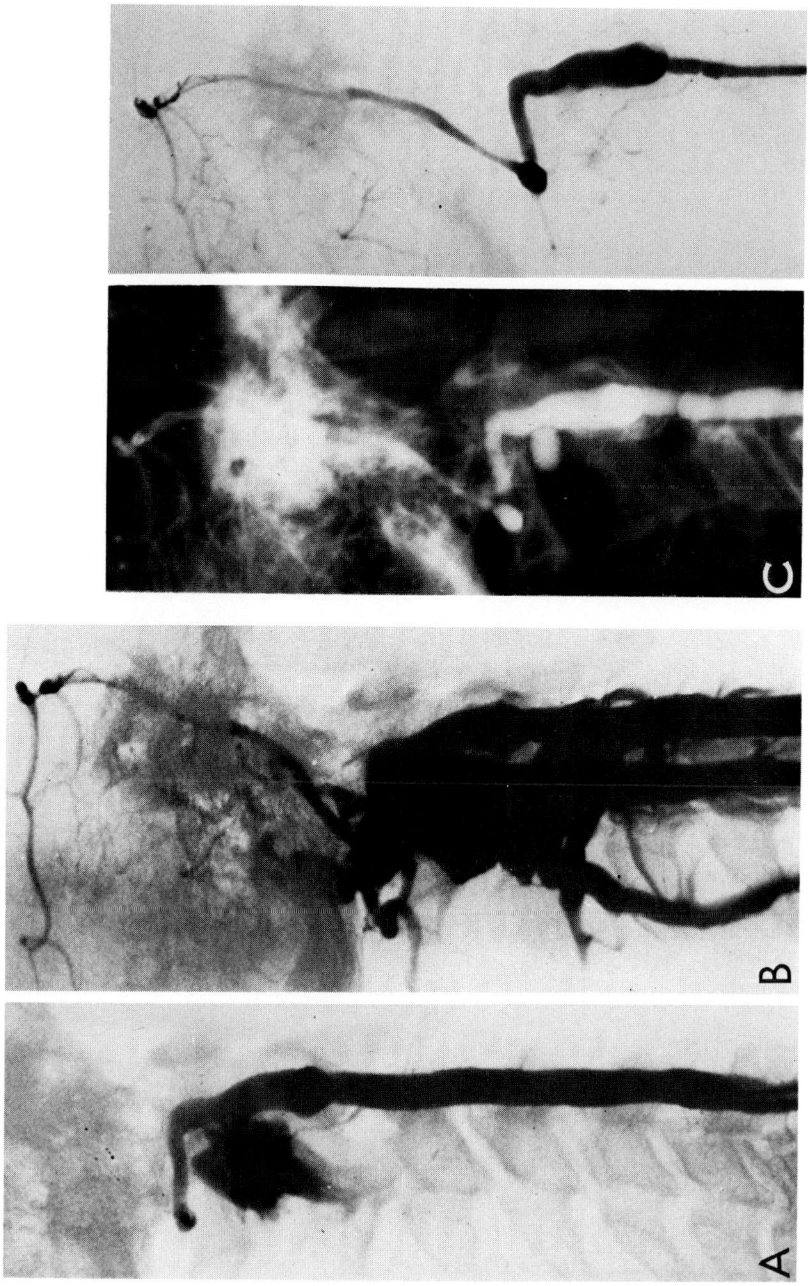

Fig. 5-15. **A.** and **B.** Congenital vertebrovertebral fistula at C1-C2. **C.** The balloon has been released in the fistula and is still opacified 8 days later. The fistula is occluded. The vertebral blood flow is preserved.

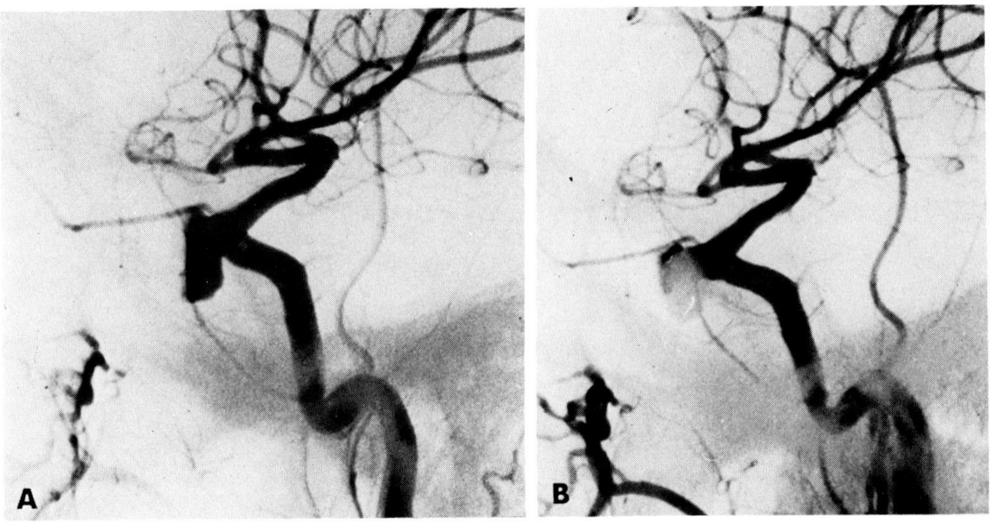

Fig. 5-16. A. Aneurysm of the carotid siphon in the cavernous sinus. **B.** One balloon has been released in the aneurysmal pouch, which is occluded.

The balloon was very difficult to advance because of the slow blood flow. However, we succeeded in reaching the neck of the aneurysm, but the balloon would not enter it. Ten millimeters of isotonic glucose infusion were injected into the carotid artery with a syringe to make the balloon enter the aneurysm, but the latter ruptured at this stage, and the patient died. Thus, we do not advise treatment of inoperable aneurysms with spasm by the balloon technique.

In a second case, a young man with a small aneurysm of the right middle cerebral artery in the sylvian fissure, we could enter the sac and inflate the balloon with contrast, but the moment the balloon was released, it moved back and occluded the sylvian artery. The patient was operated upon and the sylvian artery disobliterated, but a left hemiplegia resulted and some days later the patient died.

Without doubt this complication should have been avoided. It was properly a surgical case, the aneurysm being too small and too distal.

Minor complications occurred in 2 cases of carotid cavernous fistulas when we used iodinated contrast medium only. In the case of the balloon that deflated progressively (2 to 4 weeks) there was a false aneurysm pouch, which was occluded by a second balloon inflated with silicone, with good results.

Conclusions

1. The inflatable, detachable balloon technique is particularly indicated in the treatment of post-traumatic carotid-cavernous fistulas.
2. Our experience is too small to determine whether the technique will be useful in the treatment of inoperable brain angiomas.
3. The treatment of aneurysms is difficult, dangerous, and must be reserved to certain anatomic situations and inoperable aneurysms.
4. Since the volume of iodine-filled balloons does not remain constant, use of a polymerizing substance, that does not leak out of the balloon, is more satisfactory.

Summary

A technique is described in which an inflatable, detachable balloon is used to treat some intracranial vascular lesions, particularly post-traumatic carotid cavernous fistulas.

In this technique, a small finger-shaped latex sleeve, attached to the end of a catheter by an elastic thread, closes the aperture of the balloon at the time it is released. The balloon is detached by using a coaxial catheter.

The first patients were treated using an iodinated contrast medium to fill the balloons; but gradual resorption of the iodine solution tends to occur within the following weeks. Hence, balloons inflated with a polymerizing substance that does not leak from the balloon is preferred.

REFERENCES

1. Serbinenko FA: Balloon catheterization and occlusion of major cerebral vessels. *J Neurosurg 41*:125-145, 1974.
2. Debrun G, Lacour P, Caron JP, et al: Experimental approach of carotid-cavernous fistula with an inflatable and isolated balloon—Application in man. *Neuroradiology 9*:9-12, 1975
3. Debrun G, Lacour P, Caron JP, et al: Inflatable and released balloon technique—experimentation in dog—application in man. *Neuroradiology 9*:267-271, 1975
4. Debrun G, Lacour P, Caron JP, et al: Traitement de fistules artério-veineuses et d'anévrysmes par ballon gonflable et largable. Bases expérimentales. Application à l'homme. *Nouv Presse Méd 4*:2315-2318, 1975
5. Debrun G, Lacour P, Caron JP, et al: Technique endovasculaire de ballonnet gonflable et largable. *Ann Radiol 3*:313-315, 1975
6. Debrun G, Lacour P, Caron JP, et al: Traitement des lésions vasculaires carotido-caverneuses par ballonnet gonflable et largable. *Nouv Press Méd 5*:1294-1296, 1976
7. Debrun G, Lacour P, Caron JP: Balloon arterial catheter techniques in the treatment of arterial intracranial diseases, *Advances and Technical Standards in Neurosurgery. 4*:131-145, 1977

CHAPTER 6

Surgical Therapy of Tumors of the Glomus Jugulare

Gale Gardner
James T. Robertson
Edwin W. Cocke, Jr.

FOLLOWING STACY GUILD'S DESCRIPTION of the glomus jugularis in man in 1941 and Rosenwasser's classic paper of a tumor of the middle ear and mastoid arising from the glomus in 1945, the correct therapy for these lesions has been a continual therapeutic problem.[1,2] Glomus tumors in the middle ear can usually be cured by total removal, either through the ear canal or mastoid. Treatment of glomus tumors, which arise from the jugular bulb, however, is controversial.[3-5] Although these tumors are usually benign, they are malignant by virtue of their localization. The authors believe that these tumors should be considered as arising, and remaining for an indefinite period, as extradural tumors. Tumors arising from the jugular bulb extend into the mastoid and middle ear, anteriorly to the carotid artery and carotid canal, and inferiorly as a local soft tissue mass as well as an intravascular jugular mass. They extend posteriorly and medially to involve the nerves of the jugular foramen and clearly lie extradural, medially more than posteriorly. The tumors have a rich vasovasorum, which, viewed from the posterior fossa, creates a red, vascular, angry pulsating mass that invaginates the dura before invading it. Careful pathologic studies on nonoperated specimens are sparse. This lack of pathologic studies has interfered with the true understanding of the surgical pathology of these peculiar growths.

Since neurosurgeons and otolaryngologists have been responsible for the treatment of these lesions, we have used a combined otolaryngology-neurosurgical team approach to their treatment.[3,4] Presently, our therapeutic approach involves careful radiologic definition of the site and size of the lesion, radiotherapy to the growth, and a subsequent surgical approach involving radical exposure of the inferior and lateral aspects of the tumor. This procedure is followed by a mastoidectomy-suboccipital craniectomy, extratumoral exposure with rerouting of the facial nerve, and finally excision of the jugular vein, bulb, and inferior sigmoid and/or lateral sinus intravascular portion of the tumor. Every effort is made to adhere as closely as possible to the oncologic principle of exposure around the tumor before the mass is excised. In addition, the emphasis is to remain extradural during the process of tumor excision. This approach, in our hands, has been highly successful and has considerably reduced surgical morbidity and blood loss associated with the procedure.[3,4]

Department of Otolaryngology and Maxillofacial Surgery and the Department of Neurosurgery, University of Tennessee, Memphis, Tennessee 38103

Historical Review

Surgical Therapy–Radiation Therapy

Gardner[4] elsewhere has reviewed the history of the therapy of glomus tumors. Since this historical review is so complete, it will be repeated with minimal modification. The location of the glomus tumor at the base of the skull, in a relatively inaccessible site, and the previous frustrating and disappointing surgical approaches utilized have led to the conclusion that this particular tumor should be treated by either limited surgery combined with irradiation therapy or with irradiation therapy alone.[3-7] The controversy involving treatment arises because our knowledge of the natural history of a particular glomus tumor is unknown. These tumors can be diagnostic problems.[8] Usually they grow slowly and untreated cases have been recorded, which existed for 42 years.[9] In other cases the tumors grew rapidly, and in a short period destroyed the interior of the temporal bone and the base of the skull, extended into the neck, involved the cranial cavity, and, on occasion, metastasized to other parts of the body.[10] Mortality has been reported to be between 9.4% and 22% in major studies.[9-11] It is difficult to determine if radiation therapy alone is curative.[5,11-13] At the same time, since these tumors may grow very slowly, the results of partial surgical excision are probably questionable, if reported with less than a 10-year followup.[14] We have never observed death secondary to increased intracranial pressure. It is probable that death occurs from secondary causes because of cranial nerve involvement; for example, inanition and aspiration pneumonia.

A review of therapeutic approaches to the glomus tumor emphasizes the vascular frustrating nature of this lesion.[5-7,10,15-20]

In 1949 Lundgren[15] suggested removing or coagulating the jugular bulb in those instances in which a glomus tumor arose from the bulb. He was influenced by Seiffert,[21] who, in 1934, reported a case in which an apparent glomus jugulare tumor, originating in the bulb, produced a jugulare foramen syndrome. Seiffert[21] explored the bulb and found intraluminal tumor. Weille et al.[16] believed these tumors originate from the dome of the jugular bulb and emphasized the difficulty of their surgical removal. He recommended removing bone from around the tumor so as to avoid tumor trauma. The danger of serious hemorrhage prevented his recommending that the jugular bulb be removed. Semmes[17] reported the successful removal of a 2.0-cm glomus jugulare tumor from the jugular foramen through a suboccipital approach. The patient had hearing loss and tinnitus, a red discoloration of the involved tympanic membrane, and involvement of cranial nerves IX through XII. The tumor removal was considered to be complete, as regards the posterior fossa, but no tumor could be removed from the temporal bone. He did not remove the tumor from the middle ear or mastoid, and used irradiation therapy postoperatively.

Albernaz and Bucy[18] reported a case in which the patient had symptoms of a jugular foramen syndrome and hearing loss. They approached the tumor suboccipitally and found that cranial nerves IX to XII were abnormal, but no tumor was visualized. A cardiorespiratory arrest occurred and the patient expired. A careful autopsy study revealed a 1.0- to 2.0-cm tumor within the jugular foramen, involving all structures of the foramen. This was not recognized as a glomus jugulare tumor. Bucy acknowledges that this tumor was a probable glomus jugulare tumor.

In 1952 Capps[6] reported 5 cases of glomus jugulare tumors. In one case he described mobilizing the facial nerve, packing-off the lateral sinus, ligating the upper end of the internal jugular vein, and attempting to remove the jugular bulb. The postoperative course was stormy. He had used radiation therapy, and in 4 other cases believed the tumor responded to irradiation.

Williams et al.,[5] in 1955, emphasized that x-ray therapy should be added to any form of surgical treatment and that radiation therapy alone may well be sufficient to control the lesion.

Subsequent advances in neuroradiologic technique allowed arteriography to become commonplace.[13] X-ray subtraction technique was introduced in 1961.[22] Valvassori[23,24] reported on the use of polytomography in 1963. Retrograde jugular venography in the diagnosis of this tumor was introduced by Gejrot in 1964.[25] Subsequent authors advocated careful assessment of the size and extent of glomus tumors to select the most appropriate form of therapy, be it surgery, x-ray, or both.[10,19]

In 1958 Meacham and Capps[17] and Thoms[20] reported the removal of glomus jugulare tumors through a suboccipital approach. Meacham and Capps felt the opportunity to remove such a tumor successfully was unusual. Thoms preferred the posterior fossa approach and reported a case with surgical excision. If extensive bone invasion, particularly of the temporal bone, had occurred, however, Thoms believed surgery was probably not feasible and preferred radiation therapy.

In the 1960s, with the aforementioned advances in neuroradiology, advocates of surgical therapy returned. Gastpar[26] advocated bulbectomy, if the jugular bulb was involved, and was willing, if necessary, to sacrifice the facial nerve and the labyrinth.

In 1962 Michelson and Connolly[27] reported a case in which they used cerebrovascular occlusion with hypothermia to allow removal of a recurrent glomus jugulare tumor adherent to the wall of the internal carotid artery. Cerebrovascular occlusion was employed for a period of 10 minutes. This technique was advocated as an adjunct to intracranial procedures. We became very interested in the use of profound hypothermia in 1964. The problems inherent in this technique were many, but the most serious was the hemorrhagic diathesis that occurred when the patient was warmed. The authors[28] used profound hypothermia in 8 patients with intracranial aneurysms. During the period between 1965 and 1969, limited hypothermia and hypotension were used in one case of glomus jugulare tumor and resection attempted. Our interest during this period was in a closed-chest extracorporeal technique and, although we finally solved the problem of hemorrhagic diathesis, the complicated nature of profound hypothermia with circulatory arrest has prevented its use in glomus tumor surgery.

In 1963 Shapiro and Neus[29] reported a case of recurrent glomus jugulare with previous radical mastoidectomy in which they used an extended excision, rerouted the facial nerve, exposed the hypotympanum and bulb, and accomplished complete tumor removal with minimal blood loss.

Gejrot[30] was aware of the frequency of intraluminal jugular bulb extension by these tumors. In 1965 he described a procedure in which he performed a radical mastoidectomy, rerouted the facial nerve, exposed and opened the internal jugular vein, jugular bulb, and sigmoid sinus, and removed the tumor tissue in and around the bulb. He believed the jugular bulb was involved when a glomus tumor was present in the hypotympanum and felt removal of the jugular bulb portion was necessary for cure. He described packing the sigmoid sinus superiorly and removing the lateral wall of the sinus inferiorly toward the bulb, thereby preserving the medial wall of the sinus and avoiding an opening into the subarachnoid space. With the sigmoid sinus exposed above, the internal jugular vein below, and the jugular vein centrally, he described removing the tumor from both directions.

In 1968 House[31] emphasized removal of glomus jugulare tumors without sacrificing the bony ear canal. He recognized the need for greater exposure at the base of the skull. Gardner,[14] a strong advocate of a team approach, has been the stimulus to our successful effort. This has contributed the disciplines of neurosurgery and otolaryngology to the enhancement of both specialties and to better results.

Portmann,[32] in 1968, described removing a large glomus jugulare tumor having intracranial extension in two stages, using a team approach. Kempe[33] described en block excision of tumors, arising in the jugular foramen, with involvement of both the temporal bone and posterior fossa. This procedure was similar to those developed by Shapiro and Neus[29] and by Gejrot[30] but, in addition, included a suboccipital craniectomy with ligation of the sigmoid sinus. He did not mention transposition of the facial nerve. With very large tumors, it was necessary to resect dura in his cases. Hilding and Greenberg[34] used a combined suboccipital and transtemporal approach in glomus tumor removal. They performed a radical mastoidectomy, rerouting the facial nerve, and removed bone anteriorly from over the internal carotid artery and posteriorly from over the subocciput, with ligation of the sigmoid sinus followed by piecemeal removal of the tumor. The tenth cranial nerve was sacrificed because of tumor involvement. Preservation of near-normal hearing and normal facial function followed.

Spector et al.,[12] in 1973, analyzed the results of their treatment of 46 patients with glomus tumors. They concluded that the treatment of choice was surgical and preferred Shapiro's technique of wide excision for large tumors involving the jugular foramen and skull base. Glasscock et al.,[35] in 1974, described combining Shapiro's approach with that of House, preserving the posterior bony ear canal wall and utilizing the extended facial recess. Finally, Graham,[36] in 1975, reported House had developed a procedure for en bloc resection of glomus jugulare tumors and the jugular bulb area.

Radiation Therapy

Radiotherapy has been used extensively either as primary or adjunctive treatment following surgery.[37-40] Various doses and quantities of irradiation have been used, both preoperatively and postoperatively and as initial therapy with varying and, at times, confusing results. More recently, authors have been using megavoltage, with more predictable and higher doses of radiation, and report positive results following radiation therapy.[12,37,38,40,41] However, residual tumor vascularity with probable viable tumor is often still present following high doses of irradiation.[38,40]

Clinical Cases

Our experience includes attempted surgical resection of large glomus jugulare tumors in 17 cases, but only 10 patients with tumors originating in the jugular bulb and extending into the temporal bone have been treated surgically, using this combined team approach through the neck and skull base.[3] All of these fall into McCabe's[42] third category (petrosal and extrapetrosal) and constitute the basis of this report. In 7 of these 10 patients, tumor was limited to the area of the temporal bone and jugular foramen. In 3 cases the tumor spread into the neck. There were no instances of intracranial transdural extension or distant metastasis. The average age in this series was 42 years; tumors occurred with equal frequency in both sexes. The patients received a complete diagnostic evaluation prior to surgery. In addition to the usual otologic and neurosurgical examinations, they underwent retrograde jugular venography and cerebral arteriography. Tomography was used in selective cases. None of our cases appeared to be guilty of catecholamine secretion.[43]

Hearing loss was an initial complaint in 7 patients and had been present for an average of 39 months; tinnitus was an initial symptom in 6 patients, present for an average of 31 months; and dizziness was an initial symptom in 2 patients, being present for an average of 21 months. Hearing loss and tinnitus were present in 8 patients, dizziness in 6, pain in 5, facial nerve weakness in 3, and other cranial nerve symptoms in 2.

The tumor was visible through the ear canal at the time of initial examination in all 10 cases. Jugular venography demonstrated an obstruction of the jugular bulb in each case. The jugular foramen was enlarged in 6 cases and arteriography demonstrated a large tumor stain in 7. Cranial nerve deficit was present in 4 cases. One patient had involvement of the eighth cranial nerve alone and another patient had twelfth nerve involvement alone. A third patient had involvement of the seventh and eighth cranial nerves and the fourth had involvement of the sixth and seventh nerves. The fifth patient had involvement of cranial nerves VII, IX, X, XI, and XII. One patient had associated bilateral carotid body tumors.

All patients were treated surgically, using a combined exposure through the neck with exposure of the skull base, and removal of portions of the temporal and occipital bones so as to expose the tumor. This was done as a one-stage procedure in 4 cases and as a two-stage procedure in 6. Total tumor removal was accomplished in 7 cases and subtotal removal in 3. Four patients had had previous surgery. Three of these had been for diagnosis only and 1 patient had had a transcanal procedure with subtotal removal.

Five of these patients have been followed for less than 1 year, 2 for 1 to 2 years, 1 for 2 to 3 years, and 2 for 3 to 4 years.

Six patients in this series were treated with irradiation therapy as a preoperative adjunct in an attempt to reduce the vascularity and size of the tumor. Moderate doses of irradiation were used, varying between 4,000 and 5,000 rads given over a 4- to 5-week period. Most were treated with cobalt therapy and superior-inferior wedge pairs were utilized for beam shaping. Diagnostic studies were used to determine tumor size and field for x-ray therapy. One patient was treated postoperatively.

Surgical Procedure

This procedure is reported in illustrated detail in a previous publication.[4] However, the essentials will be described here.

Under general endotracheal anesthesia, the patient is placed on his back, with the head and neck rotated to the side opposite the tumor. The scalp is shaved so as to prepare it slightly above and back of the ear as well as anteriorly around the zygoma. Subsequently, the scalp is prepped with surgical solution, an incision is outlined, beginning in the postauricular region about 4.0 cm above the mastoid tip and extending down to just in front of the mastoid tip and, subsequently, along the anterior medial border of the sternocleidomastoid muscle to slightly below the angle of the jaw. The initial dissection is concerned with wide exposure of the inferior parotid gland and the carotid artery and jugular vein.

The superficial lobe of the parotid is reflected anteriorly and, after the facial nerve is identified posteriorly, it is followed into the parotid gland and dissected for subsequent mobilization superiorly and anteriorly.

The sternocleidomastoid insertion is resected from the mastoid tip, which is removed with the use of a Gigli saw. The carotid artery and jugular vein are identified just above the carotid bifurcation and followed superiorly to the base of the skull. Cranial nerves X, XI, and XII are identified and dissected up to the jugular foramen and skull base. All branches entering the jugular vein are ligated and divided. The dissection is followed superiorly to the carotid canal entrance, freeing the internal carotid artery anteriorly and laterally. If tumor is encountered, it is not entered at this point.

The dissection is then carried in a subperiosteal fashion to the lateral and anterior lips of the jugular foramen, with ligation, at this time, of the jugular vein below the tumor extension and subsequent transposition of the vein lateral to the spinal accessory nerve. Various branches of the external carotid artery and their branches are divided and ligated to effect this exposure. Although the regular Bovie cautery is used, when necessary, in so far as possible bipolar coagulation is preferred. The operator uses either magnified loops or the operative microscope, as indicated, to effect dissection around the jugular foramen.

The greater auricular nerve is identified and divided during this dissection and tagged. It may be used, if necessary, for later facial nerve grafting. The mastoid and adjoining suboc-ciput is exposed widely. Care is taken to avoid damage to the vertebral artery. A circumferential incision is then made in the external ear canal at the bony cartilaginous junction. The ear is turned forward and, using a high speed drill, a simple mastoidectomy is effected with subsequent skeletonization of the facial nerve and sigmoid sinus.

If tumor is encountered in the mastoid cells, an attempt is made to remain around the tumor until the facial nerve is finally exposed. The facial nerve is carefully dissected away from tumor, under microscopic control, and elevated anteriorly. Bone is now removed from the temporal bone, as necessary, to extend medially, inferiorly, and anteriorly around the tumor. It may be necessary to remove portions of the tumor piecemeal during this dissection. Final bony removal along the sigmoid is effected, with removal of the lateral wall of the jugular foramen and portions of the anterior wall. At this point, the jugular vein has been ligated and is seen in continuity with the jugular bulb and sigmoid sinus. The carotid artery is exposed up to the carotid canal. A suboccipital craniectomy is effected, exposing the lateral dura of the posterior fossa as well as the anterior lateral sinus and its junction with the sigmoid sinus. A small incision is made in the lateral sinus or upper end of the sigmoid sinus above the tumor.

Using a pursestring suture, with 4-0 or 5-0 proline arterial suture, a Fogarty catheter of appropriate size is passed superiorly into the lateral sinus and inflated. Another Fogarty catheter is passed inferiorly toward the tumor and inflated. The lateral sinus is opened and carefully sutured to its medial wall above the tumor and the proximal Fogarty catheter is removed with final closure. Then proceeding inferiorly, the remaining lateral sinus and sigmoid sinus are packed with Surgicel gauze quite tightly. This allows occlusion of the petrosal veins entrances into the sinus. The Fogarty catheter can then be deflated and removed.

The lateral wall of the remaining lateral sinus and sigmoid sinus is excised very carefully, using pressure on the Surgicel to control bleeding from petrosal veins. Using a combination of inferior and superior dissection, the jugular vein and bulb are removed in continuity with the lateral wall of the sigmoid and/or lateral sinus and intravascular tumor is removed. Care is taken to use as much sharp dissection as possible to remove the vein from the adjoining cranial nerves. The remaining tumor, which is usually not in direct continuity with the intravascular portion, is then carefully removed extradurally from the remaining mastoid or temporal bone extension. If it extends anteriorly around the carotid, the tumor is removed as completely as possible under microscopic control.

If the patient has no nerve-loss hearing and if the posterior bony wall canal is either intact or can be reconstructed, it may be possible to repair the ossicular chain and tympanic membrane. If, on the other hand, the hearing loss is severe and sensorineural, the residual canal wall and tympanic membrane are excised and the meatus closed primarily.

We have used abdominal fat to fill the cavity created by this procedure and to support the membranous ear canal, on occasions. Bleeding is meticulously controlled and the facial nerve returned to its original position. Attention is given to the repair of any dural laceration that was created. If a large section of dura requires resection, it should be meticulously grafted with fascia or preserved dura. Routine wound closure follows, with the use of a Hemovac for 3 to 4 days. If prophylactic antibiotics are used, they should be started prior to the skin incision, continued throughout the operation, and for an additional 3 to 4 days.

Postoperative care consists of meticulous attention to a patient with a facial palsy, which is usually present if the tumor has extensively involved the epineurium of the facial nerve, as well as care of a patient with a transient tenth nerve paresis.

Surgical Specimens

Primary tumors appear to be centered in the jugular bulb, with tumor tissue within the lumen of the bulb, and present a smooth and capsulated lobulated surface. The tumor is shaped like a cigar. In only one instance, did the primary tumor fail to be present, as described. Usually, the specimen was removed as a single specimen. An effort was made to remove the specimen so as to retain its attachment to the lateral wall of the sigmoid sinus superiorly and to the inferior jugular vein inferiorly. In no instance was the primary tumor that involved the bulb removed in multiple pieces.

The 3 cases of incomplete removal resulted from residual tumor firmly adherent to the internal carotid artery. After the tumor was removed, it was hard to correlate its arteriographic appearance with its actual size, and this may well have been due to the extensive collateral vascularity present. The appearance of the smooth lobulated primary tumor situated within the jugular bulb is quite different from its extensions into air cells of the mastoid and middle ear. A puzzling problem is our failure to note a single well-defined connection between the primary mass in the jugular bulb and extensions of tumor into the temporal bone or anteriorly around the carotid. This almost suggests that the origin of the tumor is multicentric. In one patient, who clearly had a tumor preoperatively by examination as well as radiographic studies, the surgical specimen did not contain any tumor tissue. This patient had been treated preoperatively with 5,000 rads and may well be a radiation cure.

The effects of irradiation preoperatively were delineated by comparing irradiated with nonirradiated specimens. Swelling of the endothelial cells, lining vessels that contain thrombi, was the most consistent change distinguishing the irradiated from the nonirradiated series. Swelling of endothelial cells, however, was seen frequently in specimens not receiving irradiation therapy. In one of the irradiated specimens, a portion of the tumor was necrotic as a result of an infarction, implying interference with blood supply to the tumor. Two of the irradiated specimens showed changes in the tumor cells themselves. These changes consisted of focal disappearance of cells and the appearance of pyknotic nuclei and granular cytoplasm. The degree of fibrosis present in both the irradiated and nonirradiated cases failed to show any significant difference between the two groups. This may be due to the fact that surgery followed irradiation in 4 to 6 weeks, rather than wait for fibrosis to occur as a result of irradiation. Irradiation appeared to exert its primary effect on endothelial cells, with a subsequent reduction in tumor vascularity.

Presently, only the short-term status of these patients can be reviewed. All patients are alive. There are no instances of long-term central nervous system complication or disability, except for a single case. This patient underwent total removal of a large tumor after 4,500 rads. The posterior bony canal wall was sacrificed and an effort made to reconstruct the conductive system of the middle ear, which was unsuccessful. Postoperatively, a postauricular fistula, a large cavity, and chronic drainage developed. This patient is emotionally unstable and, at one time an irradiation effect upon the central nervous system was considered but never proved. No definite, recurrent disease has been found in this individual, nor in any of the other cases. Two other patients had difficulty when a cavity developed in the mastoid due to a lack of bony canal support. One required revision surgery and another was managed conservatively.

Three of this series of 10 patients had significant sensorineural loss preoperatively. Of the remaining 7 patients, 2 had a pure-tone average, postoperatively, within 5dB of the preoperative levels; 1 patient has had a 40-dB improvement; 1 patient, who had normal hearing preoperatively, sustained a short-term 50-dB loss postoperatively; and in 3 additional patients primary closure of the external auditory meatus was performed with planned sacrifice of hearing function. Five patients experienced an improvement in their tinnitus; none felt that it was worse, but two described it as unchanged. Four patients described an improvement in the degree of their dizziness.

The most serious complication occurred as a result of a spinal fluid leak leading to meningitis, which was treated successfully. Facial nerve paresis or palsy followed the surgical procedures. Three patients had preoperative facial palsy. The facial nerve was mobilized from the anterior genu to the first bifurcation and transposed anteriorly in all cases. Two patients failed to regain facial function due to direct involvement of the nerve by tumor.

Three losses recovered with minimal, if any residual, weakness. The 5 additional patients were all operated upon within the past year and, in all of these residual facial weakness is still present but is expected to clear.

On the 6 instances of postoperative loss of cranial nerves V through XII, 5 of these cleared within a few weeks or up to 4 months. Residual deficit is present in 1 patient who was operated upon recently.

Discussion

The present surgical approach modified by preoperative x-ray therapy combines the experience of otolaryngologists and neurosurgeons over a 30-year period of attempted therapy for tumors of the glomus jugulare. We could have expedited the evolvement of our present approach with a previous careful review of the literature. Early diagnosis of tumors of the glomus jugulare should be emphasized; tumors limited to the middle ear are surgically curable. Tumors involving the jugular bulb, emphasized in this presentation, require detailed diagnostic studies. If confined to the jugular bulb and the temporal bone, without extensive extension around the carotid artery, they are surgically curable. The adjunctive benefits to be gained from computerized axial tomography and/or posterior fossa myelography await further study. Clearly the increasing use of sophisticated techniques, such as computerized axial tomography, will revolutionize the early diagnosis of tumors in and about the jugular foramen and their extension.

Preoperative x-ray therapy should be given strong consideration in the surgical approach to these tumors. A combined team approach allows a one-stage procedure with minimal blood loss, although the operative time will probably continue to be between 8 and 10 hours. Proximal vessel ligation, such as external carotid artery or ascending pharyngeal artery ligation, probably should be abandoned except in the most unusual cases. We have not found this to be of benefit.

Transposition of the facial nerve is required for the controlled removal of these tumors. Wide peritumoral exposure is essential to control bleeding and for tumor removal. In very large tumors it will probably continue to be necessary to remove the posterior bony canal wall. The extradural approach to these tumors must be emphasized repeatedly. In those occasional cases in which intradural extension has occurred, extradural removal should be the primary procedure. Until a method of providing reliable support to the membranous ear canal can be developed, in those cases in which the bony canal is sacrificed, it is recommended that the ear be closed primarily rather than risk the cavity, cyst, and fistula that will occur.

Tumor extending around the carotid artery remains a problem that can only be solved by further exposure and meticulous microscopic dissection. Sacrifice of the carotid, with or without bypass surgery, is feasible. The small portion of tumor that may not be removed around the internal carotid artery may have a benign course. This possibility is unknown, as is the necessity of absolute removal of all tumor remnants.

Summary

We have described a satisfactory procedure, using a combined team approach with preoperative x-ray therapy, for the removal of tumors of the glomus jugulare, which deserves trial and offers, in our opinion, the best opportunity for complete tumor removal.

REFERENCES

1. Guild R: A hitherto unrecognized structure, the glomus jugularis, in man. *Anat Rec 79:Suppl 2*:28, 1941.
2. Rosenwasser H: Carotid body tumor of the middle ear and mastoid. *Arch Otolaryngol 41*:64-67, 1945
3. Robertson JT: The surgical treatment of tumors of the glomus jugulare. Presented at the Meeting of the Society of University Neurosurgeons, Atlanta, Georgia, May 1974
4. Gardner G, Cocke EW, Robertson JT, et al: Combined approach surgery for removal of glomus jugulare tumors. *Laryngoscope 87*:655-688, 1977
5. Williams L, Childs S, Jr, Parkhill EM, et al: Chemodectomas of the glomus jugulare (nonchromaffin paragangliomas) with especial reference to their response to roentgen therapy. *Trans Am Otol Soc 43*:264-290, 1955
6. Capps FCW: Glomus jugulare tumours of the middle ear. *J Laryngol Otol 66*:302-314, 1952
7. Meacham WF, Capps JM: Intracranial glomus-jugulare tumor with successful surgical removal. *J Neurosurg 17*:157-160, 1960
8. Berg NO: Tumours arising from the tympanic gland (glomus jugularis) and their differential diagnosis. *Acta Pathol Microbiol Scand 27*:194-221, 1950
9. Bickerstaff ER, Howell JS: The neurological importance of tumors of the glomus jugulare. *Brain 76*:576-593, 1953
10. McCabe BF, Fletcher J: Selection of therapy of glomus jugulare tumors. *Arch Otolaryngol 89*:156-159, 1969
11. Rosenwasser H: Long-term results of therapy of glomus jugulare tumors. *Arch Otolaryngol 97*:49-54, 1973
12. Spector GJ, Maisel RH, Ogura JH: Glomus tumors in the middle ear. I. An analysis of 46 patients. *The Laryngoscope 83*:1652-1672, 1973
13. Riemenschneider, PA, Hoople GD, Brewer D, et al: Roentgenographic diagnosis of tumors of the glomus jugularis. *Am J Roentgenol Rad Ther Nucl Med 69*:59-65, 1953
14. Rosenwasser H: Glomus jugulare tumors, long-term tumors. *Arch Otolaryngol 89*:160-166, 1969
15. Lundgren N: Tympanic body tumours in the middle ear—tumours of carotid body type. *Acta Otolaryngol 37*:366-379, 1949
16. Weille FL, Lane CS, Jr: Surgical problems involved in the removal of glomus-jugulare tumors. *The Laryngoscope 61*:448-459, 1951
17. Semmes RE: Discussion of paper by Alexander E, Jr, Adams S: Tumor of the glomus jugulare. Follow-up study two years after roentgen therapy. *J Neurosurg 10*:672-674, 1953
18. Albernaz JG, Bucy PC: Nonchromaffin paraganglioma of the jugular foramen. *J Neurosurg 10*:663-671, 1953
19. Kohut RI, Lindsay JR: Glomus jugulare tumors (new techniques for determining operability.) *The Laryngoscope 75*:750-762, 1965
20. Thoms OJ, Shaw DT, Trowbridge WV: Glomus jugulare tumor. Report of a case with surgical removal. *J Neurosurg 17*:500-504, 1960
21. Seiffert A: Cited by Lundgren
22. Ziedes des Plantes. Cited by Kohut and Lindsay
23. Valvassori GE: Lamingography of the ear—normal roentgenographic anatomy and pathologic conditions. *Am J Roentgenol 89*:1155-1178, 1963
24. Compere WE, Valvassori GE: *Radiographic Atlas of the Temporal Bone.* Book I, The Radiologic Examination of the Petrous Portion of the Temporal Bone. HM Smyth Company, St Paul, Minnesota, 1964
25. Gejrot T: Retrograde jugularography in the diagnosis of abnormalities of the superior bulb of the internal jugular vein. *Acta Otolaryngol 57*:177-180, 1964
26. Gastpar H: Die Tumoren des Glomus Caroticum, Glomus Jugulare-Tympanicum und Glomus Vagale. *Acta Otolaryngol Suppl* 167:1961
27. Michelson RP, Connolly JE: Removal of glomus jugulare tumor utilizing complete occlusion of the cerebral circulation. *The Laryngoscope 72*:788-805, 1962
28. Morgan HW, Dugdale M, Robertson JT: Hemorrhagic studies with hemodilution technique during profound hypothermia and cardiorespiratory arrest. *J Surg Res 14*:459-464, 1973
29. Shapiro MJ, Neus DK: Technique for removal of glomus jugulare tumors. *Arch Otolaryngol 79*:219-224, 1964
30. Gejrot T: Surgical treatment of glomus jugulare tumours. With special reference to the diagnostic value of retrograde jugularography. *Acta Otolaryngol 60*:150-168, 1965
31. House W: Panel Discussion, McCabe BF, Moderator, Rosenwasser H, House W, Witten RM, Hamberger C-A: Management of glomus tumors. *Arch Otolaryngol 89*:170-178, 1969
32. *Disorders of the Skull Base Region.* Edited by CA Hamberger, J Wersall. John Wiley, New York, 1969, pp 297-298

33. Kempe L, VanderArk GD, Smith, DR: The neurosurgical treatment of glomus jugulare tumors. *J Neurosurg 35*:59-64, 1971
34. Hilding DA, Greenberg A: Surgery for large glomus jugulare tumor. *Arch Otolaryngol 93*:227-231, 1971
35. Glasscock ME, Harris PF, Newsome G: Glomus tumors. Diagnosis and treatment. *The Laryngoscope 84*:2006-2032, 1974
36. Graham MD: The jugular bulb. Its anatomic and clinical considerations in contemporary otology. *Arch Otolaryngol 101*:560-564, 1975
37. Silverstone S: Radiation therapy of glomus jugulare tumors. *Arch Otolaryngol 97*:43-48, 1973
38. Maruyama Y: Radiotherapy of tympanojugular chemodectomas. *Radiology 105*:659-663, 1972
39. Rosenwasser H: Glomus jugulare tumors. VI. Follow-up of cases. *Arch Otolaryngol 88*:35-40, 1968
40. Spector GJ, et al: Glomus jugulare tumors: effects of radiotherapy. *Cancer 35*:1316-1321, 1975
41. Walsh, TE: Discussion of paper by Williams HL, et al: Chemodectomas of the glomus jugulare (nonchromaffin paragangliomas) with especial reference to their response to roentgen therapy. *Trans Am Otol Soc 43*:264-290, 1955
42. McCabe BF, Fletcher, MM: Transtympanic approach to extratympanic (jugular bulb) chemodectoma. *Trans Am Acad Ophthalmol Otolaryngol 69*:827-831, 1965
43. Guild SR: The glomus jugulare, a nonchromaffin paraganglion, in man. *Ann Otolaryngol 62*:1045-1071, 1953

CHAPTER 7

Intracranial Pressure Measurement: Current Techniques and Role in Clinical Management

Edward Tarlov

THE RELATIONSHIPS BETWEEN INTRACRANIAL pressure (ICP), cerebral blood flow, and neurologic status are difficult to define in patients. Studies have shown no consistent relationship between these variables, except at very high levels of ICP.[1] Nevertheless, a sustained increase in ICP indicates compensatory mechanisms have failed. Therefore ICP measurements in neurologic patients might be expected to provide a warning, before cerebral damage occurs, to guide medical therapy and to provide useful prognostic information.

To assess the possible usefulness of ICP monitoring in clinical management, we measured these levels in about 100 patients with head injuries during 1972 to 1976. Although clinical ICP monitoring was introduced in 1951,[2] it has not become a routine technique in clinical practice. Our experience with ICP monitoring began about 1 year before computerized tomography (CT) scanning became available to us for the study of patients with head injuries and covered a period of several years, during which CT scanning became a routine admission study on all patients with serious head injuries. The availability of noninvasive CT scanning, a paramount technique in diagnosing and managing many intracranial disorders and in determining effects of therapy, has reduced the usefulness of invasive ICP measurement in our hospital.

CT scanning facilities are however not yet generally available at hospitals where many patients with head injuries are first evaluated. Consequently ICP measurement may sometimes be useful. In contrast to the apparent value of CT scanning, we are still in a fact-gathering stage regarding the value of ICP measurement in everyday neurologic problems. Hence, careful investigative studies of ICP are to be welcomed. If a reliable noninvasive method could be devised, ICP measurement would find wider application.

Neurological Service, Massachusetts General Hospital and the Harvard Medical School, Boston, Massachusetts 02114

Methodology

A continuous record of ICP should ideally be started as soon after admission as possible, although concern about infection in long-term recordings has led us to defer measurements until a day or two after admission in patients who do not have an elevated ICP at admission. The record should either be made directly by a strip chart recorder or read from an oscilloscope and recorded by nursing personnel at frequent intervals. Nurses should be instructed to look for trends of continued high pressure and to record the frequency, height, and duration of sustained increases in pressure. Changes in ICP should not be considered alone but in connection with neurologic changes, such as extensor posturing. Arterial pressure and respiratory changes in relation to changes in ICP should also be recorded. Increased hydration and body temperature, which can increase ICP, should be considered. Artifacts due to movement should clearly be marked on the record. It should be emphasized that low or normal ICP is never a guarantee that no space-occupying mass is present.

Sites From Which ICP Can Be Measured

Pressure Gradients

Since herniation of cerebral tissue occurs from higher to lower pressure regions, it is relevant to consider the possible significance of ICP gradients. ICP measured at one site may not accurately reflect ICP in other intracranial locations.

Between intracranial and spinal compartments. When displaced brain tissue obstructs the subarachnoid space at the foramen magnum or at the tentorial hiatus, pressure gradients develop between the adjacent supratentorial posterior fossa and spinal compartments. The clinical studies of Kaufmann and Clark[3] showed that when a pressure differential of 10 mm Hg between the ventricle and spinal subarachnoid space was present, significant transtentorial or tonsillar herniation had occurred. Such gradients can experimentally be abolished if the subarachnoid space is reconstituted.[4] Here, displacement of brain tissue causes the gradient. This phenomenon is the principal reason lumbar puncture may not accurately measure ICP.

Within a single compartment. It is particularly clear on CT scans and on conventional contrast studies as well, that local pressure gradients must occur at some stage during the expansion of an intracranial mass. The structures nearest to a mass are shifted by a greater degree than those further away (Fig. 7-1). The experimental confirmation of such gradients depends on the technique used, and while gradients may not be apparent from extracerebral measurements,[5] the experimental studies of Schulman and his colleagues,[6] using multiple special wick catheters filled with wet cotton wool and implanted into the cerebrum near and far from an expanding mass, have shown local pressure gradients up to 35 mm Hg around acutely expanding intracranial lesions. These gradients were shown to subside 2½ to 4 hours after the lesion expanded. Safe clinical methods of measuring such gradients are not yet available, and pressure in the frontal region has been taken as an indicator of the *general* intracranial pressure.

Specific Sites At Which ICP Can Be Measured

Extracranial. Measurement of intracranial pressure via the anterior fontanel in infants, using a special tonometer, has been reported.[7-8] Construction of a false fontanel has been suggested.[9] In patients in whom a bony decompression has been carried out, a nonquantita-

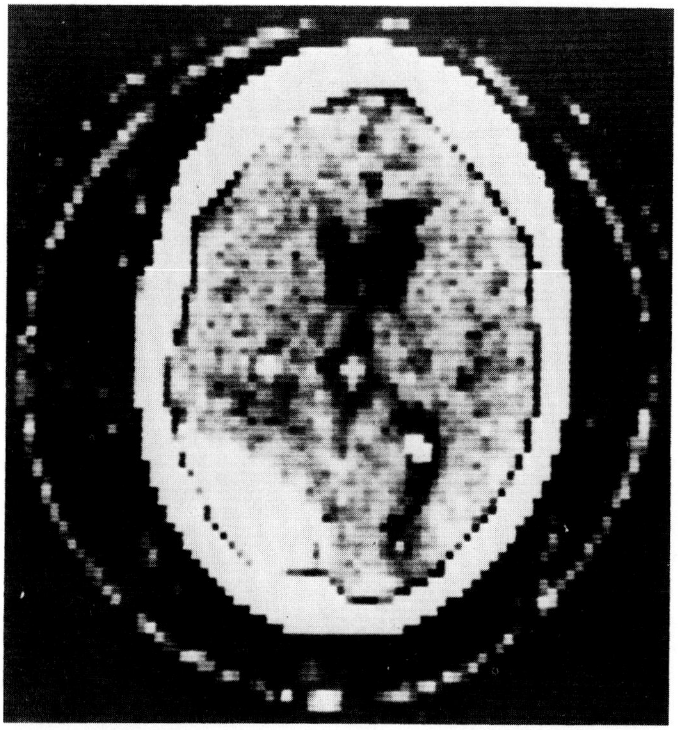

Fig. 7-1. CT scan, left occipital epidural hematoma. Existence of local intracompartmental pressure gradient here is attested by considerable anterior shift of left glomus of choroid plexus near the mass and minimal shift of the more distant pineal gland and right glomus of choroid plexus.

tive but useful judgment of intracranial pressure can be made from palpation of the scalp overlying the defect. The use of a rubber sponge gauge to test flap tension has been reported,[10] but scalp swelling, the size of the flap, and the presence of subcutaneous fluid all affect the reliability of such methods, especially in the important acute phases of illness.

Extradural. Epidural pressure monitoring is the least invasive of presently available techniques, one of the main benefits being a reduction in the risk of intracerebral infection if the dura remains intact. This can conveniently be carried out using an epidurally placed transducer.[11] For accurate measurements, it is important that the measuring surface be coplanar with the dura. This eliminates the effects of changes in the tension of the dura that accompany changes in intradural pressure. These forces, dural elastic tension and intradural pressure, are acting at right angles to each other. If the dura is not deformed by the sensor, the vector of dural tension force will be zero and dural tension will not influence measurements of intradural pressure. If, however, the dura is inwardly deformed, the forces due to dural tension may become very significant. Studies have shown[11] that the measured epidural pressure is usually 5 to 10 mm Hg higher, but can be up to 20 mm Hg higher than intraventricular pressure, the difference increasing at higher pressures. Depending on the configuration of the recording system, scalp edema and fluid accumulation in the wound may also alter the pressure recorded and, although small artifacts may not be significant at high pressures, they may be highly significant at low or normal pressure.

Subdural. Because subdural placement of pressure measurement devices eliminates the possible pressure distorting effect of dural elasticity, this has become a commonly used extracerebral site for pressure measurement. Subdural and cisterna magna pressure closely parallel each other.[8]

Intraparenchymal. Pressure within cerebral tissue can be measured through special wicks[6] placed into the cerebral substance. The principal usefulness of this method has been in the experimental investigation of intracranial pressure gradients, clinical usefulness being restricted by the need for puncturing the cerebrum.

Intraventricular. Direct pressure measurements within the ventricles via a catheter formed the basis for early clinical studies of intracranial pressure. The principal advantages of the ventricular catheter technique are its simplicity and the possibilities of withdrawing cerebrospinal fluid for decompression and injecting gas for radiologic studies. Its disadvantages are the potentially serious consequences of infection in this location, blockage of the catheter, and occasional difficulty in puncturing a small or displaced ventricle. Using a low frontal approach however, as described below, some portion of a lateral ventricle can usually, but not always, be entered.

Lumbar subarachnoid. Except in special circumstances, measurements of lumbar subarachnoid pressure may not be useful in following the course of elevated intracranial pressure. In occasional instances, including certain patients suspected of pseudotumor cerebri such as the one illustrated below, continuous lumbar subarachnoid pressure measurements through a percutaneously placed catheter has been helpful in recognizing intermittently increased intracranial pressure.

Devices for Measuring ICP

A large number of devices for measuring intracranial pressure are presently available. The ideal method would be inexpensive, simple, noninvasive, accurate, stable, and capable of being calibrated in situ. No such device is presently available, but the devices in use are relatively safe. Each has its own advantages and disadvantages, which may make it most suitable for a particular situation.

The devices available fall into three general groups: (a) those in which a fluid column is in contact with the intracranial contents, connected to an external sensor and recording device; (b) those in which an implanted sensor transmits a signal through a wire or tubing to an external recording device; and (c) telemetric devices that do not depend on wire or tubing passed through the skin. The latter group and noninvasive methods may offer the greatest promise for the future, but the development of their reliability continues to be a problem.

Fluid Column Devices

The simplicity and reliability of devices based on this principle are their major advantages.

Ventricular catheter. A catheter placed in the ventricle can be connected to a standard blood pressure transducer and intraventricular pressure recorded continuously. In addition to ICP measurement, the catheter can be used to drain ventricular fluid to abort pressure waves, and to instill gas for radiologic contrast studies. We use a ventricular catheter kit in the emergency room and the operating room, which includes a No. 8 pediatric feeding tube, a K wire, and a 5/32 inch twist drill. A twist drill opening is made low in the right frontal region,

3 cm from the midline and 2 to 3 cm above the supraorbital ridge. A subcutaneous tunnel is then made to the forehead on the contralateral side and a ligature passed through this. The feeding tube is placed over the K wire, and the assembly passed posteriorly and slightly medially into the ventricle. The K wire is withdrawn and the end of the catheter drawn through the subcutaneous tunnel. The tubing is connected to rigid pressure tubing and, after the system has been filled with saline, connected via a stopcock, for flushing, to a strain gauge. The wounds are sutured and the catheter fastened to the skin. To reduce the incidence of infection inherent in an externally connected fluid-filled system, a variation of this technique has been reported, using a ventricular catheter attached to a subcutaneous Ommaya reservoir.[12] A small gauge butterfly needle is inserted percutaneously for pressure recording and the needle changed daily. Meticulous daily care of the wound, with all devices, is critical to prevent infection.

Tightly fitting fluid column devices placed into skull opening, connected to subdural space. A simple effective method for subdural ICP recording is the placement, through a 0.422 cm (0.166 inch) twist drill hole after the dura has been opened, of the male end of a plastic three-way stopcock or the plastic tip of a pressure monitoring tubing.[13]

Since the above device can be dislodged by a restless patient, a modification has been devised.[8] A self-threading hollow metal bolt, firmly threaded into the skull, is used (Fig. 7-2). A skull opening is made with a ¼ inch drill. The thickness of the skull is measured off on the threaded portion of the bolt so as to place the end of the bolt 1 mm below the dura. The dura and arachnoid are opened sharply, or by electrocoagulation, and the opening irrigated until clear. The bolt is placed with a special wrench and connected via its Luer-lock fitting to rigid tubing and thence to a strain gauge. A stopcock is attached near the strain gauge for irrigation.

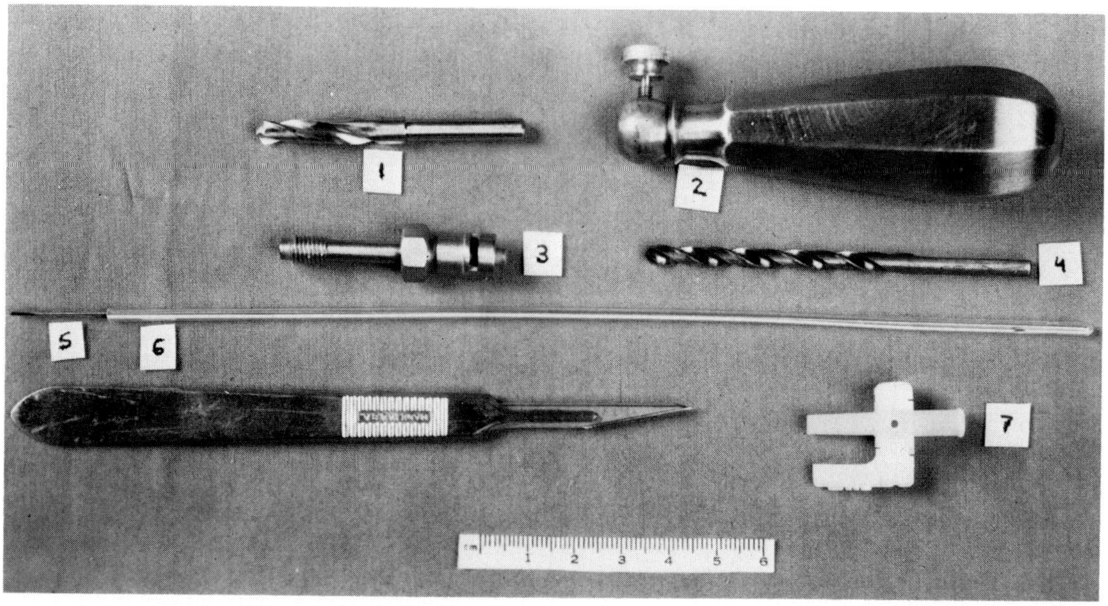

Fig. 7-2. Equipment for three simple methods of ICP monitoring: hollow bolt method (3), ventricular catheter (6) and stopcock method (7). To insert hollow bolt a ¼-inch twist drill hole (1 and 2) is made and after opening the dura and arachnoid, hollow bolt (3) is screwed into drill hole using wrench. Male end of plastic stopcock (7) can also be used, forced into 0.422 cm drill hole. Ventricular catheter, made up from a No. 8 pediatric feeding tube (6) over K wire (5), can be inserted through drill hole as described in text.

Both of these methods have advantages over ventricular catheterization in that they do not require cerebral puncture or the introduction of a device into a small or displaced ventricle. Although not as reliable as the ventricular catheter for decompressive cerebrospinal fluid drainage, they can be used for this purpose.

With any of the fluid column devices, from time to time recorded pressure fluctuations may be dampened because the lumen becomes plugged with debris or cerebral tissue. This often may be corrected by irrigating the system with 0.25 to 0.5 ml of sterile saline. Such irrigation may be made a part of tests of intracranial elastance, as described below. As with all devices passing through the skin, meticulous daily attention to dressing changes, in a manner such as that outlined below, is essential to prevent intracranial infection, which, in our experience, occurs in a large number of cases no matter which method is used, unless the same attention now given to subclavian and hyperalimentation lines is given to these devices. In a busy general hospital careful daily dressing changes and wound care can most effectively be given by trained nursing personnel, as is customary for subclavian and hyperalimentation lines.

Other Devices

An extradurally implanted transducer is advocated by Dorsch and Symon.[11] Such a device, which they recalibrate by moving it away from the dura and which has given stable recordings in their hands, can be fabricated in an instrument shop and lends itself to extradural recording, where fluid column devices do not perform well.

An ingenious device devised by Numoto and Donaghy,[14] referred to as the *Numoto switch*, is a pressure-indicating bag that can be implanted in the epidural or subdural space and is connected through the scalp, via an enclosed fluid column, to an extracranial sensor. Since the fluid column is isolated from the intracranial space, the risk of infection is reduced. The extracranial part of the device adds fluid to the bag, until ICP is just exceeded, and withdraws fluid until ICP just exceeds pressure in the bag, providing a low frequency reading of average ICP. Another similar device uses a fiberoptic coupling. Although the low frequency response is barely able to resolve the pulsatile component of intracranial pressure, this may be of little practical significance. The equipment is still relatively costly.

A simpler device, based on the same principle described by the same group, consists of a mineral-oil filled silastic bag connected, via a tube, to a saline-filled syringe via a pressure gauge. A zero point is marked on the tube. The ICP is taken to be the pressure necessary to move the oil-water interface back to the zero point.

Several totally implantable devices have been described, but are not presently available for general use. They would be advantageous for long-term recording, with a very low risk of infection. A device whose passive resonance frequency was pressure dependent could be implanted in the ventricle,[15] but lacked reliability. Another device was reported by Walker;[16] its stability is under study. An implantable induction-powered oscillator-transducer has been devised[17] and may prove to be promising. In another completely implantable ICP monitoring device, a change in pressure causes a small amount of radioisotope to go from one chamber to another, the movement being detected by an external sensor and correlated with pressure levels.[18] Its reliability is being tested. Zervas and his colleagues[19] have devised a telemeter method that can be calibrated in vivo. This will be a major advance, as the problem of drift of the baseline has been the major difficulty with these and other devices, and the problem of rechecking the zero point in situ remains a major one. Small variations from the baseline are relatively unimportant at very high pressure, but are likely to be extremely important in the normal to slightly elevated pressure range. None of these devices is presently commercially available. On the whole, in the past the reliability of commercially available products of this kind has been less than that of the prototypes. It remains to be seen whether the incentives to

Table 7-1: Advantages and Disadvantages of ICP Monitoring Devices

Device	Availability	Reliability	Risk of infection	Feasibility of long term implantation
Fluid column devices	Readily available	High	Relatively high if used for prolonged periods—can be lowered by special techniques	No
Transducers	Obtainable	Fair, depending on model, ability to recheck zero point essential	Relatively low	No
Telemeters	Not yet commercially available	Probably high but presently being investigated	Very low	Yes

the manufacturers are sufficient to allow the production of a reliable instrument. The pros and cons of each of the above types of devices are represented in Table 7-1. A potentially promising technique might be developed with the use of ultrasound. Jeppson[20] has used a decrease in the rise time of the echo pulsation as an indicator of increased ICP. Richardson[21] has correlated the presence of plateau waves with a decrease in the magnitude of the echo wave. The method indicated a change in pressure, but at present does not seem capable of providing quantitative information.

Recording Devices

In most instances, the subdural, epidural, or intraventricular devices are connected to a strain gauge, mounted at the bedside at the level of the ventricular system. Such a device is then connected to an oscilloscope or strip chart recorder, from which readings can be taken directly. A considerable mass of data accumulates, even in a relatively short period of time. Systems of data display and retrieval have been devised;[10] the practical value of these is not yet certain.

Hysteresis

A major technical problem in all transducers is the tendency of transducer circuits to drift, so that over a period of hours, days, or longer the zero point is no longer a true zero and consequently the recorded ICP may be quite inaccurate. This tendency, called *hysteresis*, results from instabilities in available circuits. The capacity to recheck the zero point in situ is thus a highly desirable adjunct to the manufacturer's assurance that zero drift is low. Small recording errors may not be significant at high pressures, but in the normal to slightly elevated range, in which most patients are found, they may be highly significant. Barometric pressure changes, which commonly reach 150 mm H_2O in magnitude, are another possible source of error in obtaining accurate readings of ICP. To compensate for barometric pressure changes and to reduce the problems of hysteresis, the ability to recalibrate any ICP measuring device in situ is an important feature.

Interpretaion of Pressure Elevation and Volume-Pressure Relationships

Sustained severe elevations in ICP do not present difficulty in interpretation. An abrupt sustained elevation in ICP, referred to as a plateau wave, signifies intracranial vasomotor decompensation and may precede longer sustained elevations of ICP. Other forms of intermittent ICP elevation (Lundberg B and C waves[22] described below) usually have less dire significance. Studies of intracranial volume-pressure relationships, as measured by pressure changes induced by adding a small increment to intracranial volume, may also add significantly to the value of ICP recordings in clinical management.

Pressure Waves

Plateau Waves

Episodic increases in ICP, usually beginning from an elevated baseline, reaching 50 to 100 mm Hg and lasting 5 to 20 minutes or longer have, because their steep rise and abrupt fall give them a plateau-shaped appearance, been referred to as *plateau waves*.[22-23] In some circumstances, as in pseudotumor cerebri, they may be unaccompanied by any change in neurologic function, while in others, including occasional cases of severe head trauma, they may be associated with brainstem dysfunction.[22-23] Because they are intermittent, sometimes separated by many hours, sporadic measurement of lumbar pressure or ICP may not reveal their presence, particularly in the occasional cases, such as case 3 below, in which they do not arise from an elevated baseline. Numerous studies of the pathogenesis of plateau waves have been made. They usually arise in a *tight* situation within the intracranial space when most of the displaceable volume has been exhausted. A possible sequence of events in which low-amplitude pressure waves might be transformed into plateau waves has been hypothecated by Langfitt:[24] resistance vessels dilate, producing increased intracranial blood volume, with a resulting decrease in flow and an increase in pressure. As waves become larger in amplitude, ischemic damage to resistance vessles occurs. They may fail to contract as ICP increases, resulting in a further increase in ICP and further damage to surrounding areas. Clinical measurements of regional cerebral blood volume during plateau waves[25] showed that these waves are correlated with increased intracranial blood volume, a finding that would be consistent with a part of the proposed mechanism. Plateau waves seem to signify cerebral vasomotor decompensation, and therapy to reduce intracranial pressure when they are observed, particularly if correlated with clinical changes, is usually warranted.

Other Waves

Little clinical attention has been paid to the B and C waves described by Lundberg,[22] as they are so frequently seen under normal circumstances. The B waves, rhythmic ½ to 2/min waves up to 50 mm Hg, are seen in normal patients but can also occur during periodic breathing. They usually disappear when the patient is placed on a respirator.[22] The C waves, small rhythmic oscillations 4 to 8/min, up to 20-mm Hg amplitude, seem to reflect the normal Traube-Hering variations in blood pressure.[22]

Intracranial Volume-Pressure Relationships

Evidence[26-28] points to an exponential relationship between small rapid additions to intracranial volume and intracranial pressure (Fig. 7-3). At low ICP, small rapid additions to intracranial volume produce little change in intracranial pressure; at higher ICP levels, the

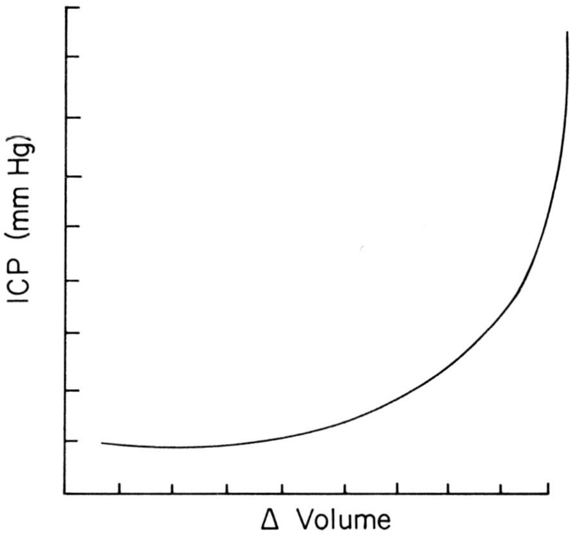

Fig. 7-3. Theoretical volume-pressure curve, indicating the degree to which successive increments added to intracranial volume may increase intracranial pressure. The purpose of volume-pressure response tests, described in the text, is to determine the extent to which intracranial compensatory mechanisms have been exhaused. On the leftward portion of the curve, little rise in pressure is expected to result from additions to intracranial mass, whereas on steeper portion of curve to right, small increments cause greater rise in ICP.

same increments may produce large rises in ICP. Miller[26-28] has brought attention to the possible value of a simple clinical test to determine the adequacy of reserve ICP compensatory mechanisms. Based on the assumption of an exponential relationship between intracranial pressure and volume and a positive correlation between resting ICP and the response of ICP to a uniform change in volume, the test consists of measuring the change in ICP resulting when a 1-ml volume of fluid is injected intracranially in 1 second. This, theoretically, may determine whether a patient is at a point on the intracranial pressure response curve where a small increase in volume will cause a large increase in pressure. The result, expressed as change in pressure (mm Hg)/change in volume (ml) is referred to as cerebral elastance, the inverse of cerebral compliance. A rise in pressure of 0 to 2 mm Hg/1 ml injected, is felt by Miller[28] to be in the normal range, while an increase in pressure of 3 mm Hg/ml or greater is felt to be significantly abnormal. Miller's studies[26-28] have shown a relationship between intracranial elastance and ICP, except in patients with large ventricles. In such patients, high levels of ICP may not be associated with increases in cerebral elastance.

Miller's studies of the effects of therapy on cerebral elastance[28] indicate that although hyperventilation and hypocapnia effectively lower raised ICP, the change in arterial Pco_2 does not alter the volume-pressure relationship. The advantages afforded by hyperventilation will thus, according to Miller,[28] be negated if an additional equivalent volume is added. Mannitol, on the other hand, may act in a different way, reducing cerebral elastance to a much greater extent than intracranial pressure.[29] Steroids, in patients with cerebral tumor, may have an even greater differential effect on cerebral elastance.[29] At a stage when these agents have produced little or no decrease in ICP, elastance may be much reduced.

Miller has suggested that measurements of intracranial pressure and elastance may prove to be clinically useful in the following four ways:[28]

1.	Low ICP < 15 mm Hg Low elastance < 2 mm Hg	This is a safe situation with adequate intracranial reserve. If the patient has a severe neurologic deficit, it suggests the presence of severe primary cerebral damage.
2.	Low ICP < 15 mm Hg High elastance > 3 mm Hg	Such patients should be screened carefully for the possible presence of an intracranial mass.
3.	High ICP > 15 mm Hg High elastance > 3 mm Hg	Such a situation may demand urgent treatment.
4.	High ICP > 15 mm Hg Low elastance < 3 mm Hg	This situation is seen in patients with large ventricles.

It may be necessary to evaluate large numbers of comparable cases to confirm the above findings. Although our own experience with this test, in a small number of cases, has not yet demonstrated the extent of its value to us, it seems possible that it may prove to be more valuable than ICP measurements alone.

Many variables are at play in determining volume-pressure relationships. The basic assumption that volume and pressure are related exponentially may not be true under all circumstances. Nakatani and Ommaya[30] found experimentally that an expanding intracranial mass, enlarging at a rate at or below 0.02 ml/min, produced cerebral death with only moderate elevation of ICP. More rapidly expanding masses produced a steep rise in ICP, with a concommitant Cushing response. Their results indicate that increased arterial blood pressure, accompanying the Cushing reflex, is the determining factor for a rapid rise in ICP in the later phases of expansion of an intracranial mass. These results are important, not only in that they confirm that cerebral death due to an intracranial mass can occur with a minimal rise in ICP, but more important, the intracranial volume-pressure relationship may not be exponential if the rate of increase in the size of a mass is considered, and further, that a steep late rise in ICP may, under certain conditions, be a consequence of arterial hypertension.

Clinical Applications of ICP Measurement

Except when the value is dramatic and the technique entirely safe, as in CT scanning, documentation of the usefulness of a method of clinical situations may be difficult. Proponents of a technique may convince each other of its value, without bringing about a shift in the main stream of clinical practice. Since the introduction of clinical ICP measurement in 1951,[2] observations have indicated that: (a) the clinical state of the patient is not always a reliable indication of the level of ICP; (b) ICP elevations may be episodic so that isolated measurements may be misleading; (c) normal ICP does not exclude the possible presence of a large intracranial mass, of traumatic or other etiology; and (d) all available methods of measuring ICP carry a certain risk.

Head Trauma

In the approximately 100 patients in whom we continuously measured ICP for durations of a few hours to 10 days, levels could be considered to have had some clinical usefulness in about 10% of the patients. In most it cannot be stated with any certainty that ICP measurement influenced the outcome. In some cases it provided a more rational basis for the use of hyperosmolar therapy or hyperventilation, or indicated the advisability of CT scan or other study for assessing the cause of increased ICP. It will be apparent, from the following clinical examples, how difficult it is to quantitate the value of ICP measurement; by contrast the value of CT scanning, serially if necessary, in head injury and other disorders was easily apparent.

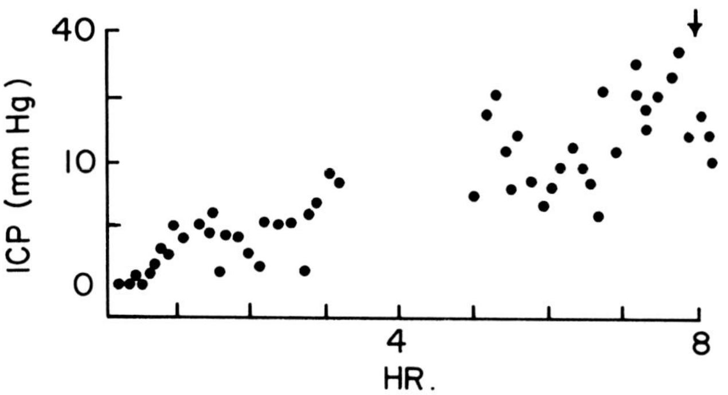

Fig. 7-4. ICP recording in case 1, brainstem injury. Ordinate mm Hg; abscissa in days. Highest pressure during each 3-hour period is recorded by dot. Note late rise in ICP on days 5 to 8 in spite of vigorous hyperosmolar therapy. CT scan showed no mass. Neurologic changes led to frontal decompression (arrow) which effectively lowered ICP.

Illustrative Cases

Case 1. An 11-year-old boy with brainstem injury, pulmonary contusions, and tibial fractures, was decerebrate with skew ocular deviation and a poorly reactive left pupil. Admission bilateral carotid angiography showed no intracranial mass. Muscle relaxants and treatment on a respirator hampered serial neurologic examinations. ICP monitoring (Fig. 7-4) was discontinued on day 4 to avert infection but, because of respiratory irregularity, was reinstituted on day 5. Progressive moderate elevation of ICP occurred on days 5 to 8 despite hyperosmolar therapy. When pupillary dilation and fixation on the left occurred, craniectomy was carried out on day 8. ICP monitoring documented the effectiveness of decompression in lowering ICP. A partial recovery to partial self care status occurred over a 2-year period.

Comment: ICP monitoring provided a form of neurologic monitoring during therapeutic muscle paralysis for the treatment of chest injury and was helpful, in a negative sense, in showing no elevation of ICP. ICP monitoring warned of the delayed development of generalized cerebral swelling, which might not have been predicted from initial findings. The efficacy of medical and surgical therapy in lowering ICP was disclosed by monitoring. The outcome, however, probably did not differ significantly from the natural history of this injury in a child treated with modern respiratory support and other standard therapy. ICP monitoring in this case helped the doctors, but it is uncertain whether it helped the patient.

Case 2. A 36-year-old woman with brainstem and frontal lobe contusions and cervical fracture had a marked decerebrate posture, left third nerve palsy and a right pupil briskly reactive, with full movement of the right eye. A CT scan on admission showed small left parietal contusion without mass effect. ICP monitoring (Fig. 7-5) showed a normal ICP during the first day after injury. Hypertension and respiratory irregularity led to lumbar puncture on day 5, showing normal pressure. On day 16, because of further similar episodes, a CT scan was carried out (Fig. 7-5), showing bifrontal contusions. The ICP monitoring bolt was reinserted. ICP rose slowly over a 3-day period, during the development of left subdural hematoma. As ICP rose a CT scan was carried out. No new abnormality was recognized because of a CT artifact due to the ICP device. The rise in ICP preceded neurologic deterioration, which prompted removal of the ICP measuring equipment in order to obtain a satisfactory CT scan. This showed a frontal subdural hematoma on the side where the ICP monitoring device had been inserted (Fig. 7-6). Subdural hematoma removed. Partial recovery to a severely incapacitated but conscious state after 1 year.

Comment: A slow rise in ICP preceded the increase in severe neurologic deficit. ICP elevation occurred during the development of a subdural hematoma, which was a complication of ICP measurement. ICP measurement also hindered CT scanning, but might be considered somewhat helpful, although it was the cause of a complication. It is doubtful that ICP measurement influenced the outcome in any beneficial way.

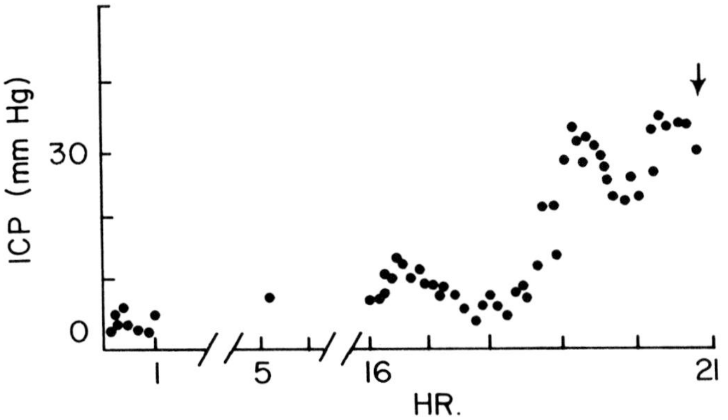

Fig. 7-5. ICP recording in case 2. Ordinate mm Hg; abscissa in days. Highest ICP in each 3-hour period indicated by dot. Recording shows pressure changes during formation of subdural hematoma on days 18 to 21. ICP recording, although it was in this patient the cause of intracranial bleeding (Fig. 7-5), demonstrated rise in ICP prior to clinical changes. Pupillary dilation occurred at arrow, at which time CT scan carried out and hematoma removed.

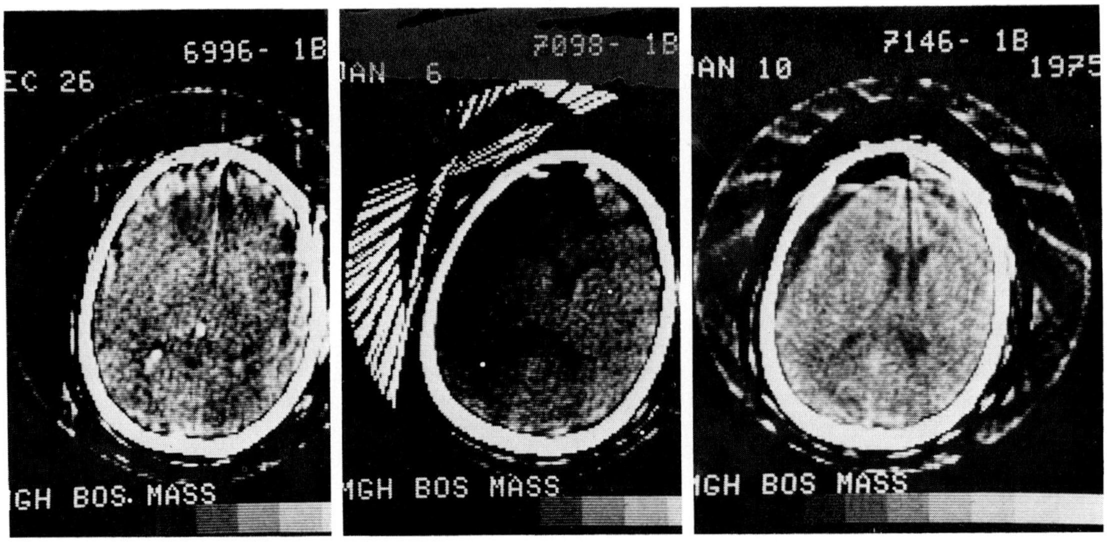

Fig. 7-6. CT scans in case 2. On day 6 (scan at left) CT shows bifrontal contusions in small ventricles. On day 15 (middle scan) scan shows extensive CT artifact over left side of scan, due to metallic monitoring device (hollow bolt). Subdural hematoma could not be seen because of this artifact. On day 21 (right scan) chronic subdural hematoma visualized after ICP monitor removed.

Hyperosmolar Therapy

Intracranial pressure measurement seems to have been useful in guiding the need for hyperosmolar therapy. It has been our practice, in managing trauma patients with elevated ICP and serious neurologic deficits, to use intravenous 20% mannitol, 3 g/kg initially, then 1 g/kg every 6 to 8 hours, or saturated glycerol solution up to 60 ml every 4 hours, instilled into the stomach to reduce intracranial pressure, reducing the doses if serum osmolarity exceeds 320 mOsm/liter. In some patients ICP measurements indicated that such therapy should be intensified or showed that it could be discontinued, avoiding the risks, however small, inherent in the use of these agents.

External Decompression

Prophylactic and therapeutic wide bony decompression has been suggested as routine treatment of patients with acute subdural hematoma[31] or with severe neurologic deficits.[32] Such procedures, which were carried out in our clinic relatively often before we began to use ICP measurement, are now being used much less frequently. ICP measurements showed us that the development of significant brain swelling was not reliably predicted on clinical grounds alone, and numerous patients were spared craniectomy. In this area, ICP measurements were helpful to us in showing the wide bony decompression is infrequently necessary to lower ICP.

Prognostic Application of ICP Measurements in Head Injury

A theoretical reason for carrying out ICP measurements in patients with a head injury is their possible value in clarifying prognosis. Although several groups[33-34] have felt that ICP measurements increased the accuracy of clinical prognosis, this has not been the experience of others,[35] except at very high levels of ICP. In fact it has been suggested[36] that in the presence of severe neurologic deficit, normal ICP may signify cerebral damage, with a high likelihood of giving rise to a persistent vegetative state. Our own experience would support the contention[35] that ICP measurement does not aid in prognosis, except at prolonged, extremely elevated levels of ICP. The possible clinical value of measurements of intracranial elastance, as opposed to simple measurement of ICP, in prognosis has yet to be determined.

Current Policy

It is our current impression that there are some patients whose management may be aided by ICP monitoring. However, now that CT scanning is readily available we use it routinely to assess, on admission, all patients with significant neurologic deficit after head injury. In complex cases, including most patients with prolonged deficits, one or more further scans are carried out for reassessment. In many instances the CT scan demonstrates lesions not suspected on clinical grounds, guiding therapy and perhaps providing some prognostic data.[37] At the present time we consider carrying out ICP measurements in head trauma patients with serious neurologic deficits in whom studies do not indicate the presence of any lesion requiring definitive intracranial operation, particularly if slowing of angiographic circulation time, ventricular compression or midline shift on CT scan, funduscopic examination or in some cases LP pressure suggest that intracranial pressure is or is likely to become elevated. Our present practice is to place a subarachnoid screw in the frontal region. We have in a number of instances, since the duration of recording in our experience bears on the incidence of infection, deferred the placement of such a device for a day or two after the initial injury, so as to be able to pick up late elevations of intracranial pressure that may occur due to delayed brain swelling in patients who do not have elevated ICP initially. It is difficult to be certain how much ICP monitoring adds to the management of patients with head injuries, who can easily be noninvasively assessed by CT scanning, repeated if necessary. With more experience with tests of intracranial volume-pressure responses, the value of ICP monitoring may be increased. At present we feel the available data do not justify routine ICP measurements in most patients with head injury.

Other Clinical Applications of ICP Measurement

As more reliable, less invasive, safer methods of ICP measurement are developed, a wider range of clinical uses will be found. At present, ICP measurement may play a part in the diagnosis and/or treatment of the conditions that follow.

Postoperative Care After Elective Craniotomy

Postoperative measurement of ICP after craniotomy has been advocated.[22] Although postoperative elevation of ICP may provide additional warning of intracranial complications, not suspected on clinical grounds in some patients, it does not seem advisable to recommend its widespread use in this area now. Although knowledge of the presence of high ICP might be clinically useful, the presence of normal ICP does not exclude a mass, such as a postoperative clot. When available, CT scanning of patients who deteriorate after elective craniotomy may provide more definitive information than ICP measurement.

Benign Intracranial Hypertension

The diagnosis of benign intracranial hypertension is based on the presence of increased ICP for which no cause can be identified. In certain cases, such as the one described below, relation of increased ICP to symptoms may be unclear.

Case 3. A 20-year-old woman was admitted because of severe headache, progressive for 1 year, and papilledema. She gave a history of oral contraceptive therapy. Examination 1 week previously had disclosed no papilledema and an LP pressure of 175 mm H_2O and normal cerebrospinal fluid. A pneumoencephalogram, bilateral carotid and vertebral angiography, and a CT scan were all normal. The patient was placed on steroids and glycerol, with initial disappearance of her headache. LP pressure was 30 mm H_2O, and the severe headache recurred. Over the ensuing 5 weeks, severe headache and visual blurring developed while a program of medical management with steroids, oral glycerol, Diamox, and intravenous mannitol was developed. Intermittent lumbar puncture revealed a variable relationship between headache and high cerebrospinal fluid pressure. On the first day headache was severe and LP pressure was 175 mm H_2O. On hospital day 21 headache was severe and LP pressure was 280 mm H_2O. On day 29 LP pressure was 60 to 70 mm H_2O, although severe headache and bradycardia were present. On day 34 headache was severe and LP pressure was 125 mm H_2O. Accordingly, to clarify the relationship between intracranial pressure changes and her symptoms, continuous recording of ICP was carried out via lumbar subarachnoid catheter (Fig. 7-7). This revealed episodes of markedly elevated ICP in the 50 to 80 mm Hg range, correlating with severe headache and interspersed with periods of no symptoms. Overnight drainage of cerebrospinal fluid relieved her symptoms, which recurred when the catheter was removed. A lumboperitoneal shunt abolished her headaches and papilledema, which had been refractory to maximal medical management. Over the succeeding year, several shunt revisions were carried out. Thirteen months later, bilateral subtemporal craniectomy was necessary to control ICP and 2½ years later she is asymptomatic and working.

Comment: Continuous monitoring of subarachnoid pressure clarified the etiology of severe headache in this lady with severe intermittently raised ICP in whom several measurements of pressure at lumbar puncture had not revealed elevated ICP. Johnston and Paterson[38] reported that ICP monitoring clarified the diagnosis of benign intracranial hypertension in their series of 20 patients with suspected papilledema and suspected raised ICP. Continuous ICP measurement via an intraventricular catheter revealed that the clinical suspicion of raised ICP was incorrect in up to 25% of their cases. A lumbar subarachnoid catheter may be a preferable means of assessing ICP continuously in patients without intracranial masses.

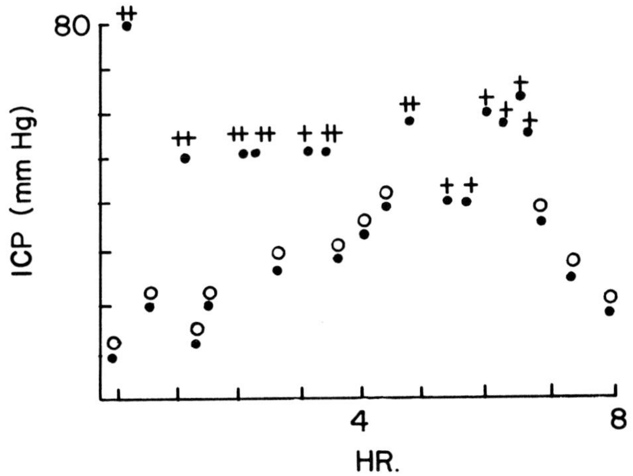

Fig. 7-7. Case 3. Lumbar subarachnoid pressures recorded via catheter in case 3, pseudotumor cerebri. ICP in mm Hg; time scale in hours and signifies headache. + signifies mild headache; ++ signifies severe headache; 0 signifies no symptoms. Note intermittent nature of cerebrospinal fluid pressure increase and close correlation between high pressure and symptoms.

Investigation of Hydrocephalus

The syndrome of *normal* pressure hydrocephalus (NPH)[39] with dementia, gait disturbance, and frequent incontinence remains difficult to diagnose, the only entirely certain method being improvement in signs following ventricular shunting. Preoperative isotope scanning and pneumography have been the usual preoperative tests, but a high proportion of patients, as many as 76%[40] judged, by these tests and on clinical grounds, to have NPH have not benefited from shunts, so that any improvement in preoperative selection would be welcome. The detection of intermittent elevation of ICP in adults suspected of NPH has been advocated as a useful test for symptomatic hydrocephalus. Symon and Dorsch[41] have been able to identify two groups of patients among 27 candidates for shunts on the basis of 2 to 41 days of continuous ICP measurement via an epidural transducer. In one group in whom shunts were carried out mean pressure was 22 mm Hg, whereas in the other group not shunted mean pressure was 16 mm Hg. Plateau and B waves were seen more frequently in the shunted group, averaging 1.58 A waves in shunted patients versus 0.14 per day in nonshunted patients; B waves were similarly more frequent in the shunted group. Among the 13 patients shunted, 8 showed some improvement, but improvement was marked in only a few. Postoperative pressure measurements showed the pressure elevations corrected by shunting. In Symon's hands the ICP monitoring technique improved on the predictive accuracy of benefit from shunt. No complications of Symon's extradural monitoring technique occurred. Nevertheless, the modest clinical response to shunting reported in Symon's series leaves an element of doubt as to the degree to which hydrocephalus was present, even in the patients in whom ICP elevations were demonstrated. Further evaluation is needed to know the value of ICP measurement in the diagnosis of NPH.

Serial measurements of lumbar subarachnoid pressure during infusion of normal saline at a rate of 0.76 ml/min, about twice the normal rate of formation of cerebrospinal fluid, has been suggested as a test of cerebrospinal fluid malabsorption[42] to identify patients with symptomatic hydrocephalus.[43] We have carried out cerebrospinal fluid infusion tests in dozens of patients suspected of NPH and concur with Wolinsky et al.[44] that no available test, including cerebrospinal fluid infusion, can accurately predict the response of these patients to shunting.

Reyes Syndrome

Reyes syndrome of encephalopathy with fatty infiltration of the viscera occurs in children and is frequently associated with elevated ICP. Monitoring ICP to guide therapy in this condition has been reported.[45-46] The level of maximal ICP did not correlate with survival,[44] but it is possible that hyperosmolar therapy increased the survival rate of the patients studied. As the skull is thin in children, the most effective method for recording ICP may be a tightly fitting stopcock placed in a small drill hole in the skull,[13] or an intracranial catheter.

Complications

Until noninvasive methods of recording pressure are developed, complications of ICP recording will occur. The most frequent complication, when part of an ICP measuring device passes through the scalp, is infection. The consequences of infection are more frequently significant if the device is implanted beneath the dura. Hemorrhage occasionally occurs. Equipment failure and plugging of the devices lumina with debris does occur, but these usually interrupt recordings only transiently.

Infection

Criteria for Occurrence of Infection. Daily cultures and cell counts of cerebrospinal fluid from devices implanted beneath the dura are routinely taken. In some patients positive cultures are obtained without cerebrospinal fluid pleocytosis. In such cases the positive cultures may represent contaminants. Concern about infection usually leads us to remove the device and, if necessary, replace it in another location if ICP recording seems to be helpful. We usually consider patients with positive cultures and positive cell counts to have infections.

Incidence of Infection. Sundbarg and his colleagues[47] have reported the incidence of infection in a 10-year experience with 1,061 ICP recordings, averaging 8 days duration. Clinically significant infections occurred in 1.1% of their patients. In an additional 3.6% positive cultures and positive cell counts occurred "without clinical signs of infection." An additional 5.1% had positive cultures without other signs of infection, for an overall percentage of 9.8%. In this Lund series, no patients were judged to have had significant sequalae of intracranial infection, although several patients are mentioned to have been severely ill. *Staphylococcus albus* was the most frequent infecting organism, with *Staphylococcus aureus, Pseudomonas,* and *E. coli* also being present. Although Sundbarg[47] reported no increase in the incidence of infections with prolonged recordings, Wyler and Kelly[48] reported the incidence of infection of ventriculostomies rises in proportion to the length of time the device is in place, a significant increase in incidence occurring at 3 days, an experience that coincides with our own. Like Wyler and Kelly, we have usually used prophylactic antibiotic coverage in patients in whom ICP measurement devices are left in place longer than 3 days. Our own experience with infection has been that clinically significant infection occurs in about 10% of patients and laboratory evidence of infection without clinical significance in an additional 10%.

Prevention of Infections. It is clear that careful attention to daily wound care and dressing changes is a most important factor in preventing infections. The daily dressing change program we have adopted includes the following: cleaning the skin at the site of the device with acetone and alcohol followed by bacitracin solution and clean occlusive dressings. We change all stopcocks and tubing each day. We have found that the use of a heavy antibiotic paste may discourage the nursing staff from cleaning this area, which, after a few days, can provide a culure medium. Fastening all connections so that they cannot become disconnected is important as well. The dressing changes are carried out by trained nursing personnel. Manipulations of the system are carried out with aseptic precautions.

Hemorrhage

Occasional instances in which ventricular puncture has caused intracranial bleeding have been reported.[47] In our experience with CT scanning we have frequently seen contusion or minor bleeding along the tract of a ventricular puncture (Fig. 7-8), but this has seldom been of clinical significance. Its occasional occurrence makes us favor the less invasive subdural and epidural methods of recording. It is our impression that intracranial hemorrhage may be less frequent with the hollow bolt technique than with ventricular catheters.

Epilepsy

There is no evidence that the incidence of epilepsy is higher after ICP monitoring devices, including ventricular catheters, have been placed.[47]

Scalp Lesions

A slough of the scalp has occasionally occurred at the site where a subarachnoid bolt was placed, apparently related to burning of the skin when the underlying dura was coagulated. Minor wound revisions have been necessary in several instances.

Failure of the Recording System

A damping of the recorded pulse waves after a ventricular catheter or subarachnoid screw has been in place for a few days has occurred rather frequently. This may give a falsely low recording of intracranial pressure. Irrigation of the catheter has clarified the presence of

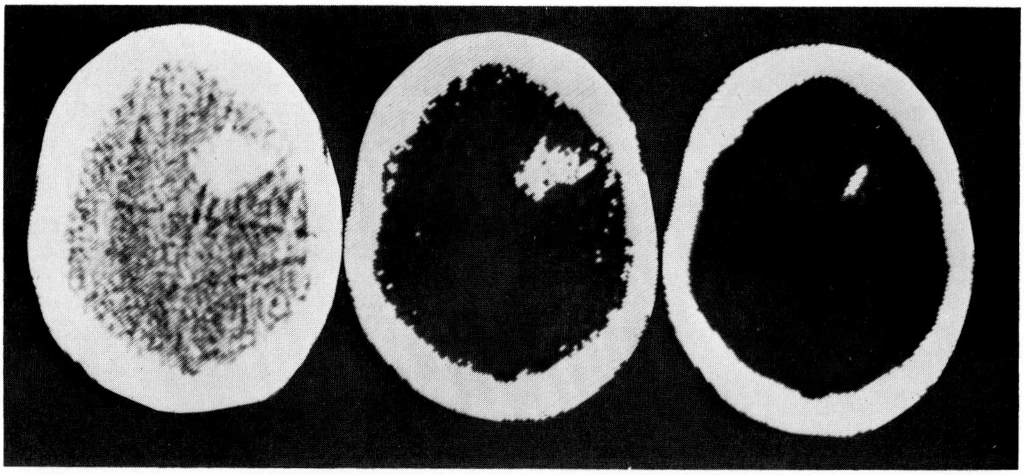

Fig. 7-8. CT scans at three settings, showing right frontal hematoma at site of ventricular catheter. Catheter seen in scan at right. No new signs resulted from right frontal hematoma in this patient with ruptured anterior communicating aneurysm. Hematoma resolved over a 3-week period.

this problem. Placing the screw too far beneath the level of the inner table may, by allowing cerebral tissue and blood clot to plug its end, increase the incidence of this problem. Because technical failures of transducers and other recording equipment are frequent, these should be checked and recalibrated at least daily.

Interference with Other Studies, Particularly CT Scanning

The subarachnoid bolt, as mentioned above, clearly may, by the large metallic artifact it casts on CT scans, interfere with the correct interpretation of scans (Fig. 7-5). The ventricular catheter may similarly obscure the CT scan appearance of adjacent cerebral tissue.

Summary

A multitude of devices and techniques have been used to make direct measurements of intracranial pressure. At present the simplest, most reliable, least invasive of these is the placement, through a small trephine, of a device connected via a fluid column to a transducer to measure subdural pressure. A significant risk of infection from such devices exists, but can probably be kept low by careful attention to details. The recording of plateau waves signals impending or existing intracranial vasomotor decompensation. These waves are infrequently seen following head injury. Measurement of elastance may, in the future, prove useful. The value of ICP measurement in clarifying prognosis in head injury and other conditions is uncertain. CT scanning, where available, has, from the practical standpoint, largely supplanted ICP measurement in diagnosing intracranial complications of head injury. ICP measurement may be helpful in some patients, but its routine clinical application is not advocated by presently available data. As experience with the use and interpretation of CT scanning increases and as less invasive techniques are perfected, it seems probable that the risks inherent in present intracranial pressure measurement techniques may be bypassed.

REFERENCES

1. Bruce, DA, Langfitt TW, Miller JD, et al: Regional cerebral blood flow, intracranial pressure, and brain metabolism in comatose patients. *J Neurosurg 38*:131-144, 1973
2. Guillaume J, Janny P: Manometrie intracranienne continue. *Rev Neurol 84*:131-142, 1957
3. Kaufman GE, Clark K: Continuous simultaneous monitoring of intraventricular and cervical subarachnoid fluid pressure to indicate development of cerebral or tonsillar herniation. *J Neurosurg 33*:145-150, 1970
4. Langfitt TW, Weinstein JD, Kassell NF, Simeone FA: Transmission of increased intracranial pressure. 1. Within the craniospinal axis. *J Neurosurg 21*:989-997, 1964
5. Symon L: Distribution of pressure within the cranial cavity and its significance, *Head Injuries*. Proceedings of the Second Chicago Symposium on Neural Trauma. Edited by R McLaurin. Grune and Stratton, New York, 1975, pp 249-261
6. Shulman K, Marmarou A, Shapiro K: Brain tissue pressure and focal pressure gradients, *Head Injuries.* Proceedings of the Second Chicago Symposium on Neural Trauma. Edited by R McLaurin. Grune and Stratton, New York, 1975, pp 279-285
7. Davidoff LM, Chamlin M: The "Fontanometer." Adaption of the Schiotz tonometer for the determination of inracranial pressure in the neonatal and early periods of infancy. *Pediatrics 24*:1065-1068, 1959
8. Edwards J: An intracranial pressure tonometer for use on neonates: Preliminary report. *Develop Med Child Neurol 16*:Suppl 32:38-39, 1974
9. Forrest DM, Tsingoglou S: The false fontanelle as a practical method of long term testing of intracranial pressure. *Develop Med Child Neurol 10*:Suppl 16:17-20, 1968
10. McGraw CP: Continuous intracranial pressure monitoring: Review of techniques and presentation of method. *Surg Neurol 6*:149-155, 1976
11. Dorsch NWC, Symon L: The validity of extradural measurement of intracranial pressure. *Intracranial*

Pressure II. Proceedings of the Second International Symposium on Intracranial Pressure. Edited by N Lundberg, U Ponten, M Brock. Springer-Verlag, New York, 1975, pp. 403-408
12. Fleischer AS, Patton JN, Tindall GT: Intraventricular pressure monitoring using an implanted reservoir in head injured patients. Technical note. *Surg Neurol 3*:309-311, 1975
13. Gosch HH, Kindt GW: Subdural monitoring of acute increased intracranial pressure. *Surg Forum 23*:405-406, 1972
14. Numoto M, Donaghy RMP: Pressure indicating bag (PIB), *Intracranial Pressure II.* Proceedings of the Second International Symposium on Intracranial Pressure. Edited by N Lundberg, U Ponten, M. Brock. Springer-Verlag, New York, 1975, pp 382-383
15. Atkinson JR, Shurtleff DB, Foltz EL: Radiotelemetry for the measurement of intracranial pressure. *J Neurosurg 27*:428-432, 1967
16. Walker AE, Viernstein L, Chubbuck JG, et al: Intracranial pressure monitoring. Presented at Annual Meeting of the American Association of Neurological Surgeons, 1975
17. Rylander HG, Taylor HL, Aissinger JP, et al: Chronic measurement of epidural pressure with an induction-powered oscillator transducer. *J Neurosurg 44*:465-478, 1976
18. Meyer GA, Lyon WC, Bustard TS: A new device for long term intracranial pressure measurement. *Child's Brain 1*:217-227, 1975
19. Zervas N: Intracranial pressure monitor. *J Neurosurg,* in press
20. Jeppson S: Echoencephalography V: A method for recording the intracranial pressure with the aid of the echo encephalographic technique: a preliminary report. *Acta Chir Scand 128*:218-224, 1964
21. Richardson A, Eversden ID, Sternbergh WCA: Detecting intracranial pressure waves with ultrasound. *Lancet 1*:355-357, 1972
22. Lundberg N: Continuous recording and control of ventricular fluid pressure in neurosurgical practice. *Acta Psychiatr. Neurol Scand 36*:Suppl 149:1-193, 1960
23. Lundberg N, Troupp H, Lorin H: Continuous recording of the ventricular-fluid pressure in patients with severe acute traumatic brain injury. *J Neurosurg 22*:581-590, 1965
24. Langfitt TW: Pathophysiology of increased ICP, *Intracranial Pressure, Experimental and Clinical Aspects.* Edited by M Brock, H Dietz. Springer-Verlag, Berlin, 1972, pp 361-364
25. Risberg J, Lundberg N, Ingvar DH: Regional cerebral blood volume during acute transient uses of the intracranial pressure. *J Neurosurg 31*:303-310, 1969
26. Miller JD, Garibi J: Intracranial volume/pressure relationships during continuous monitoring of ventricular fluid pressure, *Intracranial Pressure, Experimental and Clinical Aspects.* Edited by M Brock, H Dietz. Springer-Verlag, Berlin, 1972, pp. 270-274
27. Miller JD, Leech PJ, Pickard JD: Volume pressure response in various experimental and clinical conditions, *Intracranial Pressure II.* Proceedings of the Second International Symposium on Intracranial Pressure. Edited by N Lundberg, U Ponten, M Brock. Springer-Verlag, New York, 1975, pp 97-100
28. Miller JD: Clinical aspects of intracranial pressure-volume relationships, *Head Injuries*, Proceedings of the Second Chicago Symposium on Neural Trauma. Edited by R McLaurin. Grune and Stratton, New York, 1975, pp 239-245
29. Miller JD, Leach PJ: Effects of mannitol and steroid therapy on intracranial volume pressure relationships. *J Neurosurg 42*:274-281, 1975
30. Nakatani S, Ommaya AK: A critical rate of cerebral compression, Intracranial Pressure, Experimental and Clinical Aspects. Edited by M Brock, H Dietz. Springer-Verlag, Berlin, 1972, pp 144-148
31. Ransohoff J, Benjamin MV, Gage EL, et al: Hemicraniectomy in the management of acute subdural hematoma. *J Neurosurg 34*:70-76, 1971
32. Kjellberg RM, Prieto A: Bifrontal decompressive craniotomy for massive cerebral edema. *J Neurosurg 34*:488-493, 1971
33. Vapalahti M, Troupp H: Prognosis for patients with severe brain injuries. *Br Med J 3*:404-407, 1971
34. Becker DP, Vries JK, Sakalas, et al: Early prognosis in head injury based on motor posturing, oculocephalic reflexes, and intracranial pressure, *Head Injuries.* Proceedings of the Second Chicago Symposium on Neural Trauma. Edited by R McLaurin. Grune and Stratton, New York.
35. Tindall G, Fleischer AS: Intracranial pressure (ICP) monitoring and prognosis in closed head injury, *Head Injuries.* Proceedings of the Second Chicago Symposium on Neural Trauma. Edited by R McLaurin. Grune and Statton, New York, 1975, pp 31-34
36. Jennett B, Johnston IH: The uses of intracranial pressure monitoring in clinical management, *Intracranial Pressure. Experimental and Clinical Aspects.* Edited by M Brock, H Dietz. Springer-Verlag, Berlin, 1972, pp 353-356
37. Merino de Villasante J, Taveras J: Computerized tomography in acute head trauma. *Am J Roentgenol 126*:765-778, 1976
38. Johnston I, Paterson A: Intracranial pressure monitoring in patients with benign intracranial hypertension, *Intracranial Pressure II.* Proceedings of the Second International Symposium on Intracranial Pressure. Edited by N Lundberg, U Ponen, M Brock. Springer-Verlag, New York, 1975, pp 500-502

39. Adams RD, Fisher CM, Hakim S, et al: Symptomatic occult hydrocephalus with "normal" cerebrospinal fluid pressure: a treatable syndrome. *N Engl J Med 273*:117-126, 1965
40. Stein SC, Langfitt TW: Normal pressure hydrocephalus: Predicting the results of cerebrospinal fluid shunting. *J Neurosurg 41*:463-470, 1974
41. Symon L, Dorsch NWC: Use of long term intracranial pressure measurement to assess hydrocephalic patients prior to shunt surgery. *J Neurosurg 42*:258-273, 1975
42. Katzman R, Hussey F: A simple constant-infusion manometric test for measurement of CSF absorption. 1. Rationale and method. *Neurology 20*:534-544, 1970
43. Hussey F, Schanzer B, Katzman R: A simple constant-infusion manometric test for measurement of CSF absorption. 2. Clinical studies. *Neurology 20*:665-680, 1970
44. Wolinsky JS, Barnes BD, Margolis MT: Diagnostic tests in NPH. *Neurology 23*:706-713, 1973
45. Chandler WF, Kindt GW: Monitoring and control of intracranial pressure in nontraumatic encephalopathies. *Surg Neurol 5*:311-314, 1976
46. Pizzi FS, Schut L, Berman W, et al: Intracranial pressure monitoring in Reye's syndrome. Paper presented at the American Association of Neurological Surgeons, Miami, Florida, 1975
47. Sundbarg G, Kkallquist, Lundberg N, et al: Complications due to prolonged ventricular fluid pressure recording in clinical practice, *Intracranial Pressure, Experimental and Clinical Aspects.* Edited by M Brock, H Dietz. Springer-Verlag, Berlin, 1972, pp 348-352
48. Wyler AR, Kelly WA: Use of antibiotics with external ventriculostomies. *J Neurosurg 37*:185-187, 1972

CHAPTER 8
The Surgical Removal of Acoustic Neuromas

William A. Buchheit   Craig H. Johnson

A DISCUSSION OF THE OPERATIVE management of acoustic tumors requires a brief historical review of the surgical techniques that have evolved since the first cerebellopontine angle tumor was operated upon Ballance[1] in 1894.

The 70% to 80% mortality rate testifies to the difficulties encountered with excision of these tumors at the turn of the century. Because it was impossible to diagnose these tumors early, surgical procedures were performed exclusively on patients with large tumors. In addition, finger enucleation with resultant edema, hemorrhage, and compromise of brainstem circulation were responsible for these dismal results.

Advocating incomplete removal of acoustic tumors by intracapsular gutting of the tumor mass, Cushing[2] was the first surgeon to significantly reduce the operative mortality. Cushing's approach involved a large bilateral suboccipital craniectomy which, besides gaining access to the tumor, provided palliative decompression of the posterior fossa. He made no attempt to dissect the tumor capsule from the brainstem, the cranial nerves, and the important vascular structures.

The technique for total removal of acoustic tumors was developed by Dandy.[3,4] Initially through a bilateral and later through a unilateral suboccipital craniectomy the tumor was exposed, an intracapsular decompression of the tumor mass was performed, and the remaining capsule with residual tumor was excised with careful dissection. With this approach Dandy[5] was able to accomplish total excision with an exceedingly low mortality rate.

Early tumor recurrence after incomplete removal and increased mortality associated with reoperation were reported by Horrax and Poppen[6] in 1939. In Olivecrona's series,[7] the 5-year total tumor mortality rate was 44% after partial removal as compared to 20% after complete removal. These reports emphasized the importance of total extirpation.

Complete tumor removal with sparing of the facial nerve has become the focus of attention during the last two decades.[8,9] With smaller tumors coming to surgery and with the development of microsurgical techniques, surgeons have been able to spare the facial nerve in most cases. In those cases in which this has not been possible, the operating microscope has permitted intracranial anastomosis of a divided seventh nerve, with or without a graft.

Four basic operative approaches are used for the excision of acoustic tumors: (a) the translabyrinthine, (b) the combined suboccipital translabyrinthine, (c) the middle fossa, and (d) the suboccipital.[10]

Department of Neurosurgery, Temple University Hospital, Philadelphia, Pennsylvania 19140

The translabyrinthine operation was originally described by Panse[11] in 1904, and recently perfected by House.[12] Hitselberger and House[10] have advocated this procedure for the removal of moderate size tumors. Unfortunately, with this approach, any preoperative auditory function is destroyed.

Borchardt[13] in 1905 described an approach to acoustic tumors which combined the suboccipital and translabyrinthine approaches and included division of the sigmoid sinus. Hitselberger and House[10,14] in 1966 revived this procedure using microsurgical techniques and have suggested it be used for the excision of large tumors.

The middle cranial fossa operation involves an extradural, subtemporal approach with microsurgical unroofing of the internal auditory canal. This approach is only applicable for the excision of small intracanalicular tumors that have not yet escaped the confines of the internal auditory canal.[10,15]

The suboccipital approach has already been discussed.

In 1964 Rand and Kurze[16,17] modified the suboccipital operation by adding a transmeatal microsurgical dissection. With their modification, the posterior and superior aspects of the internal auditory canal are removed permitting dissection of the tumor within the canal. Following this, dissection of tumor from the brainstem and adjacent cranial nerves is carried out. This operation has an advantage in that it is applicable to tumors of all sizes, and permits intracranial anastomosis of the facial nerve when necessary.

Anatomy

Although most agree that acoustic tumors originate within the internal auditory canal, there is controversy regarding the cell of origin. Most favored is the hypothesis that it originates from the Schwann cell, as opposed to the perineurothelial cell.[18-20] The Schwann cell is commonly believed to be derived from the neuroectodermal germ layer, specifically, the neural crest cells.[18,19]

The nerve roots are covered by pia along their subarachnoid course with axonal support provided by neuroglial cells.[18,20,21] With penetration of the pia, the neuroglial support ceases and each axon in the nerve root acquires a sheath composed of reticulin and Schwann cells.[18,20] The point at which the nerve roots penetrate the pia and the axons acquire the reticulin and Schwann cell sheaths varies considerably among different cranial and spinal nerve roots. This point is a considerable distance from the brainstem along the eighth cranial nerve and is usually found within the internal auditory canal. In addition, this junction is more distal along the vestibular nerves than along the cochlear nerve.[18] In summary, most acoustic tumors originate within the internal auditory canal, since the Schwann cell sheath does not exist medial to the porus.

Acoustic tumors usually arise from the vestibular nerve,[18,22] most often the superior, although up to 10% may develop from the cochlear nerve.[23] Generally, as the tumor increases in size, it assumes an eccentric or peripheral position on the nerve, characteristic of Schwannomas, rather than splaying out nerve fibers over a fusiform central mass, as in neurofibromas.[18,22]

Inasmuch as the tumor originates within the internal auditory canal, knowledge of the normal anatomic relationship of the seventh and eighth nerves within the canal is important in understanding how the tumor displaces these nerves. The porus can be divided conceptually into four quadrants when viewed from inside out (Fig. 8-1). The anterior-superior quadrant is occupied by the facial nerve, the anterior-inferior quadrant by the cochlear division of the eighth nerve, the posterior-superior quadrant by the superior vestibular nerve, and the posterior-inferior quadrant by the inferior vestibular nerve. As most acoustic tumors arise from the vestibular nerves located in the posterior quadrants of the porus, continued growth displaces the facial nerve anterior and inferior to the tumor.[24-26] The facial nerve may be displaced superiorly by a tumor arising from the cochlear nerve.[25]

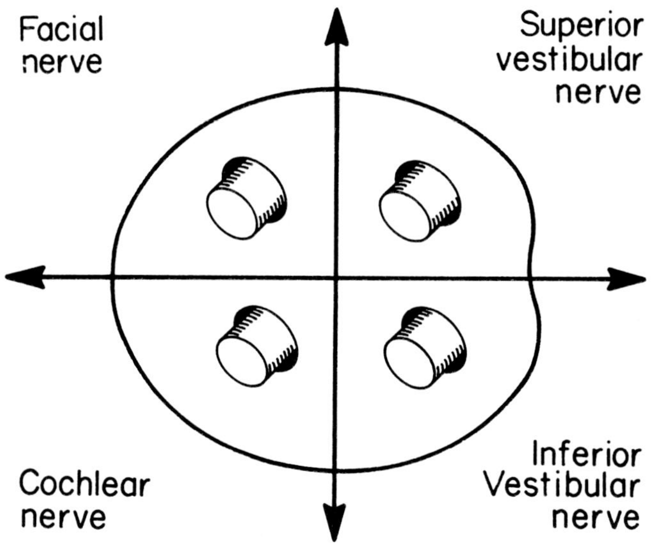

Fig. 8-1. The right internal acoustic meautus as seen from the suboccipital approach.

The cerebellopontine angle cistern is a pyramidal-shaped cerebrospinal fluid space bounded medially by the brainstem, posterolaterally by the cerebellum, anterolaterally by the posterior surface of the petrous bone, and superiorly by the tentorium. This cistern adjoins the lateral medullary cistern and the cisterna magna inferiorly, the pontine and interpeduncular cisterns medially, and the ambiens cistern superiorly and medially.[22]

Normally, the subarachnoid space of the cerebellopontine cistern extends as a diverticulum into the internal auditory canal. As the tumor grows and extends out of the porus it invaginates the arachnoid ahead of itself and forms the cyst commonly seen capping the tumor.[24,26] Ultimately, this arachnoid invagination becomes a tissue plane between the tumor and the brainstem, which permits their separation at the time of surgery.

Venous structures essentially encircle the cerebellopontine cistern. Connecting the cavernous sinus with the transverse sinus, the superior petrosal sinus extends along the superior lateral aspect of the cistern running within the edge of the tentorium at its junction with the petrous bone. Within the base of the cerebellopontine cistern the inferior petrosal sinus connects the cavernous sinus with the jugular vein at the jugular foramen. Posteriorly and laterally within the cistern the sigmoid sinus connects the transverse sinus and the jugular vein by running inferiorly down the posterior lateral aspect of the petrous ridge and then anteromedially in the petro-occipital junction to the jugular foramen. The petrosal vein crosses the cerebellopontine cistern as it leaves the anterolateral edge of the cerebellar hemisphere and courses anterolaterally to join the superior petrosal sinus. The point of entry into the superior petrosal sinus varies but is usually within the medial one-third adjacent to the fifth nerve. The petrosal vein, although it contributes to the venous drainage of the cerebellar hemisphere and brainstem,[27] is not a vital structure.

The seventh and eighth cranial nerves pass anteriorly, laterally, and superiorly through the cerebellopontine angle cistern as they pass from the brainstem to the internal auditory meatus. Although the cochlear and vestibular divisions of the acoustic nerve course as a single bundle within the cistern, they enter the brainstem separately (Fig. 8-2). The larger cochlear division enters the pontomedullary junction lateral, posterior, and inferior to the vestibular nerve.[21,28,29] The fibers of the acoustic nerve spiral in their subarachnoid course in order to assume the configuration previously described at the level of the porus, with the vestibular nerves being located posteriorly and the cochlear nerve anteriorly.[22] The origin of

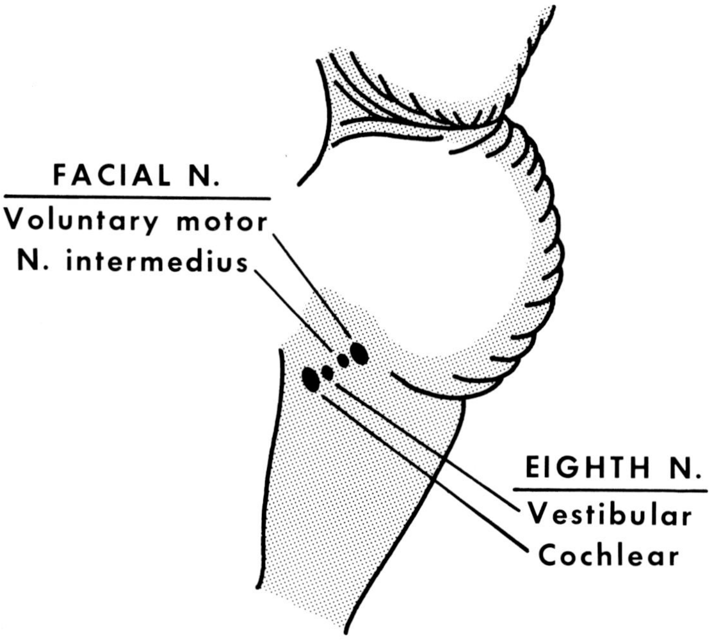

Fig. 8-2.

the motor root of the facial nerve is located anterior, medial, and superior to the vestibular nerve. The nervus intermedius (the nerve of Wrisberg) enters the brainstem between the origin of the motor root of the facial nerve and the vestibular nerve. The nervus intermedius usually is adherent to the vestibular nerve for a variable distance prior to its entrance into the brainstem. Rhoton[25,30] reported that in 20% of cases the nervus intermedius cannot be identified within the cerebellopontine angle as it remains adherent to the acoustic nerve throughout its entire course and joins the facial nerve only within the internal auditory canal.

The motor and sensory roots of the trigeminal nerve are located at midpons level and pass anterolaterally through the upper portion of the cerebellopontine angle cistern to the anterior-superior-medial edge of the petrous ridge. The petrosal vein is generally located along the lateral edge of the trigeminal nerve.[21]

The anatomy of the arteries of the cerebellopontine cistern is vitally important. Occlusion of these vessels leads to brainstem infarction and loss of neural and end-organ function in areas not involved directly with tumor. The most important vessel is the anterior-inferior cerebellar artery which has a variable relationship with divisions of the acousticofacial bundle within the cerebellopontine angle as well as within the internal auditory canal. The anterior-inferior cerebellar artery, or a branch of this vessel, forms a loop near or within the internal auditory canal. This vessel or loop may in its course pass anterior, posterior, or between the seventh and eighth nerves.[21,22,30] The anterior-inferior cerebellar artery supplies the lateral aspect of the brainstem and the cerebellum and is the origin of the labyrinthine artery except when the latter arises from the basilar artery.[21] The labyrinthine artery is variable in its relationship with the neural structures. This artery may even supply the brainstem by way of recurrent branches. Immediately adjacent to the brainstem the circumferential branches, arising directly from the basilar or from the anterior inferior cerebellar artery, pass among the components of the acousticofacial bundle and supply the posterolateral aspect of the brainstem.[30]

Diagnosis and Selection of Cases

Acoustic tumors constitute 8% to 10% of intracranial tumors and account for 71% of cerebellopontine angle tumors. Patients are primarily in the middle-age group. These tumors tend to occur more commonly in women than in men; some claim the ratio is as high as 2:1. Four percent of acoustic tumors are bilateral; these usually occur in patients with von Recklinghausen's disease, which is inherited as a Mendelian dominant.[18,22]

Since acoustic tumors originate within the internal auditory canal on one of the vestibular or the cochlear nerves, the initial symptoms result from the dysfunction of these structures. With tumor extension into the cerebellopontine angle, the cerebrospinal fluid protein becomes elevated in most cases. Continued expansion in the cerebellopontine angle results in symptoms and signs attributable to the compression of the trigeminal nerve, the brainstem, the middle cerebellar peduncle, and the cerebellum. With very large lesions, signs of increased intracranial pressure due to hydrocephalus can occur.

Early diagnosis is essential to minimize the morbidity and the mortality of surgery. All patients with unilateral hearing loss, tinnitus, or fullness in the ear should be considered as acoustic tumor suspects. If pure tone audiometry indicates a sensory-neural hearing loss, then a more complete evaluation of eighth nerve function should be obtained including examination of cochlear and vestibular components. Special audiometric tests indicate whether the sensory-neural hearing loss is due to end-organ dysfunction (cochlear) or to neural dysfunction (retrocochlear). An acoustic tumor is a retrocochlear lesion and audiometric testing in these patients most often demonstrates a retrocochlear pattern of hearing loss. There are excellent reviews of the special audiometric tests and their application in the diagnosis of acoustic tumors.[31-35] Reference to them is encouraged.

In addition to audiometric analysis of eighth nerve function, vestibular function should be investigated. Nystagmus and a reduced or absent caloric response should be sought on the side of the suspected lesion. An abnormal caloric response has been noted unilaterally in 95% of patients with acoustic tumors.[22] Electronystagmography and more sophisticated forms of quantitative vestibulo-ocular testing are useful.[36]

All patients with unilateral sensory-neural hearing loss or vestibular dysfunction should undergo routine radiologic examination of the skull, including Stenver's and base views, as well as tomograms of both temporal bones. Taveras and Wood[37] indicate that it is possible to diagnose 65% of acoustic neuromas by plain films alone and 70% of cases by tomography. Ojemann et al.[38] have reported plain film abnormalities in 70% and abnormal tomograms in 82% of their cases of acoustic tumor. Valvassori[39] established the relative significance of various internal auditory canal tomographic abnormalities in an excellent study. These will not be reviewed here, but reference to the classification of these abnormal findings and their significance is suggested.

Positive contrast cisternography with iophendylate is the most definitive test presently available for acoustic tumors. Both cerebellopontine angles are examined in each patient. This study is performed when temporal bone tomography is distinctly abnormal, when the results of tomography are indefinite, or when the tomograms are unremarkable but there is strong clinical and audiometric evidence for an acoustic tumor. In addition to demonstrating lesions of the cerebellopontine angle clearly, positive contrast cisternography contributes quite significantly to the early diagnosis of acoustic tumors since small intracanalicular tumors can be demonstrated readily by this method.

Failure to fill the internal auditory canal with iophendylate, however, is not always specific for intracanalicular tumor. Wright and Turner,[41] in 1973, reported 7 cases of false-positive cerebellopontine angle myelograms and reviewed the literature concerning this problem. They reported a 7% incidence of false-positive angle myelograms in their series of 100. Valvassori,[40] in 1969, proposed five possible explanations for false-positive angle myelograms: (a) arachnoidal adhesions, (b) neural edema, (c) foreshortening of the meningeal lining of the internal auditory canal, (d) tight fit of a normal neurovascular bundle within a narrow internal auditory canal and (e) inability to fill the internal auditory canal with high-viscosity iophendylate by gravity alone.

Vertebral angiography is of limited value in the early diagnosis of acoustic tumors. In large tumors it assumes more importance by demonstrating vascular displacement and tumor vascularity. The latter may require subtraction techniques.

The importance of computerized axial tomography (CAT) of the brain in the early diagnosis of acoustic tumors is likewise limited since acoustic tumors smaller than 1.5 to 2.0 cm are difficult to demonstrate. Patients who are undergoing CAT scanning as acoustic tumor suspects should be studied after contrast enhancement. An additional method of enhancement of cerebellopontine angle mass lesions, not universally available at the present time, combines computerized axial tomography (CAT scan) with positive contrast cistern enhancement using water soluble contrast material (metizamide). If the CAT scan is to be obtained, it should be done before iophendylate cisternography since residual contrast will interfere significantly with the study.

Preoperative Preparation

The successful removal of an acoustic tumor begins with meticulous attention to details during the preoperative period. Inasmuch as most of these cases do not constitute a surgical emergency, ample time is available for complete and detailed evaluation of the cardiac, pulmonary, renal, and hematologic systems. This is particularly important in patients over 50 years of age.

During the day prior to surgery, provided there is no medical contraindication, dexamethasone, 6 mg, or methylprednisolone, 32 mg, every 6 hours is begun orally. At the same time a prophylactic antibiotic is administered orally. The evening before surgery all patients receive a hexachlorophene shampoo.

Prior to surgery the patient is taken to the anesthesia induction room where the head is shaved completely, the legs are wrapped with elastic bandages from the toes to groin, and a right atrial catheter is inserted. The patient is then moved to the operating room where general endotracheal anesthesia is administered. A Foley catheter is inserted into the bladder, and an intraarterial cannula is placed to facilitate blood pressure monitoring. A doppler stethoscope is attached to the precordium to aid in the detection of air emboli. Recording electrode pads are placed on the face, ipsilateral to the tumor, for electromyographic (EMG) monitoring of facial muscles with intracranial stimulation of the facial nerve. With these measures complete, the patient is ready for the sitting position (Fig. 8-3). Frequently there is a drop in blood pressure with a change from the supine to the sitting position; consequently, it must be done with care. It is important that this change be accomplished by two people aside from the anesthesiologist. One person should be responsible for maintaining the position of the head and the second for movements of the table. As the table is being flexed the footplate must be dropped so as not to *jackknife* the patient in the straight-leg position. Although stretching of the sciatic nerve will be tolerated transiently, if prolonged, it can result in stretch neuropathy. Once the table has been maximally flexed, the headpiece from the operating table is dropped backward and the head held in the position in which it is to be stabilized for surgery. It is our policy to position the head and then attach the headholder, rather than the opposite. We prefer the head be rotated 20° to 30° toward the side of the tumor and carefully flexed maximally. The scalp is then prepped with povidone-iodine and the three-point Gardner headholder attached with the single-pointed side of the headholder ipsilateral to the tumor; this facilitates subsequent attachment of a self-retaining retractor in a position that allows the retractor arms to coil around the head out of the field of the surgeon and the scrub nurse. The headpiece from the operating table is then moved to a horizontal position to serve as an armrest during the operative procedure.

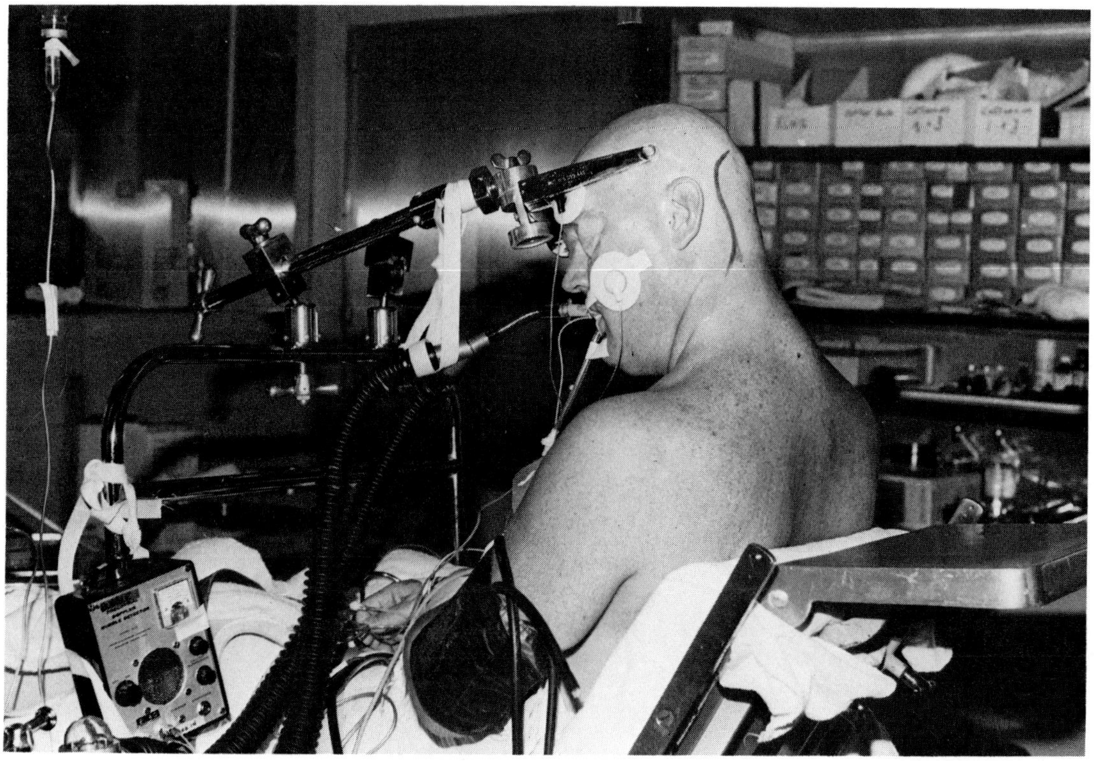

Fig. 8-3.

Once these steps have been taken, incisions are outlined with a surgical marking pen. In most cases a large "S"-shaped incision over the lateral aspect of the occipital bone is adequate (Figs. 8-3 and 8-4). For larger tumors, a horseshoe-shaped incision is preferred (Fig. 8-5). In all cases, an occipital burr hole is outlined. The skin is surgically scrubbed and then prepped with povidone-iodine. Drapes are sutured in place. The surgical field and the headpiece of the operating table, now being used as an armrest, are covered with Steri-Drapes. In patients with no cardiovascular problems, the surgical incision is infiltrated with 1:200,000 epinephrine solution to facilitate hemostasis.

Surgery

Surgery is begun by placing a burr hole in the occipital area. We prefer a site 7 cm above the external occipital protuberance and 4 cm lateral to the mid-sagittal plane (Figs. 8-4 and 8-5). In patients with small tumors and no increased intracranial pressure, the burr hole is placed but the dura is not opened. In those with increased intracranial pressure, the dura is opened, the underlying cortex is coagulated, and the lateral ventricle is cannulated with a metal brain cannula. This cannula is replaced with a Scott cannula or a No. 8, red-rubber catheter onto which a one-way stopcock has been secured. With the catheter in place, intraventricular pressure is slowly reduced to normal. Once the pressure has equilibrated, the stopcock is closed and surgery is directed to the posterior fossa.

In patients with small tumors a sigmoid incision is preferred (Fig. 8-4). With this incision, few difficulties are encountered. A large emissary vein at the base of the mastoid tip may bleed briskly, but bleeding is easily controlled with bone wax. In addition, one must be

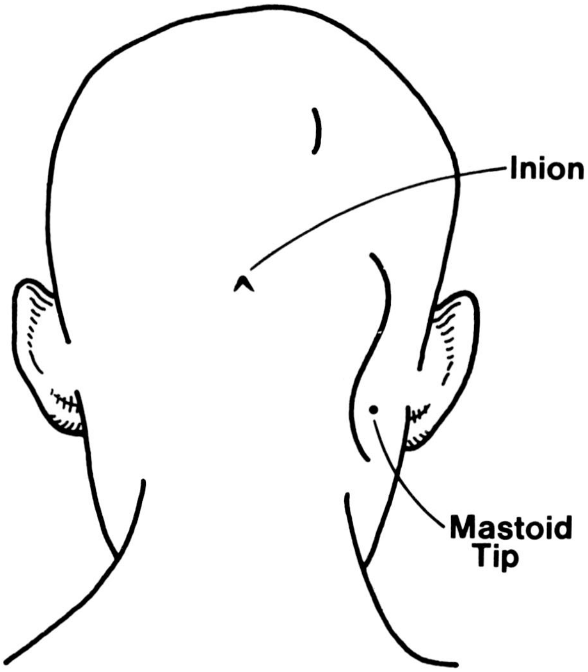

Fig. 8-4.

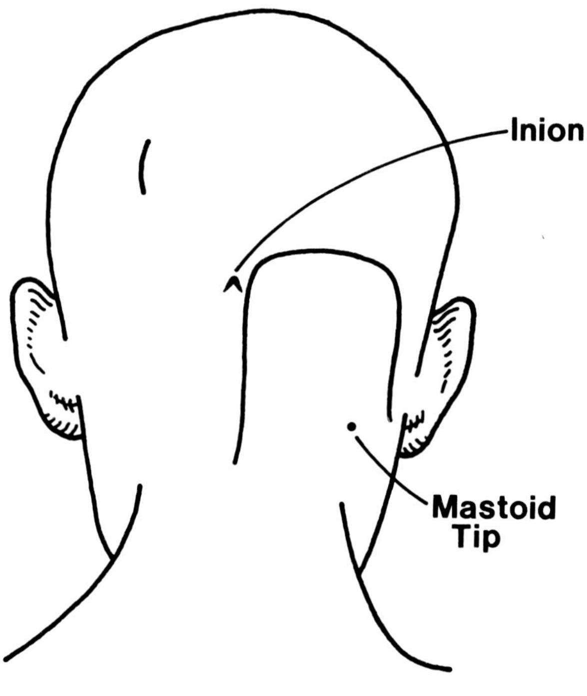

Fig. 8-5.

cautious not to dissect too far forward in the region of the stylomastoid foramen, deep to the medial aspect of the mastoid tip, where the seventh nerve may be injured as it exits the skull. Undercutting muscle origins along the superior nuchal line is necessary, both medially and laterally. With the aid of a Weitlaner self-retaining retractor, adequate exposure can be obtained without difficulty. It is important that the exposure include the posterior and lateral aspects of the mastoid process and the lateral third of the squamous portion of the occipital bone.

In patients with large tumors a horseshoe-shaped incision is preferred. With this incision (Fig. 8-5), the lateral limb is subject to the same concerns as the sigmoid type incision. In addition, it is necessary that the medial limb of the incision be exactly in the midline. This plane is easily identified and permits an avascular dissection.

With either incision the object is to expose and remove the bone overlying the angle created by the transverse and sigmoid sinuses. This is accomplished by placing a single burr hole and removing the squamous portion of the occipital bone, as well as the medial third of the mastoid bone, with a rongeur. The mastoid air cells that have been opened must be immediately sealed with bone wax. By removing bone laterally, a view of the tumor may be obtained without an overhanging ledge of bone obscuring the exposure. This is the same principle that applies to a low-placed frontal bone flap in the subfrontal approach to the pituitary fossa. The total craniectomy should be 5 cm in diameter. For larger tumors, it may be necessary to carry the craniectomy medially through the foramen magnum and remove the arch of the atlas.

In the event that the dura is not slack, its opening should be delayed and the intraventricular pressure should be measured. In most cases the pressure in the posterior fossa will respond favorably to a reduction in intraventricular pressure. If this is unsuccessful, administration of intravenous Lasix, 40 to 60 mg, usually is associated with a reduction in pressure within 20 to 30 minutes (the purpose of the Foley catheter).

Initially the dura is opened in the midportion of the craniectomy. The dural incision is then extended upward toward the angle between the sigmoid and transverse sinuses and downward toward the foramen magnum. To facilitate the identification of the sinuses and to provide safety in opening the last few millimeters of dura, a fiber optic light is inserted intradurally and the operating room lights dimmed. This transillumination of the dura allows the dural incisions to be made exactly to the venous sinuses without lacerating them. The dura is opened maximally by incising it at right angles to the original opening. The dural flaps are then sutured to muscle to increase exposure and to control epidural bleeding.

Once the dura is opened, a small, flat-bladed, Cushing brain retractor is used to elevate the cerebellum and expose the cisterna magna. With sharp forceps this cistern is opened, and the cerebrospinal fluid is allowed to escape, rapidly decreasing the volume of the posterior fossa. The small, flat-bladed, Cushing retractor is then replaced with a 3-cm retractor which is inserted laterally and inferiorly so that the cerebellum can be elevated and the presence of a tumor confirmed. The retractor is then incorporated into the self-retaining apparatus and held in position so that the tip of the retractor is in the junction between the overlying cerebellum and the superior-posterior aspect of the tumor (Fig. 8-6). It is unwise to retract forcibly against the cerebellum. If adequate exposure is not available with reduction of intraventricular pressure, Lasix, and opening of the cisterna magna, then the bony exposure along the lateral aspect of the craniectomy should be reevaluated. If this is adequate, the only alternative is resection of the lateral third of the cerebellum. In most cases this is not necessary.

Once the self-retaining retractor is secured, the operating microscope is positioned and the tumor resected with the aid of this instrument. We prefer a 300-mm lens with a 12.5-mm eyepiece for acoustic surgery. This combination of lenses has a 16-inch focal length that permits the use of standard microneurosurgical instruments and yet provides adequate distance between the microscope and the operative field. We prefer to place the binocular assistant tube on the surgeon's right side, the same side on which we prefer the nurse. The

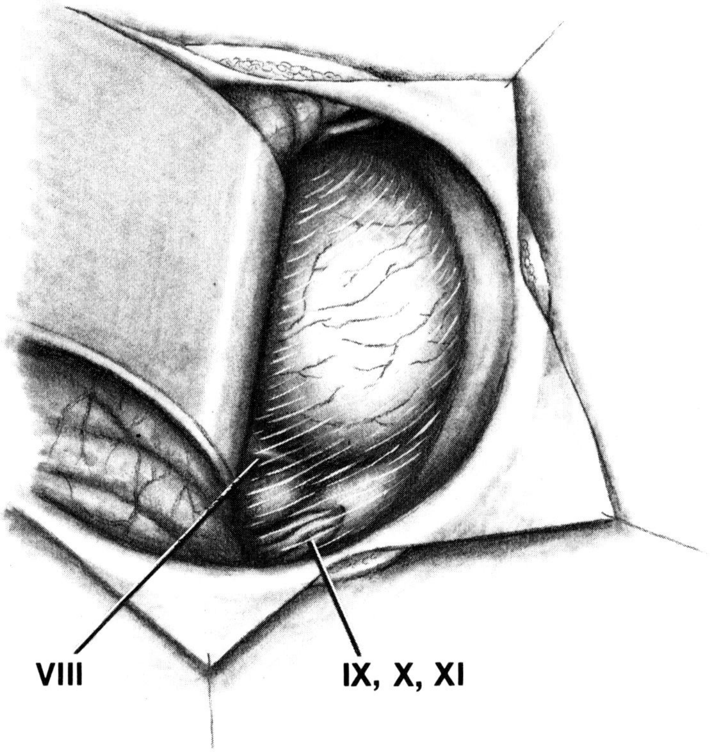

Fig. 8-6.

photographic equipment, or a second assistant's monocular viewing scope, is located on the surgeon's left.

Through the microscope the cerebellopontine angle and its contents are then inspected. The arachnoid covering of the tumor is easily seen (Fig. 8-6). In large tumors it is this arachnoid that forms the capping cyst over the dome of the tumor. In smaller tumors drainage of cerebrospinal fluid from the cisterna magna permits the arachnoid to settle onto the tumor making its identification more difficult. In either circumstance it is necessary to pick up and open the arachnoid with sharp dissection. Once this has been carried out, the tumor is clearly exposed (Fig. 8-7). The petrosal vein can be seen above the upper pole of the tumor entering into the superior petrosal sinus. We prefer to coagulate and transect the petrosal vein at this early stage of the operation so as to prevent the troublesome bleeding that occurs if the vein is torn from its entrance into the superior petrosal sinus. At the lower pole of the tumor, the ninth, tenth, and eleventh cranial nerves may be seen entering the jugular foramen. These should be isolated and protected, with either a cottonoid or a rubber drain.

Completion of these preliminary steps sets the stage for tumor removal. At the inferomedial aspect of the tumor, the glistening, white, medial portion of the eighth nerve can be seen merging with the tumor (Fig. 8-7). This nerve serves as the base of a triangular space whose medial boundary is the cerebellum and whose lateral boundary is the tumor. This triangular acoustic space identifies two important landmarks: the arachnoid plane between the tumor and the pons, and the origin of the seventh nerve at the brainstem. The arachnoid plane is the key to dissection of the medial aspect of the tumor and permits total tumor removal without injuring the pons or its circumferential arcade of vessels. This plane is easily identified in smaller tumors that have not abutted against or indented the lateral pons. In the case of large tumors it is usually necessary to open the tumor capsule and morsellate the center with small ring curettes. During the morsellation, bleeding is controlled with two-point

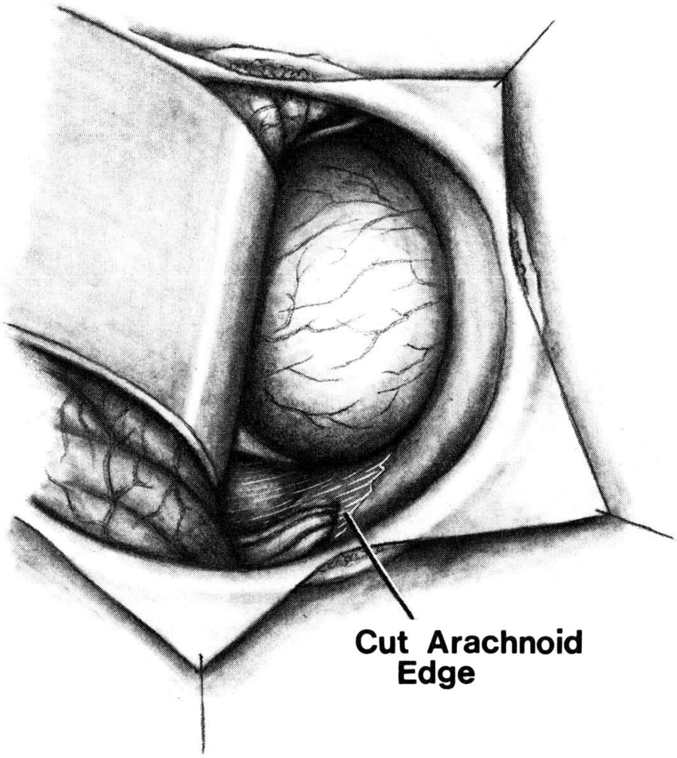

Fig. 8-7.

coagulation under direct vision and small cotton packs soaked in topical thrombin. Reduction in the bulk of the lesion and lateral retraction of the capsule facilitate the identification of the acoustic triangle. As the medial plane is further developed, the origin of the seventh nerve, anterior and superior to the termination of the eighth nerve, can be seen. Stimulation of the seventh nerve affords functional confirmation of the anatomy. The identification of the nerve, before it becomes thinned and stretched anteriorly around the tumor, is critical. Once the seventh nerve has been identified and confirmed by stimulation, its preservation depends upon meticulous dissection. In larger tumors morsellation is important to allow retraction of the capsule away from the brainstem and ultimately the seventh nerve. As the tumor is rolled laterally, additional surface tumor vessels become visible and should be coagulated in turn. While coagulating these vessels, it is extremely important that the circumferential blood supply of the brainstem, the posterior and anterior-inferior cerebellar arteries and their related branches, be preserved. The superior pole of the tumor must be managed likewise. Morsellation and retraction downward, associated with dissection in the arachnoid tissue plane between the tumor and the fifth nerve, gradually bring the latter into view. It is not uncommon to find the anterior-inferior cerebellar artery at the junction of the tumor and the pons near the root entry zone of the fifth cranial nerve.

Similar technique is applied to the lower pole of the tumor. With gradual morsellation and upward traction, the bulk of the tumor is reduced facilitating extracapsular dissection at the lower pole. Gradually the tumor is involuted on itself to a point where it is possible to see around the medial, superior, and inferior poles. During this dissection it is important to continually stimulate the seventh nerve. The bulk of the free portion of the tumor can be removed with sharp dissection without danger. One is then left with residual tumor in the porus acousticus. In many instances the porus is eroded allowing direct visualization simply by moving the microscope toward the midline and looking laterally. In smaller tumors, however, this may not be the case, and it is necessary to remove the posterior lip of the porus with either a fine punch or an air drill. We prefer the latter. To do this a small flap of dura is raised adjacent to the porus, and the air drill used to grind down the posterior lip. Enough bone must be removed to adequately visualize the contents of the porus. If petrous air cells are encountered, these must be sealed with bone wax to prevent cerebrospinal fluid leak. Alternatively, one can visualize the internal auditory canal with a 5-mm laryngeal mirror. Often the nubbin of tumor extending into the porus can be removed with judicious blunt dissection, or piecemeal with a fine microsurgical biopsy forceps. If bleeding occurs in the porus, it is important not to use coagulation. A piece of Gelfoam soaked in topical thrombin controls the bleeding in most instances. Once residual tumor is removed from the porus, the seventh nerve can be seen along its entire course from the brainstem to the porus.

As soon as the tumor is removed completely, the anesthesiologist should be asked to elevate venous pressure by transient jugular compression to reconfirm hemostasis. Following this, the dura is closed primarily. If necessary, a small autogenous graft is used to complete the dural closure. The wound is closed in standard multiple-layer fashion.

Postoperative Care

The patient is removed to the recovery room and soon thereafter to the Neurosurgical Intensive Care Unit. Vital signs are monitored carefully. Attention to central venous pressure, arterial pressure, intracranial ventricular pressure, and fluid and electrolyte balance is mandatory. Immediately after surgery, neurologic examination should be performed with particular attention to the fifth, seventh, ninth, tenth and eleventh cranial nerves. In patients with evidence of trigeminal and/or facial nerve dysfunction, an air-tight eye shield should be applied in the recovery room. With suspected injury to the ninth, tenth, or eleventh cranial nerves, the endotracheal tube should be left in place until it can be removed safely or, if necessary, a tracheostomy can be performed. Fortunately these patients tolerate endotracheal tubes extremely well. The ventriculostomy tube is removed after 48 hours provided intracranial pressure is normal. During the first 48 hours, fluids are restricted to 900 to 1200 ml/day. Fluid composition is generally 0.45% saline in 5% dextrose. Wearing antiembolic stockings, the patient is kept at absolute bedrest with 15° to 30° elevation of the head for the first 2 to 3 days postoperatively. Steroids (dexamethasone, 6 mg, or metylprednisolone, 30 mg, every 6 hours) are continued parenterally for 3 to 4 days postoperatively and are then tapered gradually and administered orally over the next 5 to 6 days. Prophylactic antibiotic coverage is provided parenterally until 48 hours after the ventriculostomy has been removed and then maintained orally until all sutures have been removed from the operative wound. Patients are generally out of bed and beginning to ambulate after the fourth postoperative day.

Complications

Details regarding preoperative and intraoperative complications have been previously considered.

Postoperative hemorrhage in the form of subdural, epidural, or intracerebellar hematomas can occur. These problems must be identified early and surgically corrected. Recognition of these problems depends on close monitoring of vital signs, intracranial pressure, and neurologic status. Postoperative angiography or CAT scanning are capable of confirming clinical suspicions.

Pontomedullary infarction occurs when the blood supply to the brainstem is disrupted. Occlusion of the anterior-inferior cerebellar artery is thought to be responsible for this fatal complication in most cases. Circumferential and recurrent vessels supplying the lateral aspect of the brainstem may also be injured during dissection of the tumor capsule leading to irreversible brainstem infarction.

Postoperative cranial nerve dysfunction results in undesirable problems. Aside from the emotionally disabling effect of facial nerve palsy, the potential danger of exposure keratitis is a serious concern. To prevent corneal dessication in those patients the eye must be covered with an air-tight seal until tarsorrhaphy can be performed. With dysfunction of the ninth, tenth, and eleventh cranial nerves the possibility of aspiration pneumonitis exists. The loss of residual auditory and vestibular function can occur even with the most careful microsurgical tumor removal.

The most common wound complications include cerebrospinal fluid leaks and infections. The escape of cerebrospinal fluid from the operative wound itself is usually the result of increased intracranial pressure and improper wound closure. In these cases the cause of the elevated intracranial pressure must be sought. Possibilities include cerebellar edema secondary to retraction, intracerebellar hemorrhage, subdural hematomas, hydrocephalus, and meningitis. Restoration of normal intracranial pressure and revision of the operative wound are necessary to control cerebrospinal fluid leaks. Rarely will the mere placement of a few sutures across the incision at the site of the leak, suffice. Cerebrospinal fluid rhinorrhea also occurs. This complication usually results from the inadequate sealing of mastoid or petrous air cells exposed at the time of surgery. In most cases the surgical wound will have to be reexplored to correct this problem.

Infectious processes directly related to the operative procedure include soft tissue wound infection and postoperative meningitis. A high index of suspicion is often required for the early diagnosis of postoperative meningitis since the onset of this problem may be insidious due to the use of prophylactic antibiotics and steroids. Sterile meningitis, perhaps related to the tumor itself, is seen more often than bacterial meningitis, and usually occurs between 7 to 10 days postoperatively. Since urinary tract infections secondary to catheter drainage are a potential problem, routine culture and sensitivity tests of urine should be obtained pre- and postoperatively. The bladder catheter should be removed as soon as the clinical condition permits.

With the use of pre- and postoperative steroids, gastroduodenal stress ulcers occasionally occur. Since these ulcerations tend to be superficial erosions, bleeding is more common than perforation. An attempt should be made to prevent these by neutralizing gastric acid with antacids and oral alimentation as soon as the patient's postoperative condition permits. Iced saline lavage, whole blood transfusions, subtotal and even total gastrectomy may be required in some circumstances.

Late complications include hydrocephalus and tumor recurrence. The hydrocephalus is communicating in nature and probably due to postoperative subarachnoid adhesions. This problem usually resolves spontaneously but occasionally requires a cerebrospinal fluid shunt. The difficulties encountered with tumor recurrence have been mentioned previously.

REFERENCES

1. Ballance C: *Some Points in the Surgery of the Brain and its Membranes.* Macmillan and Co, London, 1907
2. Cushing H: *Tumors of the Nervus Acousticus and the Syndrome of the Cerebellopontine Angle.* WB Saunders, Philadelphia, 1917
3. Dandy WE: An operation for the total extirpation of tumors in the cerebellopontine angle. A preliminary report. *Bull Johns Hopkins Hosp 33*:344-345, 1922
4. Dandy WE: An operation for the total removal of cerebello-pontile (acoustic) tumors. *Surg Gynecol Obstet 41*:129-148, 1925
5. Dandy WE: Results of removal of acoustic tumors by the unilateral approach. *Arch Surg 42*:1026-1033, 1941

6. Horrax G, Poppen JL: Experiences with the total and intracapsular extirpation of acoustic neuromata. *Ann Surg 110*:513-524, 1939
7. Olivecrona H: Acoustic tumors. *J Neurosurg 26*:6-13, 1967
8. Drake CG: Surgical treatment of acoustic neuroma with preservation or reconstruction of the facial nerve. *J Neurosurg 26*:459-464, 1967
9. Drake CG: Total removal of large acoustic neurinomas. A modification of the McKenzie operation with special emphasis on saving the facial nerve. *J Neurosurg 26*:554-561, 1967
10. Hitselberger WE, House WF: Surgical approaches to acoustic tumors. *Arch Otolaryngol 84*:286-291, 1966
11. Panse R: Ein Gliom des Akustikus. *Arch f Ohrenh 61*:251-255, 1904
12. House WF: Monograph: Transtemporal bone microsurgical removal of acoustic neuromas. *Arch Otolaryngol 80*:597-756, 1964
13. Borchardt M: Zur operationen der tumoren des Kleinhirnbruckenwinkels. *Berl Klin Wchnschr 42*:1033-1035, 1905
14. Hitselberger WE, House WF: A combined approach to the cerebellopontine angle. *Arch Otolaryngol 84*:267-285, 1966
15. House WF: Surgical exposure of the internal auditory canal and its contents through the middle cranial fossa. *Laryngoscope 71*:1363-1385, 1961
16. Rand RW, Kurze T: Micro-neurosurgical resection of acoustic tumors by a transmeatal posterior fossa approach. *Bull LA Neurol Soc 30*:17-20, 1965
17. Rand RW, Kurze T: Facial nerve preservation by posterior fossa transmeatal microdissection in total removal of acoustic tumors. *J Neurol Neurosurg Psychiat 28*:311-316, 1965
18. Nager GT: Acoustic neurinomas. Pathology and differential diagnosis. *Arch Otolaryngol 89*:252-279, 1969
19. Rubinstein LJ: *Tumors of the Central Nervous System.* Armed Forces Institute of Pathology, Washington, DC, 1972
20. Russel DS, Rubinstein LJ: *Pathology of Tumours of the Nervous System.* Third edition. Williams and Wilkins, Baltimore, 1972
21. Hollinshead WH: *Anatomy for Surgeons, vol 1, The head and neck.* Second edition. Harper and Row, New York, 1968
22. Portmann M, Sterkers JM, Charachon R, et al: *The Internal Auditory Meatus, Anatomy, Pathology and Surgery.* Churchill Livingstone, Edinburgh, 1975
23. Pulec JL: Comments on translabyrinthine approach to acoustic neuromas. *Arch Otolaryng 83*:592-594, 1966
24. Malis LI: Microsurgical treatment of acoustic neurinomas, *Microneurosurgery.* Edited by H Handa. Igaku Shoin Ltd, Tokyo, 1975
25. Rhoton A: Microsurgery of the internal acoustic meatus. *Surg Neurol 2*:311-318, 1974
26. Yasargil MG, Fox JL: The microsurgical approach to acoustic neurinomas. *Surg Neurol 2*:393-398, 1974
27. Wilson M: *The Anatomic Foundation of Neuroradiology of the Brain.* Second edition. Little, Brown and Company, Boston, 1972
28. Goss CM: *Gray's Anatomy*. Twenty-eighth edition. Lea and Febiger, Philadelphia, 1966
29. Truex RC, Carpenter MB: *Human Neuroanatomy.* Sixth edition. Williams and Wilkins, Baltimore, 1969
30. Rhoton A, Kobayashi S, Hollinshead WH: Nervus intermedius. *J Neurosurg 29*:609-618, 1968
31. Dirks DD: Audiologic problems associated with eighth nerve tumor, *Microneurosurgery.* Edited by RW Rand. CV Mosby, St Louis, 1969, pp 104-114
32. Green DS: Modified tone decay test (MTDT) as screening procedure for eighth nerve lesions. *J Speech Hear Disord 28*:31-36, 1963
33. Jerger J: Bekesy audiometry in analysis of auditory disorders. *J Speech Hear Res 3*:275-287, 1960
34. Johnson EW, Sheehy JL: Audiological aspects of the diagnosis of acoustic neuromas. *J Neurosurg 24*:621-628, 1966
35. Tillman TW: Audiologic diagnosis of acoustic tumors. *Arch Otolaryngol 83*:574-581, 1966.
36. Baloh RW, Konrad HR, Dirks D, et al.: Cerebellar-pontine angle tumors. *Arch Neurol 33*:507-512, 1976
37. Taveras JM, Wood EH: *Diagnostic Neuroradiology.* Second edition. Williams and Wilkins, Baltimore, 1976
38. Ojemann RG, Montgomery WW, Weiss AD: Evaluation and surgical treatment of acoustic neuroma. *N Engl J Med 287*:895-899, 1972
39. Valvassori GE: The radiological diagnosis of acoustic neuromas. *Arch Otolaryngol 83*:582-587, 1966
40. Valvassori GE: The abnormal internal auditory canal: the diagnosis of acoustic neuroma. *Radiology 92*:449-459, 1969
41. Wright RE, Turner JS: Positive angle myelograms without acoustic neuroma. *Laryngoscope 83*:733-746, 1973

CHAPTER 9

Surgery of Epilepsy—Current Technique of Cortical Resection

Robert R. Hansebout

DESCRIPTIONS OF THE FALLING SICKNESS are found in man's writings since the dawn of recorded history. Fortunately, attempts at cures for epilepsy have been elevated from those with an aura of mysticism and superstition to more medically oriented forms, due to the greater understanding of brain physiology during the past 100 years.

Although the earliest attempts and successes at reducing seizures appear to have been surgical, the advent of modern drug therapy has allowed many epileptics to become productive. Still, current drugs may be toxic or not tolerated by some,[1] and may fail to control seizures in another 20% of epileptics.[2] It is estimated that about 1 in 200 persons today has epilepsy and that 10% of the population would be amenable to surgery.[2]

Among the surgical procedures used in the treatment of epilepsy, selective cortical resection has earned its place and has been used at an increasing number of neurosurgical centers during the past few years.[3] The following will illustrate salient features of that procedure.

Overall Conception of the Technique

In 1870 J. Hughlings Jackson first recognized that epilepsy could be due to a sudden excessive discharge of a focus of grey matter in the brain. The experimental demonstration of functional localization in the cortex by Fritsch and associates, confirmed Jackson's observations. In his book, published in 1881, William Gowers indicated that cerebral seizures could either be secondary to structural lesions of the brain or idiopathic, in which case there was no visible lesion.[4]

Otfrid Foerster, after World War 1, successfully carried out a number of cortical resections in post-traumatic epileptic patients with focal lesions.[5] Wilder Penfield's scholarly elaboration of cortical function by electrical stimulation, during a large series of operations for epilepsy, coupled with Herbert Jasper's neurophysiologic expertise fully established the usefulness of cortical resection in the neurosurgical armamentarium.[6] Theodore Rasmussen's meticulous surgical technique and analytic observations have broadened the scope and safety of the procedure.[3,7]

Causes of the focal seizure discharge range from tumors and vascular anomalies to scars and atrophic lesions, both in adults and children. Such atrophic cortex was most often found

Department of Neurology and Neurosurgery, McGill University, Montreal, Quebec, Canada

in the medial temporal lobe.[8] This *incisural sclerosis* of the Montreal school was thought to be due to birth injury, while Falconer associated this *mesial sclerosis* mainly with febrile illness and infantile seizures.[8,9] The seizures could be alleviated by removing abnormal brain tissue.[10]

In early series discrete cicatrical lesions were surgically removed in nontumoral cases of epilepsy,[5] but subsequently, it became clear that the area of epileptogenic brain tissue was usually larger than the structural abnormality and was often composed of several areas of varying epileptogenicity. When cortex in the region of maximum electrographic abnormality is removed, seizures often cease completely. In other cases seizures can then arise from adjacent cortex, again with lower than normal thresholds for epileptogenicity. It was found that the more complete the removal of epileptogenic brain tissue, the greater the likelihood the seizure tendency would be abolished.[3] Moreover, initial operation abolished or reduced seizures, which later recurred or increased in frequency in a few patients. After reoperation and the removal of more epileptogenic cortex, one-half of these patients became seizure-free or had a reduced seizure tendency.[3]

Therefore, in patients with drug-refractory focal seizures the current philosophy is to localize the epileptogenic area clinically, by electroencephalogram and ancillary methods. Operation may be considered if this area is deemed resectable. The epileptogenic brain tissue is mapped visually, electroencephalographically, and by stimulation at operation. As much abnormal epileptogenic cortex as possible is then removed, compatible with the least risk of causing or increasing a neurologic deficit.[3]

Criteria for Patient Selection

Seizures are a symptom of brain dysfunction, and therefore other entities, such as metabolic disturbances and brain tumor, must be excluded before it is presumed the patient has a static lesion that requires treatment for the seizure tendency alone. Surgical treatment is then considered, according to the following criteria:

1. The patient must have had an adequate trial of maximally tolerable doses of medications, without a degree of control adequate to lead a fairly normal life, or must be intolerant to medications. The seizures may interfere with psychologic and intellectual development, preclude employment, or be sufficiently severe to pose a threat of mental deterioration to warrant surgical consideration. Surgery is considered only when all potentially epileptogenic areas have matured, the seizure tendency is stable, and furthermore, there is no tendency toward spontaneous regression, especially in post-traumatic epilepsy.[11,12] Operation is rarely advisable until recurrent seizures have been present for 3 to 4 years and the patient is at least 15 to 16 years old. However, with newer anesthetic techniques more patients are now being operated in late childhood and their early teens.
2. Clinical and electroencephalographic studies should show that attacks are focal in origin and arise from a dispensible portion of brain. The more consistent the attack pattern, the better the chances that surgical extirpation will succeed. The patient must be strongly motivated to cope with an exhaustive diagnostic regimen and a lengthy operative procedure under local anesthesia.[13,14]

Investigation

Clinical

A careful history, especially regarding evidence of birth trauma, seizures early in life, and other potential causes of epilepsy, is necessary. Whether other family members have epilepsy should be known. Handedness should be ascertained. Questioning as to what the patient feels at the beginning of attacks and what observers see may indicate the area of lowest seizure threshold. Phenomena such as transient dysphasia or postictal paresis are of considerable lateralizing value.

The neurologic examination, including visual fields, may be normal in temporal lobe epilepsy or show minimal to marked deficits, especially when other lobes are involved.[14]

Radiologic

Stereoscopic plain x-ray films of the skull may show smallness or asymmetry of one side, indicating brain atrophy from early life. Pneumoencephalography is the most useful method of evaluating subtle atrophic brain changes. Angiography is done if the previous studies are normal or a vascular malformation is suspected. The computed tomogram may show a brain tumor or area of atrophy not demonstrated on previous studies.[14]

Electroencephalographic

The electroencephalogram gives the most useful information as to the location and size of the epileptogenic area.[13] An interictal epileptiform abnormality repeated on several occasions may be significant. Recordings with pharyngeal or sphenoidal electrodes are useful in temporal lobe epilepsy.[15]

Activation procedures, such as medication withdrawal, hyperventilation, or drug-induced sleep may enhance abnormalities or even provoke a seizure, the recording of which may elucidate the focus if there is not too much muscle artifact. Intravenous methohexital may enhance the epileptiform abnormality in temporal lobe epilepsy, while intravenous pentylenetetrazol may provoke the patient's habitual seizures.[15]

The intravenous injection of thiopental (technique of Lombrosa and Erba) may permit the differentiation of primary (corticoreticular) and secondary bilaterally synchronous epileptiform abnormalities due to a unilateral lesion.[16] The intracarotid injection of amobarbital and pentylenetetrazol may lateralize the unilateral lesion. In patients with bitemporal foci, stereotactic depth-electrode studies may identify the most active side, when conventional recordings have failed.[15]

Telemetric recordings allow the patient freedom of movement while undergoing prolonged recording to increase the likelihood of seeing interictal epileptiform activity or to document an attack. Computer assistance may increase the effectiveness of recording, using telemetry or chronic implanted depth electrodes, by reducing the recording time of ictal events.[15]

Neuropsychologic

Such tests help to confirm the location of the focus, since they usually corroborate clinical and electroencephalographic evidence by elaborating deficits, which vary with the lobe involved and the dominance of the hemisphere. Any discrepancy between psychologic and clinical localization may indicate unusual lateralization of speech or bilateral temporal lobe lesions.[17] The intracarotid Amytal speech test[18] is done preoperatively when lateralization of speech is uncertain, as in left-handers, ambidextrous persons, and right-handers who have had left hemisphere injury in infancy.[13,17] Preoperative lateralization of speech areas adds to the safety of the cortical resection, since electrical stimulation at the time of surgery may give a false-negative response.

Memory testing is also done during the carotid Amytal speech tests. This is especially important in temporal lobe epilepsy when there is independent epileptiform activity or evidence of injury on the side opposite that of the proposed removal. This test identifies the patient in whom surgery carries a risk to memory dysfunction, since one hippocampus can only be removed when the other is functional.[13,17,19]

Preoperative Preparation

When operation is indicated and the patient accepts, it is desirable to have the epileptogenic cortex as active as possible during surgery. Thus, whenever possible, doses of most antiseizure medications are gradually reduced the week prior to surgery. In patients who have many attacks, an effective, but short-lasting anticonvulsant may be continued until the evening before operation, or the patient stops all oral intake. Glucocorticoids are begun 24 hours preoperatively. Should an attack occur preoperatively, phenobarbital (Luminal sodium, 240 mg) may be given by injection, intramuscularly, or paraldehyde 10 ml, orally or 20 ml rectally.[20]

Anesthesia

Whenever possible, local anesthesia, potentiated by analgesic drugs, is used so that motor, speech, and sensory areas can be mapped readily during surgery, a better electrocorticogram can be obtained, and occasionally, auras can be reproduced by stimulation. Under such conditions, motor and speech functions can be periodically tested to assure maximum safety during the removals.[10,13,21]

Atropine (0.4 mg) is given preoperatively. Uncooperative adults and children may require an endotrachial tube and general anesthesia consisting of nitrous oxide, intravenous sodium methohexital (Brietal), fentanyl, and a curariform agent.[22] The nitrous oxide is discontinued before the electrocorticogram, since it obliterates epileptiform activity.[20]

Nupercaine (dibucaine hydrochloride) has proved to be an excellent local anesthesia agent but is no longer available. Lidocaine (Xylocaine) is suggested as a substitute.[22] Unless there is a medical contraindication, 0.5 ml of 1:1000 epinephrine is added per 125 ml of local anesthetic solution.[20] Xylocaine, 125 ml of a 1% solution, is injected into the superficial skin, using a 25-gauge needle, along the area of proposed incision, with maximum saturation in the supraorbital, temporal, and occipital regions (Fig. 9-1). Then 125 ml of 0.5% Xylocaine is injected down to the periosteum and in the temporalis fascia and muscle, using a 20-gauge needle.[22]

This local anesthesia, fortified by intravenous fentanyl and droperidol, is effective throughout the opening. Other intracranial structures are insensitive to pain, except the dura along the larger meningeal vessels. Here local anesthetic can be injected intradurally, using a 27-gauge needle.[10] The patient is usually alert and comfortable throughout the procedure, with additional intravenous injections of fentanyl and droperidol as required. If drowsiness ensues, the patient must be roused to check motor and speech functions during cortical resection. Brietal is given intravenously should a seizure develop at any time.[22] A general anesthetic may become necessary if the patient becomes unruly, especially after a seizure. A blind transnasal intubation may then be required,[10] and followed by nitrous oxide administration and intravenous fentanyl and droperidol for balanced anesthesia.[22]

Special Aspects of Surgical Technique

Surgical techniques for cortical resection are described in detail elsewhere.[7,8,10,20,21,23-25]

Positioning

The patient is postured comfortably on the side, with a Stryker pillow under the hip and pads protecting other boney prominences. The face is slightly inclined toward the side of the incision. The head of the table is somewhat elevated to reduce venous oozing (Fig.9-2). The

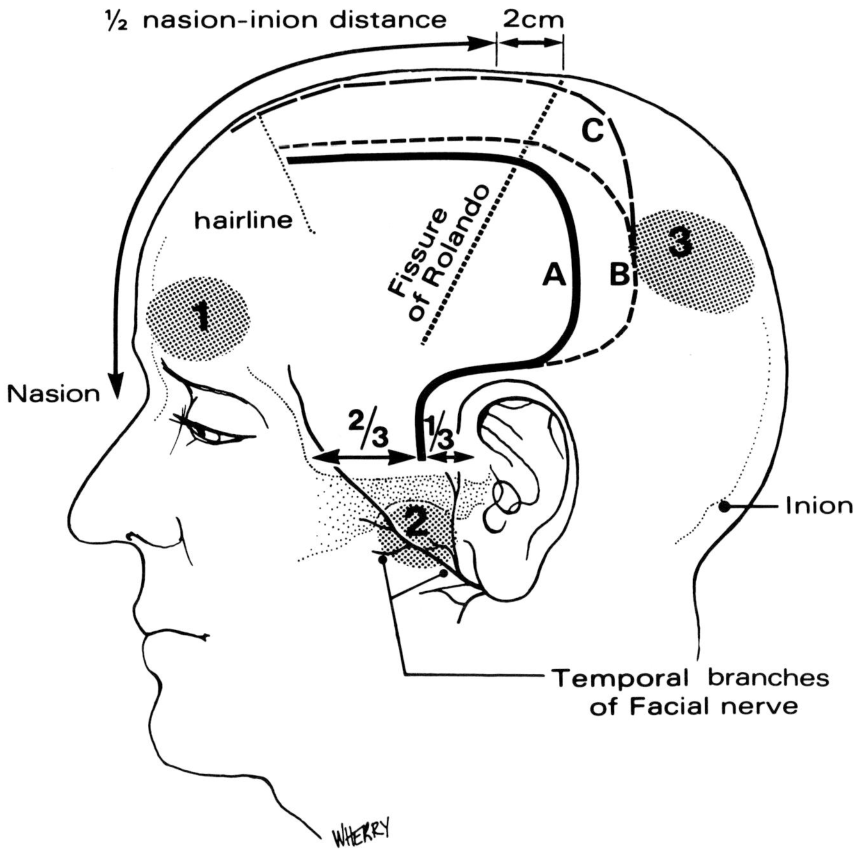

Fig. 9-1. Skin incisions for **(A)** dominant, **(B)** nondominant temporal, and **(C)** frontotemporal exposures. 1, 2 and 3 denote points of maximum local anesthetic infiltration for major sensory nerves. Note external landmarks for Rolandic fissure.

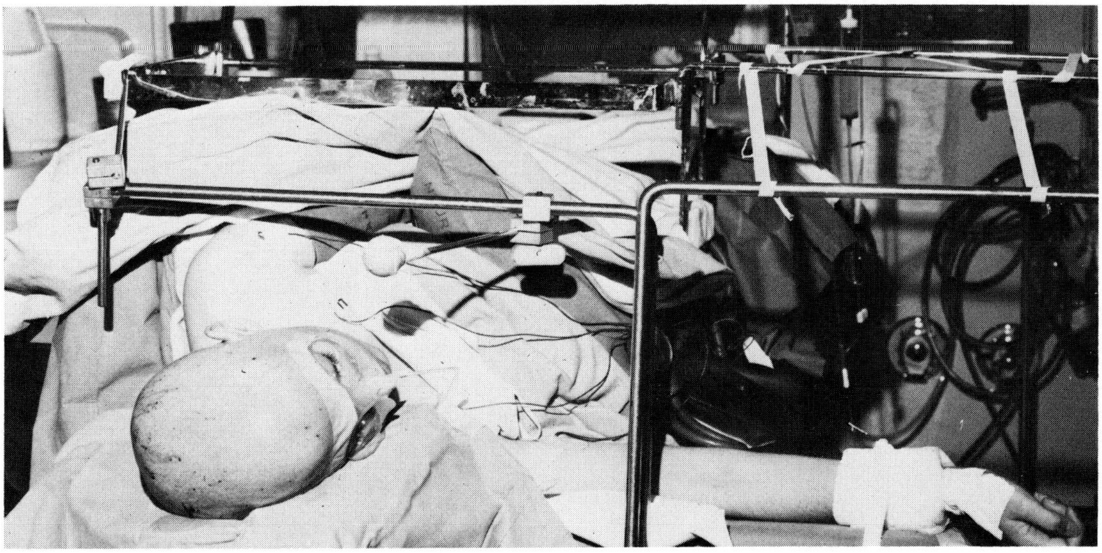

Fig. 9-2. Position for left frontotemporal exposures.

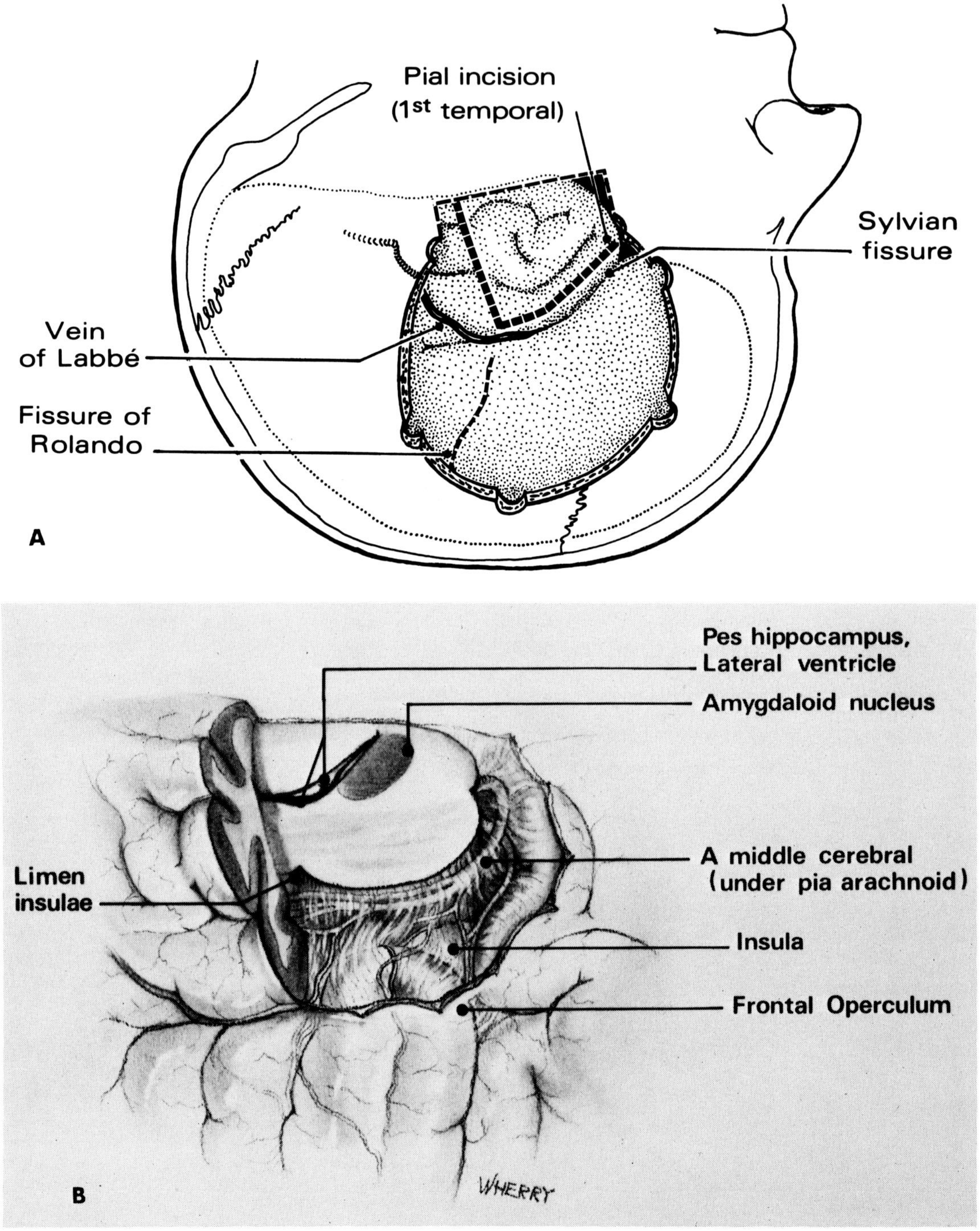
Pial incision
(1st temporal)
Sylvian fissure
Vein of Labbé
Fissure of Rolando
A
Pes hippocampus,
Lateral ventricle
Amygdaloid nucleus
Limen insulae
A middle cerebral
(under pia arachnoid)
Insula
Frontal Operculum
B
WHERRY

Fig. 9-3.

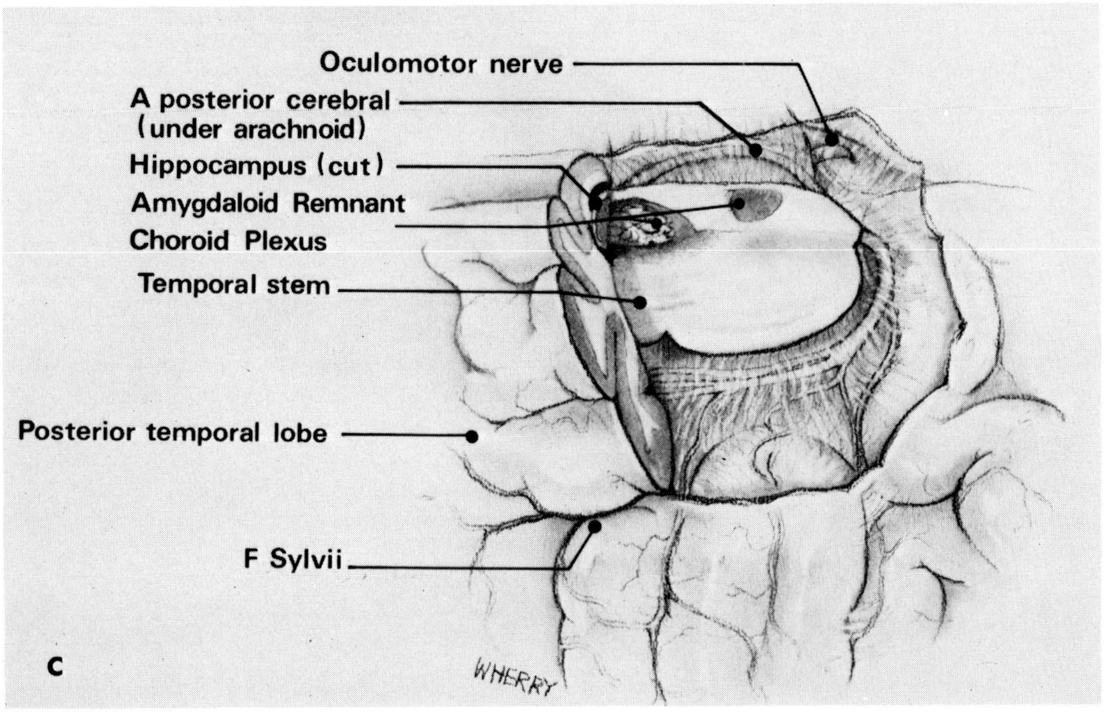

Fig. 9-3. Dominant temporal lobectomy, surgeon's view. **A.** Left temporal exposure showing line of proposed cortical resection. **B.** Superficial temporal lobe removed, exposing lateral temporal horn and lateral amygdaloid. **C.** Following removal of pes hippocampus and most of amygdaloid. Note blood vessels and third nerve protected by pia-arachnoid.

skin is sterilized and a plastic sheet (Pliofilm) placed around the line of incision. Towels are sutured into place in the anesthetized skin so they do not become dislodged if the patient moves. The anesthetist always has access to the patient's face.

Incisions

A generous-sized opening is necessary to afford adequate exposure to map the epileptogenic area and to note it's relationship to the central region on either side and the speech areas in the dominant hemisphere. A question-mark incision is the most useful for temporal lobectomy.[9] Adequate incisions for temporal and frontotemporal removals are shown in Figure 9-1. To expose the frontal lobe alone, a C-shaped incision is suggested, with the superior portion at the midline extending up to 2 cm above the frontal sinus,, and the posterolateral limb extending downwards to the level of the zygoma.[20] If the epileptogenic focus is posterior, a C-shaped incision is made with its medial limb in the midline and the lateral limb curved downwards to expose the central region.[20]

The Opening

A detailed description for the most common cortical resection, partial temporal lobectomy, will follow. The principles are easily modified for cortical resection elsewhere.

The question-mark incision is begun at the superior aspect of the zygoma at the junction of its anterior two-thirds and posterior one-third (Fig. 9-1). If the lowest part of the incision is made too anteroinferior, temporal branches of the facial nerve may be damaged, causing a frontalis muscle palsy. The superficial temporal artery is coagulated early. The galea is separated from the temporalis fascia for application of skin clips. The superior portion of the incision is made down through the periosteum. The temporalis muscle and fascia are divided to the periosteum, using electrocautery. With a periosteal elevator, the skin and muscle are reflected forward over a roll of gauze, and muscle *fishooks* are applied for retraction. Burr holes are made, as in Figure 9-3A. It is important to rongeur away the sphenoid between the two burr holes to expose the anterior temporal lobe. Moreover, if a trough is rongeured inferiorly, from each of the two temporal burr holes, access to the inferior temporal region is easier and cosmetic restoration will ultimately be better. A free bone flap provides better exposure and more comfort for the patient than a hinged flap.[20] The edges of the bony opening are waxed. A hole for the electrode post is made along the superior edge of the craniotomy (Fig. 9-7). Dural traction sutures are placed to decrease venous oozing.[7]

The middle meningeal vessels are coagulated and divided. The dura is opened a few millimeters from the bone edge. It is then pulled into a small Penrose drain and reflected anteroinferiorly over the temporalis muscle, along its remaining 2 cm of attachment. The patient raises his head every 2 hours so the anesthetist can massage the downward side to prevent pressure burns.

The Electrocorticogram

Electrocorticography and depth electrode recording have proven very useful to map epileptogenic regions during surgery.[15,23]

A steel post is screwed into the hole at the superior craniotomy edge and a 16-channel electrode holder attached. One montage for both monopolar and bipolar recording is shown in Figure 9-4. Wire electrodes can be substituted for the usual contact electrodes for recording on the undersurface of the temporal lobe, frontal lobe, and medial aspect of the hemisphere. Small lettered tags are placed at any site of electrographic abnormality (Fig. 9-7).

In temporal lobe cases, the inferior eight electrodes are removed and needle, four-step, depth electrodes are inserted, perpendicular to the surface of the second temporal convolution, to a depth of 3.5 cm at distances of 3 and 5 cm from the tip of the temporal lobe (Fig. 9-5A). The deepest contact of the anterior depth electrode records from the amygdaloid nucleus, and the posterior electrode from the pes hippocampus. The superficial contacts record from the surface grey matter. The intermediate two contacts of the anterior depth electrode record from circuminsular cortex, and the middle two contacts of the posterior depth electrode from the grey matter in the depths of Heschl's gyri.[23] The superior eight contact electrodes retain their former position. A further electroencephalographic recording is obtained.

Electrical Stimulation Study

The brain is then electrically stimulated to determine the position of the pre- and post-central gyri. A 2-msec square wave pulse at 60 Hz, starting a 1 and increasing by 0.5-V increments is used until a motor response is seen by the anesthetist, or a sensory change felt by the patient. Positive stimulation points are marked, using numbered tickets (Fig. 9-7). The Rolandic fissure is thus identified. In the dominant hemisphere the speech areas are stimulated while the patient carries out simple verbal tasks.[23] The frontal speech area is indicated by speech arrest, while the posterior temporal area is identified by arrest or a dysphasic reaction during stimulation. A negative stimulation does not always exclude the presence of speech function in the convolution stimulated.[21]

Areas of after-discharge (rhythmic electroencephalographic activity different from the

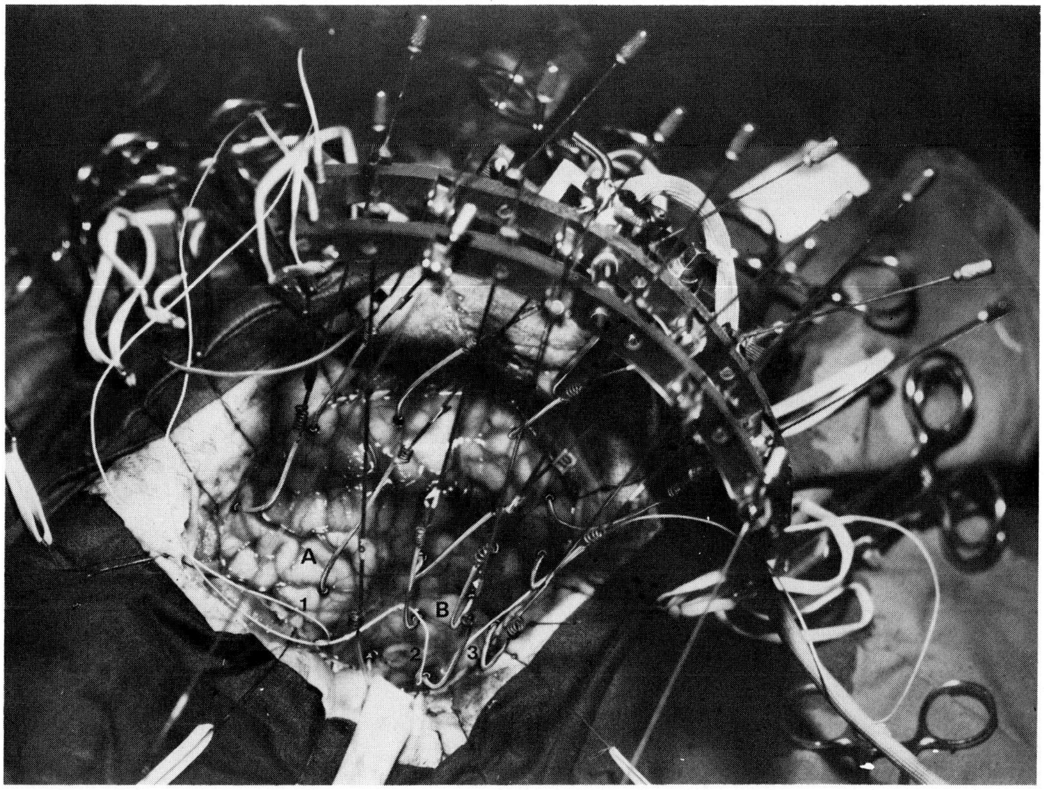

Fig. 9-4. Electrode holder and electrodes over **(A)** left frontal, **(B)** temporal and central regions. Wire electrodes for recording from (1) undersurface of frontal and (2,3) temporal lobe.

prestimulation activity) may develop at the stimulation site or in adjacent regions. These may indicate areas of hyperirritable cortex,[10] although the clinical significance of this has not yet been documented.[23]

Other areas of the exposed cortex and the depth electrodes may then be stimulated, endeavoring to reproduce the patient's aura. A stimulating voltage more than 3 V higher than that required to elicit motor or sensory responses is dangerous. Above such levels, a nonspecific, full-blown seizure may develop, which precludes the patient's cooperation for some time.[23]

Anatomic Considerations—Plan of Removal

The frontal (Broca) and posterior speech areas in the dominant hemisphere, as determined by stimulation studies and ablations around these areas, are shown in Figure 9-6.[26] The speech areas are indispensable and their removal is never justified.[10] The pre- and postcentral face area can be removed if pial barriers are respected so the blood supply to the Rolandic and speech areas is preserved. This results in contralateral facial paresis, which subsequently improves but may leave some mild facial underaction.[25] Removal of the postcentral arm or leg area causes some persistent astereognosis and is rarely indicated unless markedly epileptogenic cortex in this area is causing a severe seizure tendency.[25] Removal of the precentral arm or leg area produces contralateral spastic hemiparesis and is not indicated unless marked preoperative hemiparesis is present.[27]

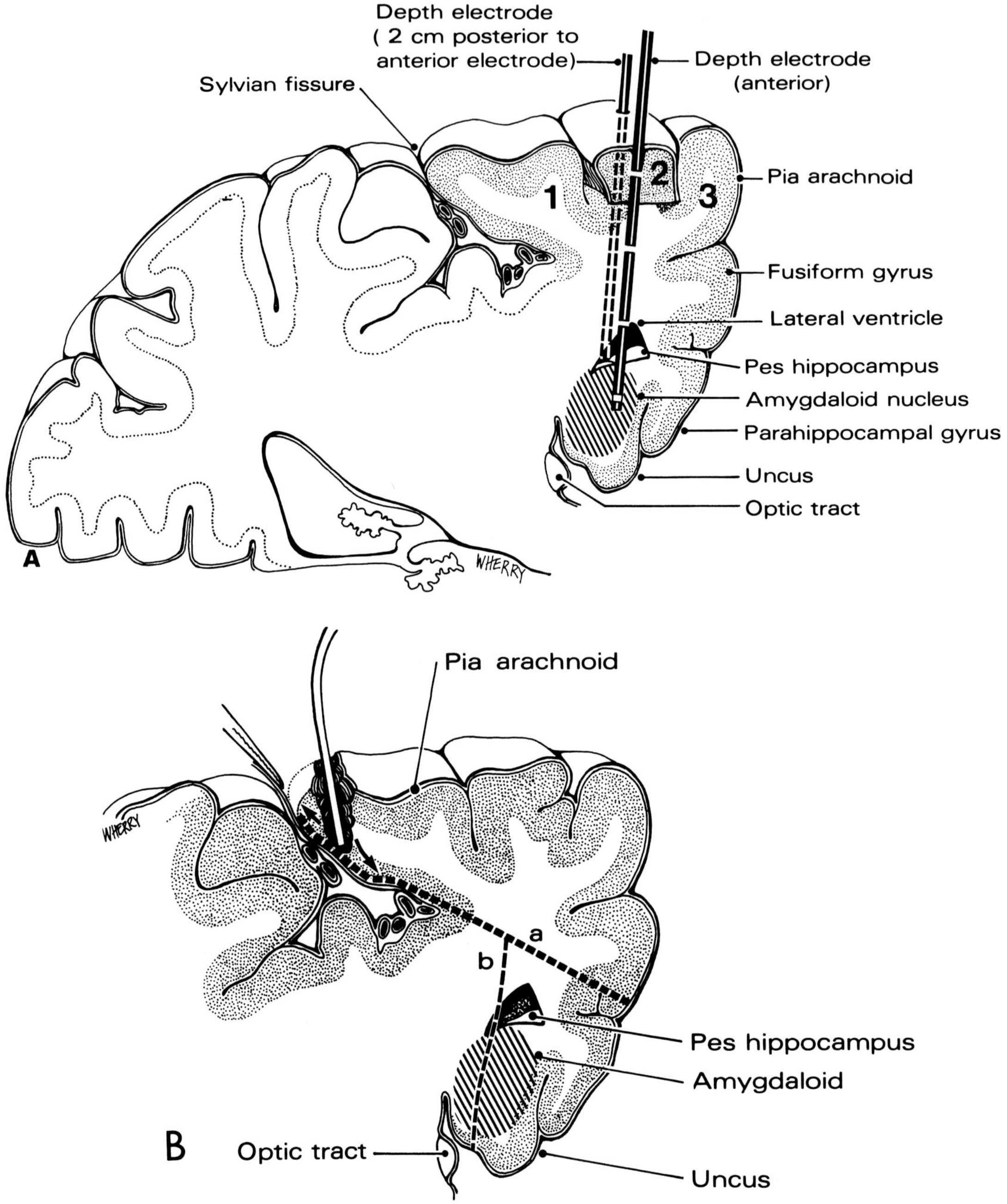

Fig. 9-5. Coronal section of left hemisphere at the tip of the temporal horn. **A.** Depth electrodes in place in amygdaloid (anterior) and hippocampus (posterior). **B.** Subpial dissection in first temporal convolution while retracting pia-arachnoid. (a) Line of superficial temporal resection. (b) Line of removal of medial temporal structures.

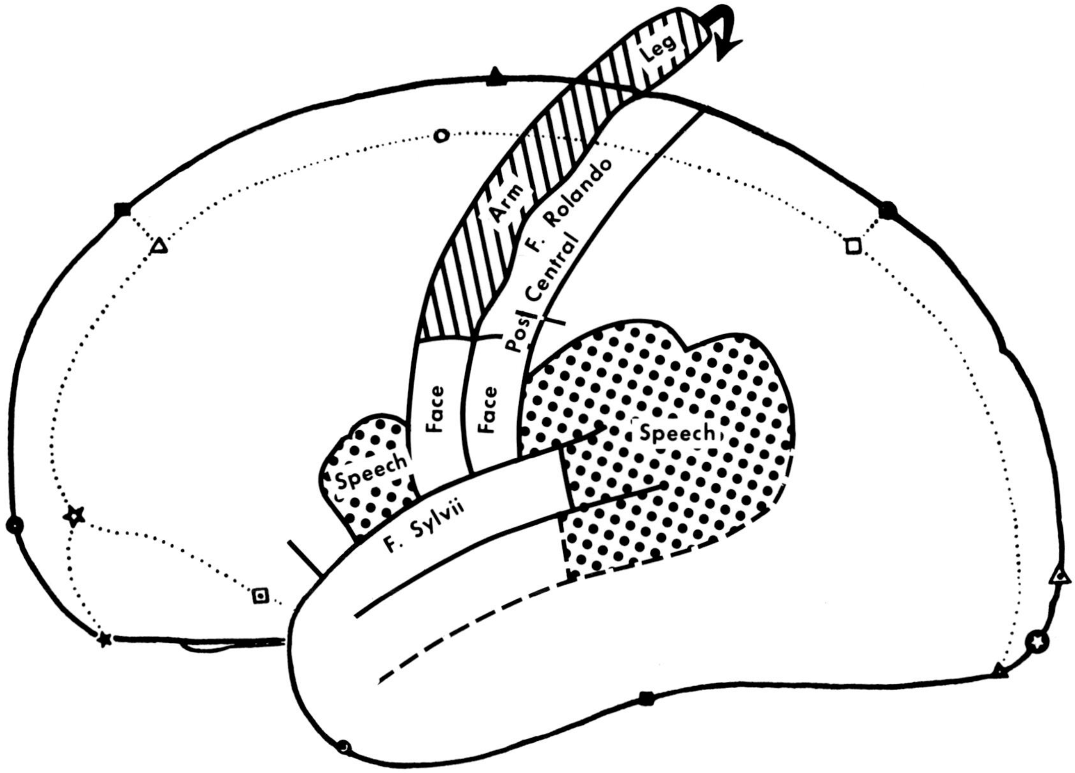

Fig. 9-6. Most common position of pre- and postcentral gyri and speech areas in dominant hemisphere.

Originally it was suggested that the anterior 5 to 6 cm of the dominant temporal lobe could be removed,[21] the resection being carried out along the vein of Labbé[8-10] without producing dysphasia. However, due to variability in the position of this vein and the size of the temporal lobe, the best landmark to use is the junction of the Rolandic and Sylvian fissures. Removal of the dominant first and second temporal convolutions posterior to that point carries the risk of permanent dysphasia.[20]

The parietal speech zone extends superiorly 1 to 4 cm above the Sylvian fissure and from 2 to 4 cm behind the postcentral sulcus. The frontal speech area occupies one or both frontal opercular convolutions anterior to the precentral gyrus.[26]

In the Montreal Neurological Institute series, a number of epileptic patients without evidence of early damage to the left cerebral hemisphere underwent the carotid Amytal speech test. In right-handers 96% had speech in the left hemisphere and 4% in the right hemisphere. In left-handed or ambidextrous individuals 70% had speech on the left, 15% on the right, and 15% had some representation of speech in each hemisphere. Similar studies of speech lateralization in individuals with early left hemisphere damage shows more variability, with larger numbers having speech in the right hemisphere than those without early damage.[26] Thus in epileptic patients, any hemisphere is considered dominant unless the carotid Amytal speech test provides otherwise.

When the speech and precentral regions are avoided, *unilateral* removals of frontal, parietal, and temporal cortex are possible without significant additional deficits. When possible, it is best to leave one gyrus between the cortical removal and indispensable areas of cortex. As much white matter as practicable should be left beneath the cortical removal to reduce any neurologic deficit.

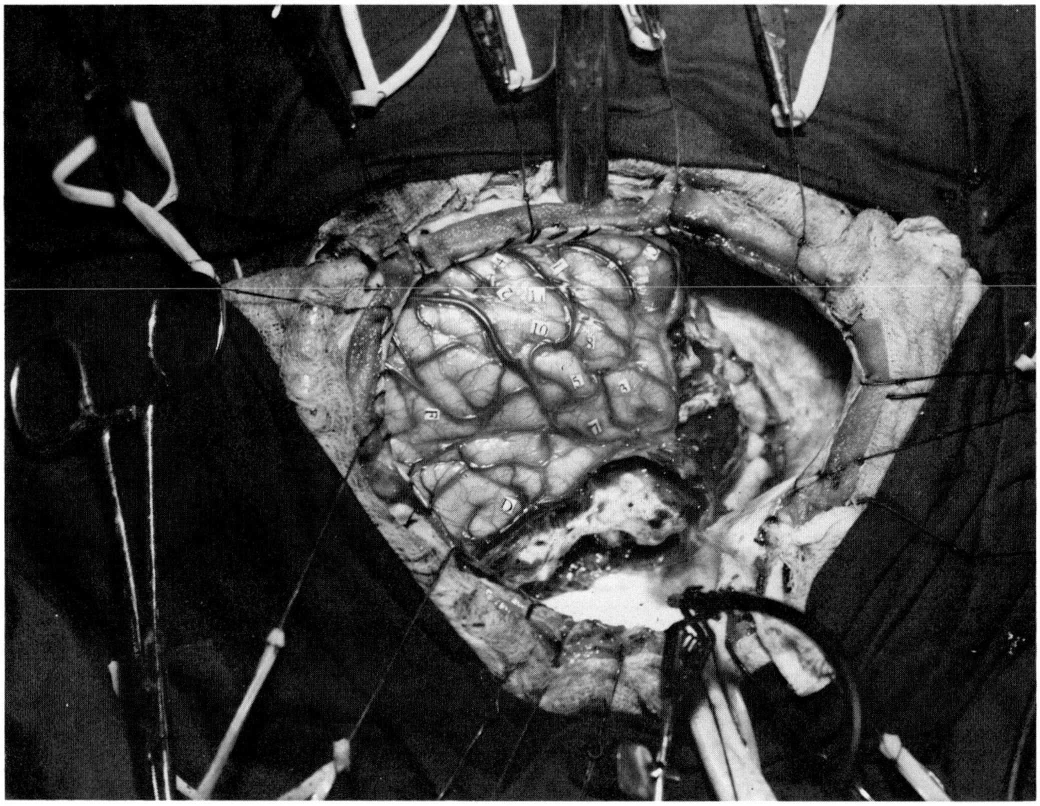

Fig. 9-7. After right frontal and temporal lobectomies with cortical incision following sulci and leaving untraumatized convolutions at removal edge. Note steel post for electrode holder at edge of superior bone margin, and *fishooks* retracting dura.

Following temporal lobectomy, a visual field defect is rarely seen, if resection is limited to the anterior 5 cm of a normal-sized temporal lobe,[8] or not posterior to the intersection of the Rolandic and Sylvian fissures in any temporal lobe.[23] If the temporal horn opening is confined to the anterior 1 cm and white matter lateral to the ventricle is preserved, geniculocalcarine tract damage is minimized and a superior quadrantanopsia may be avoided even in removals 7 to 8 cm posterior to the temporal tip.[23]

Bilateral removal of the temporal lobes is never justified due to the profound memory loss produced.[28]

Cortical Resection

Bearing the above principles in mind, the area of proposed cortical resection is outlined, using a piece of thread. The brain is irrigated at intervals and kept moist, especially during recordings. The thin nonadhesive transparent Pliofilm is placed over cortical areas to be preserved to prevent brain drying and postoperative edema.[10]

In temporal lobectomy, as elsewhere, subpial dissection is stressed. The pia at the summit of the first temporal gyrus is coagulated and incised with a scalpel (Fig. 9-3A). Using a small-bore suction, grey matter is meticulously pulled away from the pia to expose the white matter. The incision line is lengthened anteroposteriorly. The pia-arachnoid is coagulated and divided, using scissors, and the incision deepened by the suction technique. Gradually, sufficient grey matter along this gyrus is removed to expose the pia-arachnoid covering the insula (Fig. 9-5B). The superior grey matter of the first temporal convolution is suctioned away from the pia. Deeper grey matter is suctioned away from the intact pia-arachnoid, as illustrated to expose the insula. Meticulous hemostasis is necessary and brain movement must be avoided. Great care must be taken not to traumatize the middle cerebral vessels situated beneath this protective pia-arachnoid in order to prevent postoperative hemiparesis[7] (Figs. 9-3B and 9-5B). At the posterior margin of the incision, in the first temporal gyrus, the line of incision is carried inferiorly toward the base of the temporal lobe (Fig. 9-3A). Cotton pledgets are placed in the incision, as dissection proceeds distally, and are subsequently removed so that the incision can be deepened using the suction. Only that brain tissue to be removed is retracted away from tissue to be preserved. Larger vesesls are coagulated and divided.

When the insular surface is exposed, the incision is carried through the white matter of the temporal stem medially, at an angle of about 45° to avoid deep structures in the basal temporal lobe (Figs. 9-3B and 9-5B). The posterior end of the incision is then carried forward along the fusiform gyrus and the anterior end of the first temporal gyral incision is carried anteroinferiorly until the two meet on the inferior surface of the temporal lobe. The superficial temporal lobe is lifted out, leaving white matter overlying the lateral ventricle and amygdala (Fig. 9-5B). When extremely gliotic brain is encountered, scissors may be used to incise the brain tissue.

The white matter of the anterior temporal lobe inferior to the insula is removed by suction until the ventricle is entered. The pes hippocampus can then be visualized and the amygdala is evident (Fig. 9-3B). All but the medial rim of the amygdaloid nucleus and most of the uncus are removed. The remaining portion protects the subjacent optic tract (Fig. 9-5B).[23]

If preoperative studies and depth-electrode recordings indicate hippocampal involvement and the opposite hippocampus is functional, the pes hippocampus is then removed together with the anterior parahippocampal gyrus (Fig. 9-5B).[23] Great care must be exercised to preserve the pia-arachnoid, separating these structures from the third nerve, posterior cerebral artery, and cerebral peduncle (Fig. 9-3C). Heschl's convolution on the dominant side are not removed, unless necessary, since this increases the risk of decreasing the blood supply to the posterior speech area.

Postremoval Recording

Wire electrodes are placed on the undersurface of the posterior temporal lobe and orbital surface of the frontal lobe. Cortical electrodes are put on the temporal convexity, insula, amygdaloid, and hippocampal remnants. The remaining cortical electrodes are placed on the dorsolateral convexity of the hemisphere above the Sylvian fissure. Persistent spiking from the hippocampus or posterior temporal lobe may require further excision, if no severe neurologic deficit will be produced. In the nondominant hemisphere, excisions are sometimes carried out to 8 cm posterior to the temporal tip. Epileptiform abnormality, recorded from the insular surface, is ignored, since further removal of cortex from that structure does not increase the success rate.[29,30] When spikes or sharp waves persist in dispensable cortex above the Sylvian fissure, the subpial removal of these convolutions is carried out one by one. Preservation of the pial *barrier* protects the adjacent gyri and sulcal blood vessels supplying those gyri and other portions of the brain.[7] Several such additional excisions may be made before a clear electroencephalographic tracing is obtained, or an effort to achieve this is abandoned.[20]

Closure

A Penrose drain is left beneath the bone flap. Gelfoam is placed over the dural closure. The bone flap is wired into position and burr hole covers installed. After the galea and skin have been approximated, a wet Sulfadiazine-soaked gauze is placed over the incision. Pliofilm is placed over this and a full, head dressing used, covering the ear on the side of temporal lobectomy. The drain is removed on the first postoperative day.

Postoperative Care

An intravenous solution of glucose and saline, containing 250 mg diphenylhydantoin, 240 mg phenobarbital, and 100 mg hydrocortisone per 100 ml, is given until oral intake begins. Fluids are restricted to 1500 ml daily for the first 5 postoperative days to decrease edema. Dexamethasone (6 mg every 6 hours) is given the first 5 days and the dose then tapered over the next 7. Ambulation begins the third or fourth day. The sutures are removed on the fifth day.

Unless another medication has proven superior, diphenylhydantoin (100 mg, three times daily) and phenobarbital (60 mg, twice daily) are given the first postoperative year.[20] If the patient is then seizure-free, with a nonepileptiform electroencephalogram, the medications are gradually reduced at 6- to 12-month intervals. Should seizures recur, the original anticonvulsant doses are restarted and reduced only after 2 seizure-free years.[20]

Complications

An aseptic meningitis, accompanied by fever up to 40°C, probably due to breakdown products of blood in the subarachnoid space, may follow large cortical resections.[31] This syndrome clears spontaneously over a 10- to 20-day period.[20]

Cerebral edema after long procedures may cause transient cortical dysfunction and seizures during the first 7 to 10 days.[10] Such *neighborhood* seizures usually originate from cortex adjacent to the removal and have no bearing on the ultimate prognosis.[20] These complications are reduced by the cortisone regime.[32]

An increasing, marked, superior quadrantanopsia occurs when the temporal lobe resection is carried progressively further behind the Rolandic-Sylvian junction,[13] or if care is not taken to preserve white matter lateral to the temporal horn.[23] When the occipital lobe has been removed, complete contralateral homonymous hemianopsia has resulted.[25] The memory loss that may occur when the remaining functional hippocampus is removed[33] has been avoided since 1958 by preoperative bilateral administration of the Amytal speech and memory test, when indicated.[23] Of the 250 dominant, partial, temporal lobectomies done from 1958 to 1975, only 2 patients had mild persistent dysphasia.[23] Mild deficits in verbal fluency may increase after dominant temporal lobectomy,[17,33] but later, verbal fluency often improves compared with preoperative levels, if seizures are reduced.[17] Transient dysphasia may follow cortical removal from the dominant hemisphere.[24,26]

In an earlier series of dominant temporal lobectomies, especially with cortical resections above or medial to the Sylvian fissure, a contralateral hemiplegia, homonymous hemianopsia, and dysphasia were sometimes noted. These were felt to be due to manipulation of the middle cerebral arteries over the insula. They can be prevented by preserving the pia-arachnoid over these vessels, avoiding arterial traction, and leaving insular cortex despite electrographic spiking.[7] Such manipulative hemiplegia has been avoided in temporal lobectomy, since 1958. Cortical removals above the Sylvian fissure have an incidence of hemiparesis or dysphasia of 0.5%, unless the sensorimotor cortex is involved, in which case the risk becomes greater.[20]

Of the total 1,497 operations for nontumoral lesions, from 1928 through 1974, the operative mortality was 1%. From 1957 through 1975, in 820 consecutive operations there were 2 postoperative deaths, ie., 0.2%. In 700 temporal lobe operations, from 1950 through 1973, there was no postoperative death.[20]

Results and Discussion of Experience

Histopathologic examination of specimens from 506 consecutive cases operated at the Montreal Neurological Institute, from 1961 through 1970, showed varying etiologies for focal epilepsy. One-third had discrete lesions, a further third had essentially normal findings, while the rest had extensive lesions, such as cortical atrophy, hippocampal sclerosis, and chronic encephalitis.[34]

Cortical resection for nontumoral epilepsy was performed in 1,267 patients from 1928 through 1971, with a median followup of 10 years in 1,145 patients (Table 9-1). The seizure tendency was abolished in 36%, while in another 28% seizures were substantially, although not completely reduced. Variable results were obtained in the remaining 36%, with some experiencing a 90% reduction in seizures and a few essentially unchanged.[20]

In the temporal lobe series (653 patients) seizures were completely or almost completely reduced in 71%; in the frontal group (212 patients), in 55%; in the parietal group (80 patients), in 59%; in the central (sensorimotor) group (63 patients), in 57%; in the occipital lobe group (19 patients), in 68%; and in the group undergoing total or subtotal hemispherectomy for large destructive lesions (77 patients), in 50%.[20,23-25]

To 1971 repeat operations were performed on 129 patients who had inadequate seizure reduction. After additional epileptogenic cortex was removed, 25% became seizure-free and 29% had a reduced seizure tendency.[3]

Tumors and arteriovenous malformations, the prime symptom of which was epilepsy rather than increasing neurologic deficit or increased intracranial pressure, were removed in an additional 347 patients. When the causative lesion and surrounding epileptogenic cortex were removed as completely as possible, the reduction in seizure tendency compared favorably with the nontumor group, until neoplasia recurred.[35]

Thus the efficiency of seizure reduction correlates with the completeness with which the causative lesion and epileptogenic cortex are removed, rather than with the nature of the lesion or the length of time the patient had seizures.[3] About one-fourth of the patients had some postoperative seizures during the first 2 years, but these subsequently ceased. Medica-

Table 9-1. Results of Cortical Excision for Focal Epilepsy in Patients with Nontumoral Lesions Operated on During the Years 1928 Through 1971

	Patients			
			Totals	
Results	No.	(%)	No.	%
Seizuure free since discharge	237	21		
Became seizure free after some early attacks	179	15	416	36
Free of seizures 3 or more years then rare or occasional attacks	122	11		
Marked reduction in seizure tendency	198	28	320	28
Moderated or less reduction in seizure tendency			409	36
Total patients with follow-up data of 2 to 41 years: median 10 years			1145	
Inadequate follow-up data	85			
Deaths in 2 years	22			
Postoperative deaths	115			
Total patients	1267			

Data compiled from Rasmussen.[35]

tions were stopped after 2 years in about one-half of the patients. A further one-fifth are controlled with medication, whereas, this was not possible preoperatively. In addition to the decrease in seizure tendency, there may be psychologic improvement, in that the patient can often hold a responsible job.[36]

In one center the temporal lobe, including hippocampal and amygdaloid regions, is removed en bloc for optimal histologic study, but the removal is then somewhat more complex than in the stages above.[9] Moreover, the contribution of the first temporal convolution to a seizure tendency has been questioned.[1,9] In the present series the best results have been obtained when as much abnormal cortex as possible is removed in addition to the hippocampus and amygdala, when feasible.[36]

Although cortical resection, as applied above, is highly successful and safe, its application is limited to about 10% of epileptics, where a focus exists in a resectable area of cortex.[2] Failures in operated cases are attributable mainly to involvement, by epileptogenic tissue, of subcortical structures, nondispensable areas of cortex, or a significant focus in the opposite hemisphere, particularly the temporal lobe.[3]

Stereotactic ablative procedures may someday solve the problem of dealing surgically with generalized, bilateral, or multifocal seizure disorders. To date, targets and methods are not standardized and usually these techniques have been reserved for especially intractable and complicated seizure problems.[37] Similarly, the results of commissurotomy, cerebral cooling, and cerebellar stimulation await longer followup.[37] The latter two procedures are of particular interest in that there is no ablation.

Although current medical management, using anticonvulsants and controlled drug levels, has been extremely effective, such medications may have toxic effects or may fail to control the seizures. In such instances a place remains for cortical resection in selected epileptic patients, until an ideal medication has been developed.

Acknowledgment

I wish to thank my preceptor and colleague, Dr. Theodore Rasmussen for his helpful advice and for the use of his detailed records.

REFERENCES

1. Walker AE: Critique and perspective: neurosurgical management of the epilepsies, *Advances in Neurology,* vol 8. Edited by DP Purpura, JK Penry, RD Walter. Raven Press, New York, 1975, pp 333-349
2. Robb P: Focal epilepsy: the problem, prevalence, and contributing factors, *Advances in Neurology,* vol 8. Edited by DP Purpura, JK Penry, RD Walter. Raven Press, New York, 1975, pp 11-12
3. Rasmussen TB: Surgical treatment of epilepsy: the clinical neurosciences, *The Nervous System,* vol 2. Edited by DB Tower. Raven Press, New York, 1975, pp 277-286
4. Penfield W, Jasper H: Historical introduction, *Epilepsy and the Functional Anatomy of the Human Brain.* Little, Brown, and Company, Boston, 1954, pp 3-20
5. Foerster O, Penfield W: Structural basis of traumatic epilepsy and result of radical operation. *Brain 53*:99-120, 1930
6. Penfield W, Jasper H: *Epilepsy and the Functional Anatomy of the Human Brain.* Little, Brown and Company, Boston, 1954
7. Penfield W, Lende RA, Rasmussen TB: Manipulation hemiplegia, an untoward complication in the surgery of focal epilepsy. *J Neurosurg 18*:760-776, 1961
8. Penfield W, Baldwin M: Temporal lobe seizures and technique of subtotal temporal lobectomy. *Ann Surg 136*:625-634, 1952
9. Falconer MA, Hill D, Meyer A, et al: Treatment of temporal lobe epilepsy by temporal lobectomy: Survey of findings and results, *Lancet 1*:827-835, 1955
10. Penfield W, Jasper H: Surgical Therapy. *Epilepsy and the Functional Anatomy of the Human Brain.* Little, Brown and Company, Boston, 1954, pp 739-817

11. Caveness WF: Onset and cessation of fits following cranio-cerebral trauma. *J Neurosurg 20*:570-583, 1963
12. Walker AE, Erculei F: Post-traumatic epilepsy 15 years later. *Epilepsia 11*:17-26, 1970
13. Rasmussen TB: The role of surgery in the treatment of focal epilepsy. *Clin Neurosurg 16*:288-314, 1969
14. McNaughton FL, Rasmussen TB: Criteria for selection of patients for neurosurgical treatment: Neurosurgical management of the epilepsies. *Advances in Neurology,* vol 8. Edited by DP Purpura, JK Penry, RD Walter. Raven Press, New York, 1975, pp 37-48
15. Gloor P: Contributions of electroencephalography and electrocorticography to the neurosurgical treatment of the epilepsies. *Advances in Neurology,* vol 8. Edited by DP Purpura, JK Penry, RD Walter. Raven Press, New York, 1975, pp 59-105
16. Lombroso CT, Erba G: Primary and secondary bilateral synchrony in epilepsy. A clinical and electroencephalographic study. *Arch Neurol 22*:321-334, 1970
17. Milner B: Psychological aspects of focal epilepsy and its neurosurgical management: Neurosurgical management of the epilepsies. *Advances in Neurology*, vol 8. Edited by DT Purpura, JK Penry, RD Walter. Raven Press, New York, 1975, pp 29-321
18. Wada J, Rasmussen TB: Intracarotid injection of sodium amytal for the lateralization of speech dominance. Experimental and clinical observations. *J Neurosurg 17*:266-282, 1960
19. Milner B, Branch C, Rasmussen TB: Study of short-term memory after intracarotid injection of Sodium Amytal. *Trans Am Neurol Assoc 87*:224-226, 1962
20. Rasmussen TB: Cortical resection in the treatment of focal epilepsy: neurosurgical management of the epilepsies, *Advances in Neurology*, vol 8. Edited by DP Purpura, JK Penry, RD Walter. Raven Press, New York, 1975, pp 139-154
21. Rasmussen TB, Jasper H: Temporal lobe epilepsy: indication for operation and surgical technique, *Temporal Lobe Epilepsy.* Edited by M Baldwin, P Bailey. Charles C Thomas, Springfield Illinois, 1958, pp 440-460
22. Trop D: Personal communication
23. Rasmussen TB: Surgical treatment of patients with complex partial seizures, *Advances in Neurology*, vol 11. Edited by JK Penry, DD Daly. Raven Press, New York, 1975, pp 415-449
24. Rasmussen TB: Surgery of frontal lobe epilepsy: neurosurgical management of the epilepsies, *Advances in Neurology*, vol 8. Edited by DP Purpura, JK Penry, RD Walter. Raven Press, New York, 1975, pp 197-205
25. Rasmussen TB: Surgery for epilepsy arising in regions other than the temporal and frontal lobes, *Advances in Neurology,* vol 8. Edited by DP Purpura, JK Penry, RD Walter. Raven Press, New York, 1975, pp 207-226.
26. Rasmussen TB, Milner B: Clinical and surgical studies of the cerebral speech areas in man, *Cerebral Localization.* Edited by KJ Zulch, O Creutzfeldt, GC Galbraith. Springer-Verlag, New York, 1975, pp 238-257
27. Penfield W, Rasmussen TB: Excision of cortical regions, *The Cerebral Cortex of Man.* Macmillan, New York, 1950, pp 183-201
28. Scoville WB, Milner B: Loss of recent memory after bilateral hippocampal lesions. J Neurol Neurosurg Psychiatr 20:11-21, 1957
29. Ajmone-Marsan C, Baldwin M. Electrocorticography. *Temporal Lobe Epilepsy.* Edited by M Baldwin, P Bailey. Charles C Thomas, Springfield Illinois, 1958, pp 368-395
30. Silfvenius H, Gloor P, Rasmussen TB: Evaluation of insular ablation in surgical treatment of temporal lobe epilepsy. *Epilepsia 5*:307-320, 1964
31. Jackson IJ: Aseptic hemogenic meningitis. *Arch Neurol Psychiatr 62*:572-589, 1949
32. Rasmussen TB, Gulati DR: Cortisone in the treatment of a postoperative cerebral edema. *J Neurosurg 19*:535-544, 1962
33. Milner B: The memory deficit in bilateral hippocampal lesions. *Psychiatr Res Publ 11*:43-58, 1959
34. Mathieson G: Pathologic aspects of epilepsy with special reference to the surgical pathology of focal cerebral seizures: neurosurgical management of the epilepsies, *Advances in Neurology*, vol 8. Edited by DP Purpura, JK Penry, RD Walter. Raven Press, New York, 1975, pp 107-138
35. Rasmussen TB: Surgery of epilepsy associated with brain tumors, *Advances in Neurology,* vol 8. Edited by DP Purpura, JK Penry, RD Walter. Raven Press, New York, 1975, pp 227-239
36. Feindel W: Factors contributing to the success, or failure of surgical intervention for epilepsy, *Advances in Neurology,* vol 8. Edited by DP Purpura, JK Penry, RD Walter. Raven Press, New York, 1975, pp 281-298
37. Ojemann GA, Ward AA, Jr.: Stereotactic and other procedures for epilepsy, *Advances in Neurology*, vol 8. Edited by DP Purpura, JK Penry, RD Walter. Raven Press, New York, 1975, pp 241-263

CHAPTER 10

Surgery of the Peripheral Nerves and Brachial Plexus

Robert D. Leffert

"I would like to see the day when somebody would be appointed surgeon somewhere who has no hands, for the operative part is the least part of the work." Harvey Cushing
November, 1911[1]

ACCOMPLISHMENTS IN PERIPHERAL NERVE SURGERY in the 65 years since this was written are undeniable proof that it cannot be accepted verbatim. However, it is immediately apparent to anyone with more than trivial clinical experience that reestablishment of axonal continuity with the end organ, although of major importance to functional recovery, cannot guarantee it. Restoration of function of the paralytic or sense-deficient part depends on a variety of operative and nonoperative techniques involving such nonneural tissue as skin, muscle, bone, and joint. To achieve optimal functional results from the nerve operation, a surgeon must be familiar with these as well as their indications and timing so that alternatives can be evaluated and proper decisions made. Above all, these must be relevant to the patient and his particular needs.

The focus of this symposium is on current neurosurgical operative techniques, so these will be described in detail and context. Since a thorough and all-inclusive discourse on the subject is impossible in the space available, the reader may avail himself of an extensive array of pertinent literature, including several major texts and monographs devoted to the subject.[2-5] The advances since Cushing's day have come largely from the carefully documented clinical experience of two World Wars[3,6] (and several lesser ones) as well as laboratory research. Technologic improvements in optics and suture material have made microsurgery possible. Without it, the current state of the art would be severely lacking.[7,8]

Many of the peripheral nerve techniques are identically applicable to the brachial plexus, but the specialized nature of this area makes certain individual considerations of diagnosis and treatment necessary. These will be described later.

Before proceeding further, a brief comment should be made on some anatomic, physiologic, and pathologic features of the peripheral nervous system that define it from the central nervous system. The unique potential, under optimal circumstances, for regeneration in the periphery makes successful surgical manipulation possible. However, this phenomenon primarily depends upon survival of the cell body, without which new axoplasm cannot be

Department of Orthopaedic Surgery and the Department of Rehabilitation Medicine, Massachusetts General Hospital and the Harvard Medical School, Boston, Massachusetts 02114

synthesized. Then if the supporting stroma of the injured nerve is in continuity, or if alignment of the severed distal segment can be restored and scar does not unduly obstruct the juncture, regeneration can take place. The metabolic background within which this occurs is complex and only partly understood.[9] In addition to the interdependence of the cell body and axon, the complex structure of the peripheral nerve itself contributes to the difficulty of repair. Although the axon is the conducting medium for the nerve impulse, the supporting fibrous elements and myelin sheathing are of great importance, both under normal and pathologic conditions (Fig. 10-1).

Unfortunately, the simplistic comparison of peripheral nerve with telephone cable has led to many illogical and unsuccessful attempts at surgical repair of damaged nerves. The monumental work of Sunderland[5] in demonstrating the intraneural topography of major peripheral nerves has provided an anatomic substrate within which the surgeon may work (Fig. 10-2).

The constantly changing pattern of groups of fibers within a nerve, as it traverses the limb, helps to explain why long gaps due to injury, even if they can be overcome, often lead to poor operative results. Since the pattern does not remain constant for more than 1.5 cm, this imposes a limit on just how many potential axon-bearing sheaths may be reunited following a lengthy resection.

Furthermore, even though peripheral nerves are abundantly supplied with blood vessels at all structural levels (Fig. 10-3) and these are arranged both segmentally and longitudinally, it cannot be assumed that extensive mobilization will not have an adverse effect on their nutrition, or that destruction or ligation of adjacent vessels will not prejudice the ultimate result.

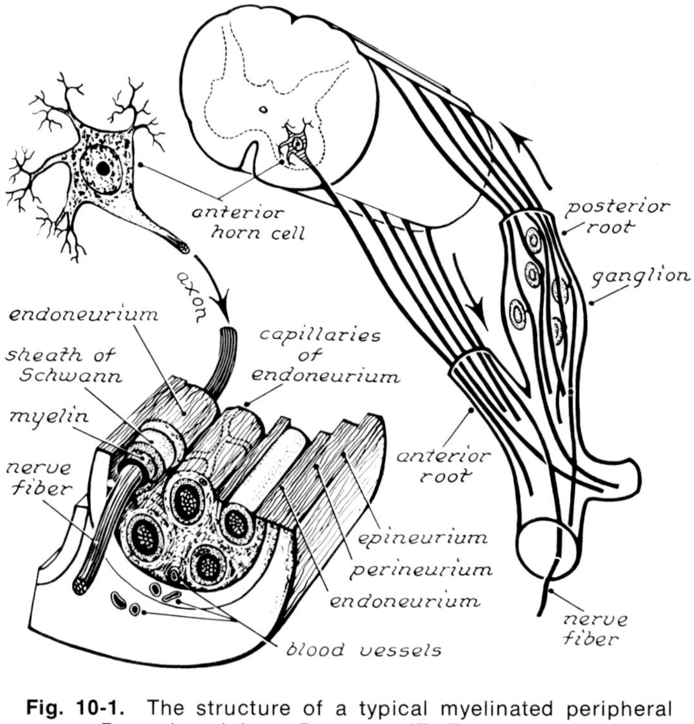

Fig. 10-1. The structure of a typical myelinated peripheral nerve. Reproduced from Bateman JE: *Trauma to Nerves in Limbs* with the permission of the author and publisher.

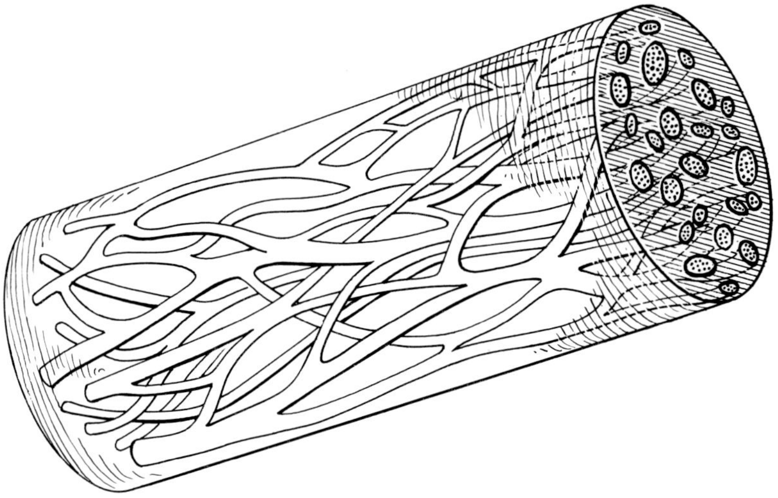

Fig. 10-2. The intraneural topography of a peripheral nerve, adapted from Sunderland.

There are two specific situations wherein the presence of an intraneural artery may prove troublesome. Both the sciatic nerve and the median nerve have well-developed and relatively constant arteries. In the sciatic, a laceration of the intraneural artery that leaves the bulk of the nerve intact can cause catastrophic pressure necrosis of the surrounding fascicles, if it is not promptly relieved. A suture of the median nerve under tourniquet ischemia may rupture once arterial flow is reestablished, if the artery is not microcoagulated and the epineural closure is tight.

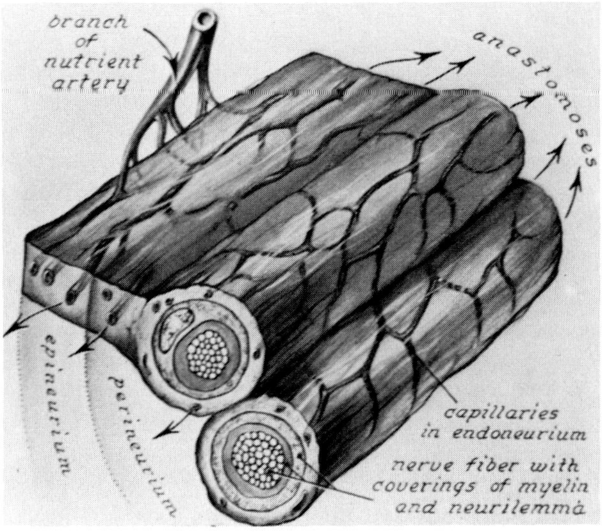

Fig. 10-3. The blood supply of a peripheral nerve. Reproduced from Bateman JE: *Trauma to Nerves in Limbs,* with the permission of the author and publisher.

Mechanism of Injury

The peripheral nerves may be injured by a variety of types of trauma, which can act singly or in combination (Table 10-1).

These may not only involve different components of the nerve, but different lengths as well. For example, knife wounds are characteristically discrete and involve small segments, while traction injuries usually involve longer lengths and are harder to delineate.

In addition the injury may be immediate, such as a gunshot wound, or delayed, as in the traction-friction neuritis presenting as a tardy ulnar palsy years after an elbow fracture. Therefore, an almost infinite variety of clinical presentations of nerve injury is possible, leaving the surgeon with a very difficult-to-define state of pathology on which to attempt to define rational management. Fortunately, however, traumatized nerves react in a reasonably predictable fashion. Although a number of classifications and descriptions of the type of nerve injury have been advanced, that of Seddon,[10] who defined three basic varieties of nerve injury, has, in my opinion, proved most workable (Table 10-2).

Table 10-1. Mechanism of Injury

Compression	Ischemia
Traction	Chemical injury
Laceration	Thermal or cold injury

Degeneration and Regeneration

A brief discussion of the sequence of events involved in the process of degeneration of a transected nerve and regeneration following repair will serve as a physiologic background against which to interpret the technical procedures available.

Within 4 days after the nerve is severed, all conductivity in the distal segment is lost. Axons and myelin sheaths disintegrate and are ingested by macrophages and Schwann cells. This active process is called *Wallerian degeneration*. A proliferation of Schwann cells and endoneurial fibrocytes causes the cut end of the distal stump to swell, with the result that it is initially enlarged. With time, the cellular population diminishes, endoneurial tubes shrink, and collagen is laid down around them so that the whole distal part of the nerve shrinks. The proximal segment undergoes similar changes in its distal stump, over a very short segment, without shrinkage, but significant effects of the injury are also recorded in the parent cell body. Depending on the severity and proximity of the injury, the neuron may undergo complete destruction, or more usually, begin manufacturing increased amounts of RNA in preparation for regeneration. The axoplasm streams out of the tangle of Schwann cells and collagen to form a randomly arranged and bulbous neuroma. If, however, with a primary suture, the supporting elements of the nerve have been accurately aligned and opposed, vigorous proliferation of Schwann cells and fibroblasts of the distal segment causes them to reach proximally, in an orderly fashion, and align themselves longitudinally. With correct orientation, then, more of the axons may find their way into the proper distal endothelial tubes. Suture within 3 months of injury is called *early secondary suture*. The cellular hyperplasia is then at its highest level and the epineurium is thickened, so that if epineurial sutures are used, they will hold solidly. The extent of scarring is more easily delineated than immediately post injury, but greater resection is usually necessary. Beyond 3 months, suture will be *late secondary*, and although Schwann tubes may remain open for longer than 6 months, there is proportional diminution in their available number and size, with decreased quality of the end result.

Table 10-2. Three Types of Nerve Injury

	Neurapraxia	Axonotmesis	Neurotmesis
Common causes	Compression Traction Freezing Ischemia Missiles	Compression Traction Missiles Ischemia Freezing Friction	Lacerations Missiles Traction Injections Ischemia
Pathology (may involve all or part of anatomical nerve circumference)	Local Demyelination, *no* axonal interruption	Axonal interruption, supporting stroma (Schwann sheaths intact)	Axonal and sheath interruption
Clinical findings	Complete motor paralysis, incomplete or lesser sensory loss	Complete motor and sensory loss	Complete motor and sensory loss
EMG	Rare fibrillations, no voluntary action potentials	Fibrillations > 3 wk. No voluntary action potentials	Fibrillations > 3 wk. No voluntary action potentials
Operative findings	Continuity preserved	Continuity preserved. Occasional neuromatous swelling	Anatomic gap or scar in continuity
Spontaneous recovery and timing	Usually by 4-6 wk, in no regular order of innervation	1 mm/day in order of innervation	None unless surgically repaired, then 1 mm/day with delays
Quality of recovery	Normal	Usually normal	Never completely normal even after surgical repair

Adapted from Seddon.[10]

Diagnosis of Peripheral Nerve Injury

"When in doubt, do a history and physical. . . ." Anon.

Although this maxim would seem both inappropriate and unnecessary, many nerve injuries escape initial detection in a massively traumatized patient or one wherein a surgeon caring for an injured extremity is introduced to a patient already under anesthesia. The implications of first noting the nerve deficit after treatment are obviously unfortunate. Careful notation of when the neurologic loss occurred is mandatory, both in fresh cases and those seen after a delay. Since many patients are seen late, it is necessary to establish whether motor and sensory loss have changed in the interval. The presence of associated injuries in the limb and their sequelae must be considered, since they can affect what is done to a significant degree. Information about the patient's occupation and previous function, as well as the circumstances and mechanism of injury, are pertinent parts of the record, as is the presence or absence of pain.

Physical examination in addition to discrete neurologic examination, must include an accurate assessment of the position of wounds, character of scarring, and tissue quality, as well as the range of motion of joints, the presence of contractures, and vascular status.

For peripheral nerve injuries involving the limbs, it is necessary to determine that there are no nerve lesions proximal to the obvious one and under consideration.

The assessment of motor power depends on the ability of the examiner to perform manual muscle tests accurately and with full knowledge of so-called trick and supplementary motions. Although the virtual disappearance of paralytic polio has made this technique harder to master, several available manuals are quite helpful.[11] Records should be detailed, accurate, and standardized. An acceptable scale is that of the British Medical Research Council (Table 10-3).[3]

Sensory testing in the presence of nerve injury should include determination of light touch, using a fine brush or wisp of cotton, and a pin for pain sensibility. Where applicable, in the fingertips, two-point discrimination should be tested, using a blunt caliper or two paperclips held at a constant distance between their ends. This last examination is an indication of stereognosis, a higher type of sensory function, without which the hand may have protective sensibility but still be *blind*, especially for activities where eye-hand coordination cannot compensate for deficient feedback. The *coin test*[12] provides additional data on function of the hand, which is far more informative than the standardized neurologic testing of individual modalities.

The value of Tinel's sign, eliciting paresthesias in the distribution of an injured peripheral nerve by percussion over its course, has been much debated and misunderstood.[13,14] If one taps over the point of injury, assuming the nerve is not deeply buried, a tingling sensation will be felt distally. Since it is a central phenomenon, this would happen even if the limb were amputated at that level. However, if some time has elapsed during which regeneration could have taken place, and tapping over the nerve distal to the injury produces tingling, then one can assume that at least some axons have reached this point. If, with further passage of time, the sign becomes less positive at the point of injury and more distal, this indicates that further downgrowth of axons has occurred. A persistently positive response at the site of injury and nothing distally bodes ill for recovery, but since only part of the total area of a nerve may have been injured and providing the response, an advancing Tinel's sign cannot be taken as assurance that functional recovery will ensue.

Objective electrodiagnostic testing in the form of electromyography and nerve conduction velocity determination has emerged from neurophysiological laboratory studies of nerve to provide a most useful adjunct to the management of nerve injuries.[15] Although an inexperienced or ill-advised electromyographer may serve only to obfuscate, when viewed within the perspective of the clinical situation, the test is often of critical value.

By means of small percutaneous needle electrodes, fibrillation potentials may be detected at rest in partially or completely denervated muscle after about 3 weeks, when Wallerian degeneration has taken place. Since they are entirely outside of the patient's control, they have total objectivity, dependent, of course, on the ability of the observer to correctly interpret them. The pattern, on attempted voluntary contraction, may indicate partial denervation, or sequential observations may document recovery before it can be clinically detected.

Nerve conduction velocity determination,[16] an offset of electromyelography, may be used to localize the site of a lesion of a peripheral nerve, and is particularly useful in compression lesions. Both motor and sensory components may be measured. Measurement of *evoked potentials* in the evaluation of neuromata-in-continuity at operation has greatly expanded the use of this modality.[17]

Although of historic interest, the use of chronaxie and strength-duration curves has declined with the refinement of the preceding modalities.

Since the autonomic fibers supplying the skin have the same distribution as sensory fibers, sweat secretion is a helpful objective test for integrity of sensation. Beads of sweat on

Table 10-3. British Medical Research Council Scale for Rating Muscle Power

0 = no contraction	3 = active movement against gravity
1 = trace of contraction	4 = active movement against gravity and resistance
2 = active movement with gravity eliminated	5 = normal power

the fingertips as seen with a magnifying glass can give a qualitative indication, while electrical skin resistance, measured by a micro-ohmeter, is a slightly more sophisticated way of accomplishing the same thing. Moberg's ninhydrin test[12] provides a visual and permanent record, which is quite useful but must be performed carefully.

General Operative Indications

It is most important to know when not to attempt to repair an injured peripheral nerve. Although few dicta can realistically be accepted as absolute, the following can be useful in formulating operative indications in particular cases:

When the muscles to be reinnervated are severely atrophic, fibrotic, or so distant that years would be required for recovery; if sensation is present or of much lesser importance; or if the motor lesion is partial, then restoration of deficient motor function by appropriate tendon transfers rather than by nerve repair should be done. This is particularly applicable to intrinsic muscles in the hand but is applicable in other areas as well. Lesions that have a generally poor prognosis, such as severe traction injury of the peroneal nerve accompanying rupture of the lateral knee ligaments in adults, are often better not secondarily explored to "see what happens," although individual cases may be benefited. The use of tendon transfers and/or light plastic braces may prove more satisfactory. An elderly patient with a high radial nerve lesion due to laceration will usually derive considerably more immediate and long-term functional benefit from tendon transfer to restore wrist and finger extension than from attempts to suture or graft a nerve. A patient seen years after a median nerve injury may not regain motor function after surgery, but since median nerve sensibility is so important, an attempt to restore it even partially is reasonable as long as 5 years later. If the ulnar nerve is intact, thought should be given to neurovascular island pedicle transfer to restore sensibility to the thumb, if nerve repair cannot be done or fails.[18] Extensive isolated lesions of the posterior tibial nerve low in the adult leg may, if repaired, eventuate in disabling hypersensitivity and overreaction in the sole of the foot, so that these, too, must be carefully considered.

Finally, local conditions in the limbs, such as poor soft tissue cover for the proposed repair, which will predispose to scarring, must be corrected preoperatively. If posturing of joints will be necessary to accomplish mobilization and coaptation of a nerve, then they must be mobile to allow for this maneuver.

Gunshot wounds constitute a dilemma in that often the nerve deficit is caused by a *near-miss* and the shock wave that momentarily deforms the nerve. Unless there is concomitant bone or vascular injury that requires immediate attention, or the track of the bullet, as measured by entrance and exit wounds, could not possibly have missed cutting the nerve, there is little to be gained from immediate exploration, and one should wait-out the period of neurapraxia—usually 6 weeks.

Because of the likelihood of neurotmesis when a sharp object, such as a knife or glass, has caused a significant nerve injury, these should all be explored. The timing of the procedure, however, continues to provide an ongoing controversy between those who favor immediate primary repair, and those who will electively postpone definitive surgery. Although numerous clinical theories endorsing each approach exist,[4,5,19] they generally suffer from a lack of precise statistical comparability to account for all pertinent factors. Rather than endorse one method or the other as in "voting the straight ticket," the surgeon should be aware of the advantages and disadvantages to be weighed in his or her particular case. In order to allow for primary repair, a nerve wound should be a clean laceration, without significant additional tissue damage or contamination in a patient whose general condition will not be endangered by what could be a lengthy operative procedure. An experienced surgeon and operating team should be available and the wound should not be over 18 hours old. The patient should have been on antibiotics during the interval. Children are good candidates for primary repair, since their prognosis for nerve repair is superior. Digital nerves and clean cuts of median and ulnar nerves at the wrist should be repaired primarily, since in the latter case the fascicles are readily identified. Because of the high percentage of nonfascicular tissue in the nerves at this level and the pure composition of the bundles themselves, the penalty for malrotation is severe in terms of axons that go astray.

The negative side of the primary suture, in addition to the possibly increased risk of infection because of additional surgical manipulation and time required to accomplish it, is the very real difficulty of being able to accurately assess the condition of the nerve ends in a fresh wound. Obviously, repair of compromised nerve tissue that commits the patient to a long wait, only to realize an unsatisfactory result, is to be avoided. If there is significant doubt, then one should wait and do a secondary repair when the wound has healed per primum and delineation is easier, but this usually requires greater resection of the nerve ends. The issue has become less of a problem since the operating microscope has been available; at high magnification, a more informed picture of the condition of the fascicles is possible.

Despite what might be intuitively concluded about the treatment of nerves in limbs replanted following severance, it is now generally believed by those with the greatest experience in this area, including the Chinese, that primary repair of these nerves is preferable. However documentation of these results will take years to accumulate.

The management of nerve injuries accompanying fractures and dislocations should be divided into (a) closed injuries, where a skeletal injury may be assumed to have caused the nerve injury, and (b) open injuries, where the fracture is usually incidental to the wounding agent that also injures the nerve. In the latter case indications are those of the isolated nerve injury. Closed fractures and dislocations rarely cause neurotmesis, and in most cases expectant treatment eventuates in recovery. The best example of this is a closed transverse fracture of the midshaft of the humerus with a radial palsy. The anatomic position of the nerve relative to the fracture makes it unlikely that the nerve is caught in fracture fragments. Therefore, knowing the level of fracture and nerve injury and the distance to the first motor branch, brachioradialis, calculation at the rate of 1 inch per month should set an outer limit of time allowed for spontaneous recovery. If this is exceeded, and neither electromyographic or clinical evidence of recovery is present, then the nerve should be explored. It is important to recognize that the radial palsy accompanying long oblique fractures of the humerus at the junction of the upper two-thirds and lower one-third is likely to result from the anatomic propensity of the nerve at this level to be entrapped in the fracture. These should be explored primarily and the nerve decompressed while the the fracture is fixed internally.[20]

In general sciatic nerve injury accompanying hip dislocations recovers spontaneously, while those with acetabular fractures more often require operative release. A palsy that arises after manipulation of a fracture or dislocation, when no such lesion preexisted, should, in my opinion, usually be explored.

Anesthesia

The prolonged and meticulous nature of peripheral nerve surgery makes general anesthesia preferable in most cases. Since nerve grafts may have to be obtained from the lower extremities in procedures on the upper extremity, this would necessitate a general anesthetic.

Since the continued use of muscle relaxants may interfere with intraoperative diagnostic nerve stimulation, this phase of the procedure must be discussed with the anesthesiologist in advance. Undoubtedly, there are many operations of lesser magnitude, such as carpal tunnel release or other decompressions, or even sutures, that can be performed in satisfactory fashion under regional anesthesia. However, some patients dislike experiencing additional numbness, even temporarily, in an already neurologically abnormal limb. Either interscalene, axillary block, or intravenous regional may be used in the upper limb, depending on the area of anesthesia required. However, the intravenous regional precludes a long procedure or the letting down of the tourniquet so that hemostasis may be assured before completing a neurorrhaphy or closure.

Hakstian[21] has described an ingenious technique, applying local anesthetic to explore and map the fasciculi of fresh lacerations of the median and ulnar nerves at the wrist. A microstimulator is used to identify the motor fascicles by contraction of their muscles, and sensory nerves by the patient's conscious appreciation of the stimulation. After the individual fascicles have been marked with dye, the patient is given general anesthesia and a fascicular repair is performed under the microscope. The technique is tedious, but the results are reported to be good.

Aids to Operation

Time is well spent in planning the sequence of maneuvers in an operation on a peripheral nerve, especially if it is done along with tendon, bone, or vascular repair. This will usually avoid embarrassing compromise during or after the procedure. Assuming it will not impose additional hazards to the patient under anesthesia, the position chosen should be selected for ease of surgical approach. The surgeon and operating team are comfortably seated at an absolutely steady table that will permit the surgeon to support his forearms to avoid fatigue. A number of *hand tables* have been designed and are available, but they need not be elaborate as long as they fulfill the above criteria. In addition, as a result of the technologic explosion accompanying microsurgery, a number of complicated, motorized surgeon's chairs have been suggested. We continue to use conventional operating room stools.

Prepping and draping should be done to allow for extensile exposure, and, if necessary, posturing of the limbs. Potential graft sites are covered with sterile drapes before the procedure begins so that if the sites are needed, breaks in technique will not be likely. If sural nerve grafts are to be used, the lower extremity should be prepped to the tips of the toes, and the limb draped free and mobile to avoid the aggravation of having to "stand on one's head" to harvest the grafts.

Although tourniquet ischemia and a bloodless field are not absolutely essential to peripheral nerve surgery, they can markedly facilitate exposure and identification of vital structures, especially in a scarred or previously explored area. Unless there is an anatomic or physiologic contraindication to the tourniquet, I use it routinely for at least the preliminary exposure and preparation of the nerve. Obviously it is contraindicated in the presence of significant vascular disease. In some situations in which the configuration of the part or position of the wound prevents the use of a standard pneumatic tourniquet, a pediatric-sized cuff may be used with benefit. A gas-sterilized or disposable pneumatic cuff is also a possibility, but the Esmarck or Martin bandage should be restricted to preliminary exsanguination rather than used as the definitive tourniquet in an awkward situation. If it is used, there is no way of quantitating the amount of compression excited by multiple turns of the rubber bandage at the root of the limb. The risk of tourniquet palsy, with this method, is significant but may be considered acceptable under some circumstances.

Even with commercially available pneumatic tourniquets, the presence of a pressure gauge does not insure its continued accuracy, so periodic calibration against a mercury manometer standard is a good safety measure. Recommended inflation pressures for the adult upper extremity range from 200 to 300 mm Hg, and for the lower extremity, 350 to 550. These should be adjusted according to measured blood pressure and the size of the patient for satisfactory performance and safety. There is no universally accepted time limit for tourniquet ischemia. My own practice is not to exceed 2 hours in the upper extremity, following which 30 minutes of circulation are allowed. This may be safely repeated, and by the end of this period, that part of the procedure requiring the tourniquet has usually been accomplished. It should be remembered that if electrical stimulation of the nerve is to be part of the procedure, it will have to be accomplished before 20 to 30 minutes of ischemia have passed, since nerve transmission normally ceases under these circumstances.

Use of the nerve stimulator to assess the condition of a neuroma-in-continuity is an extremely valuable technique. Even though voluntary contraction of a paralyzed muscle may not be possible, direct nerve stimulation at open operation may identify axonal continuity and prevent unnecessary resection of damaged but recovering nerves. Neurolysis in the midst of dense scar may be impossible without a stimulator. Kline[17] has described in detail the technique of evoked potentials in the evaluation of lesions in continuity. It is useful, but requires sophisticated electromyographic equipment at the operating table.

The proliferation of specialized instruments for microsurgery has created a bewildering array of available equipment that can be used for nerve suture. In addition to the usual forceps, needle holders, and scissors, which are part of the armamentarium of any neurosurgical cabinet, many new instruments have evolved from microvascular surgery. These are well suited to peripheral nerve repair, and each surgeon tends (often quite arbitrarily) to prefer one instrument type or another. In general, needle holders that can be *palmed* and do not lock are of advantage, since they encourage steadiness and do not jar when opened and closed under high magnification. Forceps, too, are almost infinite in their variety and advocates, but we tend to use the simple *watchmaker's* forceps without teeth. They are minimally traumatic to delicate tissues, but, as with all such instruments, their tips must be protected against trauma, especially during sterilization and storage, when it is wise to keep them and all microinstruments in cases specially designed for the purpose.

If a neuroma that occupies the entire circumference of a nerve is to be resected or if an epineural suture or cable graft is to be performed, then it will be desirable to cut all fascicles at the same level and at right angles to the length of the nerve. Since normal peripheral nerve fascicles have the consistency and rigidity of wet spaghetti, it is often difficult to achieve the desired neat, sharp cut by simply drawing a scalpel blade across the nerve. The nerve tends to deform as it is cut, with the result that the epineurium may shred, or fascicles may be cut on the bias or at different levels. To obviate this problem, a number of ingenious neurotomes and miniature mitre-boxes have been designed.[22] They may be helpful in achieving the desired result. In the hands of an experienced surgeon, a very sharp manual dermatome blade or a fresh razor blade can be used, while steadying the nerve against a wooden tongue depressor. The indelicate practice of pinning the nerve to the tongue blade proximal to the line of section to steady it so it can be put on tension is to be avoided. A diamond knife for microsurgical repair of nerves has been adapted from one introduced into microsurgery by Microsurgical Instrumentation Research Association.[23] This is said to be valuable in interfascicular dissection of neuromas. A simple, practical, and economic way of aiding the right-angle section of nerves prior to repair has been proposed by Clark.[24] He encloses the nerve within a paper sheath and grasps the free leaves of paper with a right-angle clamp before sectioning through it. This allows the axons to be held in a cylindric form without being crushed or rolled under the pressure of a razor blade.

Suture material has been the subject of much discussion. There are many advantages and disadvantages of various materials demonstrated in animal experiments. Although there have been great technical advances in making sutures re: uniformity, tensile strength and reactivity, there is still no ideal material. The search goes on. At the present time, 8 and 10:0 monofilament nylon with swaged-on needles are the sutures of choice for most peripheral nerve sutures. The use of plasma clot as a means of joining nerves has been shown to be effective by Tarlov and others.[25,26] However, there has been little recent enthusiasm for the method.

There is now no serious doubt that magnification must be employed in the surgery of peripheral nerves. What remains to be seen is just how much magnification is necessary, assuming a constant degree of surgical ability and visual acuity. From a purely practical point of view, most surgeons (and nurses) can barely see 10:0 suture without magnification. However, this should not lead to an immediate mandate that all sutures be done with $25,000.00 microscopes at 40× magnification. The simple devices available to achieve magnification range from loupes to operating telescopes on eyeglass frames. The former are inexpensive but rarely give more than 2×, and the operating telescopes come in various strengths up to 6×. The depth of field with these is very shallow and they do not have a focused light source. A practical compromise is the telescope with 2.5 or 3.5× magnification.

The operating microscope market can readily be compared, somewhat facetiously, to the used car market, with a bewildering array of basic models and numerous options and accessories, including power controls. Interestingly enough, the prices tend to parallel automobile prices as well. Very simply, there are less expensive models that clamp-on to the operating table and more elaborate ones with fiberoptic light sources and multiple heads as well as provisions for photography and TV.

The addition of a counterbalanced portable floor mount conveys stability, which are extremely high magnifications may be further enhanced by permanent floor or ceiling mounts.

The optical characteristics of the system, and therefore, the degree of magnification and clarity depend on the combination of ocular and objective. For most types of microsurgery, a 200 to 300 mm. focal length objective will be suitable. Then, eyepieces ranging from 10× to 20× are available.

Most microscopes have a magnification-changer setting that can be applied to a particular combination of ocular and objective to achieve a desired result. The actual degree of magnification cannot, as one would assume, be read directly from the changer setting on the microscope, but will be found by consulting the chart that comes with each instrument. Although the degree of available magnification may, in some systems, vary from 1.5 to 40×, for most purposes, sixfold magnification is sufficient. If the fascicles are less than 1 mm, then higher magnification may be required. Ease of modifying the field and magnification is greatly enhanced by motorized zoom and focusing with foot controls. Obviously this adds to the cost. Finally, the sterile draping of the microscope and stand may prove to be a logistic annoyance. To obviate this, commercial plastic microscope drapes are available, and some microscopes are designed so that they have autoclavable handles and do not require sterile draping (Fig. 10-4).

Technique

The operative approaches to major peripheral nerves in the limbs have been well illustrated in standard references.[2,4,27] Time and space will not permit their recapitulation here. The peripheral nerve surgeon must be prepared to expose a nerve throughout its length, with due regard for avoidance of vital structures and the production of hypertrophic scars and contractures, but without apology for the length of the incision, if anatomic considerations so dictate. In the presence of scarring and neuroma formation, the dissection should begin in normal tissue, both proximally and distally if possible, so that all important structures can be identified and preserved. Then, dissection is carried centripetally to expose the area of nerve damage.

If one is dealing with a compression lesion by reason of the pathogenesis, or an incom-

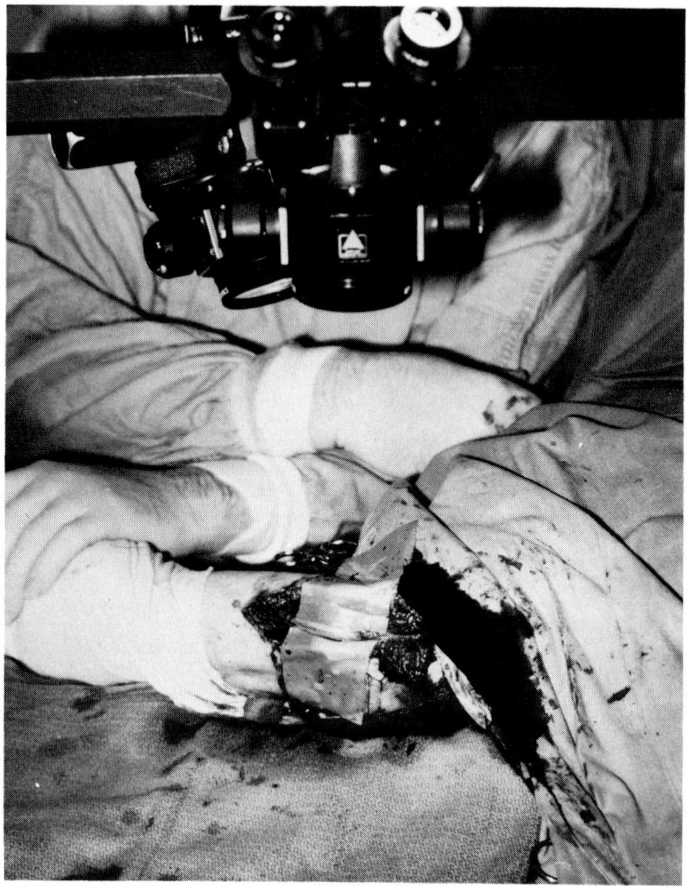

Fig. 10-4. The handles on this "two-headed" operating microscope made by Applied Fiberoptics are sterilized and allow manipulation during surgery.

plete clinical deficit, then simple decompression is indicated, and the prognosis for recovery should be favorable. A common example of this is carpal tunnel release. Even here, however, if the nerve shows evidence of epineural thickening, or the surface vascular pattern remains interrupted, then careful circumferential removal of the epineurium under magnification is indicated. I do not use saline injection under the epineurium as a test of the adequacy of decompression, or a substitute for manual neurolysis, since without relieving the constriction of tight epineurium, little would appear to be gained. Whether one should perform an additional intraneural lysis under magnification[28] is debated, since cross connections between fascicles, or the bundles themselves, could conceivably be injured during the dissection.

Neurolysis is indicated when the lesion is felt to be caused by external scar. This may present clinically as very slow recovery, plateauing, or reversal, and must be carefully documented. The procedure must be performed meticulously under magnification so as to avoid injury to intact fascicles. It may give gratifying results, but one should avoid doing it in the presence of a recovering lesion.

If the lesion is of long duration, and the neurologic defect is complete, one must attempt to differentiate axonotmesis or a mixed lesion from neurotmesis, since the latter would require resection and neurorrhaphy or graft. Direct electrical stimulation might be useful, but inspection and palpation, as in all neuromata, are most important.

Closed injuries to peripheral nerves resulting from fractures and dislocations must be evaluated in light of the magnitude and nature of the trauma that produced them as well as the pathomechanics of the lesion and its specific location. This has already been commented upon.

The management of documented complete transections of peripheral nerves is the most difficult and controversial aspect of the subject under discussion. Simply stated, the object of the procedure is to reestablish axonal continuity with the periphery in such fashion as to restore maximal neurologic function. An ecumenical and complete historical review might prove interesting (or tedious), but a series of straw men erected only to be knocked down is of little comfort to the surgeon faced with the immediate problem of managing a neurotmesis. The question of primary or secondary nerve repair has already been discussed. Having made either choice, the remaining decisions concern how to get the correct fascicles together when that part determined to be damaged has been resected after the nerve has been palpated and inspected under magnification to assure the absence of fibrosis or other impediments to regeneration. The variable gap that results may call for more than a single solution, and one ought to be prepared to consider alternatives. There is general agreement that tension is the most deleterious factor mitigating against success in nerve repair, assuming fascicular orientation is correct. In order to avoid tension at the suture line, mobilization of the nerve from its bed (and segmental blood supply) may be carried out. The question remains as to just how far this can be done before it becomes self-defeating.

The first half of this century saw the establishment of empirically determined *critical resection lengths*[4] for each nerve, limits within which one could expect regeneration following neurorrhaphy. To coapt the ends after mobilization, the adjacent joints would have to be postured accordingly and then held by external fixation, usually a cast, until healing was sufficient to allow gradual stretching. The initial period is usually 3 weeks, following which gradual resumption of full range is achieved. In general for the upper extremity, if the elbow must be flexed more than 90° or the wrist 45°, to achieve coaptation, then excessive tension will be present when full motion is required, and the prognosis for success is poor. At the knee, 90° may not be exceeded. Within these limits, epineurial suture may be performed.

The handling of the nerve must be minimized, and then only gently, with microinstruments, rubber drain retractors, or fingers. Hemostasis is essential, so the tourniquet should be down and all bleeding points stopped. A suitable background that will allow visualization of the fascicles and fine suture may be provided by a piece of sterilized, light-colored plastic, such as that used for household garbage bags.[29] Correct fascicular orientation may be aided by matching the alignment of surface blood vessels, if these are visible. Sometimes the nerve will simply lie in correct rotatory position, but it may not, especially if it has been malrotated by a previous attempt at repair. Inspection, under magnification, of the fascicular pattern at the resection surfaces is the best guide to alignment, and although exact correspondence is usually not found, major groups of bundles can be identified and approximated. Once this has been established, the epineurial repair is commenced by means of two traction sutures introduced at the edges 180° apart and left long so that they may be held by microbulldog clamps. This will permit turning the nerve so that simple interrupted sutures may be used to close the circumference of the epineurium, without deforming the fascicles. Just as many sutures as required to achieve this are used, according to the size of the nerve. It should be remembered that the suture material is foreign body that may, with remodeling, actually become incorporated within the substance of the nerve. No more than six to eight sutures, and often fewer, are needed. Despite claims that wrapping the suture line with foreign material will diminish fibrosis and improve results, there is no conclusive proof that this is so, but the list of materials so employed is long and varied. A number of these have actually proved to be deleterious on long-term evaluation. To date, there is no ideal substance for this purpose, and their use is not recommended.

For lesions that result in gaps that cannot be overcome, as described with posturing the joints or anatomic maneuvers such as anterior transposition of the ulnar nerve, grafting provides a useful alternative. After years of uncertainty, it is quite clear now that fresh autogenous grafts are the donor material of choice. Usually cutaneous nerves are preferred because they can be sacrificed with less significant residual deficit, and their smaller diameter makes central necrosis during revascularization less likely. The sural nerve has become the most popular donor, and in an average adult as much as 35 cm may be obtained by multiple transverse incisions and mobilization in the intervals. A long incision from popliteal space to lateral ankle is easier technically and may even be necessary, but it is less desirable to ultimate appearance. Cutaneous nerves in the upper extremity may be used, but it would be imprudent to sacrifice one that is providing sensation to an area adjacent to that already denervated. If a mixed nerve has been severed and is not to be reconstituted, it may serve as donor, but this situation is becoming progressively less common.

The grafts may be interposed in several ways. They may be placed side-by-side in the manner of a cable and sutured to the epineurium of the host proximally and distally, usually with one stitch per strand in a way that will cover the cross-sectional area of the nerve and preserve longitudinal orientation so that presumably the fascicles will find their way to the corresponding radial segment of the distal end of the nerve (Figs. 10-5, 10-6, and 10-7). For partial lesions or lateral neuromata, an inlay graft of this type rather than a *loop suture* may provide good results, despite the theoretical objections of two suture lines as opposed to one.

The foregoing discussion describes the general concept of nerve grafting as a salvage procedure, and although some workers devoted to meticulous technique[30] were able to document results that were satisfactory, the overall impression was not particularly favorable. The presentation of the concept of grafting *a priori*, by Millesi and his colleagues,[31,32] is a radical departure from past practice. It evolved from realization of the deleterious effects of tension at the suture line as well as their laboratory studies showing that the epineurium contributed significantly to the fibrosis that impeded regeneration past the suture. This, then, while a technique for secondary nerve repair, is an alternative to attempting mobilization,

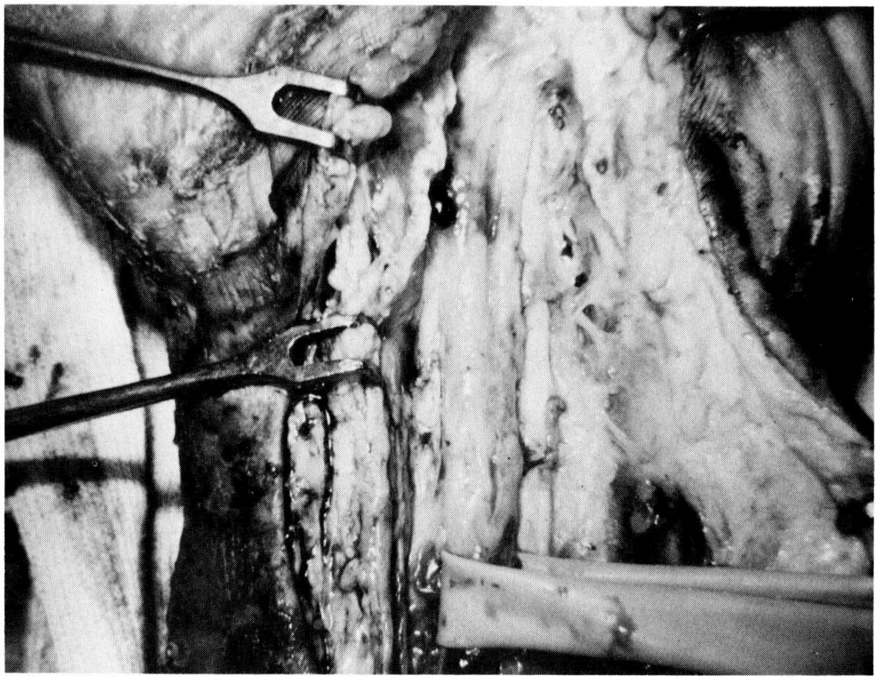

Fig. 10-5. The volar aspect of the distal forearm five months following a close range shotgun wound. The median nerve is embedded in the scar in the carpal tunnel.

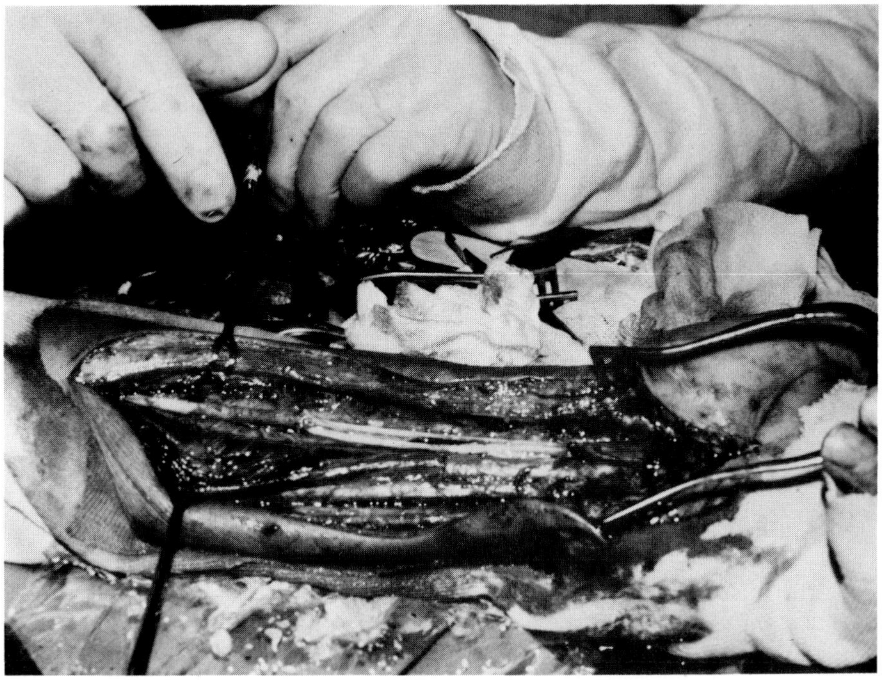

Fig. 10-6. A 10-cm segment of the scarred median nerve has been replaced by four cables of sural nerve graft.

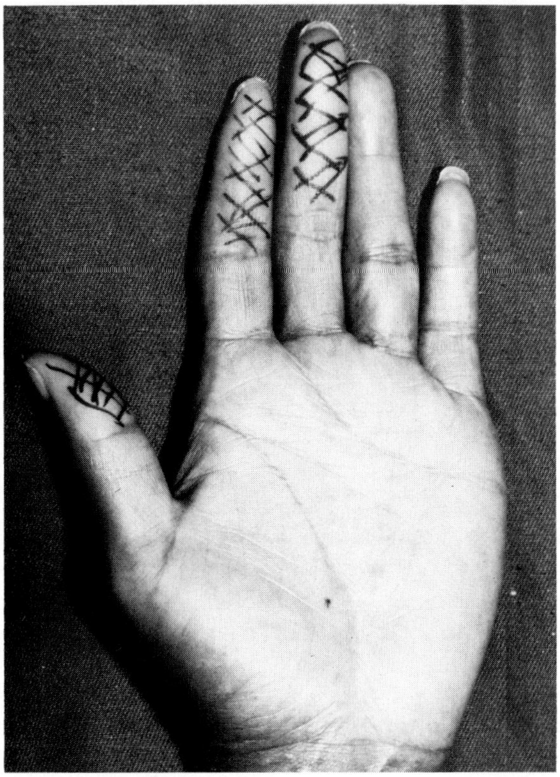

Fig. 10-7. Clinical appearance of the hand 10 months after grafting. The thenar muscle bulk had been regained and protective sensibility had returned proximal to the cross-hatched area, patient lost to followup thereafter.

and if this is not feasible, going on to graft. Millesi's criteria for the median and ulnar nerves are as follows:

All cases are grafted except:

1. if the gap in the nerve is 2 cm or less and the nerve ends can be approximated without tension with the joints of the extremity in full extension,
2. for the ulnar nerve at the elbow, gaps of up to 4 cm that can be closed without tension by anterior transposition, and
3. a nerve gap accompanying nonunion of a fracture requiring operation may be closed and sutured following shortening of the bone.

The important differences between this technique and that of the cable graft should be noted. Millesi advocates interfascicular grafting rather than epineurial bridging. Under magnification, the neuroma is approached from both ends, but rather than preserving the epineurium and transecting all fascicles at the same level, he dissects and transects each major fascicle and group of minor ones at the point of injury and then maps them before proceeding to the distal stump, where the same process occurs. The epineurium is resected from both ends, and then corresponding fascicles or groups are united by an interposed graft, usually of sural nerve, with the epineurium of the graft fixed by one fine suture to the perineurium of the host fascicles. The suture lines are, therefore, staggered as the pathology dictates. The limb is immobilized for 10 days, following which active exercises can begin. The results of this technique have been described by Millesi to be at least as good as those after epineurial suture under ideal conditions and better than those after neurorrhaphy under tension.[32]

The long-term evaluation of a strictly controlled and comparable clinical series of peripheral nerve injuries managed by these alternate methods will eventually resolve some of the controversy. In addition there are other variations in suture technique, such as the longitudinal fascicular stitch,[33] that will have to be put in proper perspective with time and experience.

A number of unusual methods of handling special situations in peripheral nerve surgery have been developed. Both nerve transfer and pedicle grafts[34] have proved useful in some cases. For details the reader may consult several excellent references.[4,5]

Postoperative Management

If a suture has been done that involves posturing of joints, immobilization is normally maintained for 3 weeks before the limb is begun on regaining range of motion. During this time, adjacent joints must be maintained mobile, and contractures must be prevented by splinting and passive exercise (Fig. 10-8). It is indeed unfortunate to regain motor power after many months of waiting for nerve regeneration only to find that it is functionally useless because the joints are stiff. Not all patients require formal physical or occupational therapy, and this must be individualized. The efficacy of electrical stimulation during the period of regeneration has not been clearly established. Many of the studies that have been done have been on animal models[35] and some have been poorly controlled. I do not believe that sufficient evidence, based on experience with humans, exists to either have my patients come to the hospital for daily stimulation or urge them to buy home stimulators.

Factors Influencing Results of Nerve Repair

A number of technical factors that influence the result of nerve repair have been mentioned. In addition there is little question that the experience and technical skill of the operator are of tremendous import.

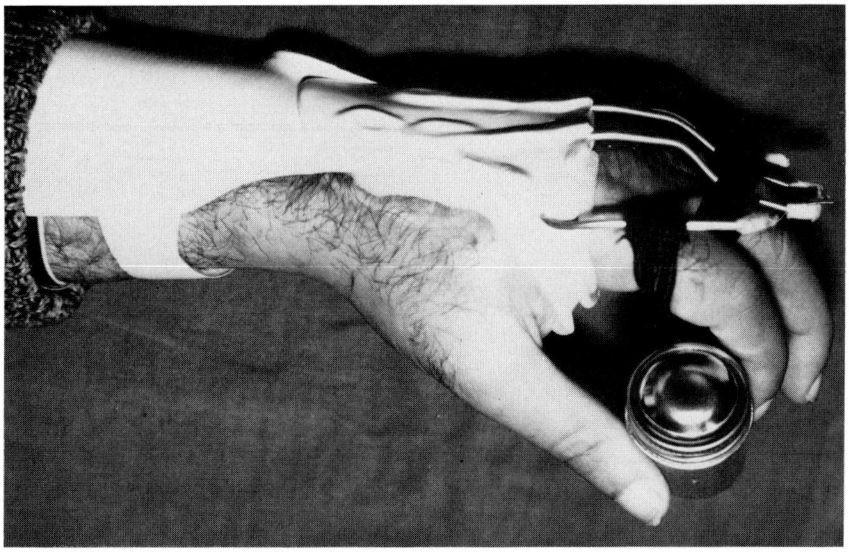

Fig. 10-8. A low-profile radial palsy splint made by Occupational Therapists at the Massachusetts General Hospital.

However, other factors independent of the operator or his control are significant determinants of the result:

1. *Age:* The power of regeneration and adaptability of children gives them considerably better results than comparable situations in adults.
2. *Mechanism of injury:* In general those wounds caused by greater trauma tend to exert a more deleterious effect on the nervous system than those of lesser magnitude, ie., blast war wounds tend to do worse than clean knife wounds.
3. *Length of resection:* In general lesions involving greater length require more elaborate maneuvers to repair, have greater dissimilarity of the fascicular pattern, and tend not to do as well.
4. *Duration between injury and repair:* Ordinarily, after 3 months, the greater the delay in repair, the poorer the result.
5. *Location of the lesion:* The closer to the spinal cord, or the more proximal the lesion, the poorer the prognosis. This may result from retrograde neurologic changes, exhaustion of axoplasm production, atrophy of the end organ with time, or a combination of all of these factors.

In the final analysis, there are many unsolved problems in surgery of peripheral nerves. Most of our efforts have been of a mechanical nature, but the greatest single impediment to success is the production of scar. It may well be that we are really very primitive in our thinking about this type of surgery, and that the ultimate solution is a biochemical or neurophysiologic one that will correctly direct the down-growing axon, preserve the waiting end-organ, and above all, prevent the formation of scar. Some interesting work is already going on in this area.[36]

Surgery of the Brachial Plexus

Many of the diagnostic and therapeutic techniques already discussed in detail are directly applicable to surgery of the brachial plexus. Sufficient specialized differences exist to merit separate consideration.

The anatomic complexity of the brachial plexus makes both diagnosis and treatment considerably more difficult than the problem posed by single or even multiple peripheral nerve injuries. If compression lesions are excluded, most of the remaining trauma can be considered under the general headings of *closed* and *open* injury. The latter will be considered first:

Open Wounds of the Brachial Plexus

Open wounds of the plexus are often accompanied by life-threatening vascular or pulmonary complications that may obscure recognition of the nerve injury or even kill the patient.[37] Surgical maneuvers to treat these problems must obviously take precedence over treatment of the nerve lesion. But what are the indications for surgical exploration of open wounds of the plexus? The answer depends, in addition to the above considerations, on several factors. The first of these is the nature of the wound. A knife or glass cut is unlikely to be anything less than a neurotmesis, so that awaiting recovery at the rate of an inch a month is pointless. If the upper or intermediate trunk or their distal outflow is injured, it is worth exploring the lesion, since a discrete injured area may be amenable to suture or graft. The muscles innervated are mainly proximal, often large, and not of great functional complexity (but not invariably). Therefore, careful neurorrhaphy has at least a chance of improving function. For the lower trunk and its terminal branches, the prognosis for recovery is so poor that in my opinion it is not worthwhile.

Gunshot wounds, however, constitute a completely different situation, much harder to assess. The passage of a bullet through the tissues causes momentary deformation that spreads like a wave through the surrounding area. Hence, the spectrum of injury may be quite broad in an individual case, and there is no way of knowing immediately which parts are actually transected, and which are going to recover. The carefully documented work of Donal Brooks,[38] in World War II, demonstrated how difficult it is to assess open wounds at surgery. He explored 54 cases, thought 16 to be amenable to surgical repair, and achieved a functional result in only 1, a lesion of an upper trunk.

The indication for the gunshot wound, therefore, is far less urgent than that of the sharp transection, although the operating microscope has brightened the outlook for treatment of open wounds.

Closed Wounds of the Branchial Plexus

These can be divided into supraclavicular and infraclavicular injuries, and since they have significantly different prognoses, they are considered separately. Infraclavicular injuries of the brachial plexus result from skeletal injuries in the region of the shoulder girdle.[39] Often accompanying shoulder dislocations or fractures, they are of lesser severity than the supraclavicular variety because the bony lesions are the cause of nerve injury by direct compression or traction, and root avulsion or postganglionic neurotmesis do not occur. The prognosis for recovery, even of hand function, is generally good, and their treatment differs considerably from the larger group of supraclavicular injuries. Criteria for their identification and management have been advanced by Leffert and Seddon.[39]

The supraclavicular injuries are usually caused by high velocity vehicular accidents, and most often by falls from motorcycles. The patient often falls so that the shoulder and neck are forced apart, and great force is brought to bear in producing a traction lesion of the plexus. The damage may vary from frank avulsion of cervical roots from the spinal cord (a preganglionic or supraganglionic lesion) to lesser or greater degrees of damage to the trunks or divisions (postganglionic), which can range from neuropraxia to neurotmesis. Differential involvement of motor and sensory components is also possible, so that an almost infinite spectrum of pathology can be observed. Detailed and accurate knowledge of the anatomy is essential. In addition to the usual techniques of clinical and electrodiagnostic evaluation, several indirect methods of study are useful in arriving at an accurate picture of the damage before surgery is considered.[40]

The presence of a Horner's syndrome usually indicates preganglionic avulsion of T1. Paralysis of the rhomboids, diaphragm, or serratus anterior are found in patients with preganglionic lesions of C5, C6, and C7, since their nerves are usually given off immediately after exit from the foramina.

Plane films of the cervical spine and shoulder girdle can provide clues as to the fate of the unseen plexus. If transverse processes are avulsed, this is a reliable indication that the nerve root at that level has suffered a like fate. If the clavicle is fractured, it almost always accompanies a supraclavicular rather than an infraclavicular injury because of the greater excursion that it allows between the head and shoulder, and the prognosis is correspondingly worse.

Cervical myelography can demonstrate root avulsion by the presence of pseudomeningoceles.[41] It should be performed not sooner than 2 to 3 months following injury to allow the meninges to retract at the site of avulsion and form pockets that will allow the dye to pool and be seen on x-ray (Fig. 10-9).

The use of the axon reflex by studying the response to intradermal histamine can provide an additional indicator of the level of the lesion.[42] Yeoman's excellent article evaluating these methods can be consulted for details.[43]

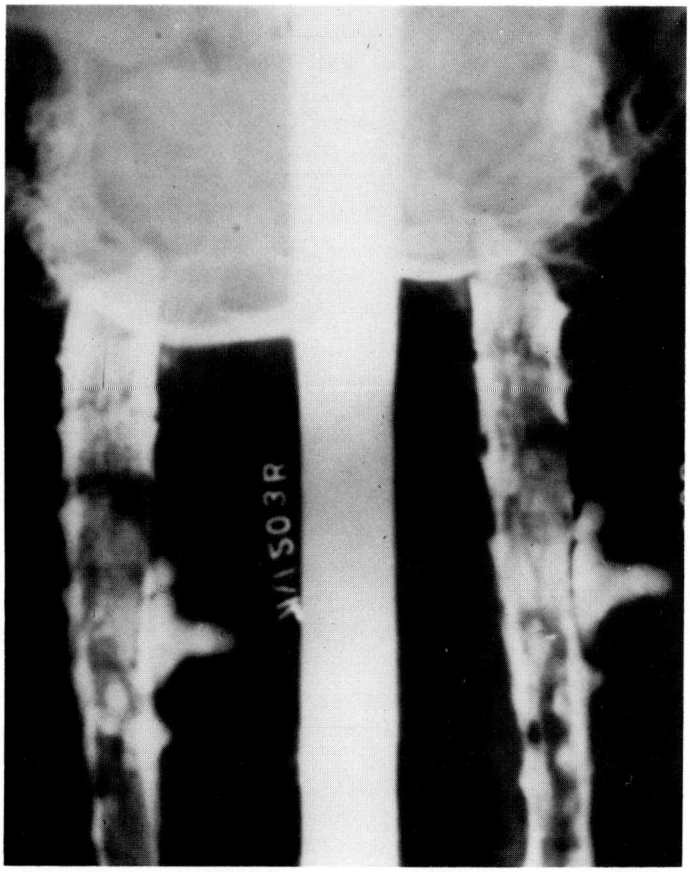

Fig. 10-9. Traumatic pseudomeningoceles seen on the cervical myelogram of a patient who has sustained avulsion of three roots in a traction injury.

All of these methods of evaluation, used in conjunction with the clinical and electromyographic studies, make cervical laminectomy absolutely unnecessary in determining the presence of root avulsion, which, in the present state of technology, is not amenable to surgical repair.

Surgical exploration of the plexus in the supraclavicular fossa is indicated, however, for diagnostic purposes in the presence of a flail anesthetic arm, when myelography shows two or fewer traumatic meningoceles and they are of the lowest roots.[4] The alternative is to wait years for recovery or its failure. If the nerves are found to be torn apart, although they are usually not amenable to direct suture, they might be candidates for grafting if sufficient proximal root stock is preserved.

The operative approach is extensile, starting at the posterior border of the sternocleidomastoid at the junction of its upper one third and lower two thirds and dropping vertically to the clavicle. If the exposure is to be carried to the infraclavicular plexus, the skin incision should take an "L-shaped" turn laterally, 1.0 inch caudal to the clavicle, and then proceed into and down the deltopectoral groove. If possible, it is desirable to avoid dividing the clavicle in the exposure, since both nonunion and osteomyelitis have been reported. Often by forward traction on the clavicle, it is possible to work around it and avoid the possibility of these complications. In the presence of massive and impenetrable scar in the area, one might consider bypassing the subclavicular region and routing the nerve grafts subcutaneously. This not only avoids much difficult dissection, but provides an unscarred bed for the grafts.

A patient with three traumatic meningoceles was considered by Seddon not to be a candidate for operative exploration, since presumably the amount of trauma necessary to produce this lesion would most certainly also cause a postganglionic neurotmesis of the remainder of the plexus.[4] The prognosis for recovery, then, was essentially hopeless. The resulting dilemma of a flail, anesthetic arm offered three major avenues of approach. If the patient could do his job one-handed and was not bothered by the presence of the arm, then nothing more had to be done. Of course it was necessary to protect the anesthetic limb from injury and support so that it was not an impediment.

Because sensory feedback is lacking, a flail arm is unlikely to be used, even if it can be postured with a brace. The same restriction pertains to the possibility of surgical reconstruction. Although Hendry[44] reported some good results with this approach, consisting of shoulder fusion, elbow bone block, and various fusions and tenodeses about the hand, I do not regard it as a viable alternative, and counsel patients against it.

The final solution, fusing the shoulder, amputating the arm above-elbow, and fitting with a prosthesis can provide a useful assistive limb in a patient who wants to remain bimanual and who is emotionally stable and mechanically inclined.[45] Of course attempting to do this more than 2 years after injury, when the patient has already adjusted to being one-handed, is probably doomed to failure. The shoulder fusion allows the arm to be voluntarily moved, since scapular control is usually retained by sparing the trapezius and serratus anterior, but the actual function obtained from this program leaves much to be desired. An alternative, even in the patient whose hand is not salvageable, is an attempt to provide an elbow under voluntary control. Hence, if the C5 root or the upper trunk is intact, even though there is neurotmesis immediately distal, a cable graft may be placed between it and the lateral cord or musculocutaneous nerve. Although it may take as long as a year to achieve active elbow flexion, the result may permit forearm amputation, prosthetic fitting, and considerably more function (Figs. 10-10, 10-11, and 10-12).

As greater experience is gained with direct surgical attack on the plexus, more patients who formerly would have either had amputations or no treatment are being considered for neurologic reconstruction or neurolysis. The latter procedure is particularly indicated in patients with documented postganglionic lesions whose recovery does not proceed as expected, or who actually experience a plateau or reversal of this process. Lusskin and

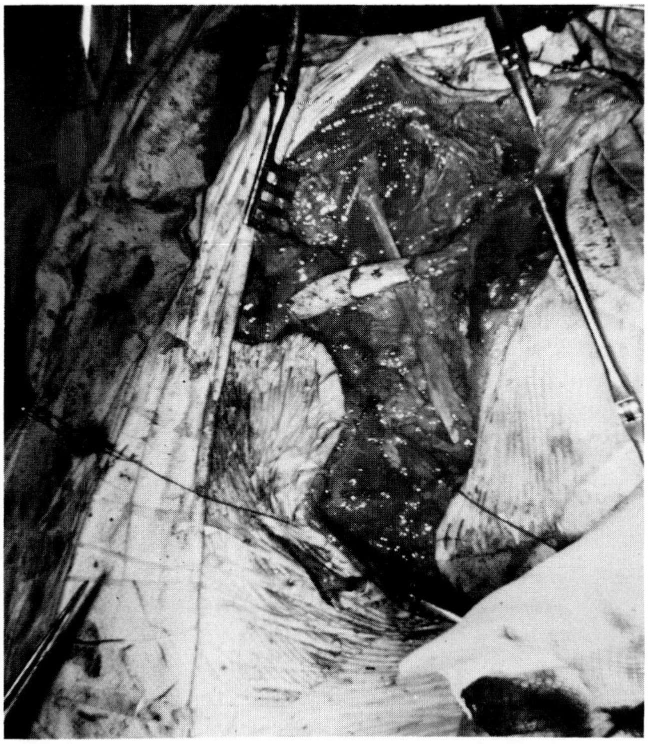

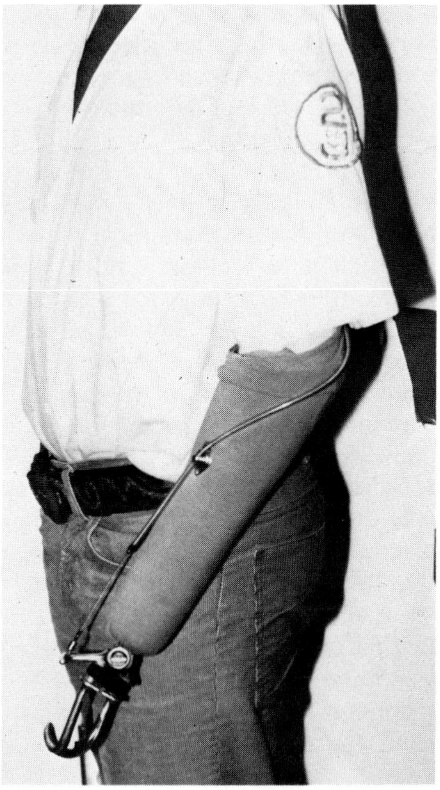

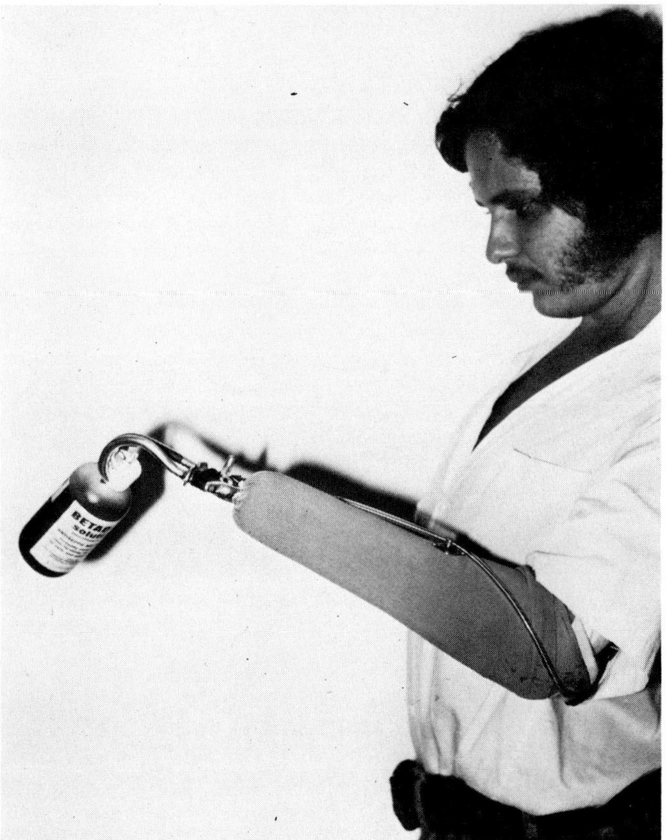

Fig. 10-10. (upper left) A 16-cm sural nerve graft of four cables from the upper trunk to the lateral cord in a patient whose C7, C8, and T1 have been avulsed. **Fig. 10-11 and 10-12.** (right) Eighteen months following nerve grafting with shoulder fusion, forearm amputation, and prosthetic fitting. The active elbow flexion is of significant benefit to the patient's ability to use the prosthesis.

Campbell[46] have reported a series of patients with plexus injuries treated surgically. Narakas[47] has also described his experience. Millesi[48] has published criteria for operations on plexus injuries, which may be used as a guide to surgical possibilities. It is obvious, then, that the management of patients with brachial plexus injuries has undergone important and ongoing changes within the past few years in response to improvements in technology. The surgeon who must advise and treat a patient with a brachial plexus injury must have a well-ordered concept of not only what is available in neurosurgical treatment, but what peripheral reconstruction can offer as well. To attempt to graft the lower trunk of the plexus when chances for restoring the intrinsics by this means are virtually nil, especially when tendon transfer in the hand is usually successful, is to ignore the goal of a functional outcome. The burden imposed on the surgeon is, therefore, one that crosses specialty borders, and must be dealt with. In patients with lesser degrees and distribution of neurologic loss, successful rehabilitation of the upper limb depends on whether a useful hand is potentially or actually present. Many of the peripheral reconstructive procedures may be adapted from their use in poliomyelitis, with the important difference that, in the latter disease, sensation is preserved. The same procedure may be employed in patients with peripheral nerve injuries, where deficits are usually less extensive than in the brachial plexus population. A detailed discussion of these operations[40] is beyond the scope of this chapter.

The problem of pain in patients with brachial plexus injuries is both major and unsolved. Many patients have severe pain, which can be unresponsive even to narcotics. Fortunately it tends to abate with time, but for some it is intractable. Neurolysis is usually not effective treatment, and although some successes for the various operative maneuvers have been recorded, the overall record is a dismal one.[49] Amputating the arm does not help to cure the pain, and may actually be contraindicated when pain is significant.[50]

REFERENCES

1. Strauss MB: Familiar Medical Quotations. Little, Brown and Co, Boston, 1968
2. Bateman JE: Trauma to Nerves in Limbs. WB Saunders, Philadelphia, 1962
3. Seddon HJ: Peripheral Nerve Injuries. Her Majesty's Stationery Office, London, 1961
4. Seddon HJ: Surgical Disorders of the Peripheral Nerves. Second edition. Churchill Livingstone, Edinburgh, London, New York, 1975
5. Sunderland S: Nerves and Nerve Injuries. Williams and Wilkins, Baltimore, 1968
6. Spurling RG, Woodhall B: Surgery in world war II. Neurosurgery. Vol 2. Office of the Surgeon General, Department of the Army, Washington, DC, 1959
7 Smith JW: Microsurgery of peripheral nerves. *J Plast Reconstr Surg 33*:317, 1964
8. Khodadad G: Microsurgical repair of peripheral nerves. *Surg Clin North Am 52*:1157, 1972
9. Ducker TB, Kempe LG, Hayes GJ: The metabolic background for peripheral nerve surgery. *J Neurosurg 30*:270, 1969
10. Seddon HJ: Three types of nerve injury. *Brain 66*:237, 1947
11. Kendall HO, Kendall FP, Wadsworth GE: Muscles, Testing, and Function. Second edition. Williams and Wilkins, Baltimore, 1971
12. Moberg E: Methods for examining sensibility of the hand, Hand Surgery. Edited by Flynn. Williams and Wilkins, Baltimore, 1975
13. Tinel J: Le signe du fourmillement dans les lesions des nerfe peripheriques. *Presse Med 47*:388, 1955
14. Henderson WR: Clinical assessment of peripheral nerve injuries. Tinel's test. *Lancet 2*:801, 1948
15. Electrodiagnosis and Electromyography. Edited by S Licht. New Haven, 1971
16. Leffert RD, Frankel VH: The value of determination of conduction velocity of peripheral nerves in orthopaedic surgery. *Bull Hosp Joint Dis 25*:32, 1963
17. Kline DG, Nulson FE: The neuroma in continuity, in symposium on operative nerve injuries and their repair. *Surg Clin North Am 52*:5, 1972
18. Littler JW: The neurovascular pedicle transfer of tissue in reconstructive surgery of the hand. *J Bone Joint Surg 38*:917, 1956
19. Michon J, Moberg E: Traumatic nerve lesions of the upper limb. Churchill Livingstone, Edinburgh, London, New York, 1975

20. Holstein A, Lewis GB: Fractures of the humerus with radial nerve paralysis. *J Bone Joint Surg 45A*:1382, 1963
21. Hakstian RW: Funicular orientation by direct stimulation. *J Bone Joint Surg 50A*:1178, 1968
22. Gabrielsson GH, Stenstrum SJ: Contribution to peripheral nerve suture technique. *Plast Reconstruct Surg 38*:68-71, 1966
23. Terzis J, Faibisoff B, Williams HB: A diamond knife for microsurgical repair of peripheral nerves. *Plast Reconstr Surg 54*:102-103, 1974
24. Clark GL: Method of preparation of nerve ends for suturing. *Plast Reconstr Surg 34*:233-235, 1964
25. Young JZ, Medawor PB: Fibrin suture of peripheral nerves. *Lancet 2*:126, 1940
26. Tarlov IM: Plasma clot suture of peripheral nerves and nerve roots. Charles C Thomas, Springfield, Illinois, 1950
27. Henry AK: Extensile Exposure. Second edition. Williams and Wilkins, Baltimore, 1957
28. Curtis RM, Eversmann WW: Internal neurolysis as an adjunct to the treatment of the carpal tunnel syndrome. *J Bone Joint Surg 55A*:733, 1973
29. Terzis J, Faibisoff B, Williams HB: Use of polyethylene bag background in microsurgical repair of peripheral nerves. *Plast Reconstruct Surg 53*:596-597, 1974
30. Seddon HJ: Nerve grafting. *J Bone Joint Surg 54A*:727, 1972
31. Millesi H, Meissl G, Berger A: The interfascicular nerve grafting of the median and ulnar nerves. *J Bone Joint Surg 54A*:727, 1972
32. Millesi H, Meissl G, Berger A: Further experience with interfascicular grafting of the median, ulnar, and radial nerves. *J Bone Joint surg 58A*:209, 1976
33. Bora FW: Peripheral nerve repair in cats—the fascicular stitch. *J Bone Joint Surg 49A*:4, 1967
34. Strange FGStC: An operation for nerve pedicle grafting, preliminary communication. *Br J Surg 34*:423, 1947
35. Gutmann E, Guttmann L: Effect of galvanic exercise on denervated and reinnervated muscles in rabbit. *J Neurol Neurosurg Psychiatr 7*:7,1944
36. Bora FW, Lane JM, Prockop DJ: Inhibitors of collagen biosynthesis as a means of controlling scar formation in tendon injury. *J Bone Joint Surg 54A*:1501, 1972
37. Nelson KG, Jolly PC, Thomas PA: Brachial plexus injuries associated with missile wounds of the chest. *J Trauma 8*:268, 1968
38. Brooks DM: Open wounds of the brachial plexus. *J Bone Joint Surg 31B*:17, 1949
39. Leffert RD, Seddon HJ: Infraclavicular brachial plexus injuries. *J Bone Joint Surg 47B*:9, 1965
40. Leffert RD: Brachial plexus injuries. *N Engl J Med 291*:1059-1067, 1974
41. Murphy F, Hartung W, Kirklin JW: Myelographic demonstration of avulsing injury of the brachial plexus. *Am J Roentgenol 58*:102, 1947
42. Bonney G: The value of axon responses in determining the site of the lesion in traction injuries of the brachial plexus. *Brain 77*:588, 1954
43. Yeoman PM: Cervical myelography in traction injuries of the brachial plexus. *J Bone Joint Surg 50B*:2, 1968
44. Hendry AM: The treatment of residual paralysis of the brachial plexus injuries. *J Bone Joint Surg 31*:42-49, 1949
45. Yeoman PM, Seddon HJ: Brachial plexus injuries: treatment of the flail arm. *J Bone Joint Surg 43B*:3, 1961
46. Lusskin R, Campbell JB, Thompson WAL: Post-traumatic lesions of the brachial plexus: treatment by transclavicular exploration and neurolysis or autograft reconstruction. *J Bone Joint Surg 55*:1159-1176, 1973
47. Narakas A: Plexo braquial terapeutica quirirgica directa. *Rev Orthop Traumatol 16*:855, 1972
48. Millesi H, Meissl G, Katzer H: Therapy of brachial plexus injuries: proposal for an integrated therapy (German). *Bruns Beitr Klin Chir 220*:429-446, 1973
49. Taylor PE: Traumatic intradural avulsion of the nerve roots of the brachial plexus. *Brain 85*:579-602, 1962
50. Fletcher I: Traction injuries of the brachial plexus. *Hand 1*:129, 1969

CHAPTER 11
Intraorbital Tumors

Edgar M. Housepian

TO APPRECIATE DETAILS OF surgical techniques, the objectives of the operation must be clearly understood. In turn these objectives are derived from a clear understanding of the nature of the pathology and detailed regional anatomy. Once achieved, the objective, advantages and limitations of a given surgical approach can be understood and a rational choice of technique made. The advantage of the transcranial neurosurgical approach to the orbit is apparent for disease processes that arise in or extend to the intracranial cavity; it also affords superior access to the apical portion of the optic nerve and to the medial and lateral superior quadrants of the orbit.

The great variety of tumors and other mass lesions, which occur behind the eye and cause proptosis, has been of interest to several surgical disciplines. Ophthalmologic surgeons can deal with many of these problems by one of a number of direct orbital approaches. The otolaryngologist can gain access to pathology arising within sinuses bordering the superior, medial, and inferior margins of the orbit. The neurologic surgeon has access to these tumors, which involve both the intracranial and intraorbital space. With the advent of modern neurosurgery, allowing safe access to the orbit by the cranial route, the neurosurgical literature began to reflect an increasing application of transcranial orbital exploration to a large number of orbital problems.[1-5] As one might expect, this encroachment on a traditionally ophthalmologic field led to a period of justifiable controversy regarding the *proper* approach to orbital problems.[6-10] Fortunately, the rapid development of diagnostic radiologic procedures has provided a means of more precisely defining the nature and extent of the problem, bringing some order to the chaos of orbital surgery.

Surgical Anatomy

The purpose of surgical anatomy is to describe and define significant anatomic interrelations and to correlate anatomy with clinical and surgical consideration.[11-14]

The Orbit

The surgeon must be oriented to the medial obliquity of the apex of the orbit (Fig. 11-1). The 5- to 10-mm long optic canal enters the intracranial cavity medial to the anterior clinoid process, beneath which lies one of the two roots of the lesser wing of the sphenoid. This root

Department of Neurological Surgery, College of Physicians and Surgeons, Columbia University, and the New York Neurological Institute, Columbia-Presbyterian Medical Center, New York, New York 10032

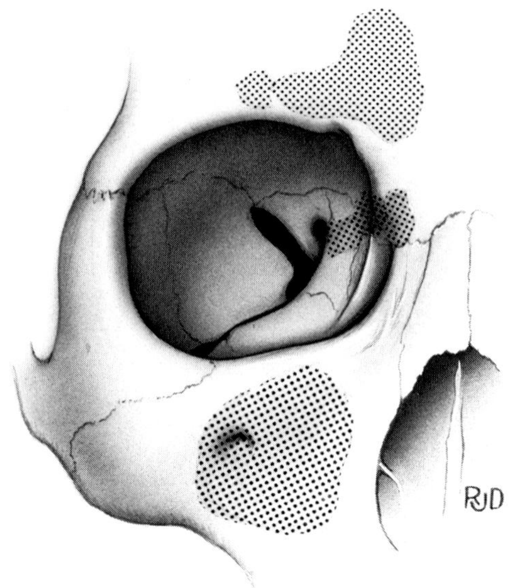

Fig. 11-1. The integrity of the bony orbit and the size and shape of its fissures and foramina may be defined by polytomography. The frontal ethymoidal and maxillary sinuses are shown in diagramatic fashion. Attention is directed to one of the two roots of the lesser wing of the sphenoid, which lies beneath the anterior clinoid and forms the lateral margin of the optic canal in the medial margin of the superior orbital fissure.

forms the lateral wall of the optic canal and the medial margin of the superior orbital fissure. The lateral margin of the superior orbital fissure is bordered by the greater wing of the sphenoid bone, and together with the frontosphenoid process of the zygomatic bone forms the lateral wall of the orbit. The roof of the orbit and the floor of the anterior cranial fossa are, of course, one and the same, and the orbital plate of the maxillary bone forms both the floor of the orbit and the roof of the maxillary sinus. The medial wall of the orbit is formed by the lacrimal bone and the fragile lamina papyracea, which covers the ethymoid sinuses, and closer to the apex, the sphenoid sinus. The frontal sinus, to a variable extent, fills that portion of the frontal bone forming the supraorbital rim.

Optic Nerve

Starting at the chiasmal end, the optic nerve has a flattened horizontal oval shape and measures approximately 4 × 6 mm (Fig. 11-2). After it enters the cranial end of the optic canal, it is 5 mm, circular, and continues to the globe as a 6 × 4 mm vertically oval structure. A pial membrane, carrying the blood supply, accompanies the nerve from the chiasm throughout its entire course to the sclera. The intracranial arachnoid, in like fashion, continues as a discrete structure through the optic canal and fuses with the pia at the globe. There are loose trabeculations in the subarachnoid space. At the apical orbital portion of the nerve however, the pia and arachnoid are fused dorsomedially and ventrally with the dura and the fibrous annulus of Zinn, tethering the optic nerve and partially occluding the subarachnoid space, but not obliterating its continuity. Normally intraocular pressure is slightly higher than intracranial pressure; it is conceivable, therefore, that the *papilledema* found in conditions producing increased intracranial pressure is directly related to this continuity of the subarachnoid space from the cranial cavity to its termination at the lamina cribrosa.

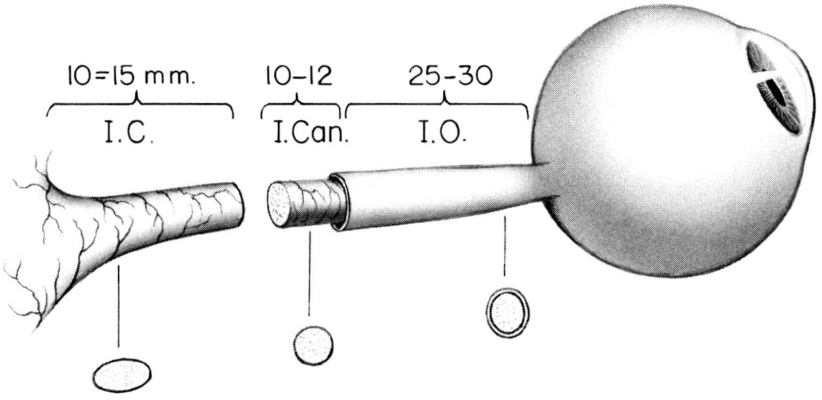

Fig. 11-2. The dimensions and contours of the intracranial, intracanalicular, and intraorbital portions of the optic nerve are shown in diagramatic fashion.

Periorbita

The intracranial dura extends into and lines the optic canal and at the orbital exit of the canal it splits into an outer periosteal (or periorbital) layer and an inner layer that accompanies the optic nerve to the globe, where it fuses with the arachnoid, pia, and sclera (Fig. 11-3). To remove the optic nerve from the globe to the chiasm, as in optic nerve glioma, it is therefore necessary to section the annulus of Zinn and its fibrous attachment to the nerve. The periorbital dura is also continuous with the intracranial dura at the superior orbital fissure and, of course, lines the inferior orbital fissure as well as the other foramina, becoming continuous with the periosteum of the skull at these sites. Anteriorly the periorbita is continuous with the periosteum at the orbital margin; structural modifications in the periorbita enclose the lacrimal gland and fix the pulley of the superior oblique tendon.

This confluence of the periorbita with the intracranial dura at the superior orbital fissure may serve as a route of entry of en plaque meningioma. Arachnoidal rests at this border zone may be the source of intraorbital meningiomas that appear to arise from the periorbita. Resection of meningioma invading the superior fissure can, of course, not be achieved without injuring the important nerves passing therein. Primary optic nerve sheath meningiomas may be defined preoperatively and safely removed by the transcranial approach. When these tumors occur at the extreme apex, where the dural sheath of the optic nerve is fused with the origins of the extraocular muscles at the annulus of Zinn, total excision can be achieved without injury to these structures if they have not been invaded by tumor.

Meningiomas may have a propensity for more rapid growth in children; thus exenteration may be advisable in children if there is microscopic residual at the annulus of Zinn or the superior orbital fissure. In older patients microscopic residual within the muscle cone may be acceptable, because the tumors grow more slowly. The annulus of Zinn provides no barrier for extension of tumor through the optic nerve (Fig. 11-4) and, serial monitoring of the canal for hyperostosis, togther with isotope and computed tomography (CT) scans will not always detect the presence of intracanalicular tumor.

Muscle Cone and Annulus of Zinn

The fibrous annulus tendineus (annulus of Zinn), previously described, serves as the origin of five of the six extraocular muscles (Fig. 11-4). Superiorly the superior rectus muscle arises from the annulus, which, at this point, is fused with the leptomeninges and dura of the

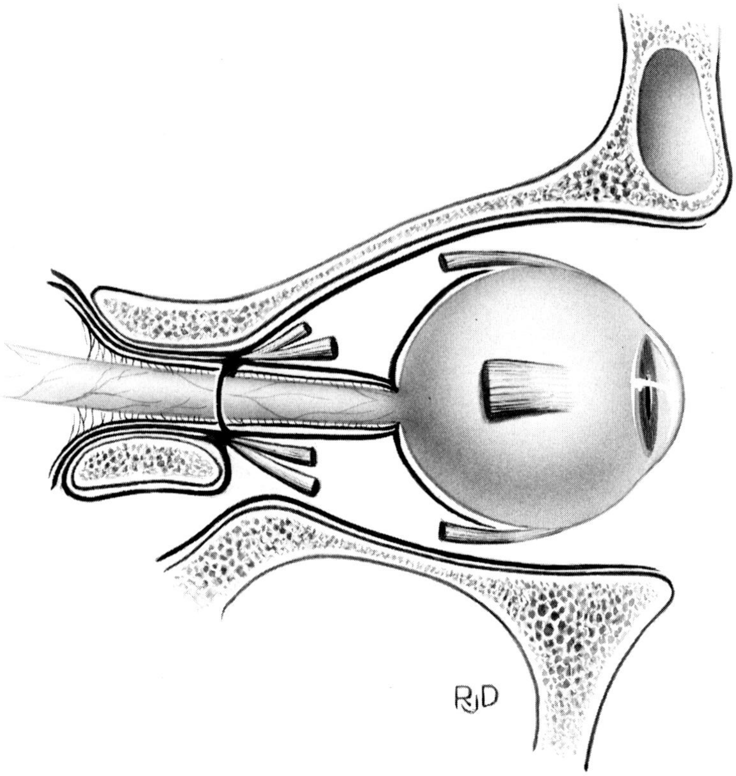

Fig. 11-3. Diagramatic representation of the membranes investing the optic nerve and lining the intracranial cavity, optic canal, and orbit. A double layered intracranial dura is seen extending through the optic canal and superior orbital fissure. The inner layer continues in the orbit as the dural sheath of Schwalb. The outer layer forms the periorbita beyond the annulus of Zinn. There is a continuous subarachnoid space that extends from the intracranial space to the junction of the pia, arachnoid, and dura at the scleral margin. This space is partially obliterated at the annulus of Zinn.

optic nerve. The levator palpebrae origin is medial and superior to that of the superior rectus muscle; more medially and inferior to this is the medial rectus origin. Although firmly fused to the optic nerve dorsally, the annulus of Zinn loops widely around the nerve, laterally and inferiorly, giving rise to the lateral rectus muscle, which has its origin from two heads: the inferior rectus derives its origin with the inferior head; the space between the two heads of the lateral rectus muscle is known as the oculomotor foramen. It is thus evident that this arrangement separates the portal of entry of the nerves, arteries, and veins into essentially three spaces: the optic foramen, superior orbital tissue, and the oculomotor foramen.

Arterial Supply and Venous Drainage

The ophthalmic artery arises from the internal carotid artery at its emergence from the cavernous sinus, passes on the medial side of the anterior clinoid, and runs in a split layer of dura beneath the optic nerves as it enters the orbital cavity through the optic foramen. Upon entering the orbit, it curves over the lateral margin of the optic nerve, gives off the central retinal branch, which perforates the dural sheath approximately 10 mm from the optic foramen, and then, within several millimeters, enters the nerve obliquely about 1.0 cm behind the globe. After giving off the central retinal branch, the ophthalmic artery crosses medially

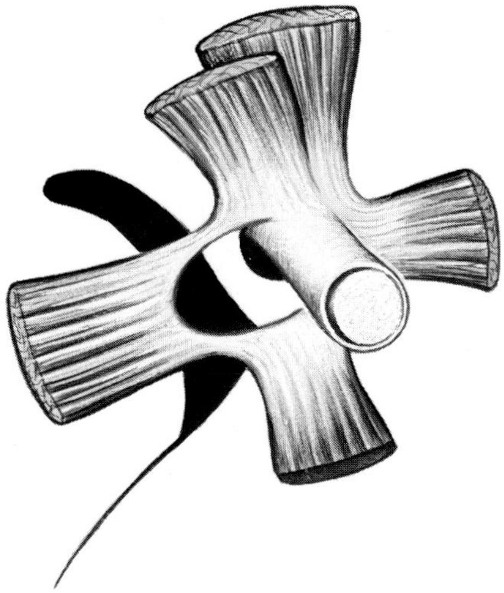

Fig. 11-4. The annulus of Zinn is a fibrous band giving rise to the origins of five of the six extraocular muscles. This fibrous tissue is in continuity with the dural sheath of the optic nerve. The two heads of the lateral rectus loop around that portion of the superior orbital fissure known as the oculomotor foramen.

forward, giving off two long posterior ciliary arteries, six or eight short posterior ciliary arteries, and then anastomoses freely with the external carotid circulation. Two small branches of the ophthalmic artery supply the ocular muscles at their origin near the annulus.[15,16]

Although obstruction of the central retinal artery results in severe loss of visual acuity, obstruction of the ophthalmic artery may not, if the arterial anastomoses are sufficient to preserve blood to the retina.

The orbital cavity is drained principally by the superior and inferior ophthalmic veins. Both of these valveless channels have extensive anastomoses with each other, as well as with external tributaries. The superior ophthalmic vein passes above the lateral rectus muscle, through the superior orbital fissure, to drain into the cavernous sinus. The inferior ophthalmic vein, which primarily drains a network of channels on the medial wall and floor of the orbit, divides, one branch draining the pterygoid plexus through the inferior orbital fissure, the other joining the superior ophthalmic vein before it enters the superior orbital fissure. These extensive communications between the pterygoid plexus and angular and deep facial veins accommodate minor alterations in venous drainage; however, occlusion of the superior ophthalmic vein may result in severe orbital venous congestion, chemosis, and proptosis.

Orbital Nerves

When the orbit is unroofed from above, the frontalis nerve is usually visible through the thin periorbita. Once the periorbita is opened, the surgeon will find the frontalis nerve overlying the levator and superior rectus muscles. In the same plane but closer to the apex lies the fine trochlear nerve. Thus the trochlear nerve, frontalis branch of the fifth nerve and its lacrimal branch pass through the superior orbital fissure in that order, and lie within the periorbita but over the extraocular muscles (Fig. 11-5). The remaining nerves traversing the superior orbital fissure enter the orbit and the muscle cone through the so-called *oculomotor foramen,* between the two heads of the lateral rectus muscle, in the following order: the superior division of the oculomotor nerve, supplying the superior rectus and levator muscles;

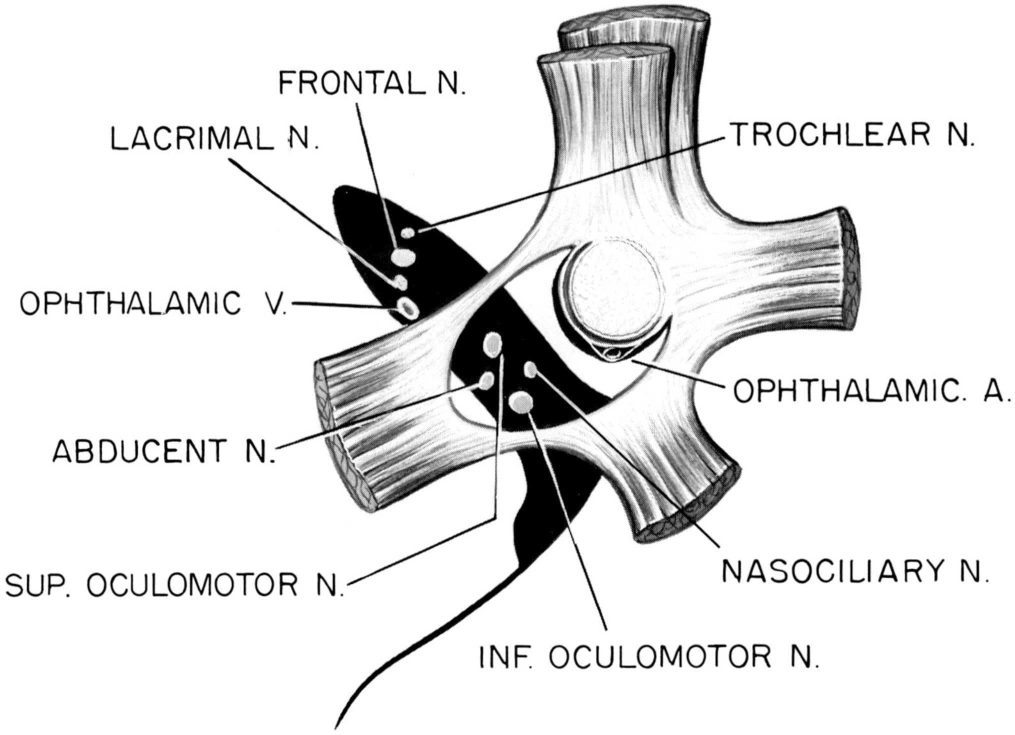

Fig. 11-5. Although partial obliteration of the subarachnoid space of the optic nerve at the annulus of Zinn is shown, the medial origin of the levator muscle is evident. The ophthalmic artery enters the orbit through the optic canal, whereas the superior division of the oculomotor nerve, the abducens nerve, nasociliary nerve, and the inferior division of the oculomotor nerve enter the muscle cone through the oculomotor foramen. The trochlear nerve, frontalis and lacrimal nerves, and ophthalmic vein enter through the superior orbital fissure and thus lie within the periorbita but outside of the muscle cone.

the nasociliary branch of the ophthalmic nerve; the sixth nerve; and the inferior division of the third nerve. The nasociliary nerve crosses over the optic nerve to reach the medial wall of the orbit. The ciliary ganglion lies lateral to the optic nerve. The inferior division of the oculomotor nerve crosses beneath the optic nerve to reach the medial and inferior rectus muscles.

Because of this arrangement, it is clear that the optic nerve can be approached directly through the medial compartment, between the medial rectus and levator muscles, without fear of injury to the nerve supply of any extraocular muscle (Fig. 11-6). The trochlear nerve can rarely be spared. When optic nerve resection is the objective, however, there is little functional or cosmetic consequence of fourth-nerve section.

Careful dissection through the lateral compartment, between the lateral and superior rectus and levator muscles, allows access to *solitary* neurofibromata, which most frequently arise from branches of the long ciliary nerves lying lateral to the optic nerve.

Tumors or mass lesions that arise external to the muscle cone are most likely to cause proptosis without limitation of extraocular movements or loss of vision. Some tumors within the muscle cone cause proptosis without neurologic or ophthalmologic findings; however, tumors that crowd the apex are most likely to lead to dysfunction of one or more of the extraocular muscles or their nerve supply, causing specific deficits.

A clear understanding of orbital apical anatomy should help the surgeon to approach safely the apical region and provides a basis for understanding the surgical limitations imposed by specific kinds of pathology. As stated, the primary advantage of transcranial explo-

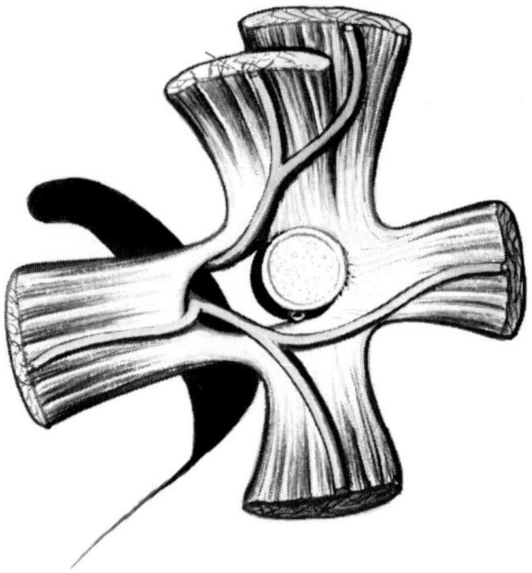

Fig. 11-6. Diagramatic representation of the nerve supply to the extraocular muscles shown entering through the oculomotor foramen. A medial superior approach to the optic nerve between the lateral and medial rectus muscles provides direct access, with minimal chance of injury to this nerve supply to the extraocular muscles.

ration is related to safe access to and preservation of function of the structures of the orbital apex. If the pathology is such that function cannot be preserved by any approach, there are other far simpler direct approaches to this region.

Diagnosis

When orbital pathology is suspected and, in particular, when unilateral exophthalmos exists, a logical sequential workup should follow the clinical examination.[15-21] This should begin with good quality radiographs of the skull, orbits, and optic canals. Calcified, hyperostosing, and grossly destructive lesions can be identified, and sinus disease may be seen.

Pleuridirectional tomography is the most critical radiographic diagnostic procedure for defining the integrity of the orbit. Polytomes provide precise definition of the bony margins of the orbit. The precise extent of a hyperostosing process may be defined in this way. Areas of dehiscence, dissolution, or destruction of bony structure can be shown that give clues to the presence of encephalocele, sinus pathology, or destructive and invasive processes.

Radioactive scanning of the orbit with mercury has helped to differentiate a number of processes. Most neoplasms found in the orbit will show positive uptake on isotope scan; nontumorous pathology, such as hyperthyroidism, is associated with a negative scan. Thus for preliminary screening, this technique is particularly useful in patients who present with proptosis and in whom plain films are normal. Isotope scanning may also be helpful in follow-up evaluation of patients who have undergone surgery for tumor. An exception to this is the patient with neurofibroma; isotope scans are usually negative in this case.

The recent availability of computerized tomography has proved extremely useful in defining orbital pathology. A well-performed study will show normal orbital anatomy, including size and portion of the globe, optic nerve, and extraocular muscles. The size and extent of meningioma, optic glioma, and neurofibroma can be defined preoperatively. Most of these tumors enhance with contrast.

Pneumoencephalography was singularly useful for defining chiasmal extension or origin of optic glioma. In this regard, although large chiasmal gliomas can easily be defined by computerized tomography, pneumoencephalography is still useful in some cases and is the more critical of the two studies in defining small chiasmal lesions.

Orbital angiography and venography have a place in defining vascular lesions in the orbit. Nevertheless they are required with less frequency now that a combination of noninvasive studies is available, which together with a clinical evaluation allows the nature and extent of intraorbital pathology to be defined with a high degree of accuracy.

Case Selection

When a thoughtful sequential diagnostic workup has been completed, the location and extent of pathology can be defined. Is a tumor present at all? If so, is it confined within the muscle cone? Does it arise from, medial to, or lateral to the optic nerve? Is the optic canal enlarged or hyperostotic? Is the bony integrity of the orbit violated? Are the fissures normal? Is the process erosive or destructive? Does the pathology extend to or from a sinus or arise from or enter the cranial cavity?

The clinical diagnosis of optic nerve glioma can be made with a high degree of accuracy. In these cases primary treatment should be the transcranial approach when clinical evidence limits the tumor to a single optic nerve. There is no disagreement that surgical excision is the treatment of choice in a patient with glioma of a single optic nerve, who presents with proptosis and poor vision in the involved eye. The rationale for the transcranial orbital approach is based on the conclusion that a wide excision, from the globe to the chiasm, is necessary to ensure total removal. A simple orbital resection too often will leave residual tumor in the apical stump of the transected, tumor-bearing nerve.

Surgical resection would not be considered when there is multicentric optic glioma or chiasmal involvement. The place of radiotherapy is not as generally agreed; however, there is good evidence, in our own large series of cases, that astrocytoma of the optic nerve is a benign but progressive process, similar to piloid astrocytoma of childhood in other locations. Our experience suggests that in many cases radiotherapy effectively arrests the course and improves proptosis and vision.

When meningioma of the optic nerve or orbit is suspected, transcranial exploration is the preferred approach. These tumors frequently involve both the cranial and orbital cavities. The transcranial approach also allows direct and safe access to the apical part of the optic nerve. Tumors arising from the lateral periorbita from arachnoidal rests near the superior orbital fissure are frequently associated with multicentric or implanted lesions on the cranial side of the superior orbital fissure.

A microneurosurgical technique is essential for the successful removal of solitary neurofibromata, usually found lateral to the optic nerve. Although the transcranial approach provides good access to these lesions, they may also be accessible to lateral canthotomy (Kroenlein operation). In view of the relative difficulty in making this diagnosis clinically, the latter approach may be advantageous.

Osteomas arising from the posterior ethmoid region can be defined and a transcranial approach selected for primary removal because of their medial epiperiorbital location. A two-stage procedure may be considered for very large lesions extending into intracranial spaces.

Obviously encephaloceles must be treated by a neurosurgical approach and some dermoids and hemangioma of the orbit may be. Lesions, such as ossifying fibroma and aneurysmal bone cyst, that border both orbit and cranial cavity can best be dealt with by the transcranial operation.

Nevertheless, a vast majority of problems arising in the orbit can more simply be dealt with by a direct approach, including mucocele, hemangioma, lymphangioma, and others.

Similarly malignant processes and nontumorous pathology must not be exposed by the cranial route for fear of seeding. Finally, the surgeon dealing with proptosis must be aware of its nonsurgical causes, such as pseudotumor and thyrotoxicosis.

Preoperative Management and Anesthesia

General anesthesia is used in all cases of transcranial orbital exploration. Principles of neuroanesthesia are adhered to and there are no special anesthesia requirements for exploring the orbit. Decadron is used as an intraoperative and postoperative adjunct to reduce postoperative edema resulting from exploration within the orbit. Mannitol is used intraoperatively to reduce intraocular as well as intracranial tension so that a suitable surgical field is obtained without major retraction of the frontal lobe.

Aids to Operation

Besides deserving credit for systematizing the preoperative workup in patients with orbital tumors, neurosurgery may also claim contributions to improved instrumentation and techniques for operating within the orbit. Thus Maroon and Kennerdell[22] recently described the advantages of neurosurgical techniques in an ophthalmologic lateral approach to the orbit. Magnification with loops and microscope is mandatory when operating on the fine and attenuated structures within the orbit. Similarly cottonoids and controlled suction are indispensable, as is the use of small malleable retractors. Bipolar coagulation has materially added to the safety of operating within the orbit by either the cranial or direct orbital approach.

Operative Procedure

After induction of anesthesia, intubation, and insertion of a Foley catheter, the patient is placed in the recumbent supine position on the operating table, with knees flexed, the back slightly elevated, and the head slightly extended. A four-hole osteoplastic craniotomy is planned (Fig. 11-7). An anteromedial trephination is located low in the midline, just above the glabella. A posteromedial trephination is marked off the midline, but covering the sagittal sinus. An anterolateral trephination is marked at the temporal side of the temporal ridge, above the lateral margin of the orbit, and a posterolateral trephination is marked at the frontal convexity, beneath the insertion of the temporalis muscle.

A coronal incision is then planned, with the lower limb toward the side of the orbit to be explored. The incision should be placed approximately 1.0 cm behind the marked trephination sites.

After the patient is prepped and draped, the scalp and galea are incised and turned as one layer, with care taken to keep from attenuating the periosteum. Hemostasis is achieved with Michelle clips or clamps. The reflected scalp and galea should be brought to within 1.0 cm of the glabella but not lower to the orbital rim. If the galeal dissection extends to the orbital rim there will be considerable postoperative ecchymosis and swelling; in addition there may be injury to the supraorbital vessel and nerve.

The periosteum is incised approximately 1.0 cm above the glabella in a horizontal direction extending from approximately 1.5 cm across the midline toward the side of the exposure and through the insertion of the temporalis fascia and muscle at the temporal ridge. Cutting current is frequently helpful for this portion of the procedure. The periosteum is then incised paramedially and along the posterior limb of the flap. It is preferable to make the periosteal

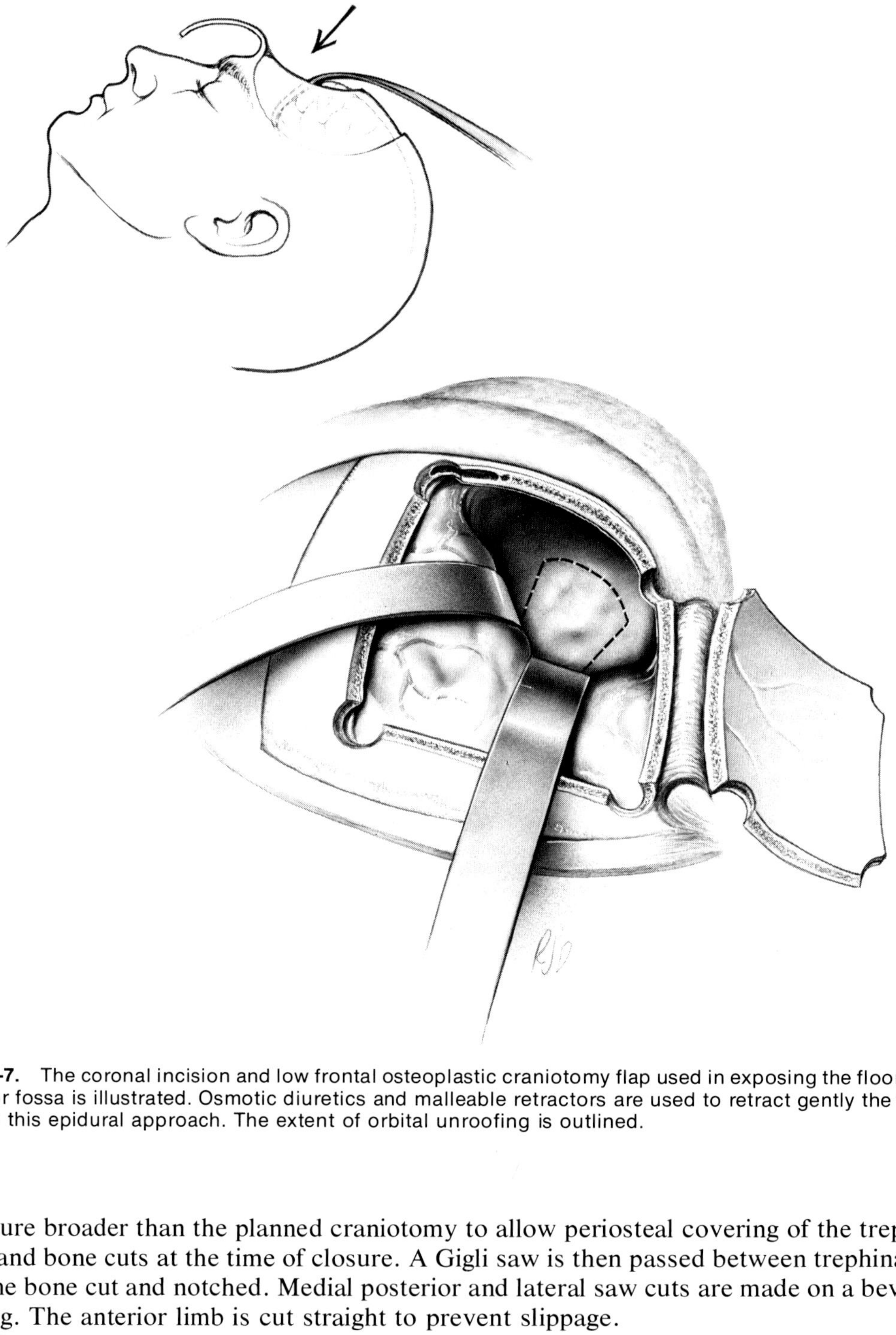

Fig. 11-7. The coronal incision and low frontal osteoplastic craniotomy flap used in exposing the floor of the anterior fossa is illustrated. Osmotic diuretics and malleable retractors are used to retract gently the frontal lobe in this epidural approach. The extent of orbital unroofing is outlined.

exposure broader than the planned craniotomy to allow periosteal covering of the trephinations and bone cuts at the time of closure. A Gigli saw is then passed between trephinations and the bone cut and notched. Medial posterior and lateral saw cuts are made on a bevel for seating. The anterior limb is cut straight to prevent slippage.

If a large frontal sinus is exposed, it is recommended that this be repaired before the dura is opened. If the mucosa is intact, Gelfoam is simply placed over this. However, if the mucosa is lacerated, the entire sinus is exenterated and the mucosa rolled and impacted into the region of the osteum. Instruments used to handle the mucosa are not reused for the cranial procedure. A piece of temporalis muscle is then placed over the rolled mucosa, and the exenterated sinus is filled with Neobacin dipped Gelfoam. A rectangular flap of pericranium is then separated from the forward edge and sutured to the dura to prevent extrusion of the muscle and Gelfoam.

After all bone margins are waxed and tenting sutures placed at the posterior and lateral dural periphery, and after the bone flap and its pedicle of temporalis muscle and fascia is covered with moist gauze, the wound is thoroughly irrigated, fresh towels placed at the margin, and all exposed surfaces, except the area of dura to be incised are covered with gauze or cottonoids.

If the orbit is being explored for optic glioma,[23] it is advisable to incise the dura and inspect the intracranial optic nerve before proceeding with the orbital unroofing. If tumor is found to extend into the chiasm, indicating that gross total resection can not be achieved, the procedure is discontinued. Once tumor is identified within the nerve, but *not* extending to the chiasm, the optic nerve is cut perpendicular to its direction at the chiasm. Hemostasis of the fine pial circulation is simply achieved with Gelfoam. If tumor is not identified in the intracranial space, the optic nerve should not be sectioned until glioma is identified intraorbitally.

Orbital exploration demands an epidural approach. This protects the underlying brain, which may require gentle retraction. In addition it protects the olfactory nerve and bulb from avulsion. Since the dura inserts at the cribriform fossa lateral to the olfactory nerve, epidural retraction avoids injury in this location. Malleable retractors are shaped and curved to expose the entire anterior fossa up to the clinoid. If properly shaped, they will serve as self-retaining retractors. Moist cottonoids are placed at the lateral margins of the exposure to advance the epidural dissection, allow irrigation, and facilitate suctioning.

The orbital unroofing is begun with a chisel or a high-speed burr. Once a small opening is made in the midportion of the floor of the anterior fossa, the remainder of the resection is facilitated by the use of fine double-action mastoid or infant Leksell ronguers (Fig. 11-8). The canal may be unroofed, if required, with infant Kerrison ronguers. The orbital unroofing does not need to come closer than 1.0 cm from the orbital rim anteriorally; it should extend approximately 1.5 cm from the medial margin and should be extended laterally to within 0.5 cm of the lateral orbital margin.

The periorbita is usually thin and transparent. When there is a significant orbital mass, the intraorbital structures are attenuated and blanched and may be difficult to see. The periorbita is incised in a cruciate fashion with a No. 11 blade. The vertical limb is placed lateral or medial to the levator and superior rectus muscles, depending on whether a lateral or medial approach to the orbit is planned. The frontalis nerve is usually visible through the periorbita, as it lies over these muscles. It serves to approximate their location. The trochlear nerve, which lies beneath the periorbita but outside of the muscle cone, is only rarely visualized. It lies close to the apex, is extremely fine, and can rarely be spared if apical pathology is encountered.

Approach to the Medial Orbit

A medial approach to the optic nerve is preferred when dealing with meningioma or optic glioma (Fig. 11-9). The primary advantage of this approach relates to the nerve supply to extraocular muscles. We are now aware that the third nerve, after it enters the orbit through the superior orbital fissure and oculomotor foramen lateral to the optic nerve, sends branches *over* the nerve to supply the under belly of the levator and superior rectus muscles and *beneath* the nerve to the inferior and medial rectus muscles. Thus a medial approach to the optic nerve can be made without traversing the course of these nerves to the extraocular muscles. Small malleable retractors are individually bent to retract the levator and superior rectus complex laterally and anteriorally. Tumor pathology is approached by blunt dissection through residual orbital fat. Magnification and gentle handling of tissues are essential to this

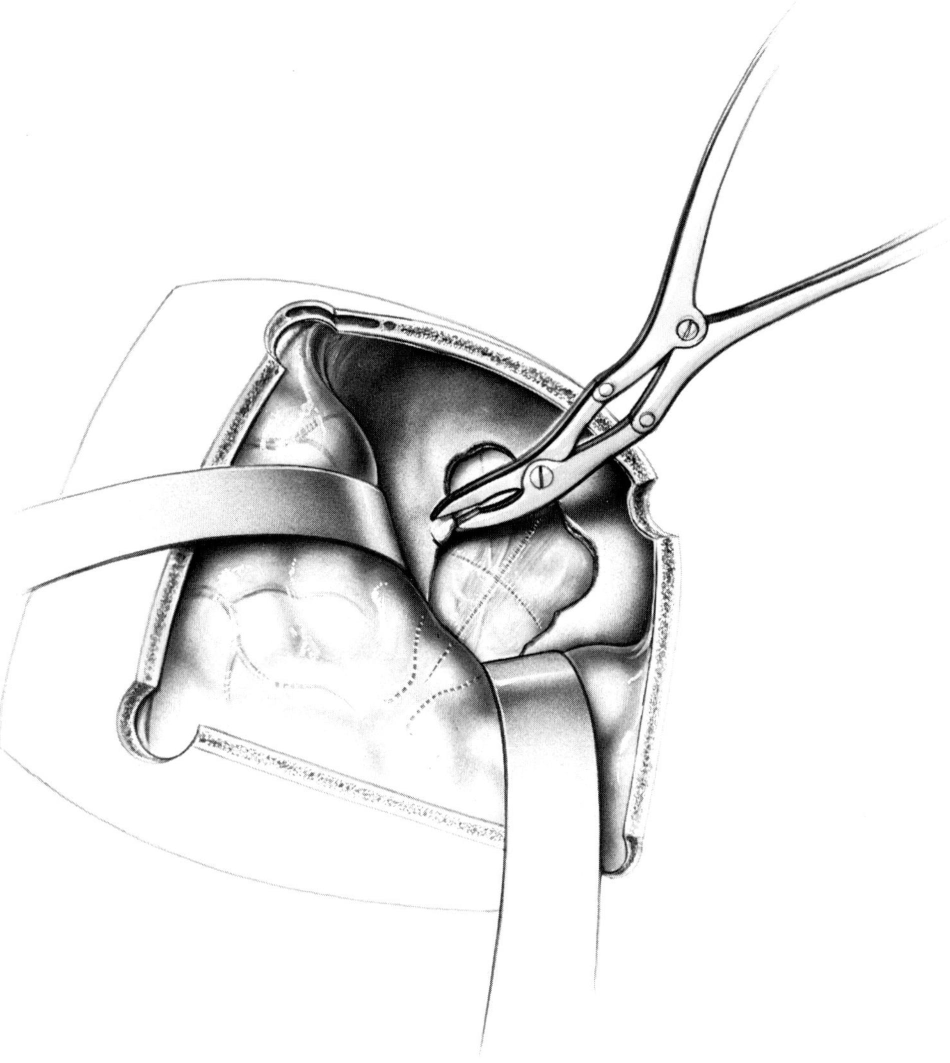

Fig. 11-8. The thin orbital roof is entered with a chisel or burr. The unroofing is completed with fine double action and Leksell ronguers. When necessary, the optic canal is opened as illustrated. The frontalis nerve may be seen through the thin periosteum and is a landmark indicating the course of the levator and superior rectus muscles which are often seen with difficulty. The dura is incised medial or lateral to these structures as indicated.

portion of the procedures. Both optic gliomas and primary optic nerve sheath meningioma are fairly firm encapsulated tumors, and a plane of dissection is started directly on the tumor capsule. Gentle retraction and the placement of moist cottonoids allows the development of a plane entirely around the tumor capsule, which is not adherent to the surrounding residual areolar tissue. This tissue separates and protects the normal neurovascular structures and which can be spared in this way during tumor removal. The junction of the tumor and the posterior margin of the globe is readily found. At this point the nerve is transected between two fine mosquito forceps used to clamp the tumor-bearing optic nerve. This technique will avoid injury to the posterior margin of the globe and the sclera. After the nerve is sectioned, the distal clamp is removed and any bleeding from the cut margin is carefully electrocoagulated with bipolar cautery. The proximal clamp may be used as a handle for further tumor dissection toward the apex.

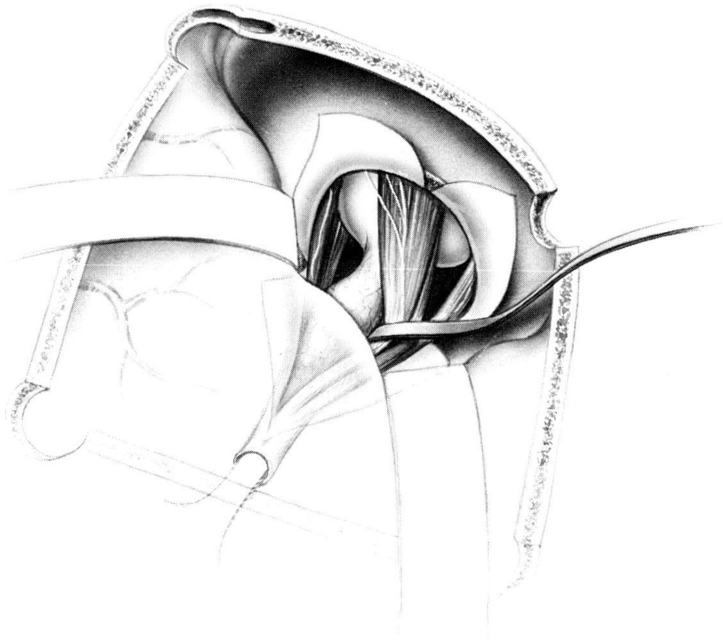

Fig. 11-9. Narrow malleable retractors and cottonoid pledgets are used to retract gently the orbital structures. The preferred approach to the optic nerve is shown.

In optic nerve glioma, to remove the tumor in one piece, from the globe to the chiasm (Fig. 11-10), the origin of the levator muscle, which inserts at the annulus of Zinn medial to the superior rectus, must be sectioned. Only in this way can the annulus of Zinn be opened from above to remove the canalicular portion of the optic nerve tethered at the orbital end of the canal. The levator origin may then be resutured after the pathology is removed. This maneuver is difficult, and in young infants structures are small and exposure limited, making the procedure difficult and unnecessary. The optic nerve can be sectioned with curved scissors at the extreme apex and the orbital specimen removed. At this juncture the ophthalmic artery is sometimes severed but the bleeding can simply be controlled with bipolar electrocautery. The intracranial portion of the nerve may then be removed as a second specimen. In order to accomplish this, epidural retractors must, of course, be removed and placed intradurally, reexposing the intracranial optic nerve so that it may now be pulled through the canal. If the surgeon feels that there may be a small amount of residual glioma at the canalicular face of the annulus, brief electrocoagulation on an angle nerve hook can safely be used. In any event a small pledget of temporalis muscle placed within the canal will prevent the flow of cerebral spinal fluid into the orbital space in the immediate postoperative period.

When dealing with primary optic nerve sheath meningioma, after the tumor has been resected, the proximal stump of the optic nerve, at the annulus of Zinn, must be inspected, preferably with the operating microscope, to determine if there is microscopic residual tumor at the annulus and origins of the extraocular muscles. Intracranial intradural inspection of the optic nerve should also be done with the operating microscope. If there is evidence of tumor at the cranial end of the optic canal, the preferred approach is to unroof the optic canal, open the intracanalicular dura, section the levator origin at the annulus of Zinn, and open the annulus. This will permit high-power inspection and gross total removal of tumor and optic nerve from the orbit close to the globe, back to the cranial end of the optic nerve near the

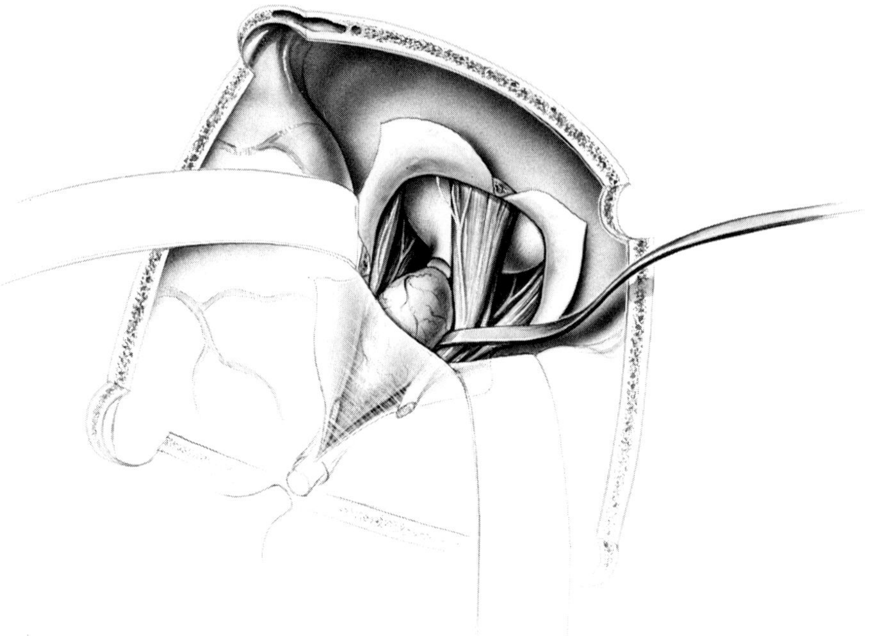

Fig. 11-10. The technique of sectioning the levator is illustrated. The annulus of Zinn cannot be opened without performing this maneuver. After resecting a tumor bearing optic nerve from the globe to the chiasm, the origin of the levator muscle is resutured. This maneuver is useful in some cases of optic glioma and meningioma.

chiasm. The annulus and levator origin should then be resutured with fine atraumatic silk or synthetic suture.

Cushing[1] has described a psammomatous meningioma arising at the sheath of Schwann and growing into the optic nerve. Though not clearly defined, it may represent the origin of some nerve sheath meningiomas. There is ample histopathologic evidence for a primary intraorbital origin of optic nerve meningioma. Meningioma of the optic nerve sheath has been found to occur in the orbit and traverse the optic canal by microscopic spread along the subarachnoid space, without producing enlargement or hyperostosis of the optic canal, though these radiographic signs are usually present.

Lateral Orbital Approach

The transcranial orbital approach to the lateral superior quadrant of the orbit is used for cases of suspected solitary neurofibroma believed to arise from the long ciliary nerves. They are thus found in a position lateral to the optic nerve. In these cases the periorbital opening is made lateral to the superior rectus insertion (Fig. 11-11), and using the techniques described for orbital exploration with malleable retractors and cottonoids, a plane is developed directly on the tumor capsule. Efforts are made to separate the loose areolar tissue from the tumor itself and minimize dissection within this tissue. To achieve lateral quadrant exposure the superior rectus is retracted medially. If the tumor is large, it may be broken into several pieces for removal. Efforts should be made to avoid the extreme apex from the lateral approach in order to minimize the chance of injury to the sixth nerve.

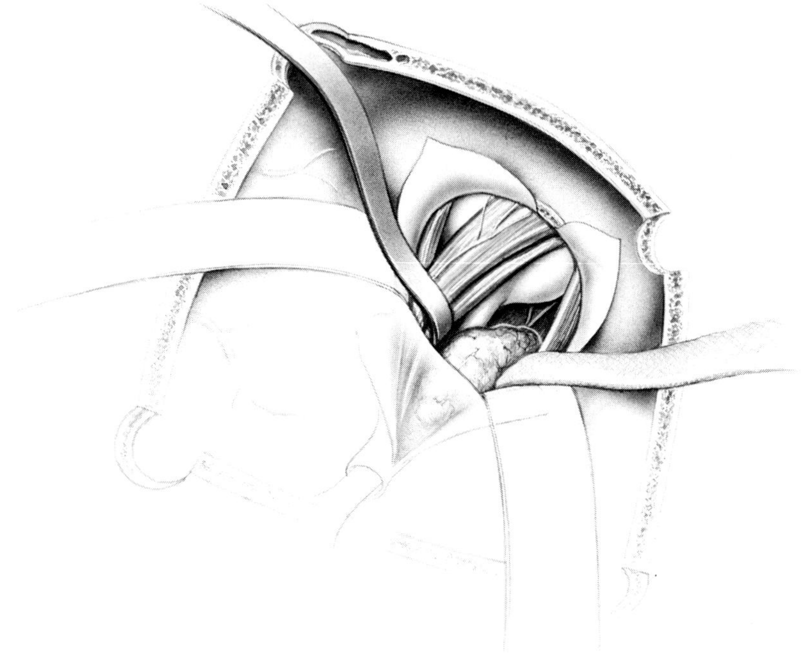

Fig. 11-11. The lateral transcranial orbital approach to an apical neurofibroma is shown. Dissection in the areolar tissue is avoided and cottonoid pledgets and shaped, narrow, malleable retractors are used to define a plane directly on the tumor capsule. Injury to the extraocular nerve supply is avoided in this way.

Closure

Once tumor removal is complete and before releasing retraction, cottonoids are carefully removed and the apical bed inspected for hemostasis. Bipolar electrocoagulation should be sparingly used to achieve this. Extensive electrocauterization behind the globe should be avoided, since it may injure the retinal blood supply as well as the sympathetic nerves and result in pupillary dilatation and corneal anesthesia. When the field is dry, all retractors and cottonoids are removed, the levator origin resutured, if sectioned, and the periorbita closed loosely by approximating the four corners. Gelfoam should then be placed over the periorbita and a piece of stainless steel screen fashioned to bridge the orbital roof defect to avoid pulsation of the globe (Fig. 11-12). No attempt should be made to close completely the entire defect. The midportion is simply bridged and the prosthesis curved to approximate the normal curve of the orbital roof. Gelfoam is then placed on the outer surface of the screen and the dura allowed to fall back after retraction is removed. Cranial dura is sutured to the pericranium; this alone holds the screen in place and no other effort need be made to secure it to the orbital roof. If the intracranial dura has been opened, it is, of course, sutured in a water-tight fashion.

Closure of the craniotomy defect should follow standard practice. Epidural and subgaleal drains are recommended; however, if the sinus has been entered, suction drainage should be avoided. Thorough irrigation during all stages of closure is recommended to remove bits of bone dust or bone wax and dry blood.

The Berke modification of the Kroenlein operation[6] may provide good access to pathology in the lateral quadrant of the orbit. The application of neurosurgical techniques, as

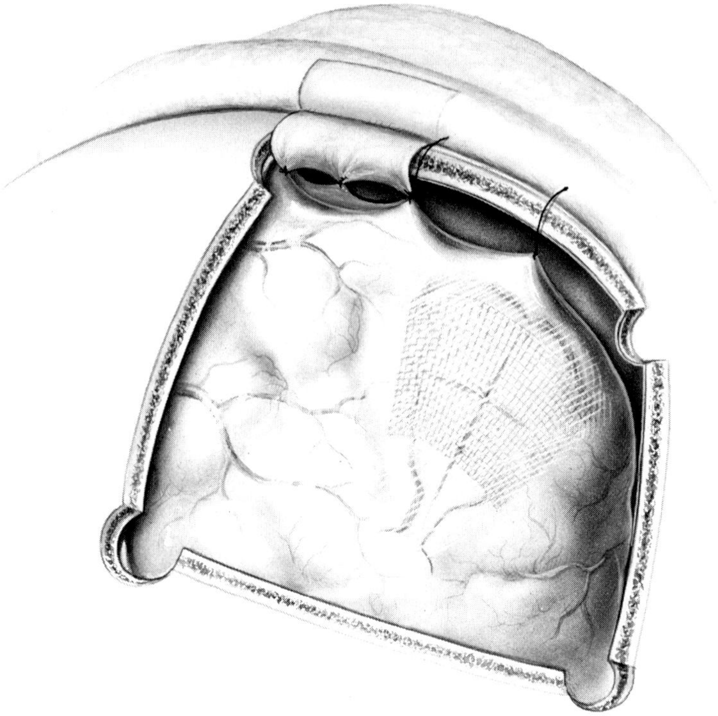

Fig. 11-12. Upon completion of tumor removal the periorbita is closed with one or several fine atraumatic sutures; Gelfoam is placed over the periorbita; a wire mesh bridge is formed and placed at the orbital roof defect to avoid postoperative pulsation of the globe. Dural tenting sutures are then placed and any defect in the frontal sinus repaired, and a flap of pericranium sutured to the dura to cover the bony defect.

described by Maroon and Kennerdell, and adherence to strict microsurgical technique should allow safe access to the lateral apex and minimize the possibility of injury to the sixth nerve. A direct approach is *not* recommended for primary optic nerve tumors, however, because of the anatomic configuration of the nerve supply to the extraocular muscles, as described previously.

Tarsorrhaphy

Prior to extubation and after the head dressing has been applied, tarsorrhaphy should be performed in all cases of orbital exploration, regardless of the route. The procedure is simple and atraumatic (Fig. 11-13). The lids are washed with a cotton ball and pHisohex solution and the cornea and conjunctiva irrigated with saline. Sterile towels are placed to keep the sutures sterile. A double-ended 6-0 suture is used to place a horizontal mattress with two rubberband bumper guards. The thin skin of the lid is protected with the bumpers and makes removal of the tarsorrhaphy simple. In principle, the suture should be placed directly over the cornea, and should pass through the grey line (tarsall plate) of both lids. Care should be taken to see that there are no inverted lashes prior to tying. When the tarsorrhaphy is completed an ophthalmic ointment is used to lubricate the cornea and conjunciva. A pledget of Adaptec gauze is placed over the eye; three small cotton balls are then used to provide gentle pressure

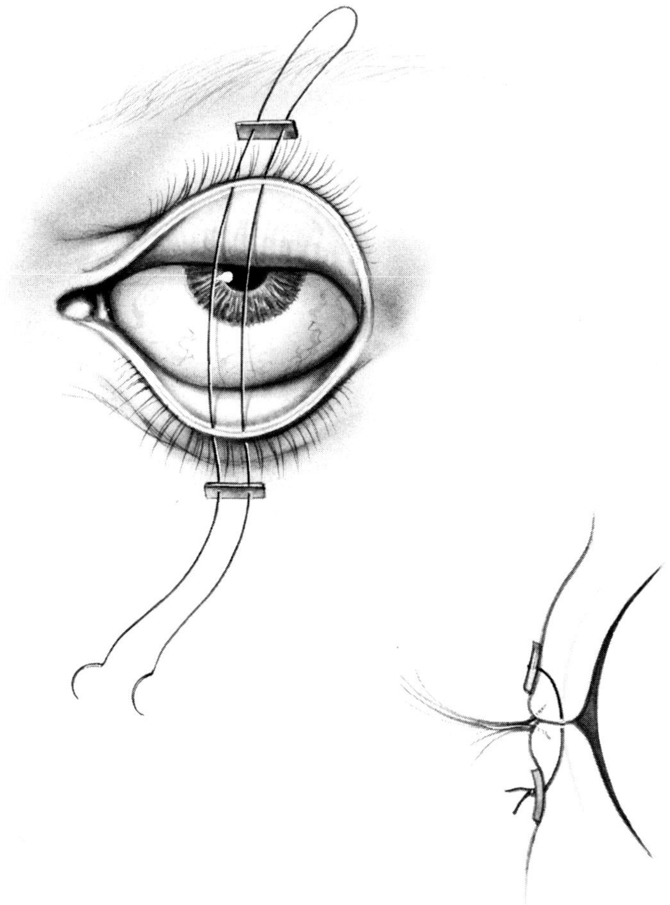

Fig. 11-13. The technique for temporary tarsorrhaphy is shown. A fine double-ended atraumatic suture is placed through the tarsal plate of each lid. Small rubber bumpers prevent maceration of the thin skin of the lid.

when taped to the head dressing. It is important for the surgeon to remove the tarsorrhaphy dressing daily to inspect the eye for signs of irritation, and ophthalmic ointment reapplied. The tarsorrhaphy is left in place until the peak edema period has passed. It is advisable to remove the pressure dressing one day before the tarsorrhaphy suture is removed. In this way, if pressure has been removed prematurely and the eye begins to bulge, the cornea will be protected.

Postoperative Care

Antibiotics are not used routinely for this procedure; dexamethasone, however, is. Antiedema doses are used through the fourth day and then tapered over the ensuing week. With some care in hemostasis, blood transfusion is usually not required. Anticonvulsant therapy may be used, although there is usually little retraction injury to the orbital brain surface.

Complications

Transcranial exploration should be a relatively benign procedure. There is, however, transient levator and superior rectus palsy in all cases. This may be complete or partial. Improvement usually is seen from within several days to 3 to 6 weeks and is complete by 3 months. Ptosis and limitation of extraocular movement could be a permanent accompaniment of orbital tumor removal by any approach. Postoperative keratitis is an infrequent but recognized complication. Seizure is almost never seen during the postoperative period.

Conclusions

Currently available diagnostic techniques have vastly improved our ability to predict the nature, precise location, and extent of tumors of the orbit. Familiarity with the variety of disease that occur in the orbit and may produce proptosis is essential to the neurosurgeon involved in the management of patients with orbital disease. A clear understanding of the regional anatomy will allow the surgeon to plan his surgical approach based on rational surgical objectives. It is not only well to know when and how to operate, but also when not to operate.

REFERENCES

1. Cushing H, Eisenhardt L: Meningiomas. Charles C Thomas, Springfield, 1938
2. Dandy WE: Results following transcranial attack on orbital tumors. *Arch Ophthalmol 25*:191-216, 1941
3. Love JG, Benedict WL: Transcranial removal of intraorbital tumors. *JAMA 121*:777-784, 1945
4. Matson DD: Unilateral exophthalmos in childhood. *Clin Neurosurg 5*:116-126, 1958
5. Van Buren JM, Poppen JL, Horrax G: Unilateral exophthalmos: a consideration of symptom pathogenesis. *Brain 80*:139-175, 1957
6. Berke RN: A modified Kronlein operation. *Trans Am Ophthalmol Soc 51*:193-231, 1953
7. Davis FA: Primary tumors of the optic nerves. *Arch Ophthalmol 23*:735-821, 957-1022, 1940
8. Jackson H: Orbital tumors. *Proc Soc Med 38*:587-594, 1945
9. Reese AB: Expanding lesions of the orbit. *Trans Ophthalmol Soc UK 91*:85, 1971
10. Spencer WH: Primary neoplasms of the optic nerve and its sheaths: Clinical features and current concepted pathogenetic mechanisms. *J Am Ophthalmol Soc 70*:490-528, 1972
11. Cunningham's Manual of Practical Anatomy. Edited by JP Brash. Oxford University Press, London, 1948
12. Duke-Elder S, Wybar KC: The anatomy of the visual system, *System of Ophthalmology,* vol 2. CV Mosby, St Louis, 1961
13. Last RJ: *Wolff's Anatomy of the Eye and Orbit.* Sixth edition. WB Saunders, Philadelphia, 1968
14. Pernkopf E: *Atlas of Topographical and Applied Human Anatomy,* vol 1. WB Saunders, Philadelphia, 1963
15. Hanafee WN, Shiu PS, Dayton GO: Orbital venography. *Am J Roentgenol 104*:29, 1968
16. Lombardi G: *Radiology in Neuroophthalmology.* Williams and Wilkins, Baltimore, 1967
17. Coleman DJ, Konig WF, Kata L: A hand-operated ultrasound scan system for ophthalmic evaluation. *Am J Ophthalmol 68*:256-263, 1969
18. Evans RA, Schwartz, JF, Chutorian AM: Radiologic diagnosis in pediatric ophthalmology. *Radiol Clin N Am 1*:459-495, 1963
19. Potter GD, Trokel S: Tomography of the optic canal. *Am J Roentgenol Radiother 106*:530-535, 1969
20. Schlesinger EB, Trokel SL, Baily S: Radioactive scanning in the analysis of unilateral exophthalmos. *Trans Am Acad Ophthalmol Otolaryngol 73*:1005-1011, 1969
21. Tenner MS, Trokel SL: Radiologic methods in neuroopthalmologic problems. *Am J Ophthalmol 68*:883-895, 1969
22. Maroon JC, Kennerdell JS: Lateral microsurgical approach to intraorbital tumors. *J Neurosurg 44*:556-561, 1976
23. Housepian EM: Surgical treatment of unilateral optic nerve gliomas. *J Neurosurg 31*:604-607, 1969

CHAPTER 12

Transsphenoidal Approach to Lesions In and About The Sella Turcica

Edward R. Laws, Jr.

IN OUR PRACTICE THE transsphenoidal approach is commonly used for the operative treatment of pituitary adenomas. It is also highly suitable for ablative hypophysectomy and for the management of certain other tumors of the pituitary area, such as craniopharyngioma. In addition, this approach may be used to remove tumors of the clivus, such as chordoma or cholesteatoma, and for the management of disease involving the sphenoid sinus, such as mucocele, carcinoma, or cyst.

The technique employed is essentially the same as that used by Cushing,[1] Hirsch,[2] and Dott,[3] with the technical advances introduced by Guiot[4] and by Hardy.[5]

The patient is placed in a semirecumbent position on an operating table, using a Mayfield headrest with horseshoe (Fig. 12-1). The patient is positioned so that the left ear is cocked downward toward the left shoulder, allowing the surgeon a more comfortable midline approach to the nose and head. If a suprasellar extension of a pituitary tumor is anticipated, an intraoperative pneumoencephalogram may be performed. This is accomplished through a malleable needle placed into the lumbar subarachnoid space. A special split mattress is used so that the needle remains undisturbed. Once the endotracheal tube is in place, the oropharynx is carefully packed with cotton gauze to prevent the accumulation of blood in the throat and eventually in the stomach. Details of anesthetic management have been described.[6]

Ordinarily, the rhinologist performs the initial portion of the procedure, up to and occasionally including the entrance into the sphenoid sinus. The rhinologic aspects of this procedure have been described in detail;[7] however the steps utilized when the neurosurgical service performs the entire operative procedure will be repeated.

Operative Procedure

After the skin of the face is prepped with an aqueous antiseptic solution, the nostrils are packed with pledgets of cotton gauze soaked in 5% cocaine and inserted with a nasal speculum and bayonet forceps. The pledgets are allowed to remain in contact with the nasal mucosa for 5 to 10 minutes, while the remainder of the draping is completed. A solution of 0.5% Xylocaine in 1:200,000 epinephrine is used for injection of the operative field. Using a

Department of Neurologic Surgery, Mayo Clinic-Foundation, Rochester, Minnesota

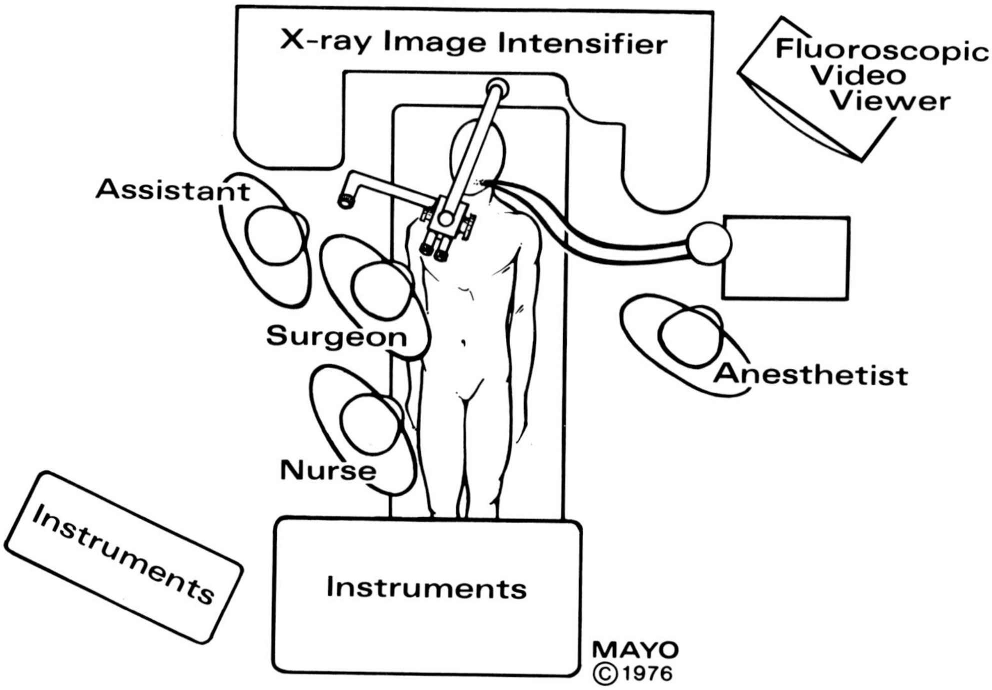

Fig. 12-1. Diagram of operating room arrangement for transsphenoidal surgery.

25-gauge needle, 10 to 20 ml of the solution are infiltrated, first along the upper gingiva, then along the inferior portion of the nasal septum, and finally along the lateral aspects of the nasal septum. A conscious effort is made to dissect the nasal mucosa away from the cartilaginous septum with the injection solution. This is done under direct vision with the aid of a nasal speculum and a headlight.

The upper lip is retracted and a transverse incision is made from one canine tooth to the other in the buccogingival fold (Fig. 12-2). The gingivae are dissected subperiosteally from the anterior face of the maxilla until the inferior aspect of the pyriform aperture is delineated. With appropriate submucous dissectors, the base of the pyriform aperture is carefully isolated and the nasal mucosa lying immediately beneath the ridge is dissected, first inferiorly, away from the face of the maxilla, and then superiorly, elevating the mucosa from the floor to the nose and the roof of the hard palate (Fig. 12-3). The base of the pyriform aperture may be enlarged, if necessary, using ronguers.

Once the inferior tunnels have been created, the lip is again retracted upward and a midline incision made along the internal aspect of the lip so as to cut down on the caudal end of the cartilaginous nasal septum. Still using sharp dissection, both sides of the cartilaginous septum are isolated anteriorly and a connection made with the inferior tunnels previously developed (Fig. 12-4). This is accomplished bilaterally and then, using a submucous dissector, the remainder of the nasal mucosa on both sides of the cartilaginous septum is carefully elevated. A long nasal speculum may then be inserted and the depths of the cartilaginous and bony nasal septum may be seen and mucosa further dissected away from them.

At this point, it should be possible to insert the transsphenoidal retractor, spreading it gently and being careful to place all tears in the nasal mucosa lateral to the retractor blades. As the retractor is opened the turbinates will fracture; it is unwise to apply a great deal of force in opening the retractor. Once the retractor is in place, the vomer should be visualized

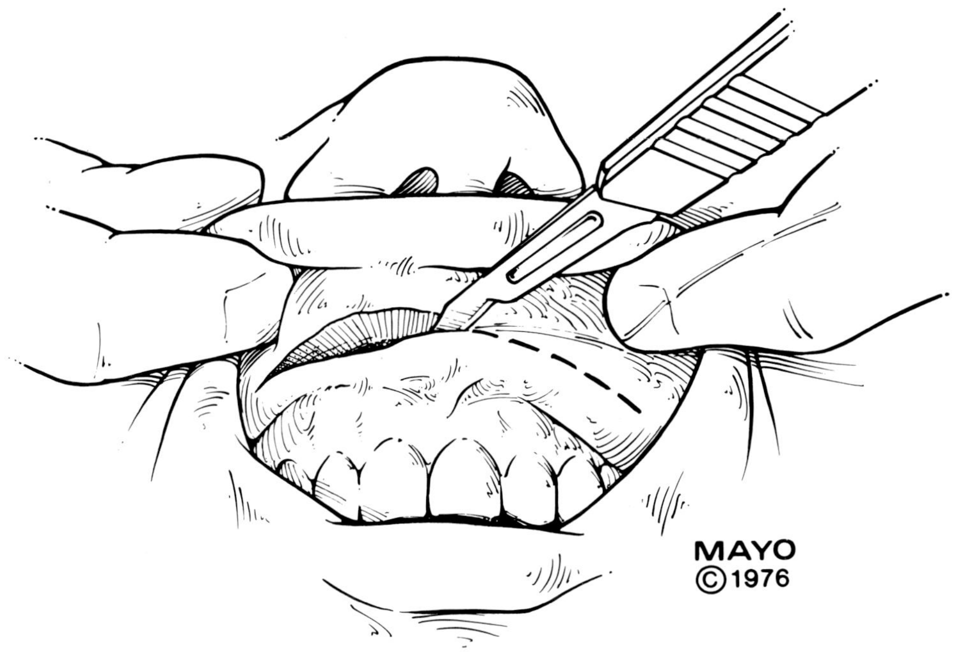

Fig. 12-2. Sublabial incision.

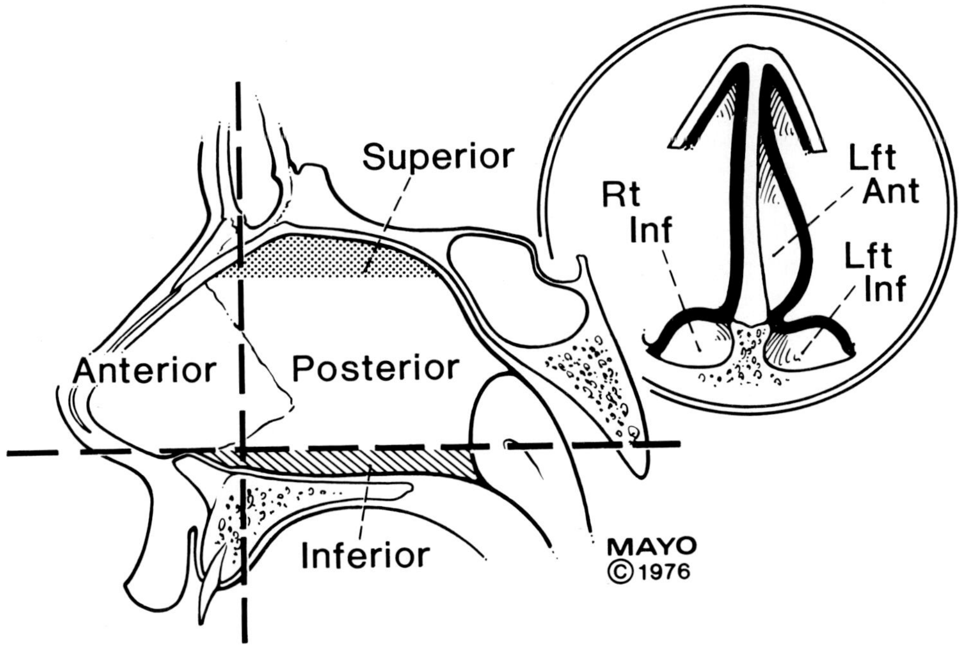

Fig. 12-3. Diagram of tunnels created by elevating nasal mucosa.

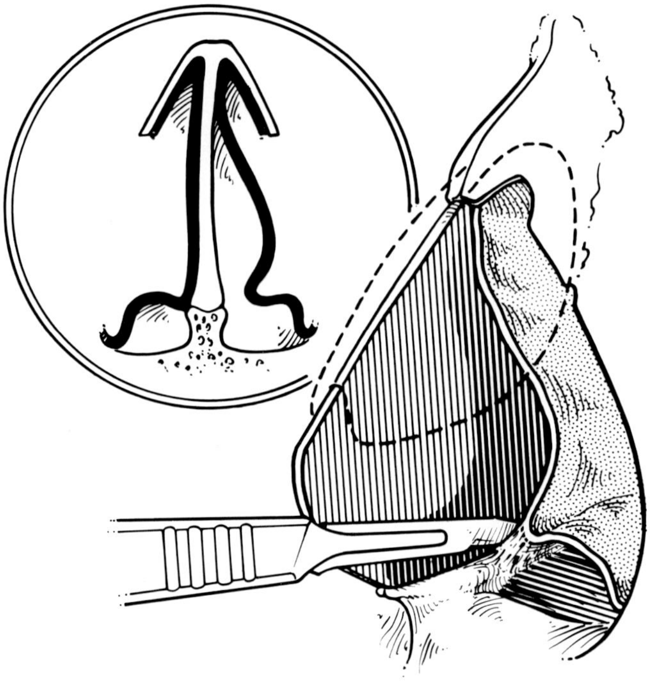

Fig. 12-4. Sharp dissection is used to connect the anterior tunnels of nasal mucosa with the inferior tunnels.

and submucous dissection then carried up to the face of the sphenoid sinus. The transsphenoidal retractor may then be repositioned and secured in place.

At a convenient point during the dissection the caudal end of the cartilaginous septum is detached from the nasal spine with a chisel. The inferior aspect of the cartilaginous septum and some of the bony nasal septum in the operative field should be resected, using a Lillie-Koffler tool or a Ferris-Smith punch (Fig. 12-5). This cartilage and bone is saved so that it may be used during the closure. With experience, the nasal spine anteriorly does not represent a major obstacle, and it is preferable, from a cosmetic standpoint, to preserve this structure rather than chisel it away.

With the transsphenoidal retractor properly positioned, the *keel* of the vomer and the face of the sphenoid sinus will be seen (Fig. 12-6). On either side of the central ridge the ostia of the sphenoid sinus may be identified.

At this point, either a lateral skull x-ray is obtained or the portable image intensifier is utilized so that bony landmarks and the relationship of the transsphenoidal retractor to the eventual pathway of operative approach can be determined. Any corrections, either mental or physical, are then made and the operating microscope is introduced.

It is usually possible to fracture into the sphenoid sinus simply by grasping the vomer with a Lillie-Koffler tool or Ferris-Smith punch. A chisel may be used, if necessary. Tomograms of the sphenoid sinus are very helpful in determining the anatomy and internal landmarks to be visualized, and the operative approach may need to be adjusted if anomalies of sinus formation are present. Once the sphenoid sinus is entered, a right-angled sphenoid punch may be utilized to complete the exposure. The mucosa within the sphenoid sinus is resected using a cup forceps. Resection of the mucosa aids in reducing bleeding and probably decreases the risk of postoperative mucocele formation.

At this point the floor of the sella should be clearly visible, and once again bony land-

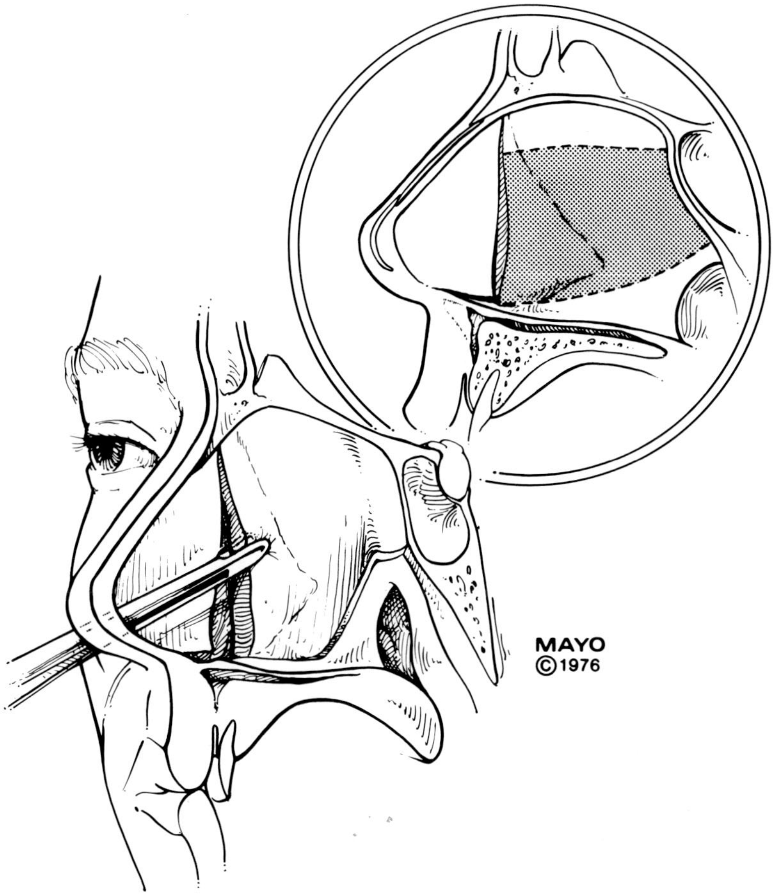

Fig. 12-5. Removal of the inferior posterior aspect of the nasal septum.

marks should be confirmed by x-ray films or with the portable image intensifier. With some tumors, the face of the sella will have been eroded away or is extraordinarily thin, so that it may be fractured with a blunt nerve hook. Occasionally a midline septum within the sphenoid sinus may be used to gain entry into the sella, simply by grasping the base of the septum where it joins the face of the sella and twisting as this bone is removed. If the floor of the sella is thick, a small chisel is used to remove a triangle or square of bone, fracturing it from the face of the sella. Exposure of the dura of the pituitary region is completed using a miniature right-angle Kerrison-type punch. In certain cases in which the floor of the sella is thick or the sphenoid bone poorly pneumatized, a high-speed air drill may be used to provide exposure.

Exposure of the sella proper is carried out utilizing the operating microscope with a 300-mm objective lens and 12.5× oculars. In most cases the magnification is set at 6 or 10×, but it is advisable to alter the magnification so that the sella fills the entire field of vision once the intrasellar portion of the operation is begun.

In some cases a pituitary tumor may have eroded through the anterior dura of the sella, but in most the dura will be intact. It is exposed as widely as feasible and careful attention is paid to its appearance. Transverse, blue intercavernous sinuses crossing the sella at the top and bottom of the operative exposure of the anterior dura are common. On rare occasions the entire anterior dura is laced with venous structures, appearing as one huge sinuous intercavernous sinus. The anterior dura may appear totally blue and very thin; this may indicate

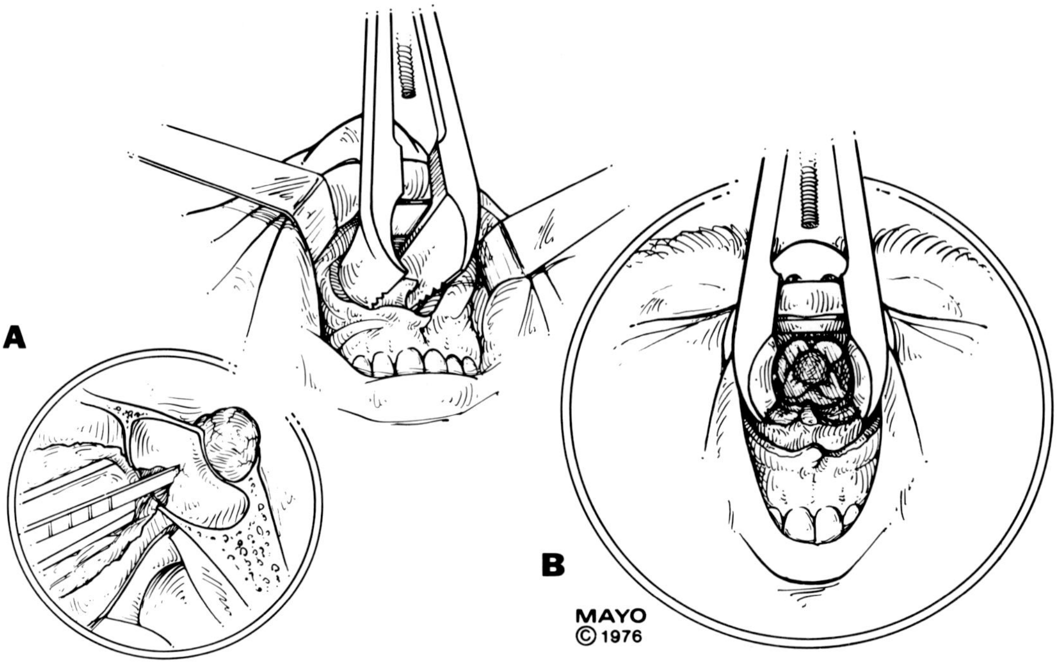

Fig. 12-6. Insertion of transsphenoidal retractor **(A)**; entrance into the sphenoid sinus **(B)**; exposure of sellar floor **(C)**.

the presence of an *empty sella*. Once the dura is exposed completely, it is cauterized with a suction-cautery device, usually around the periphery and then in a cruciate fashion where the dural incision will be made. Before the dura is opened, the sella is tapped and aspirated with a long, 19-gauge needle (Fig. 12-7). Ordinarily this procedure is monitored with the x-ray image intensifier. The goals are (a) to be certain there is no aneurysm within the sella and (b) to detect either a cystic tumor or an empty sella. After needle aspiration, the dura is opened. With a bayonet-handled knife, a horizontal incision is made between the intercavernous sinuses, if they are visualized. In most cases, a central vertical incision is then made to complete a cruciate opening of the dura. Alternatively, the incision may be performed as an "X," or an ellipse of anterior dura may be excised.[8] If possible, a blunt hook is then utilized to establish a definite subdural cleavage plane between the pituitary gland or tumor and the dura. A plane of dissection between the two layers of the dura should be carefully avoided, as this will allow entrance into the cavernous sinus and produce a great deal of venous bleeding. Once the dura has been reflected, the suction cautery device is again used to cauterize and shrink the leaves of dura so as to provide an unobstructed view into the sella.

In the case of the typical diffuse pituitary adenoma, the tumor is entered, using a ring curette, and tumor tissue is carefully loosened and removed (Fig. 12-8). This is accomplished with a relatively blunt ring curette, first cleaning tumor away from the inferior dura of the sella. Once the inferior aspect is free of tumor, dissection is continued laterally, from inferior to superior on both sides, against the medial wall of the cavernous sinus. During this portion of dissection, the carotid arteries may be seen, and injury to them must be avoided. Tissue is never pulled away from the lateral aspect of the sella, as doing so may avulse a vascular structure. It is preferable to use a ring curette to loosen tissue and to remove only loosened tissue, using a cup forceps and very little traction. With the floor of the sella and both sides cleaned of tumor, the next step is to work from the lateral walls to the superior aspect of the

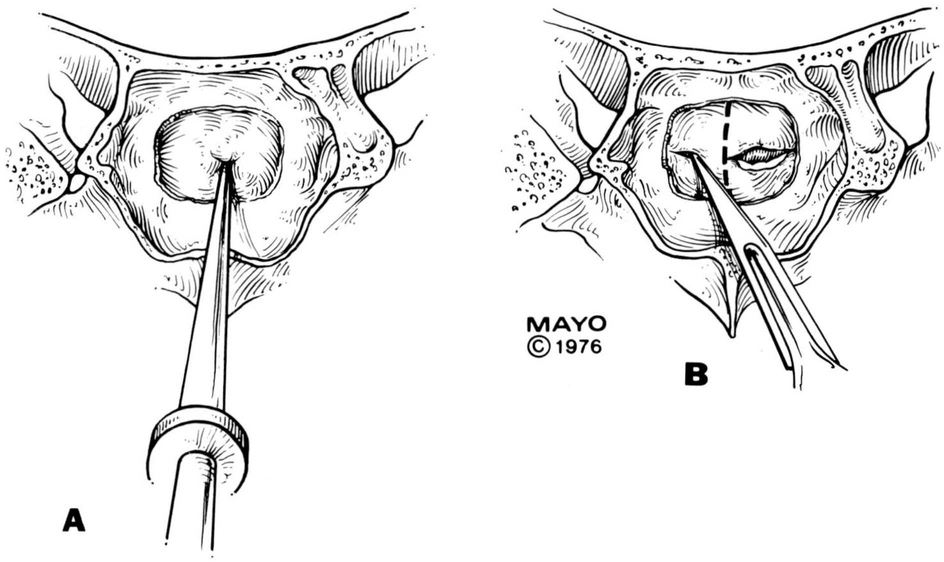

Fig. 12-7. Aspiration of sella **(A)** and incision of dura **(B)**.

tumor, starting anteriorly within the sella. Here a special effort must be made not to tear the diaphragm and thus create a cerebrospinal fluid leak. Frequently, decompression of the intrasellar portion of the tumor allows a suprasellar extension to herniate directly into view within the sella. Subsequently the diaphragma sellae or the capsule of the tumor will prolapse. If this does not occur, air injected through the lumbar malleable needle will outline the suprasellar extension of the tumor and produce a pressure differential favoring herniation of tumor into the sella. Ordinarily 15 to 25 ml of air is adequate both for x-ray visualization and to alter pressure relationships. If prolapse of the capsule does not occur, a ring curette may be used cautiously in the intracranial space, under constant x-ray control with the image intensifier. The capsule can be reexpanded, if necessary, by withdrawing cerebrospinal fluid through the lumbar needle.[9] The fact that no residual tumor is present may be confirmed by visual inspection, with the help of a dental mirror, a nasopharyngoscope, or a small flexible-tipped fiberoptic endoscope. A tantalum clip may be applied to the prolapsed diaphragm as a marker for postoperative x-ray studies.

In some cases it may be worthwhile to attempt to save normal pituitary tissue. In a large diffuse adenoma, this usually appears as a thin membrane, usually placed superolaterally. A biopsy may be taken for confirmation, but usually the appearance is typical and this tissue may be left behind with some confidence.

If a pituitary microadenoma is not visible immediately when the dura is opened, a transverse incision is made into the pituitary gland proper. Once this incision is made, subdural dissection of the lateral wings of the pituitary gland is started, first on one side and then on the other, using the Hardy dissectors. If the incision into the gland has been made deeply enough, lateral pressure with the Hardy dissector usually causes the microadenoma to herniate into the operative field. Thus, its location can be delineated, its cavity entered, and its removal completed, using a small ring curette and cup forceps. All suspicious appearing tissue is removed and the residual, presumed normal, pituitary gland is occasionally biopsied. The tumor cavity may be treated with applications of absolute alcohol or Zenker's solution, but there is no evidence that this step improves either the immediate result or the risk of recurrence.

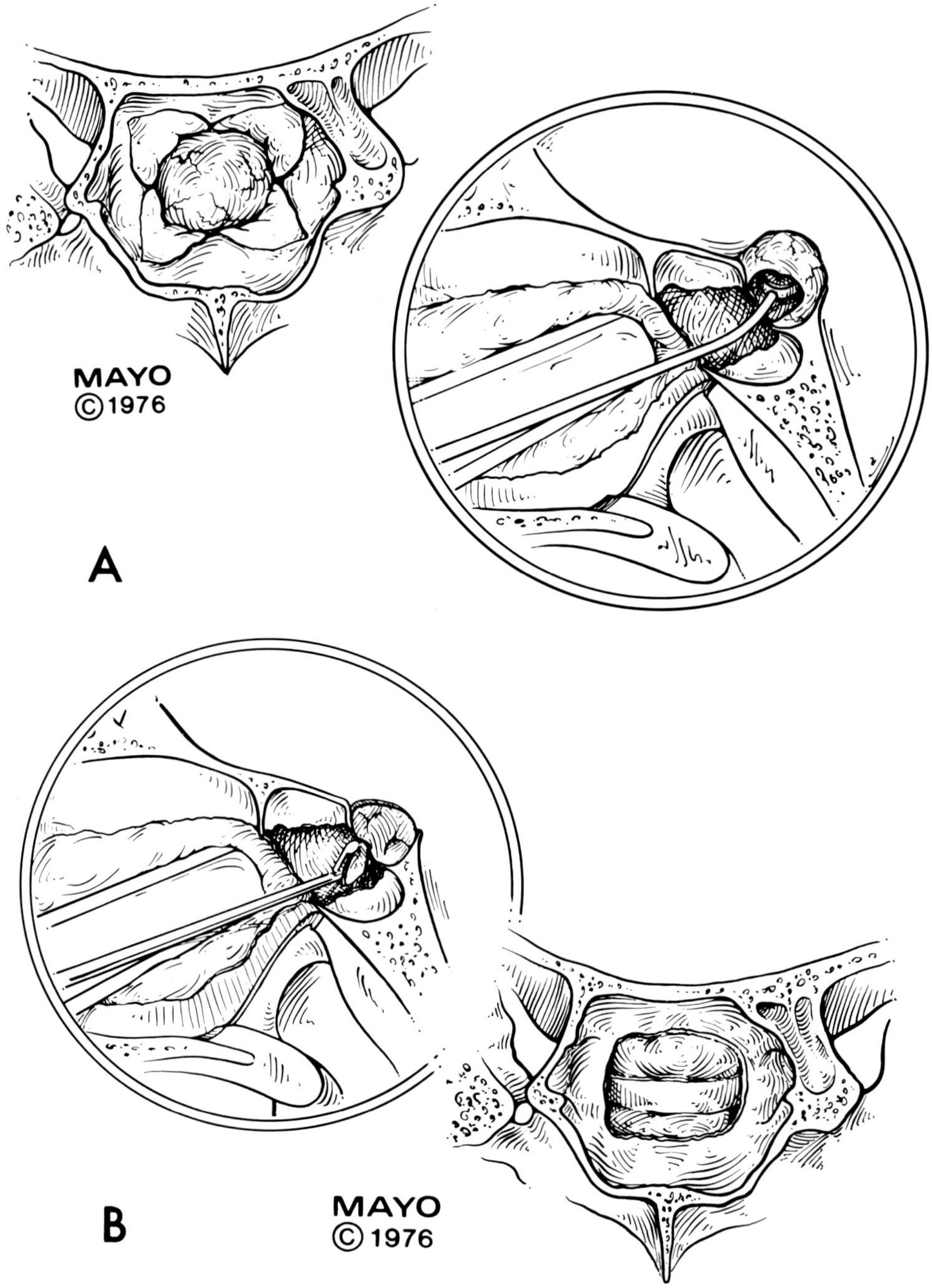

Fig. 12-8. Removal of adenoma with ring curette **(A)**; packing of sella with muscle and stent of nasal cartilage **(B)**.

The technique of hypophysectomy for metastatic carcinoma or diabetic retinopathy is similar to that described for microadenomas. The pituitary gland is dissected subdurally; the lateral wings are dissected first and then the inferior aspect of the gland. The subdural plane of dissection is maintained and considerable pressure used to strip the lateral aspects of the gland, from anterior to posterior, away from the walls of the cavernous sinus. This is done cautiously and little by little, working first on one side then the other and then on the inferior aspect of the gland, repeating this sequence many times. The gland will, in effect, shrink and once some mobility has been achieved, the superior aspect of the gland may be dissected and then depressed, permitting the pituitary stalk to come into view. The stalk is then transsected with an alligator scissors or a No. 11 blade knife. Once this has been accomplished, a Hardy dissector is placed along the floor of the sella and used to dissect behind and then over the superior surface of the gland to free it completely. In some cases the dissection does not go smoothly and the gland may have to be removed piecemeal, in which case the sella must be searched thoroughly for retained fragments of the gland. Total hypophysectomy must be achieved for optimum results.

After the tumor has been removed, or after hypophysectomy, the sella is packed, as is the tumor cavity of a microadenoma once the lesion has been removed. Most often, homograft muscle is used, taking it from another patient undergoing surgery concurrently. A piece of muscle, which has been soaked in chloramphenicol solution, is trimmed to approximate the size of the operative defect; it is tagged with a tantalum clip and placed within the sella, using the sucker and cup forceps. Once it is in place, it is secured with a piece of nasal bone or cartilage cut in the shape of a narrow rectangle or rhomboid and placed in a subdural position as a wedge to hold the muscle securely (Fig. 12-9). On occasion, more than one piece of muscle or more than one piece of cartilage or bone is employed.

If a cerebrospinal fluid leak has developed during surgery, the roof of the sella is reconstructed with a piece of homologous dural graft material or fascia lata. This step probably adds little to the security of the seal, and homograft muscle alone is usually satisfactory.

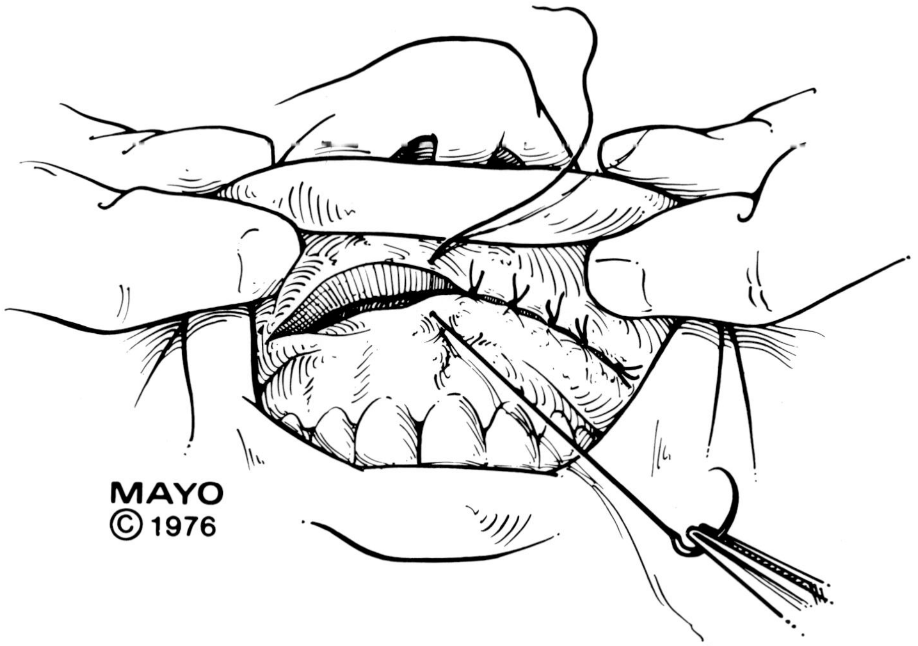

Fig. 12-9. Closure of sublabial incision.

Autograft muscle or fat from the patient's thigh may be used as well. Cyanoacrylate glue may be spread over Surgicel to seal the floor of the sella more securely.

When a cerebrospinal fluid leak has been present, usually the sphenoid sinus is also packed with muscle or fat, but in the absence of a cerebrospinal fluid leak, it is left free of packing or foreign material.

Assuming that adequate hemostasis has been achieved and the sella has been suitably packed, the nasal phase of the procedure is completed by packing the nostrils with Vaseline-impregnated gauze and closing the gingival incision with loose interrupted 4-0 catgut sutures (Fig. 12-9).

A compression dressing is applied in the form of a gauze pad placed beneath the nostrils and over the upper lip as a drip pad and the nose taped to ensure a satisfactory cosmetic result.

Prophylactic antibiotics are continued until the nasal packing is removed, usually on the fourth postoperative day. In uncomplicated cases the patient can be dismissed from the hospital on the sixth postoperative day.

The clinical entities treated in a 4-year period, along with the complications observed,[10] and the results of treatment are presented in Tables 12-1 through 12-5.

The transsphenoidal approach has proved to be safe and effective in the management of a variety of problems associated with the sella turcica. Not only have the results been as satisfactory or better than those achieved with more traditional approaches but a new group of pathologic lesions, ie., microadenomas, has become amenable to surgical correction.

Table 12-1. Clinical Entities Treated by Transsphenoidal Microsurgery (Mayo Clinic 1972–1976)

Clinical entity	No. of patients
Pituitary adenoma	234
Craniopharyngioma	15
Metastatic carcinoma (hypophysectomy)	12
Diabetic retinopathy (hypophysectomy)	3
Empty sella/arachnoid cyst	12
CSF rhinorrhea	9
Clivus chordoma	5
Miscellaneous lesions	16
Total	306

Table 12-2. Pituitary Adenomas Treated by Transsphenoidal Microsurgery

	Cases	
Clinical entity	Number	Total
Functioning adenomas		129
Acromegaly	70	
Prolactin secreting adenomas	31	
Nelson-Salassa syndrome (MSH/ACTH)	13	
Primary Cushing's syndrome	15	
Nonfunctioning adenomas		105
Malignant adenoma	1	
Total pituitary adenomas		234
Microadenomas (< 10 mm)	71	
Pituitary adenomas with visual field defect	76	

Table 12-3. Miscellaneous Lesions Treated by Transsphenoidal Microsurgery

Clinical entity	No. of patients
Mucocele	2
Nasal glioma	2
Meningioma	2
Sphenoid sinus carcinoma	2
Sphenoid sinus cyst	1
Ganglioglioma of sphenoid sinus	1
Cavernous hemangioma (parasellar)	1
Myeloma (sellar)	1
Fibrous dysplasia (parasellar)	1
Cholesteatoma of clivus	1
Tolosa-Hunt syndrome (granuloma)	1
Ectopic pinealoma	1
Total	16

Table 12-4. Results of Transsphenoidal Surgery, Mayo Clinic 1972–1976 (306 Cases)

	Cases	
	Number	Percent
Operative mortality	5	1.67
Operative morbidity (includes deaths)		
Worsening of vision	6	
Transient oculomotor or abducent palsy	4	
CSF rhinorrhea	7	
Meningitis	3	
Intracranial vascular occlusion	2	
Subarachnoid hemorrhage	2	
Nasal Septal perforation (symptomatic)	7	

Table 12-5. Results of Transsphenoidal Surgery in Patients With Preoperative Visual Field Defects[9]

Postoperative vision	Patients (%)
Improved	81
Unchanged	13
Worse	6

REFERENCES

1. Cushing H: The Weir Mitchell Lecture: Surgical experiences with pituitary disorders. *JAMA 63*:1515-1525, 1914
2. Hirsch O: Ueber Hypophysentumoren und deren Behandlung. Klin Monatsbl Augenheilkd *85*:609-640, 1930
3. Dott NM, Bailey P: A consideration of the hypophyseal adenomata. *Br J Surg 13*:314-366, 1925
4. Guiot G: Transsphenoidal approach in surgical treatment of pituitary adenomas: general principles and indications in non-functioning adenomas. Excerpta Medica International Congress Series. No. 303, pp 159-178, 1973

5. Hardy J: Transsphenoidal microsurgery of the normal and pathological pituitary. *Clin Neurosurg* *16*:185-216, 1969
6. Messick J, Laws ER, Jr: Anaesthesia for transsphenoidal surgery. *Anaesth Analg*, In press
7. Kern EB, Laws ER, Jr: Transseptal pituitary surgery: A review of 285 operations at the Mayo Clinic. *Rev Pan-Americana*. In press
8. Wilson CB: Personal communication
9. Laws ER, Jr, Trautmann JC, Hollenhorst RW, Jr: Transsphenoidal decompression of the optic nerve and chiasm: visual results in 62 patients. *J Neurosurg,* In press
10. Laws ER, Jr, Kern EB: Complications of Transsphenoidal Surgery. *Clin Neurosurg* *23*:401-416, 1976

CHAPTER 13

Transethmoidal Approach to the Pituitary

Charles W. Cummings Jonas Johnson

THE INTENT OF THIS CHAPTER is to present the advantages and disadvantages as well as a procedural description for the transethmoidal sphenoidotomy approach to the pituitary gland. This procedure, in conjunction with the transeptal sphenoidotomy approach, represents one distinct anatomical pathway to the pituitary region. The ease of approach and relatively benign postoperative course merit consideration of the procedure when approach to the pituitary is warranted.

Indications

The indications for surgical ablation of the pituitary gland have previously been discussed. Acromegaly, Cushing's Disease, and metastatic carcinoma of the breast and prostate are paramount among these indications.

Contraindications

1. This procedure should not be used with extensive suprasellar displacement of the tumor.
2. An underpneumatized sphenoid sinus, which occurs 3% of the time, is a distinct contraindication to the surgical approach because the sella is difficult to identify.
3. An overpneumatized sphenoid sinus is a relative contraindication in that the optic canal can be completely surrounded by sphenoid air cells, thus making identification exceedingly difficult, and injury more likely.
4. Chronic ethmoid sinusitis and/or sphenoid sinusitis impair surgical access because of mucosal edema, hyperemia, and potential for introducing an infection.
5. Acute sinusitis or nasal sepsis presents a high risk of contamination or infection.
6. Abnormal development of the cavernous sinus or medial displacement of the carotid arteries into the sphenoid make this surgical approach hazardous.

Department of Otolaryngology, State University Hospital, Upstate Medical Center, Syracuse, New York 13210

Advantages

The advantages of the transethmoid approach to the sphenoid, and thus to the pituitary, over other procedures are:

1. A shorter anatomic distance is traversed to enter the sphenoid sinus.
2. The procedure allows for two-plane instrumentation, ie., transnasal as well as transethmoid.
3. The operative procedure can be performed on a plane parallel to the floor of the anterior fossa.
4. It is less traumatic and is usually associated with less blood loss than the transeptal approach.
5. There is minimal postoperative discomfort.
6. Permanent septomucosal perforation is avoided by this procedure.
7. Contamination from the oral cavity is avoided.
8. Devitalization of the teeth is avoided.

Disadvantages

An external scar is necessary.

Complications

Although these complications do not represent problems specific for this surgical approach, they should be mentioned. Diabetes insipidus is by far the most frequent complication, occurring in 15% of the cases, according to Collins.[1] Usually this problem can be managed by replacement therapy, without difficulty.

Cerebrospinal fluid leak occurs in 4% to 9%[2,3] of the cases. If the sinus has been obliterated by fat, or a fascia lata and a nasal-mucosal pedical flap, a permanent leak is unusual.

Meningitis, either alone or in concert with a cerebrospinal fluid leak, is the most significant postoperative complication, and occurs less than 2% of the time.

Immediate surgical complications are:

1. Injury to the optic nerve by dissection of the superolateral aspect of the posterior ethmoidal cell or sphenoid sinus.
2. Injury to the carotid artery, as it traverses the lateral wall of the sphenoid sinus, is also a potential complication. Kirchner[3] has recommended needle aspiration of the uncapped area if there is any suspicion that the region may not be the sella.

Workup

Several special studies are necessary to obviate procedural difficulties. These should be obtained in addition to necessary diagnostic procedures.

1. Routine sinus films.
2. Tomograms of the sphenoid and sella region, both from a lateral and basilar projection.
3. Carotid arteriography to ascertain adequate intercarotid space within the sphenoid.
4. Preoperative nasal cultures.
5. Diagnostic measures to eliminate the possibility of suprasellar extension of disease (computerized axial tomography, air-contrast tomography).

Technique

The surgical technique for this procedure will be outlined in stepwise fashion. However there are several anatomic landmarks, which must be kept in mind when performing the operation.

1. *The middle turbinate.* Medial to the insertion of the middle turbinate lies the cribriform plate area. This area must be avoided to eliminate trauma to the cribriform and potential for a cerebrospinal fluid leak. The ethmoid air cells lie laterally to the insertion of the middle turbinate. These represent an area of relative safety, if the roof of the ethmoid is not violated.
2. *The cribriform area* offers superior plane orientation and is directly parallel with the floor of the anterior fossa.
3. *The anterior and posterior ethmoid arteries* form a plane at the level of the cribriform plate area and therefore represent the superior limits of surgical dissection.
4. *The posterior ethmoid artery* is the posterior limit of ethmoidal dissection. The optic foramen is 4 to 7 mm posterior to the posterior ethmoid artery and is protected by a medial rim of bone (Fig. 13-1). This artery also traverses the roof of the posterior ethmoid cell, enabling its identification. The posterior wall of this cell represents the anterior wall of the sphenoid sinus. The canal of the optic nerve intrudes upon the superiolateral aspect of the posterior ethmoid cell.
5. *The rostrum of the sphenoid* provides for location of the inferior aspect of the sphenoid sinus.
6. *The sphenoid septum* does not necessarily reside in the midline and is of no value for orientation other than by comparison to the sinus laminograms.
7. *The medial projection of the carotid canal* may be visualized within the sphenoid sinus and must not be interpreted as a sphenoid septum or the sella. As this bone is unroofed,

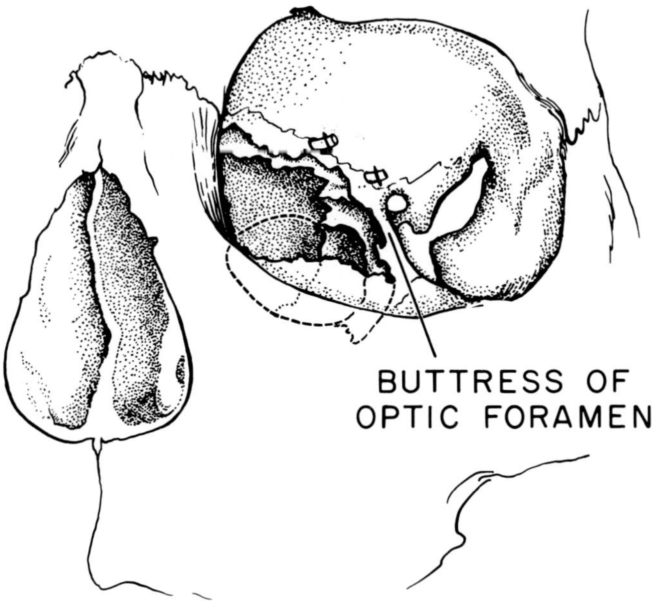

Fig. 13-1. The middle turbinate, ethmoid labyrinth, and anterior wall of the sphenoid have been removed. The medial buttress of the optic foramen is identified.

aspiration with a thin needle is advocated to rule out the contralateral carotid artery.[3] This artery will be exposed (if at all) because of the slightly off-midline approach through the ethmoid.

8. *Localization of the midline* can be performed by passing a flat instrument along the superior aspect of the nasal septum into the sphenoid sinus. This will identify the midline and the region of the sella.

Procedure

1. Head elevated 20°.
2. Protect eyes with either lid sutures or plastic eye shields.
3. Incision ½ distance from dorsum of nose and canthus, approximately 3 cm in length (Fig. 13-2).
4. Lateral retraction of inner canthal ligament; lacrimal sac.
5. Identification of anterior ethmoid artery. Clip or ligature, and divide.
6. Identification of posterior ethmoid artery.
7. Take down lamina papyraceous portion of lacrimal fossa (Fig. 13-3).
8. Incision through lateral nasal mucosa, identification of middle turbinate (Fig. 13-4).
9. Removal of middle turbinate, preserving insertion as landmark.
10. Removal of ethmoid mucosa and uncapping posterior ethmoid cell (Fig. 13-5).

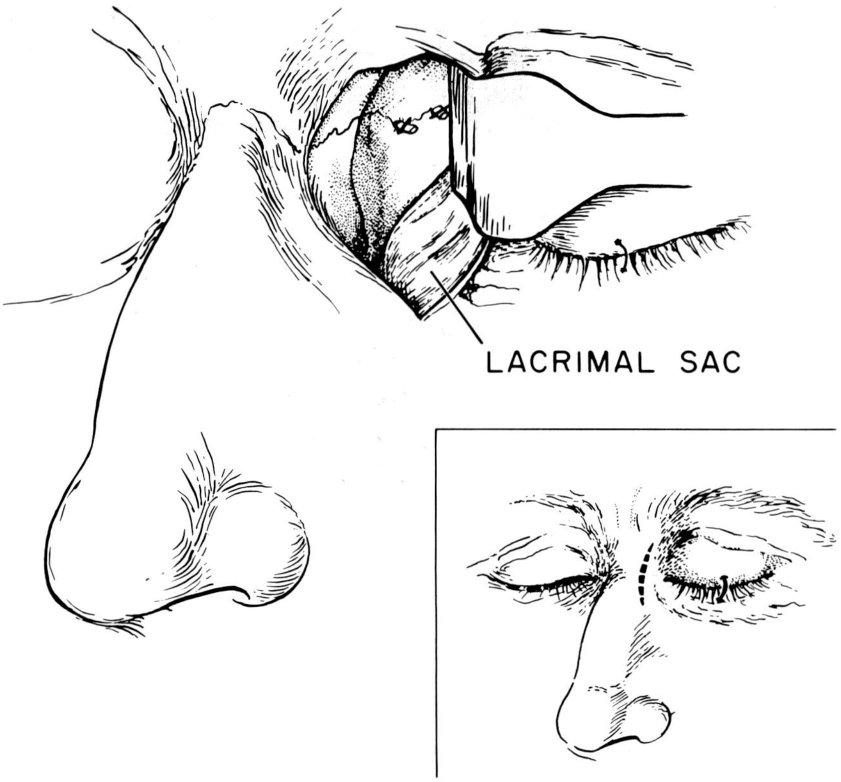

Fig. 13-2. A curvilinear incision is made one-half distance between the dorsum of the nose and the medial canthus. The periorbitum has been reflected laterally and the anterior and posterior ethmoid arteries have been divided.

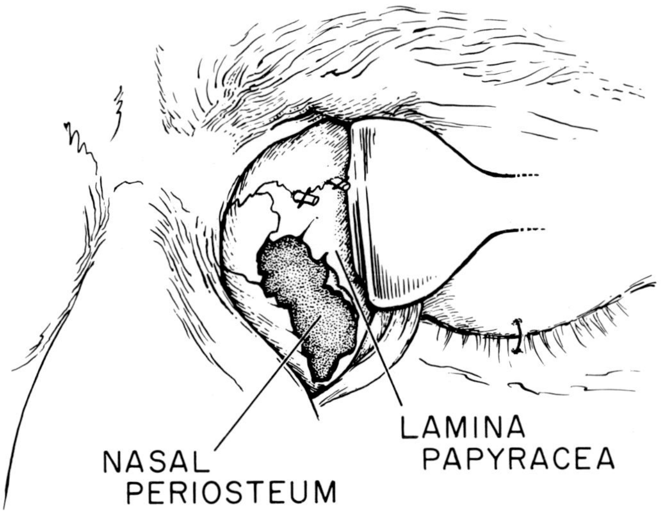

Fig. 13-3. The lamina papyracea has been partially removed.

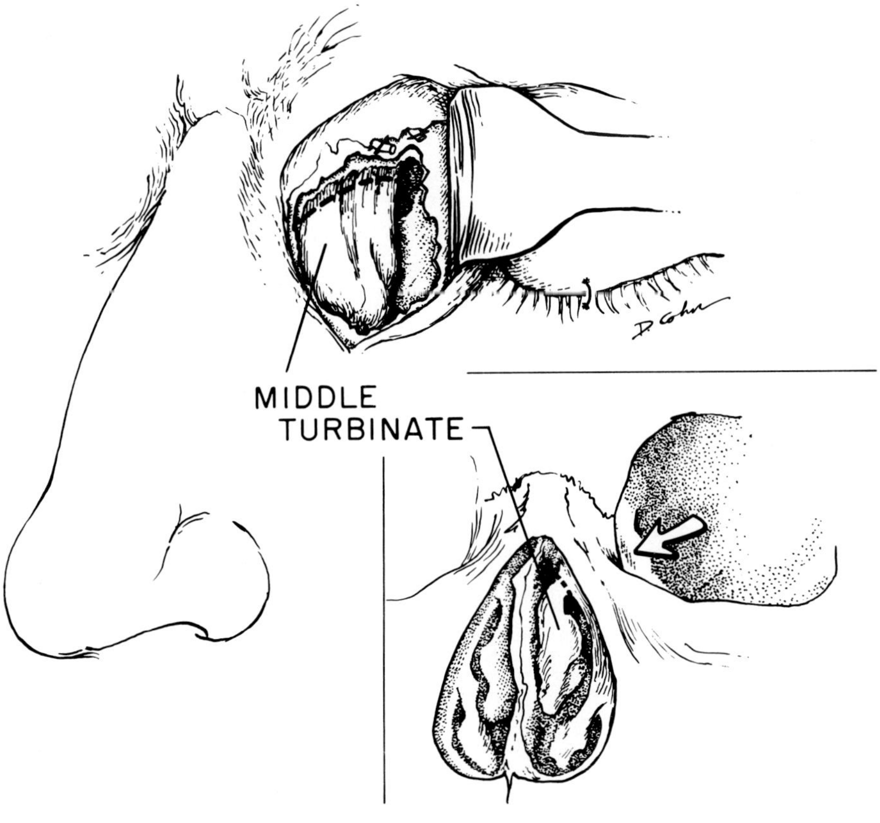

Fig. 13-4. The lateral nasal mucosa has been removed and the middle turbinate identified.

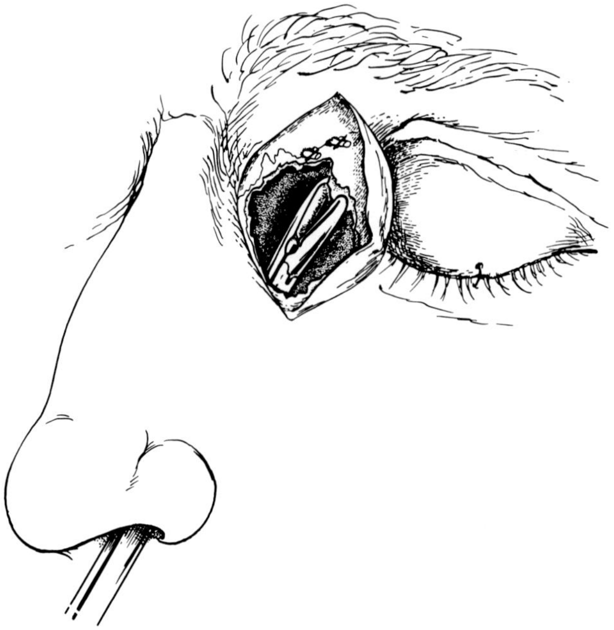

Fig. 13-5. The ethmoid air-cell mucosa is removed transnasally, under direct visualization, via the external ethmoidectomy exposure.

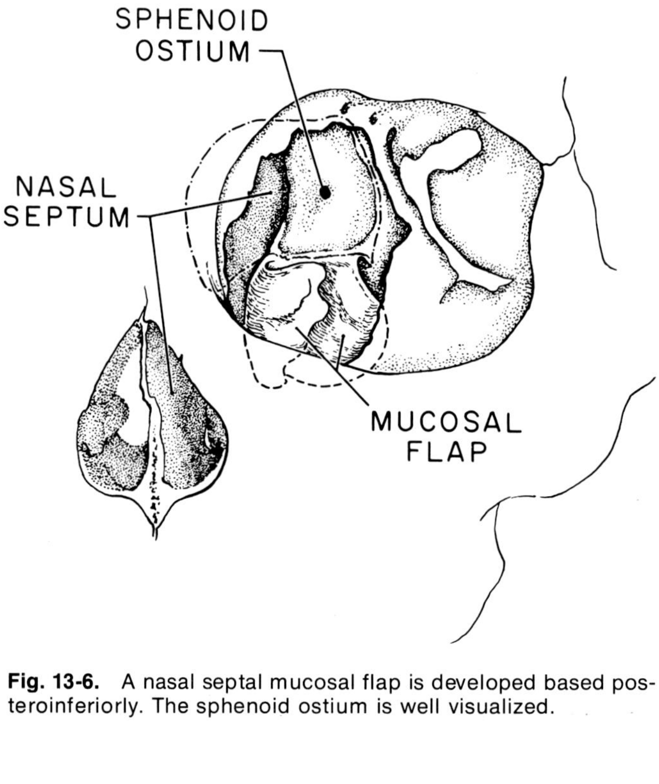

Fig. 13-6. A nasal septal mucosal flap is developed based posteroinferiorly. The sphenoid ostium is well visualized.

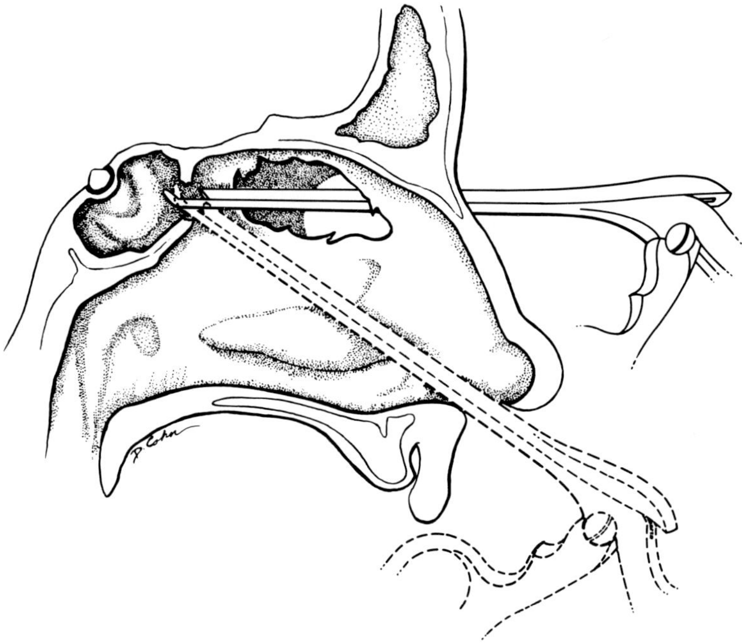

Fig. 13-7. Entrance into the sphenoid is from anteriorly adjacent to the ostium. A Cloward biting forcep can be used either transnasally or transethmoidally.

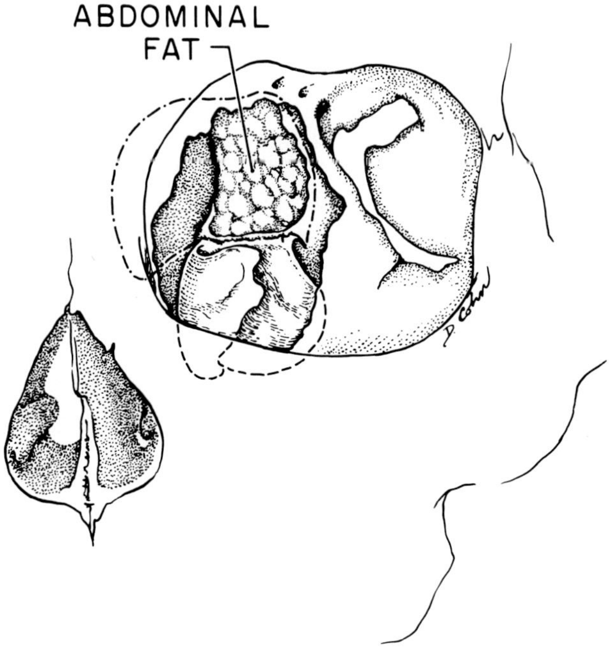

Fig. 13-8. Abdominal fat has been used to obliterate the sphenoid sinus.

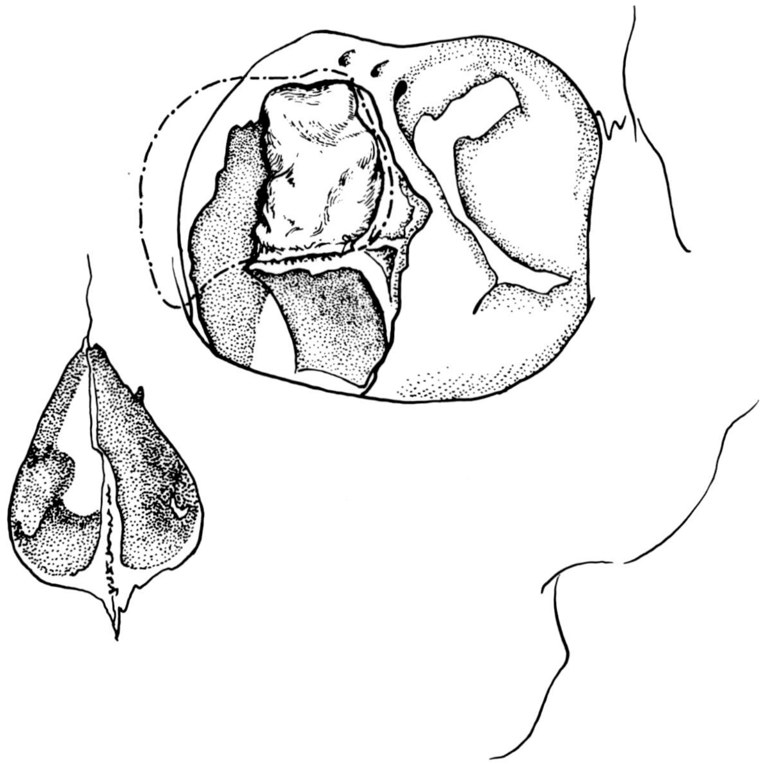

Fig. 13-9. The nasal septal mucosal flap has been placed over the fat graft.

11. Creation of inferiorly based nasal mucosal flap.
12. Identification of sphenoid ostium (Fig. 13-6).
13. Corroboration of position by image intensifying fluoroscopy with "C" arm.
14. Entrance into the sphenoid by taking down the anterior wall (Fig. 13-7).
15. Removal of sphenoid sinus mucosa. Operating microscope with 300-mm objective lens is used to aid visualization.
16. Region of the sella is uncapped from bone. The uncapped area can be aspirated with a long needle to rule out the presence of the carotid artery.
17. A cruciate incision is made in the capsule and the gland exposed.
18. The pituitary fenestration os obliterated with fat (abdominal) or fascia lata (Fig. 13-8).
19. The sphenoid is obliterated with fat, and the nasal mucosal flap is placed over the defect (Fig. 13-9). Gelfoam is placed over the flap.
20. The inner canthal incision is closed in two layers.

REFERENCES

1. Collins WF: Hypophysectomy: historical and personal perspective. *Clin Neurosurg 21*:68-78, 1974
2. Richards SH, Thomas JP, Kilby D: Transethmoidal hypophysectomy for pituitary tumors. *Proc R Soc Med 67*:889-892, 1974
3. Kirchner JA, Van Gilder JD: Transethmoidal hypophysectomy: some surgical landmarks. *Trans Am Acad Ophthalmol Otolaryngol 80*:391-396, 1975

CHAPTER 14
Stereotaxic Thermal Hypophysectomy

Nicholas T. Zervas

STEREOTAXIC HYPOPHYSECTOMY WAS INTRODUCED into the neurosurgical armamentarium by Jean Talairoch. He first employed radioactive gold to induce ablation of the pituitary gland. Since that time, radioactive yttrium, radioactive strontium, heat, cold and ultrasound have been alternate methods to induce destruction. Since 1964, we have produced heat lesions in the pituitary gland using radiofrequency current. This has proved to be a satisfactory way to bring about total destruction of the gland in most cases without the risk of damage to surrounding vascular or cranial nerve structures. Perhaps the major objection to stereotaxic transnasal procedures was the high incidence of cerebrospinal fluid rhinorrhea. This has been virtually eliminated by the tactic of packing the sella turcica with fascia lata at the end of the operation and occluding the defect in the anterior wall of the sella turcica with a silicone plug.

Methods

Preparation of the Patient

No special precautions must be taken prior to operation. A nasal culture may be indicated in patients with a previous history of sinus infections. It is essential, however, that all patients receive antibiotics before, during, and after the operation. Accordingly, the patients are given oxacillin, 1 g intravenously, beginning 6 AM the morning of operation. Also, the patients are given hydrocortisone, 50 mg intramuscularly, before operation. No other special measures are required. When the patient enters the operating room, the nasal cavity can be sprayed on either side with a vasoconstrictive agent such as neosynephrine.

Anesthesia

Radiofrequency thermal lesions can be produced in patients while they are under anesthesia because damage to visual structures has been a very rare event. In the few instances in which injury did occur, it was first manifested as anisocoria and the lesion was quickly terminated. To perform the procedure under local anesthesia is very trying for both patient

Neurosurgical Service, Massachusetts General Hospital and the Harvard Medical School, Boston, Massachusetts 02114.

and professional staff and is not necessary. Following the induction of general anesthesia, the oral pharynx is packed with a 1.0-inch moistened gauze roll.

Operation

The patient's head is fixed securely in a stereotaxic frame. We use the Todd-Wells frame (Fig. 14-1). The electrode holder should then be centered on the anterior wall of the sella turcica as close to the midline as possible. Quite obviously, it is very necessary to insure that the electrode enters the pituitary gland directly and does not go above or lateral to it. There is little security in the bony landmarks of plain films. The surgeon can never be certain where the diaphragma sellae is, nor where the lateral margins of the pituitary gland lie in an individual patient. We have not found angiography and pneumoencephalography necessary. As long as the surgeon is careful to be as close to the midline as possible and no more than 4 mm above the sella floor when entering the pituitary gland, poor placement of the electrode can be minimized. Perhaps the most variable location is the position of the diaphragma sellae. Although this should run horizontally from the tuberculum sellae to below the dorsum sellae, we have repeatedly found that it often lies quite low in the sella turcica and of course may be deficient in the midline. Accordingly, the target point on the anterior wall of the sella turcica must be kept rather low so as to avoid penetrating above the diaphragma sellae. We never enter the sella turcica more than 4 mm above the floor, regardless of its apparent configuration. If the sella turcica has a peculiar shape, one is best advised to obtain a pneumoencephalogram to be certain of the position of the diaphragma. Once the target point has been set, a nasal cannula can then be advanced into the nasal cavity on either side, whichever appears to be more expedient from the standpoint of easy advancement of the instruments. A 4-mm drill hole is then made in the anterior wall of the sphenoid sinus and a cannula inserted just short of the anterior wall of the sella turcica. The sphenoid sinus is then washed copiously with a solution of bacitracin (50,000 units/500 ml N saline). A 2.2-mm drill hole is then made in the anterior wall of the sella turcica. Care is to be taken so that the head of the drill does not extend more than 1.0 or 2.0 mm into the sella turcica. This is done so as to prevent stripping the dura away from the bone. The dura is then punctured with a series of double-ended instruments, each one larger than the other so that finally the length in the dura is larger than the diameter of the electrode tip.

The radiofrequency electrode is then inserted into the sella turcica. The electrode we employ is a totally insulated, hollow stainless steel cannula. The end is closed, but a side hole is present 1 mm short of the tip (Figs. 14-2 and 14-3). A stainless steel, coiled wire electrode, with a preformed curve, can be projected through the side hole. As this is forced through the side hole it becomes a semicircular stylet. It is quite malleable and not likely to puncture surrounding structures, such as dura or carotid artery. Within the spring, is a thermocouple, which is used to monitor the temperature at the tip. In the past we used thermister tips but these were easily broken. Thermocouples have a much longer life. The electrode is mounted on the stereotaxic frame and then advanced into the sella turcica. It is easily possible to palpate the anterior dorsum sellae with the electrode tip. At this point the electrode is withdrawn 1 or 2 mm. The lateral stylet is then advanced through the side hole until resistance can be felt as it encounters either diaphragma sellae or the floor or lateral dura surrounding the pituitary gland, depending on the angle of rotation of the outer cannula. Thus the surgeon can estimate the actual size of the gland. Passage through the gland is unimpeded, since it is rather soft. However, the dura or the diaphragma sellae offer resistance.

In order to bring about total destruction of the gland we usually place the electrode tip in the posterior and then anterior sectors of the gland. In each position, a series of lesions is made in various quadrants by alternately retracting and extending the side arm after the electrode has been turned into a new angle. It is very important to confirm the actual position of the electrode tip with a plain radiograph, since very often the malleable spring will be

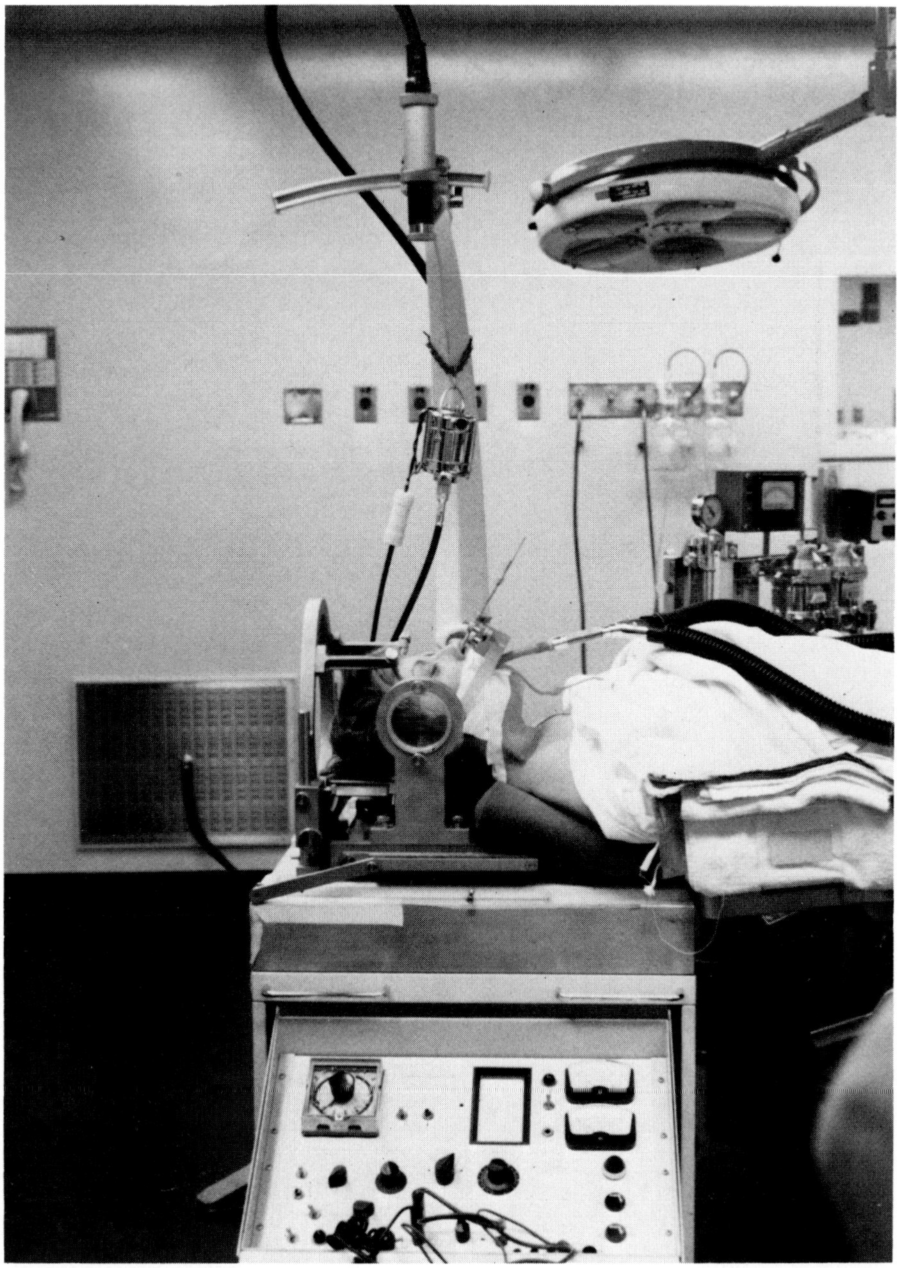

Fig. 14-1. Operative scene: the patient's head is fixed in stereotaxic frame. The electrode is in place. The miniature x-ray tubes are aligned orthogonally with frame. The RF generator is in the foreground.

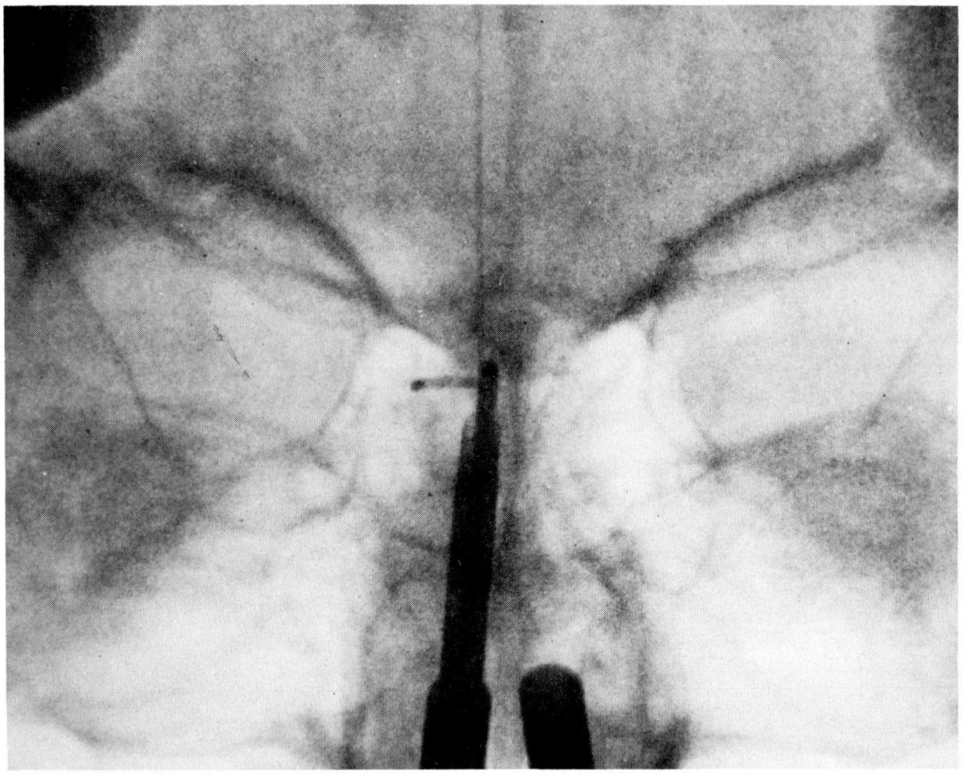

Fig. 14-2. A frontal radiograph showing the electrode in position and the sidearm projecting to the right.

diverted from its true radiant as it bumps obliquely against the diaphragma sellae or the floor of the sella. Also, if the electrode is inadvertently placed above the diaphragma sellae, the latter may catch the lateral stylet and prevent it from being directed downward into the gland. These problems can be easily detected if films are taken at each projection.

Before a lesion is made, stimulation is carried out at each lateral position of the spring electrode to detect any possible eye movements. If ocular motion is not observed at voltages less than 2 V, the lesion can then be produced. The stimulating current is 60 Hz, 2 msec.

The lesion is made with a radiofrequency generator. The ground is a 3.5-inch, 18-gauge spinal needle implanted in either deltoid. Each lesion is produced by bringing the temperature around the electrode tip as monitored by the thermocouples to 80°-90° C. The lesion duration is 120 seconds. As mentioned above a series of lesions is made in anterior and posterior positions. This usually requires turning the outer cannula 22° after each lesion. However, it is important to be certain that the electrode tip is not above the line joining the dorsum sellae to the tuberculin sellae. In most instances the diaphragma sellae can be palpated, but it should not be taken for granted that it is intact. Lesions in the midline made with the electrode are to be carefully considered and possibly avoided. We have produced bitemporal hemianopsia in 2 patients, probably related to an excessively superior positioning of the lateral spring so that it apparently came into contact with the optic chiasm a few millimeters above the sallae turcica. Such a high placement of the electrode is to be strenuously resisted.

Once the lesions have been completed, the electrode can then be removed. To prevent cerebrospinal fluid rhinorrhea, fascia lata should be packed into the sella turcica using a double pointed stylet, with a tip 1 mm in cross section. Using this double-pronged instru-

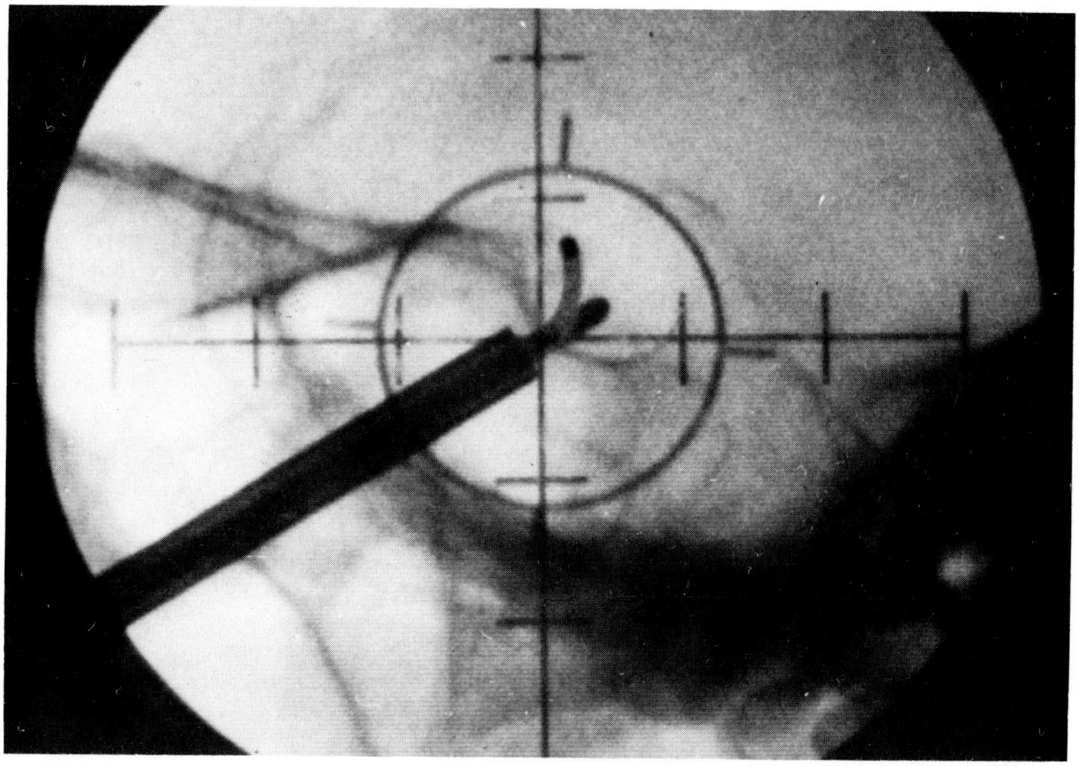

Fig. 14-3. Lateral radiographic showing sidearm projecting up.

ment, small squares of tissue can be easily carried along the cannula directly through the anterior wall of the sella into the electrode tract. As these are advanced, the surgeon can feel the tract becoming filled. In order to avoid having to remove tissue from the patient, bovine facia lata (Ethicon) can be used. This is very satisfactory material and has caused neither infection nor rejection. Once the tract appears to be filled, a dumbbell-shaped silicone plug can be impacted into the bone opening with the proper instrument. The plug we employ contains silver particles so that its proper positioning can be confirmed radiographically. The cannula in the sphenoid sinus is then partially removed and the sinus again washed copiously with bacitracin solution. The cannula is then totally removed and a Vaseline gauze pack is placed in the appropriate nostril. This can be removed 8 hours thereafter.

Following operation the patient is usually in very good condition and has few restrictions.

Postoperative Management

Replacement Therapy

Hydrocortizone is given in the postoperative period, beginning with 200 mg/day and gradually declining over a 6-day period to 30 mg/day in divided doses. Thyroid replacement can be begun at any time in the postoperative period, usually 60 mg of thyroid extract will suffice.

It is very important that antibiotics be continued in the postoperative period for 5 days. Intravenous oxycillin, 1 g every 6 hours, is used for the first 2 days and then oral dicloxacillin 1 g, every 6 hours, for the final 3 days.

Diabetes insipidus occurs in almost every patient within 2 or 3 days after operation. It generally subsides within 1 to 2 weeks. If excessive in the beginning, it can be controlled with Pitressin Tannate in oil. Thereafter, it can be minimized by giving the patient Chlorapropamide 125 to 250 mg/day. If this is not adequate, DDAVP can be given as a nasal spray twice a day. The latter virtually eliminates diabetes insipidus in all patients who require long-term therapy. In our hands 1 patient in 20 will require treatment beyond 1 month after operation. DDAVP appears to be the most satisfactory agent to control diabetes insipidus in the long term.

Complications

Cerebrospinal Fluid Rhinorrhea

This is very rare when the sella has been packed and the anterior wall defect occluded. If it does occur, it should be repaired surgically, using the open transsphenoidal method to inspect the defect quickly. Some patients complain of wetness in the nose, particularly after eating spicy food. Others worry excessively that a wet nose may mean that they have a cerebrospinal fluid leak. The surgeon should not be hastened into an unnecessary operation by concluding that wetness itself indicates rhinorrhea. The diagnosis should be confirmed by the actual collection of fluid from the nose that contains glucose on the one hand and has a higher potassium level than serum. When in doubt the diagnosis should be confirmed by radioactive isotope scanning after the introduction of intrathecal labeled isotope.

Local Infection

In over 600 cases we have not encountered an instance of infection in the sphenoid sinus or nasal cavities with exception of 1 patient who continuously complained of a greenish discharge from the nostril. However, 2 patients did develop intrasellar abscesses. Prodromal symptoms and signs were periorbital pain and fever. As the processes developed rapidly, higher fever, stiff neck with pleocytosis of the cerebrospinal fluid developed. There was no evidence of cerebrospinal fluid rhinorrhea. In both instances the sella turcica was opened stereotaxically so as to permit drainage. This tactic, together with the administration of very large doses of antibiotics, resulted in total recovery in both instances. In both cases these unfortunate complications developed in patients with diabetic retinopathy, and it is probable that the diabetic state was partially responsible for the development of the abscess. In addition 1 patient was inadvertently not given antibiotics after operation.

Hemorrhage

In none of the patients we operated upon has intraoperative hemorrhage from the sella turcica been encountered. Two patients did develop epistaxis at the very beginning of the procedure, necessitating termination of the operation. Both of these hemorrhages were the result of thrombocytopenia, caused from chemotherapy for breast cancer.

CHAPTER 15

Stereotactic Biopsy of Deep Intracranial Tumors

Louis W. Conway

RATIONAL TREATMENT OF CEREBRAL TUMORS is best served by histologic diagnosis. Typically, the neurosurgeon or radiotherapist requires tissue confirmation in order to decide upon the most suitable treatment for his patient. Certain intracranial masses, however, are often treated by external radiation following a presumptive diagnosis based on the clinical picture plus neuroradiologic studies, without confirmatory biopsy. These lesions include intrinsic tumors of the brainstem,[1] and masses in the region of the pineal and posterior third ventricle,[2-10] masses that lie within deep subcortical structures, principally the thalamus,[11-14] and tumors in or about the sella turcica.[15-17] Justified conservatism in operative exposure of these areas has been supported by one or more of the following:

1. Relative inaccessibility of the involved area.
2. A statistical knowledge of the types of tumors usually in these areas.
3. A high incidence of tumors, not surgically resectable or amenable to surgical palliation.
4. A high incidence of lesions, palliated by radiation.
5. A significant incidence of tumors, either palliated for a long period or cured by radiation.
6. An unacceptable morbidity and mortality from direct surgical approach.

Tumors of the Thalamic and Pineal Regions

Ten years ago, in a study of thalamic tumors, Cheek and Taveres[11] introduced the subject by stating: "The diagnosis of thalamic tumors was originally attempted on purely clinical grounds, but in recent years it has been based primarily on pneumoencephalographic studies, although the diagnosis may also be made by cerebral angiography." After reviewing a series of 51 cases, of which almost half (24) had open surgical biopsy, they concluded that best results were obtained if a presumptive diagnosis, based on radiographic studies, was followed by deep radiation therapy, avoiding craniotomy.

Similar approaches have been advocated for other deep and midline lesions. Thus, Posner and Horrax[7] advocated treating tumors of the pineal region on the basis of the clinical picture, including eye signs. Likewise Ward and Spurling[10] recommended that posterior third ventricular tumors be treated by subtemporal decompression and radiation. They suggested only cases that failed to respond should undergo "direct surgical attack." More recently,

Department of Neurosurgery, Arnett Clinic & Hospital, Inc., Lafayette, Indiana 47904

Suzuki and associates[9] have made a similar suggestion and advocated the use of serial Myodil ventriculography during and following radiation therapy as a guide to the effectiveness of radiation. This report, in 1969, is of interest in that Suzuki's group had previously reported a large series of surgical excisions of pineal tumors (19 cases).[19] Suzuki and associates do emphasize, however, in their earlier article, the importance of postoperative radiation, as the majority of tumors were invasive and not completely removable. The recent article by DeGirolami and Schmidek[3] reports a series of 53 cases of tumor in the pineal region, 35 of which were histologically verified, treated over a 52-year period and recommend a conservative approach. They report a 33% mortality from open biopsy in this area and a greater than 50% mortality from subtotal removal. Total removal was not accomplished. The authors review the literature on surgical mortality of operations in this area, and with notable exceptions report a mortality of between 20% and 70%. Exceptions included the Suzuki et al. report of 19 cases with an operative mortality of 10% and both Jamieson's[20] and Stein's[21] reports of little morbidity and no mortality. Each series had 6 patients. Stein resurrected the infratentorial supracerebellar technique, originated by Krause.[22] Recently Page[23] reports 9 cases, exploring this area using this technique, with one death, a patient with a glioblastoma of the left posterior thalamus. The reports of these latter four authors were published during the past 12 years and represent relatively recent surgical cases. It should be recognized that many of the studies reporting a 20% to 70% mortality either are early ones or include a series of patients dating back many years, some half a century. It is likely, therefore, that surgical mortality by modern techniques should not exceed 10%. Surgical resection is at times indicated, for not all masses are neoplastic[13] and not all neoplastic lesions are unresectable or radiosensitive.[14,19,24-26] Most studies would indicate there is approximately a 10% incidence of well-encapsulated tumors, cystic tumors, or hemangiomas, not expected to respond to radiation, plus nonneoplastic lesions, such as arachnoid cysts. At least some of these would be surgically resectable. In 1962 Sachs[26] after studying three meningiomas of the pineal region and reviewing the literature on this lesion, stated: "An excessively conservative attitude toward tumors in this region has prevailed for a long time." Thus several investigators, using modern surgical techniques, have returned to surgical exposure and biopsy or resection of masses in this area, modifying techniques described in the first third of this century by such surgeons as Krause,[22] Dandy,[27] and Horrax.[28]

In summary, it would appear that some recent investigators are willing to accept a potentially serious morbidity and mortality, probably not exceeding 10%, in order to find a resectable lesion in somewhat less than 10% of cases. Nevertheless most of these tumors are not completely excisable and are highly radiosensitive.[3,5,19] The advantages of radiation therapy on a presumptive basis however, has to be weighed against the potential hazards and, at times, inappropriateness of radiation therapy. We feel, as have others, that possibly a stereotaxic technique of biopsying these lesions might well prove to be the method of choice in obtaining, with relative safety, a histologic diagnosis by which appropriate therapy can be selected on a rational basis.

Sellar and Suprasellar Lesions

Over the years, intrasellar and suprasellar tumors have been readily approached by direct surgical means, with relatively low morbidity and mortality.[29] In recent years use of the operating microscope and recognition that a significant number of intrasellar tumors are discrete and totally resectable has led to a renewed interest in and a wide acceptance of transsphenoidal[30] and transfrontal surgery in this area. Nevertheless it would appear that most patients with sellar and suprasellar lesions are still treated with radiotherapy on the basis of clinical presentation.[15-17] Some however, have found conventional radiation therapy of limited value in pituitary adenomas[36,53] Craniopharyngiomas, although thought to be curable by external radiation by some, are best identified because of the higher doses of radiation recommended for this lesion.[15] Still other lesions should be regarded as less radiosensitive. These include cystic pituitary adenomas, nonneoplastic cysts of the pituitary,[32] intrasellar abscess,[33] mucocele of the sphenoid sinus,[34,35] meningiomas, chordomas,[36] leiomyomas,[37] granular cell myoblastoma,[38] pituicytoma,[39] enlargement of sella turcica due to dilatation of the anterior third ventricle, the empty sellar syndrome,[40,41] and intrasellar aneurysms.[42] Several of these lesions can be diagnosed by radiographic studies alone, and stereotaxic biopsy is not only unncessary but contraindicated. In others however, stereotaxic biopsy would be either useful or essential in guiding the clinician from radiotherapy to appropriate treatment.

Stereotaxic Surgery for Histologic Diagnosis

Over the past 17 years, several stereotaxic techniques have been described for obtaining tissue from deep within cerebral structures. These are instruments adapted to conventional stereotaxic machines. Most have been a form of cannula[43-46] or an adaptation of the Silverman biopsy needle.[18] Backlund[47] and Coe et al.[48] have described spiral corkscrew-like devices for holding tissue within the cannula. Waltregny et al.[49] have described obtaining specimens of neoplastic tissue using the Metzel-Wittmoser ventriculoscope forceps, introduced through a guide.

Most of the earlier biopsies were performed on nonneoplastic tissue during thalamotomy for movement disorders, to confirm the appropriateness of the target sites and to obtain tissue for histologic and histochemical study of these conditions.[43-45,50,51] Recently stereotaxic biopsy of nonneoplastic tissue has expanded. For instance, Waltregny et al.[49] report using their technique for histochemical studies of epileptic foci and Hankinson et al.[55] report biopsy of the human basal ganglia in cases of cerebral porphyria.

As early as 1947 Spiegel et al.[52] suggested that stereotaxic surgery might include the aspiration of maerial (they were thinking primarily of fluid from cysts) in the diagnosis of subcortical tumors. Over the ensuing years, little was written as regards stereotaxic biopsy of intracranial neoplastic disorders until 1969 when Conway et al.[53] and Rand et al.[36] reported an initial experience with stereotaxic biopsy of pituitary tumors during stereotaxic treatment of these lesions. The following year Lee et al.[54] reported stereotaxic biopsy of a chromophobe adenoma as a specific diagnostic step prior to external radiation therapy. Recently several authors have reported a more extensive experience with a wider group of tumors. Backlund et al.[55] report stereotaxic biopsy prior to interstitial radiation of multiple tumors, including a good success in biopsy of craniopharyngiomas[47] and a modicum of success with pineal tumors.[55] Edner,[56] in 1965, briefly reports a 5-year experience with the stereotaxic biopsy of 154 intracranial tumors, with two complications, one transient and one permanent but no mortality. Recently Waltregny et al.[49] reported the value of multiple biopsies to outline the extent of five deep-seated intracranial tumors. In 1973 we reported the value of stereotaxic biopsy in the diagnosis of 31 deep-seated intracranial tumors over an 8-year period, with a 90% positive histologic diagnosis and no significant morbidity.[31] Since that time our experience has increased to 72 cases in which positive diagnosis has been made in 68.

Clinical Material

As outlined in Table 15-1, 102 biopsies were performed on 72 patients. Thirty-four of these were tumors of the pituitary; 5 pineal lesions; 6 gliomas of the posterior thalamus; 12 tumors placed more laterally in deep structures, primarily thought to be in the thalamus, and 15 tumors deep in the parietal area, characteristically in the dominant hemisphere involving deep white matter and basal ganglia structures. The posterior third ventricular glioma group

Table 15-1. Summary of 72 Cases of Stereotaxic Biopsy

Presumptive diagnosis	No. of biopsies	No. of cases	Tissue diagnosis: Confirmatory	Tissue diagnosis: Other	
Pituitary adenomas:					
Eosinophilic	30	25	24	Nasal mucosa	1
Chromophobic	10	7	5	Craniopharyngioma	2
Basophilic	3	2		Chromophobic	2
Pinealoma	7 (9)	5 (7)	4 (5)	Blood clot	1(2)
Gliomas:					
Posterior third ventricle	8	6	4	Histiocytosis X	1
				Necrosis	1
Thalamus	21	12	12		
Deep parietal lobe	23	15	14	Gliosis	1
Total	102	72	63		9
				Diagnostic	5

includes some patients who were thought to have tumors in the posterior thalamus and corpus callosum and others that could just as well have been placed in the pineal group.

Criteria

Patients were selected for stereotaxic biopsy on the basis of the following criteria.

Lesions Relatively Inaccessible. In each case the patient would either have to be treated on the basis of a presumptive diagnosis made from clinical and neuroradiologic findings or would have had to undergo major intracranial surgery to obtain histologic confirmation. Cases in which a major neurosurgical resection or decompresssion was planned, regardless of the histologic diagnosis, were not considered candidates for stereotaxic biopsy.

Lesions Accurately Localized. This procedure was considered safe and justified only if the lesion had been accurately visualized by an appropriate combination of radioisotopic and radiographic techniques.

"Mass Effect" Minimal and Reversible. Large hemispheric tumors with clinical or angiographic evidence of tentorial herniation were not considered suitable. Patients with marked increased intracranial pressures were also excluded, unless the pressure was readily reducible. In cases with obstructive hydrocephalus, the confirmatory biopsy was either preceded or immediately followed by a ventriculoatrial shunt.

Preoperative Evaluation

The preoperative evaluation included sufficient studies to accurately localize the lesion. By carefully selecting and modifying these studies, it was often possible to obviate or minimize the need for repeat contrast studies at the time of stereotaxic biopsy.

By using identical target-to-film distances and identical positions of the patient's head and central beam of the x-ray at the time of preoperative contrast studies, as compared with these parameters at the time of stereotaxic surgery, it was possible to obtain preoperative films that could be superimposed on plain x-ray films taken during the stereotaxic procedure. Again, superimposition of studies was facilitated by the use of radiopaque markers placed on strategic areas of the patient's scalp. Alternatively, contrast studies were sometimes performed or repeated during stereotaxic biopsy. The smaller the target lesion or the more strategically the lesion was placed in relation to vital structures, the greater was the need for repeat contrast study at the time of biopsy. For all pineal lesions, for instance, ventriculography was repeated at the time of biopsy.

Although radionuclide rectolinear scanners tend to distort the shape of the skull and lesion, lengthening it in one direction, and although the radionuclide gamma camera tends to make the skull and targets more round and globular, scans can be superimposed on skull films with relative accuracy in larger lesions by techniques previously described.[57-59]

Preoperative studies varied with the lesion under consideration but have included routine and special x-ray views of the skull, nasal sinuses, and sella turcia; radionuclide imaging; computerized axial tomography; cerebral angiography; retrograde cavernous sinus angiography[60]; pneumoencephalography; and positive contrast ventriculography. Plain skull films were considered invaluable in lesions of the sella turcica to partially outline the mass and to rule out sella enlargement on the basis of erosion from below, such as from sphenoid mucocele.[34,35] Furthermore, pneumoencephalography was performed in each case with a lesion of the sella turcica to outline the superior extent of the tumor and to rule out an enlarged sella turcica on the basis of the "empty sella syndrome"[40,41] In this latter circumstance transsphenoidal violation of the floor of the sella turcica would lead to troublesome rhinorrhea. Furthermore angiography was deemed necessary in all cases to rule out a vascular lesion, such as an aneurysm,[42] in which instance needle biopsy might be expected to lead to uncontrollable hemorrhage.

Operative Procedure

With the exception of 4 children, the stereotaxic procedure was performed under local anesthesia. When the tumor was to be approached via the transcranial route, the scalp was shaved and completely prepped for surgery. For the transsphenoidal approach, no scalp hair was removed and the scalp and nose were prepared as described elsewhere.[61] The head was held firmly in the Todd-Wells stereotaxic apparatus, using positive pin fixation facilitated by infiltrating the scalp and periosteum with local anesthetic. In some cases air was introduced into the ventricular system via the lumbar theca before the patient was placed in the stereotaxic apparatus. On other occasions, either iophendylate (Pantopaque) or 60% meglumine iothalamate (Conray) was injected into the lateral ventricles through appropriately positioned burr holes to outline a lesion. Occasionally intravascular catheters were placed either in the internal carotid artery or jugular vein in anticipation of intraoperative cerebral angiography or retrograde cavernous angiography.

Subsequent to accurate localization of the lesion and positioning of the patient, needle biopsy was performed either through a cranial burr hole or, in the case of lesions of the sella turcica, through transsphenoidal drill holes in the floor or anterior wall of the sella turcica.

The equipment used for biopsy is illustrated in Figure 15-1. Trocar needles, with an outer diameter of either 2.2 or 4.7 mm, were used. These instruments are similar to those originally described by Kalyanaraman and Gillingham[45] to obtain nonneoplastic tissue from the thalamus. The outer edge of the distal portion of the needle is somewhat beveled but not sharp. A stylet fits flush with the tip of the needle. A stop can be fixed firmly at any point throughout the length of the needle by means of a thumbscrew. Additional equipment required includes soft rubber tubing with well-fitting male or female adapters on each end, a syringe, and a hemostat.

The needle, with stylet in place, is introduced through a guide toward the appropriate intracranial lesion. When the needle tip has been advanced to a point slightly short of the target, the stylet is removed. The needle tip is then advanced to or beyond the target point, thus effectively cutting a core of tissue. (The distance over which the open needle was advanced varied from 6 mm to 6 cm, depending on the size of the tumor.) Subsequently, the

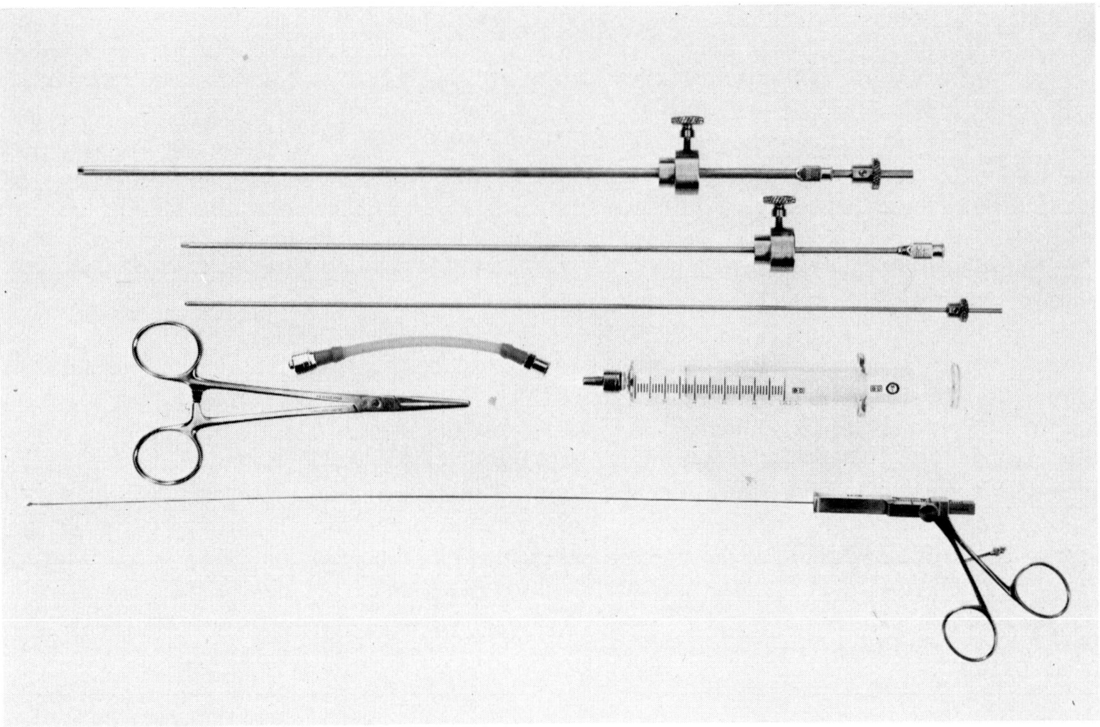

Fig. 15-1. Biopsy equipment used to obtain tissue specimens. At the top is a 4.7-mm trochar with beveled tip and stylet in place. Note the adjustable stop with thumbscrew near the proximal end of the needle. Below this is a 2.2-mm needle of similar design. The stylet has been removed from this needle and is shown immediately below. Other equipment includes a piece of soft rubber tubing that can be attached securely to the proximal end of the needle, a 10-ml syringe to be attached to the distal end of the tubing, and a hemostat. A pair of biopsy forceps is available that can be introduced to the target site through either of the above biopsy needles.

soft rubber tubing is attached to the needle hub and gentle suction applied until the tubing collapses. Negative suction is maintained by placing a hemostat on the rubber tubing; this captures the tissue specimen at the tip of the needle. The syringe is then removed, leaving the hemostat in place, and the biopsy needle is removed from the stereotaxic apparatus. A syringe filled with saline is now attached to the rubber tubing. While moderate pressure is applied to the syringe, the hemostat is removed from the rubber tubing, and the specimen gently irrigated onto a piece of moist fine mesh gauze (Fig. 15-2). Most specimens present as a cylinder of tissue. The proximal and distal ends are identified, the specimens fixed in 10% formalin, and oriented during embedding in paraffin so that longitudinal sections through the core can be obtained. These longitudinal sections can be correlated with biplane x-ray films taken during the procedure, outlining the distance and direction of travel during the coring of the biopsy specimen. By slightly altering the target point of the needle, subsequent biopsies can be obtained adjacent to the initial biopsy. Since some of the tissues biopsied are friable on occasion, only fragments of tissue are obtained. In such cases precise orientation of the specimen is not possible. Such fragments however, usually provide the histologic diagnosis.

Also available, in the event a firm mass is palpated at the tip of the needle or adequate tissue is not obtained, are a pair of biopsy forceps[62] with an adjustable stop. The forceps are introduced to the target point through either biopsy cannula and small pieces of tissue obtained. This technique is not unlike that described by Lee et al.,[54] Asenjo,[50] and Waltregny et al.[49] To date these forceps (supplied by F. L. Fischer) have proved of value in biopsying craniopharyngiomas.

Results

As outlined in Table 15-1, adequate diagnostic specimens were obtained in 68 cases (Figs. 15-2, 15-3, 15-4, and 15-5). Of these, 63 biopsies confirmed the preoperative presumptive diagnosis. In 5 cases the final diagnosis was positive but differed from the preoperative diagnosis. Two cases, thought to be nonsecreting pituitary adenomas, proved to be craniopharyngiomas. Two cases of Cushing's syndrome proved to have tumors without basophilic staining cells. One case was thought to be a posterior third ventricular glioma but proved to be a case of histiocytosis X.[63] In 4 cases, biopsy was not diagnostic. In 3 of these a pathologic process was found. The process however, was not diagnostic of a specific lesion. Subsequently, 2 of these proved to have astrocytomas. In 1 case the biopsy was of glial tissue that was thought to be not necessarily neoplastic. The other biopsy showed necrotic tissue. The latter patient, a postmortem, was found to have a largely necrotic malignant glioma of the corpus collosum. The biopsy proved representative of a large volume of the tumor. In 1 case of presumed pinealoma, with a short clinical history and rapid deterioration, the biopsy proved to be a blood clot. Although the specimen did not produce a tissue diagnosis, it did establish the diagnosis of apoplexy within the pineal region and aspiration of the clot proved of value in reversing this patient's symptoms, while on the operating table, under local anesthesia. Thereafter the patient underwent a ventriculoatrial shunt, but the immediate local decompression was clearly of therapeutic value. In only 1 case was the tissue unappropriate to the pathologic process. Nasal mucosa was obtained during transsphenoidal biopsy of a pituitary adenoma associated with acromegaly.

Two patients have undergone repeat pineal biopsy. This is so indicated in Table 15-1 by the figures in brackets. The second biopsy followed a previous stereotaxic diagnosis and external radiation therapy followed by deterioration, rebiopsy, and cryosurgery of the pineal area at the time of the second biopsy. The second was performed 18 and 36 months after the initial biopsy and radiation therapy. One of the two biopsies was productive of pineal tissue, unchanged as compared with that before therapy. The other produced white matter and fresh blood clot.

Morbidity and Mortality

Morbidity from this procedure has been minimal. One patient had a transient increase in hemiparesis, following several biopsies of a thalamic tumor. In another case the formal technique of needle biopsy was abandoned because, there was excessive bleeding through the needle as it was placed into a vascular glioma. This was treated by leaving the needle in place for several minutes while it was gently irrigated with saline. Blood and irrigation fluid were filtered through gauze and the solid tissue was submitted for pathologic study. The tissue proved to be a glioblastoma multiforme and is included among the positive biopsy specimens in Table 15-1. The patient experienced no subsequent deterioration attributable to the biopsy procedure. To date there has been no mortality associated with this procedure.

Summary and Conclusions

We have demonstrated that in appropriate cases needle biopsy offers a valuable and, at times, superior alternative, either to treatment on a presumptive basis without histologic diagnosis on one hand, or operative exposure on the other. Free-hand needle biopsy has proved to be a useful procedure.[18,64] Doubtless some of the cases reported in this study could have been so treated. Nevertheless in many, such a procedure would have been hazardous and unlikely to have provided diagnostic tissue in a significant number of cases. Clearly the larger, more diffuse, and more superficial the lesion, the less the need for the precision

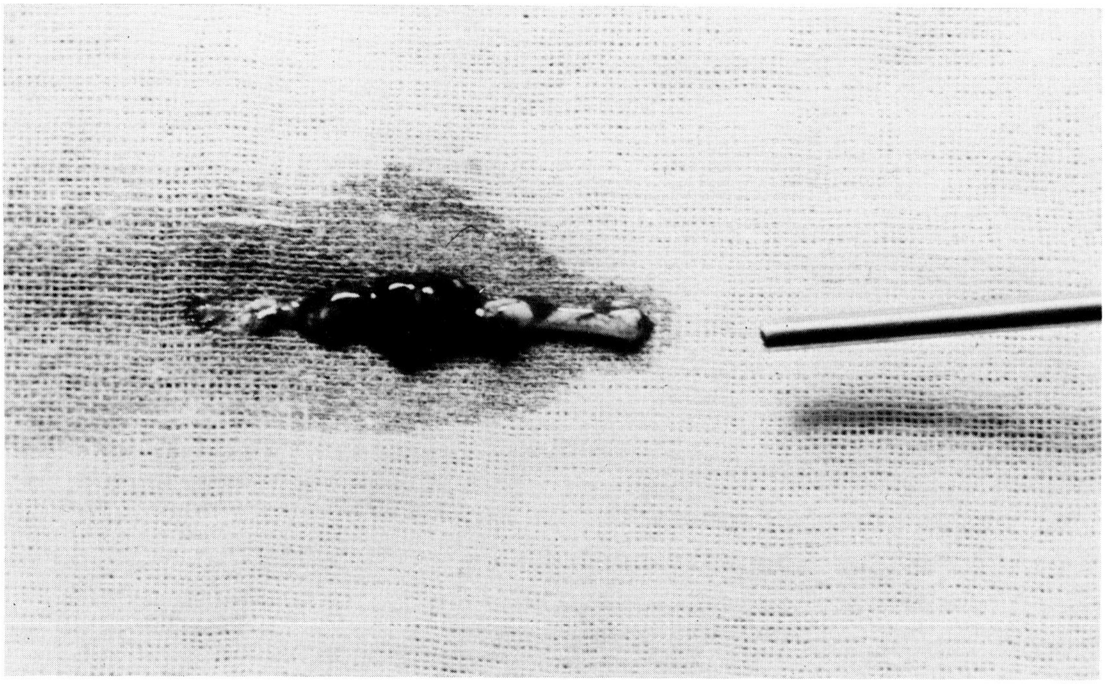

Fig. 15-2. Specimen of a glioblastoma multiforme of the lateral thalamus obtained with the 2.2-mm biopsy needle. The specimen was captured and extruded onto a piece of fine-mesh, moist gauze, as described in the text. The biopsy needle is seen to the right, the superficial end, of the specimen. The deep portion of the biopsy is cellular (Fig. 15-3); the central portion hemorrhagic necrotic tumor, and the superficial one-third white matter of the internal capsule with minimal tumor invasion.

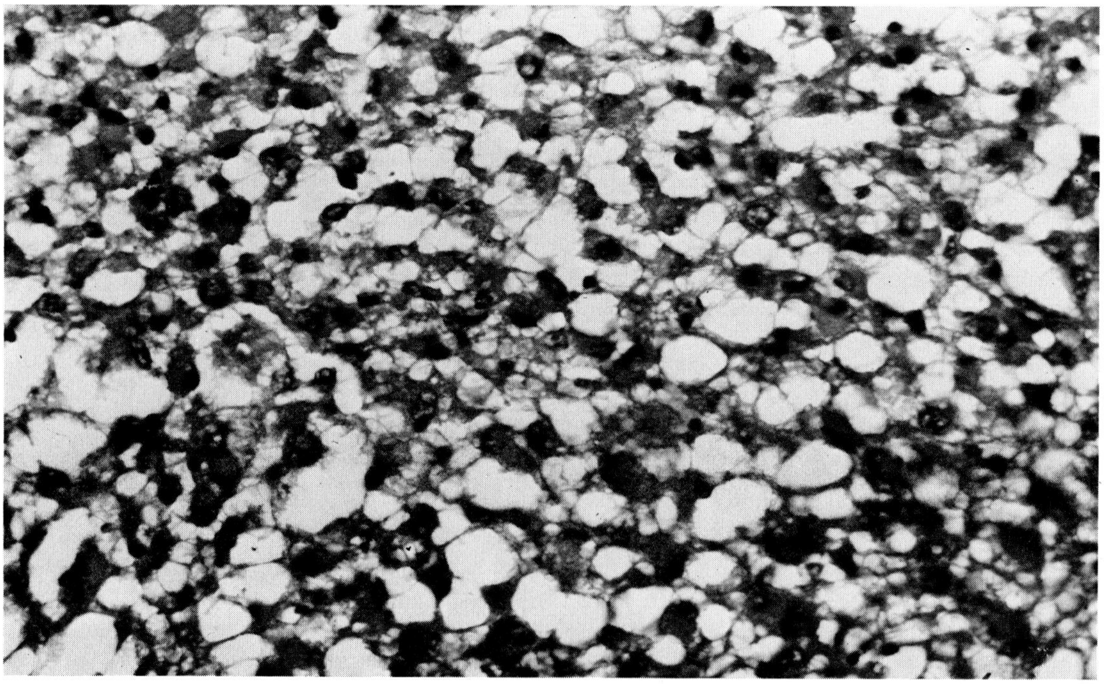

Fig. 15-3. Glioblastoma multiforme of the thalamus obtained from distal portion of the specimen in Figure 15-2 (H&E, X480).

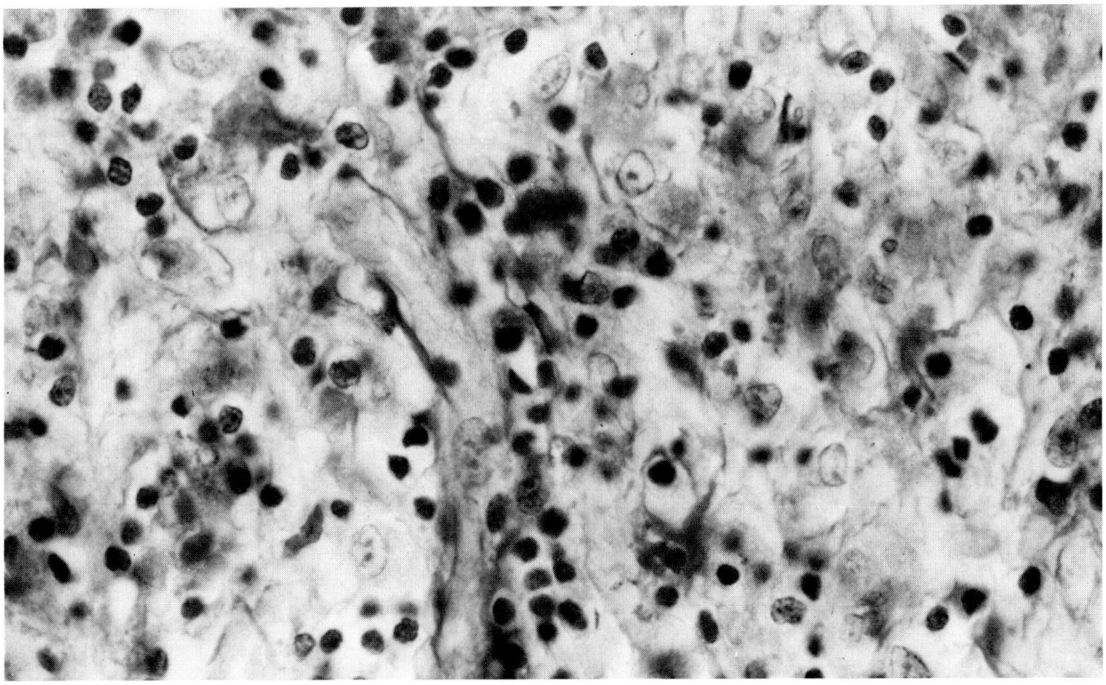

Fig. 15-4. Posterior third ventricular tumor, histologic diagnosis Histiocytosis X (PAS-PTAH, X680).

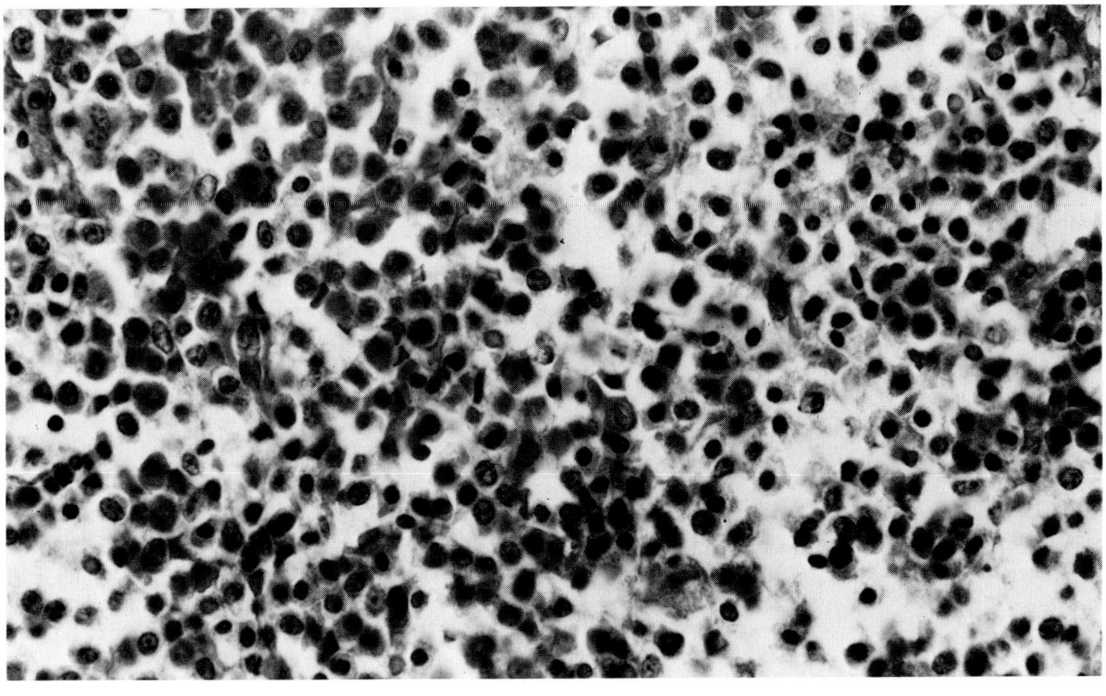

Fig. 15-5. Intrasellar chromophobe adenoma of the pituitary (H&E, X480).

afforded by stereotaxis. Conversely, therefore, particularly with the deeper less accessible and smaller tumors, provided accurate assessment of their size and position is possible, stereotaxic biopsy is the preferable and, at times, essential alternatives.

The stereotaxic technique permits biopsy of lesions otherwise inaccessible; can be expected to decrease morbidity and mortality, as compared with open surgical biopsy or freehand needle biopsy; probably increases the yield of positive biopsies; allows precise roentgenographic correlation of the site of biopsy; and allows histologic confirmation of the appropriateness of the proposed target site during stereotaxic techniques of tumor destruction.

Our experience with follow-up stereoaxic biopsy, following treatment, has been confined to 2 cases and in only 1 of these cases was the biopsy satisfactory. It is possible that stereotaxic biopsy will prove of value in the follow-up of deep-seated lesions following therapy. Others have advocated follow-up contrast studies to assess the size of deep-seated lesions following radiation therapy.[9] Certainly, while the mass is being outlined, histologic follow-up of such a lesion would be of value; the risks of obtaining such specimens may prove justified. The frequency with which follow-up histologic confirmation of the results of therapy is appropriate will increase as the number of alternate and competing modes of effective therapy increase.

REFERENCES

1. Bray PF, Carter S, Taveras JM: Brainstem tumors in children. *Neurology 8*:1-7, 1958
2. Cummins FM, Taveras JM, Schlesinger EB: Treatment of gliomas of the third ventricle and pinealomas: with special reference to the value of radiotherapy. *Neurology 10*:1031-1036, 1960
3. DeGirolami U, Schmidek H: Clinicopathological study of fifty-two tumors of the pineal region. *J Neurosurg 39*:455-462, 1973
4. Fowler FD, Alexander E Jr, Davis CH, Jr: Pinealoma with metastases in the central nervous system: a rationale of treatment. *J Neurosurg 13*:271-288, 1956
5. Minger R, Meltzer J, Botstein C: Pinealoma, a report of twelve irradiated cases. *Cancer 37*:2713-2718, 1976
6. Poppen JL, Marino R, Jr: Pinealomas and tumors of the posterior portion of the third ventricle. *J Neurosurg 28*:357-364, 1968
7. Posner M, Horrax G: Eye signs in pineal tumors. *J Neursurg 3*:15-24, 1946
8. Rand RW, Lemmen LJ: Tumors of the posterior portion of the third ventricle. *J Neurosurg 10*:1-18, 1953
9. Suzuki J, Hori S: Evaluation of radiotherapy of tumors in the pineal region by ventriculographic studies with iodized oil. *J Neurosurg 30*:595-603, 1969
10. Ward A, Spurling RG: The conservative treatment of third ventricle tumors. *J Neurosurg 5*:124-130, 1948
11. Cheek WR, Taveras JM: Thalamic tumors. *J Neurosurg 24*:505-513, 1966
12. McKissock W, Paine KWE: Primary tumors of the thalamus. *Brain 81*:41-63, 1958
13. Ng LKT, Schwarz G, Mishkin MM: Hematoma from arteriovenous malformation producing hydrocephalus and simulating a thalamic tumor. *J Neurosurg 34*:229-235, 1971
14. Tovi D, Schisano G, Liljeqvist B: Primary tumors of the region of the thalamus. *J Neurosurg 18*:730-740, 1961
15. Kramer S, McKissock W, Concannon JP: Craniopharyngiomas: treatment by combined surgery and radiation therapy. *J Neurosurg 18*:217-226, 1961
16. Roth J, Gorden P, Brace K: Efficacy of conventional pituitary irradiation in acromegaly. *N Engl J Med 282*:1385-1391, 1970
17. Svien HJ, Colby MY Jr: Pituitary chromophobe adenomas: comparative results of surgical and roentgen treatment. *Behav Neuropsychiatr 1*:35-39, 1969
18. Heath RG, John S, Foss O: Stereotaxic biopsy. *Arch Neurol 4*:291-300, 1961
19. Suzuki J, Iwabuchi T: Surgical removal of pineal tumors (pinealomas and teratomas). Experience in a series of 19 years. *J Neurosurg 23*:565-571, 1965
20. Jamieson KG: Excision of pineal tumors. *J Neurosurg 35*:550-553, 1971
21. Stein BM: The infratentorial supracerebellar approach to pineal lesions. *J Neurosurg 35*:197-202, 1971
22. Krause F: Operative Freilegung der Vierhugel, nebst Beobachtungen uber Hirndruck und Dekompression *Zentralbl Chir 53*:2812-2819, 1926

23. Page LK: Infratentorial supracerebellar exposures of tumors in the pineal area. (in print)
24. Kirsch WM, Stears JC: Radiographic identification and surgical excision of an epidermoid tumor of the pineal gland: case report. *J Neurosurg 33*:708-713, 1970
25. Russell DS: The pinealoma: its relationship to teratoma. *J Pathol Bacteriol 56*:145-150, 1944
26. Sachs E Jr, Avman N, Fisher RG: Meningiomas of pineal region and posterior part of 3rd ventricle. *J Neurosurg 19*:325-331, 1962
27. Dandy WE: An operation for the removal of pineal tumors. *Surg Gynecol Obstet 33*:113-119, 1921
28. Horrax G: Extirpation of a huge pinealomas from a patient with pubertas praecox: a new operative approach. *Arch Neurol Psychiatr 37*:385-395, 1937
29. Wirth FP, Schwartz HG, Schwetschenau PR: Pituitary adenomas: factors in treatment. *Clinical Neurosurgery,* vol 21. Williams and Wilkins, Baltimore, 1973, pp 8-24
30. Hardy J: Transsphenoidal microsurgery of the normal and pathological pituitary, *Clinical Neurosurgery*, vol 16. Williams and Wilkins, Baltimore, 1968, pp 185-214
31. Conway LW: Stereotaxic diagnosis and treatment of intracranial tumors including an initial experience with cryosurgery for pinealomas. *J Neurosurg 38*:453-459, 1973
32. Weber EL, Vogel FS, Odom GL: Cysts of the sella turcica. *J Neurosurg 33*:48-53, 1970
33. Hammann H de V: Abscess formation in the pituitary fossa associated with a pituitary adenoma. *J Neurosurg 13*:208-210, 1956
34. Doyle CS, Simeone FA: Mucocele of the sphenoid sinus with bilateral internal carotid artery occlusion: case report. *J Neurosurg 36*:351-354, 1972
35. Simms NM, Brown WE, French LA: Mucocele of the sphenoid sinus presenting as an intrasellar mass: case report. *J Neurosurg 32*:708-710, 1970
36. Rand RW, Heuser G, Dashe A, et al: Stereotaxic transsphenoidal biopsy and cryosurgery of pituitary tumors. *Am J Roentgenol 105*:273-286, 1969
37. Kroe DJ, Hudgins WR, Simmons JCH, et al: Primary intrasellar leiomyoma: case report. *J Neurosurg 29*:189-191, 1968
38. Symon L, Ganz JC, Burston J: Granular cell myoblastoma of the neurohypophysis: report of two cases. *J Neurosurg 35*:82-89, 1971
39. Liss L, Kahn EA: Pituicytoma. Tumor of the sella turcica: a clinicopathological study. *J Neurosurg 15*:481-488, 1958
40. Bernasconi V, Giovanelli MA, Papo I: Primary empty sella. *J Neurosurg 36*:157-161, 1972
41. Obrador S: The empty sella and some related syndromes. *J Neurosurg 36*:162-168, 1972
42. Cartlidge NEF, Shaw DA: Intrasellar aneurysm with subarachnoid hemorrhage and hypopituitarism. *J Neurosurg 36*:640-643, 1972
43. Housepian EM, Pool JL: The accuracy of human stereoencephalotomy as judged by histological confirmation of roentgenographic localization. *J Nerv Ment Dis 130*:520-525, 1960
44. Housepian EM, Pool JL: Application of stereotaxic methods to histochemical, electronmicroscopic and electrophysiological studies of human subcortical structures. *Confin Neurol 22*:171-177, 1962
45. Kalyanaraman S, Gillingham FJ: Stereotaxic biopsy. *J Neurosurg 21*:854-858, 1964
46. Reichert T, Gisinger MA, Molberg E: Biopsien wahrend stereotaktischer operationen beim parkinsonsyndron. *Neurochirurgia 10*:106-118
47. Backlund EO: A new instrument for stereotaxic brain biopsy. *Acta Chir Scand 137*:825-827, 1971
48. Coe JE, Dirlik P, Ommaya AK: An instrument for brain biopsy utilizing a new extraction principal. *J Neurosurg 23*:217-218, 1965
49. Waltregny A, Petrov V, Brotchi J: Serial stereotaxic biopsies. *Acta Neurochir (Wien):Suppl 21*:221-226, 1974
50. Asenjo A: Cytosiderosis and iron deposits in ventrolateral nucleus of the thalamus in Parkinson's disease: clinical and experimental study. *Johns Hopkins Med J 122*:284-294, 1968
51. Hankinson J, Hudgson P, Pearce GW, et al: A simple method for obtaining stereotaxic biopsies of human basal ganglia. A case of cerebral porphyria. *Acta Neurochir:Suppl 21*:227-233, 1974
52. Spiegel EA, Wycis HT, Marks M, et al: Stereotaxic apparatus for operations on the human brain. *Science 106*:349-350, 1947
53. Conway LW, O'Foghludha FT, Collins SF: Stereotactic treatment of acromegaly. *J Neurol Neurosurg Psychiatr 32*:48-59, 1969
54. Lee KF, Zervas NT, Horner FA, et al: Asymptomatic chromophobe adenoma in an eight-year-old child biopsied by stereotaxic technique and treated with Cobalt-60: case report. *J Neurosurg 32*:585-588, 1970
55. Backlund EO, Rahn T, Sarby B: Treatment of pinealomas by stereotaxic radiation surgery. *Acta Chir Scand 139*:237-247, 1973
56. Edner G: Stereotaxic brain tumor biopsy—five year's experience. Proceedings of the 26th annual meeting. *Acta Neurochir (Wien) 31*:261, 1965

57. Kuhl DE, Hale J, Eaton WL: Transmission scanning: a useful adjunct to conventional emission scanning for accurately keying isotope deposition to radiographic anatomy. *Radiology 87*:278-284, 1966
58. Marryat J, Bull JWD: An apparatus providing a combined radiograph and gamma scan. *Br J Radiol 37*:711-713, 1964
59. Williams JP: A simple marking device for use with the gamma camera. *J Nucl Med 12*:300-301, 1971
60. Hanafee W, Rosen LM, Weidner W, et al: Venography of the cavernous sinus, orbital veins, and basal venous plexus. *Radiology 84*:751-753, 1965
61. Conway LW: Transsphenoidal cryohypophysectomy: technique. *Int Surg 54*:192-203, 1970
62. Hallac I, Bakay L: New instrument for brain biopsy. *J Neurosurg 20*:529-530, 1963
63. Bernard JD, Aguilar MJ: Localized hypothalamic histiocytosis X. Report of a case. *Arch Neurol 20*:368-372, 1969
64. Marshall LF, Jeanette B, Langfitt TW: Needle biopsy for the diagnosis of malignant glioma. *JAMA 228*:1417-1418, 1974

CHAPTER 16

Radical Surgical Treatment of Craniopharyngioma

William H. Sweet

THERE IS A STRIKING DIVERGENCE of opinion on the management of craniopharyngioma. It was hoped in the early fifties that with the availability of cortisone and other hormones related to pituitary function many of these tumors could be totally removed. However, in the past 12 years there has been a major trend toward a minor or even minimal role of extirpative surgery. This statement will be documented in the later discussion. Matson and I appear to be the only neurosurgeons to have maintained for many years a program of radical, hopefully total removal for the great majority of these patients. Matson, noting a zero long-term survival in their patients treated by less than total removal, operated radically on nearly all of the 51 children with this tumor he saw after 1950, once good hormonal replacement therapy became available.[1] Katz' late followup of these patients treated during the last 18 years of Matson's professional life (1950 to 1968) reveals that a primary operation with presumed total excision was carried out in 34 cases without a single postoperative death—a record not yet equalled.[2] Unhappily his own death prevented him from completing the operative atlas in which he started to tell us how he did it.

Analysis of Personal Cases

This will be divided into 4 parts: (a) evidence for the extent of tumor that can be totally removed, (b) role of special glial reaction provoked by craniopharyngioma cells, (c) suggestions regarding operative management, and (d) results.

Evidence for the Extent of Tumor that can be Totally Removed

My own encouragement toward radical surgery of this tumor came from a distinguished experienced neurologist who referred to me a patient especially important to him, with the proviso that I carry out a total removal even if, as I was so doing, I estimated a mortality as high as 90%. He was led to this attitude, he said, by the relentlessly downhill course and

Department of Surgery, Harvard Medical School and Neurosurgical Service, Massachusetts General Hospital, Boston, Massachusetts 02114

unsatisfactory life of those surviving less aggressive measures. Since that time, 1954, I have sought to remove these tumors radically in all 30 patients in whom I was doing the primary therapeutic procedure and in 6 of the 7 in whom my effort was at a second or later operation.

The first 3 cases illustrate the major extent of some of the tumors removed.

Case 1. *John G,* age 7 years, showed before my first operation on him, a relatively small tumor encroaching on the anterior part of the third ventricle (Fig. 16-1A). The fluid and soft tissue part of this were readily removed, but his preoperative ataxia, to our surprise, became progressively worse. An air study 6 weeks later (Figs. 16-1B and C) revealed extreme displacement of the aqueduct and the fourth ventricle posteriorly and to the right. At suboccipital craniectomy, his giant craniopharyngiomatous cyst presented at the foramen magnum. After 56 ml of fluid had been aspirated, one could see to the left and in front of the displaced brainstem right up to the top of the dorsum sellae. The cyst wall was everywhere so thin as to be almost transparent. It seemed reasonable to leave in the shreds of cyst attached firmly to cranial nerve VII, in a few places to the brain stem, and engulfing a large vein at the fifth cranial nerve. Within 8 months the cyst wall had been reconstituted and massively refilled. The suboccipital approach was

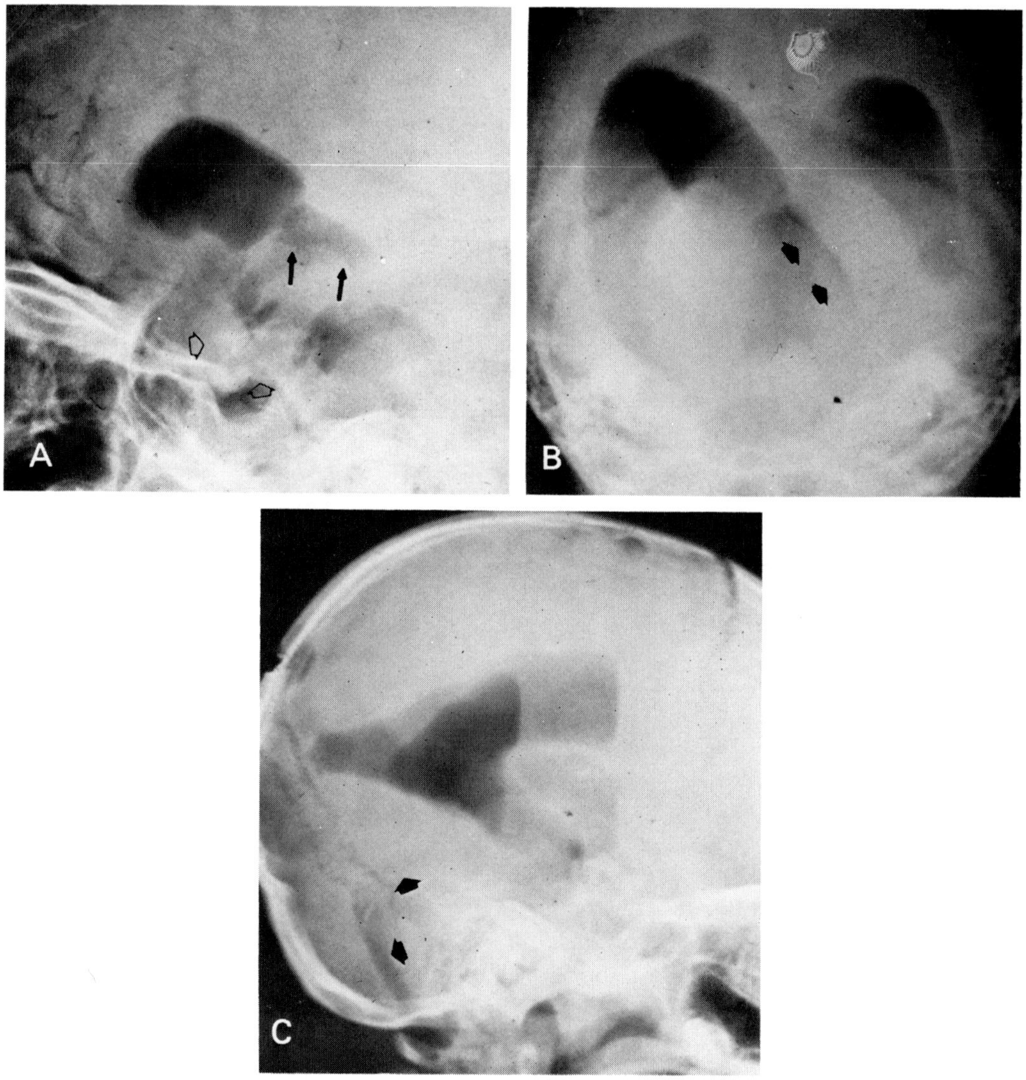

Fig. 16-1. **A.** John G. First lateral fractional pneumonencephalogram (PEG), showing moderate-sized indentation into anterior floor of third ventricle (closed arrows), rising above extensive supra- and retrosellar calcification (open arrows). **B. and C.** John G. Second PEG 6 weeks later. Lateral ventricles more dilated, fourth ventricle and aqueduct deviated to the extreme right and posteriorly (closed arrows).

repeated and all identifiable cyst removed with an ensuing paralysis of cranial nerves V and VII. The patient died 8 months later after a 4-month effort to treat subacute bacterial endocarditis. Postmortem showed no recurrent soft tissue or cystic neoplasm.

Case 2. *Joseph P,* age 8, had a huge bilateral subfrontal lesion rising straight up from the sella as shown in Figures 16-2A and B. Aspiration transsphenoidally by Dr. Hamlin with injection of air revealed (Fig. 16-2C) that there was so much solid tumor the cyst would not collapse completely. At my subfrontal operation this tumor separated with great ease from the frontal lobes but required a critical dissection from its attachment to the visual pathways. He is well 13 years later, but his preoperative mental retardation has not improved and he remains unemployable.

Case 3. *Evan D,* age 6 years, was legally blind when admitted for study. After the radiographs illustrated in Figures 16-3A and B, revealing extremely dilated lateral ventricles and marked lateral displacement of the narrow posterior crescent of the third ventricle unoccupied by tumor, he was totally blind. He has recovered only light perception after presumed total removal of his tumor, but now 11 years later he will be graduating from the Perkins School for the Blind.

Role of Glial Reaction Provoked by Craniopharyngiomatous Epithelium

My attention was forcefully drawn to this phenomenon by the following experience. Having removed the typical content and much of the capsule of this tumor lying within the third ventricle (Fig. 16-4), I brought out finally, as the last of the presumed capsule, the tissue

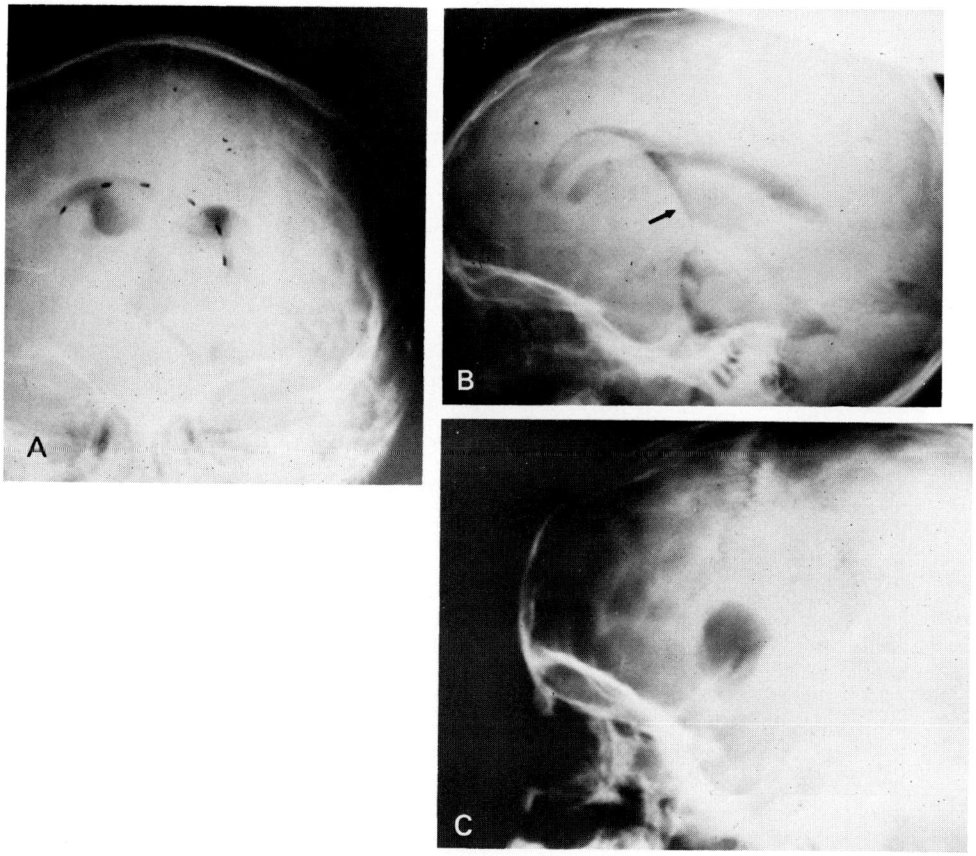

Fig. 16-2. (A and B) Joseph P. Sagittal and lateral projections showing extreme upward displacement of anterior parts of lateral ventricles right greater than left, black dashes mark upper surface dome of tumor; filling defect anterior third ventricle (arrow). No filling any basal cisterns in front of cisterna interpeduncularis. **C.** Joseph P. Lateral view after transsphenoidal aspiration of cyst by Dr. H. Hamlin and injection of air into it, showing cyst far from completely collapsed. Separation of coronal suture and increased convultional markings.

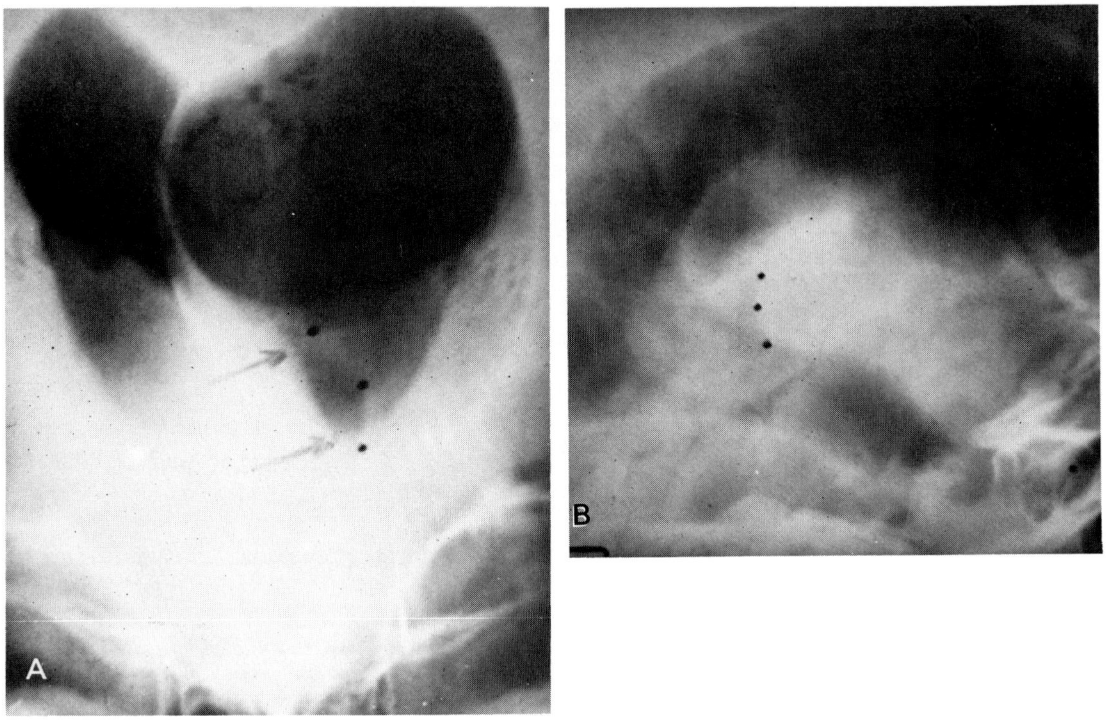

Fig. 16-3. Evan D. Ventriculogram. **A.** Sagittal view showing extreme displacement of third ventricle to the left (three black dots mark its convex left border; arrows its straight right border). **B.** Lateral view showing third ventricle as a tiny posterior crescent (three black dots mark its anterior boundary).

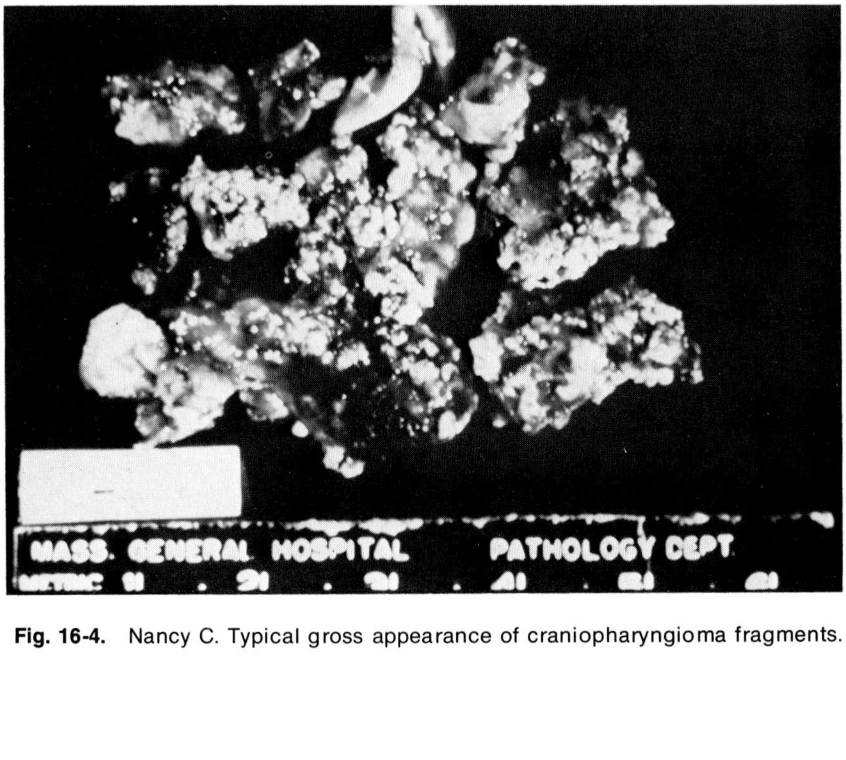

Fig. 16-4. Nancy C. Typical gross appearance of craniopharyngioma fragments.

shown in Figure 16-5A. I was aghast at this spectacle and wondered how many hypothalamic nuclei were included in it. However, the H&E stain (Fig. 16-5B) showed only astroglia with Rosenthal fibers and occasional epithelial neoplastic nests. The densely fibrous character of the glia is shown in the phosphotungstic acid hematoxylin stain in Figure 16-6. No neurones are to be seen.

As far back as 1939, Bailey, Buchanan and Bucy[3] had noted that the epithelial cells of

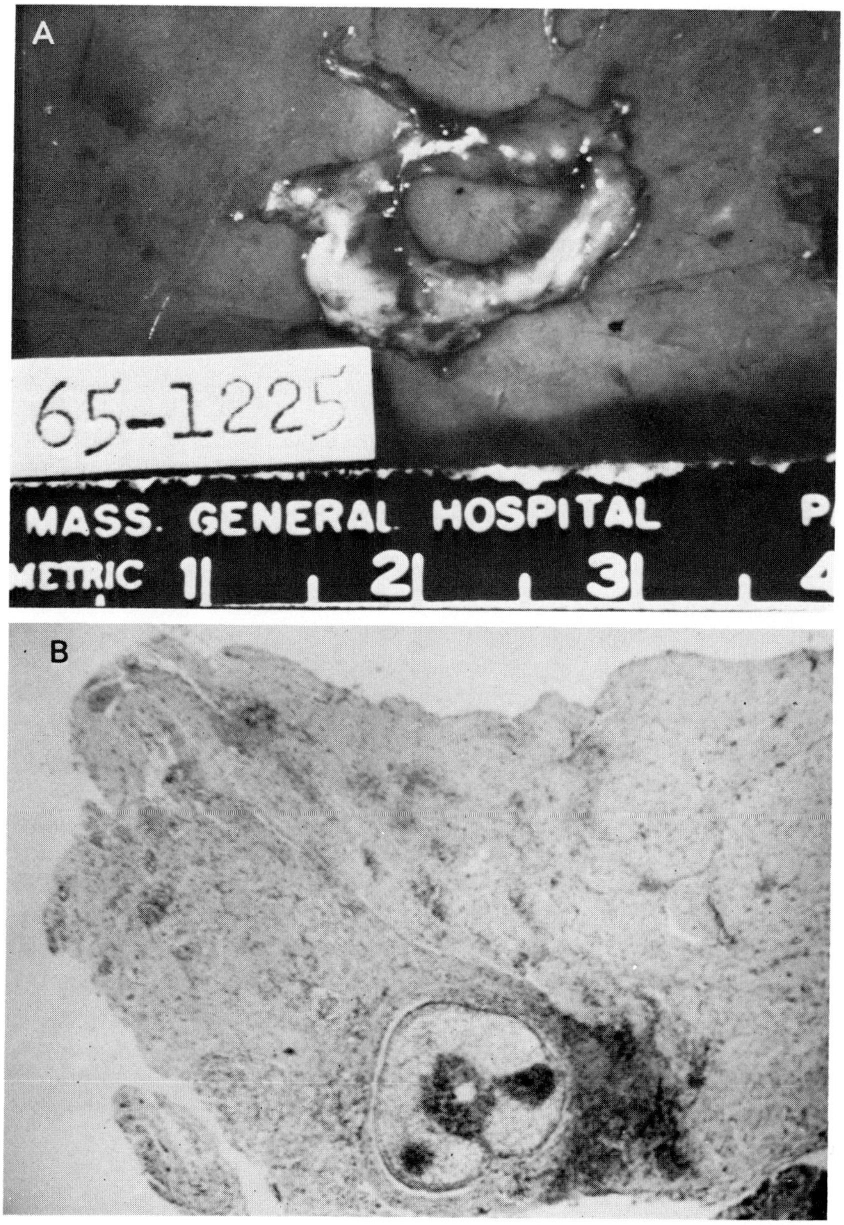

Fig. 16-5. Nancy C. **A.** Last presumed capsule with worrying resemblance to normal brain. **B.** Hematoxylin and eosin stain of same tissue showing only astroglia with many expanded tadpole-shaped denser staining "Rosenthal" bodies and one cluster of epithelial cells—no neurones or glia typical of functional brain.

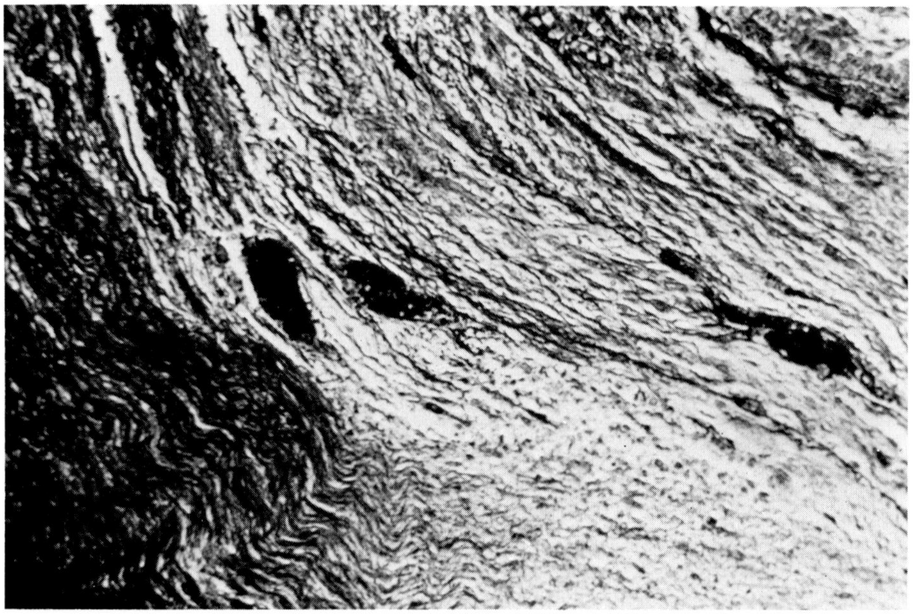

Fig. 16-6. Nancy C. Same Specimen as Figure **16-5A.** Phosphotungstic acid-hematoxylin stain showing densely fibrous nature of glia.

these tumors are imbedded in a dense gliosis surrounding the tumor and into which papillae of tumor extend. In their case 90, for example, the outer wall of the cyst was a dense mass of neuroglia with Rosenthal fibers, which "pulled free from brain tissue at postmortem." In only one of their 5 cases was there no dense gliosis; here the cyst wall was "comprised of epithelium with a small amount of supporting connective tissue." This observation of a fibrillary gliosis including abundant Rosenthal fibers at the contiguous hypothalamus in association with these tumors has been repeatedly confirmed among others by Grcevic et al.,[4] Zülch,[5] van der Bergh,[6] and Ghatak et al.[7] Timperley[8] has pointed out that this marked eosinophilia of the glial fibers, often expanded to form tadpole-shaped "Rosenthal" bodies, characterizes craniopharyngiomas, whereas an epidermoid cyst is enclosed by "an unremarkable gliosis." Incidentally, his four craniopharyngiomas and an ameloblastoma of the jaw had a high activity of alkaline phosphatase. Normal squamous epithelium from six sites and epithelium from three epidermoid cysts did not show this high activity.

"This intimate mixture of nests of tumor cells and severely altered brain tissue," to quote Ghatak and associates,[7] has been generally regarded as a major obstacle to total surgical removal of craniopharyngiomas impinging on brain tissue, the assumption being that the reactive glia adheres to the normal neural structures. My experience has led me to regard the reverse point of view as the more tenable, namely, that this glial reaction may well constitute a margin of safety between the proliferating epithelial cells we seek to remove and the functioning neurones we wish to leave behind. Happily my gentle traction on this densely gliotic tissue has nearly always yielded a trophy free of neurones. Figure 16-7A from another case illustrates this point. Figure 16-7B from the same patient shows that at other points the capsule may be much more tenuous.

One is concerned that some gliotic tissue with epithelial tongues in it may be left behind. Thus the tissue shown in Figure 16-8 was taken from the posterior edge of the chiasm 11 years ago. It looked, under the operating microscope at that time, indistinguishable from the rest of the chiasm, so I stopped. The tissue removed, as you see, contained some epithelial clumps but no nerve fibers and the patient recovered with no visual field defect. However, 10 years later his tumor recurred. He is now well 1 year after its second nearly total removal.

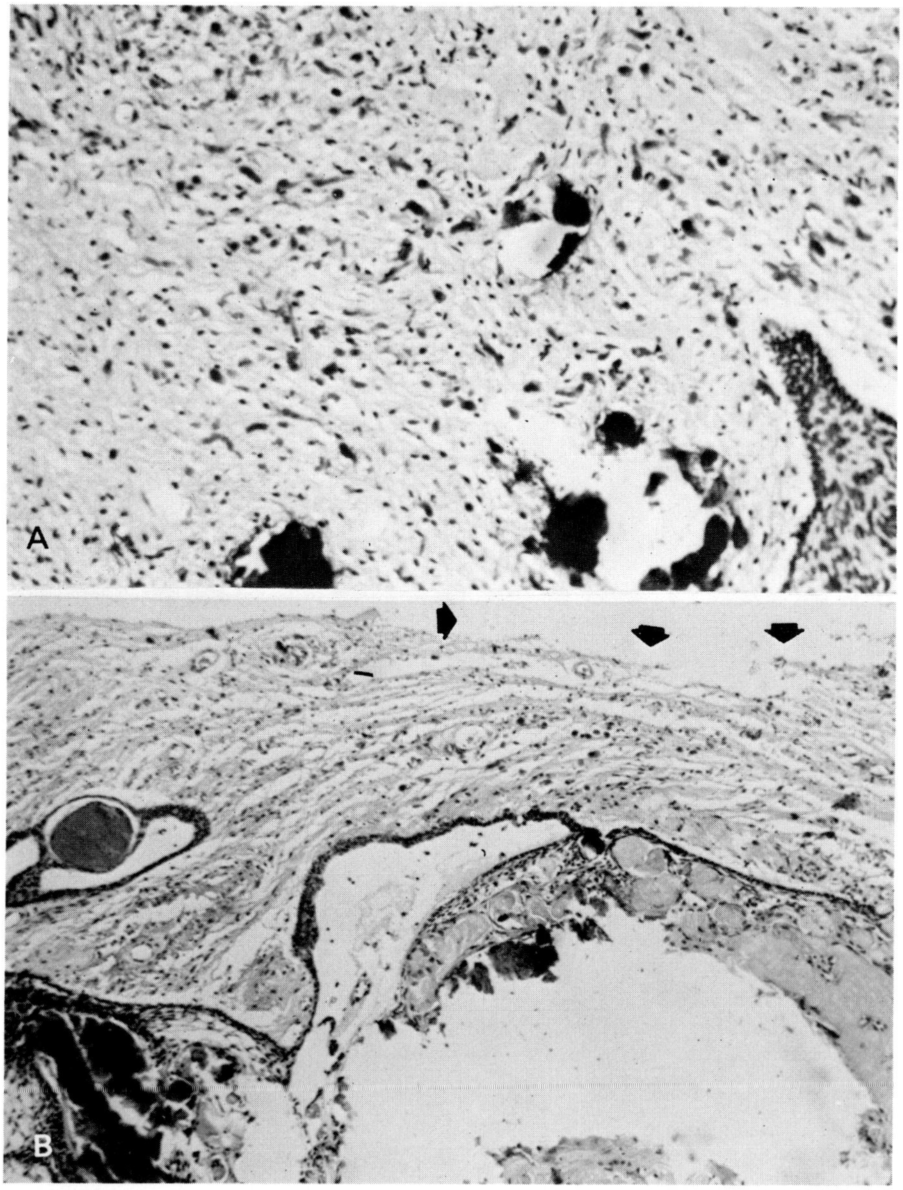

Fig. 16-7. Frederick N. Histology of tumor capsule. **A.** One area with dense astroglia, many Rosenthal bodies, one epithelial tongue, and bits of calcification (dense black blobs). **B.** Another area within thin, much less densely fibrous capsule (arrows).

The intense glial reaction can at times dominate the picture the surgeon first sees. In 2 of my cases the chiasm, the apparently grossly swollen optic tracts, and lamina terminalis seemed to be expanded by a glioma of the visual pathways or hypothalamus. In the first case the radiographs had shown no intracranial calcification; I could find no cleavage plane between the presumed medial border of optic tract and tumor, and no cyst fluid could be aspirated (Fig. 16-9). My several biopsies taken from zones halfway between the lateral borders of the two optic tracts were reported as glial tissue with a few chronic inflammatory cells. I sadly closed the wound, but Dr. E.P. Richardson sent over word, as I was taking the last scalp stitches, that he had seen one epithelial cluster characteristic of craniopharyngioma. I reopened the wound, decided the best place to find tumor surface would be in the

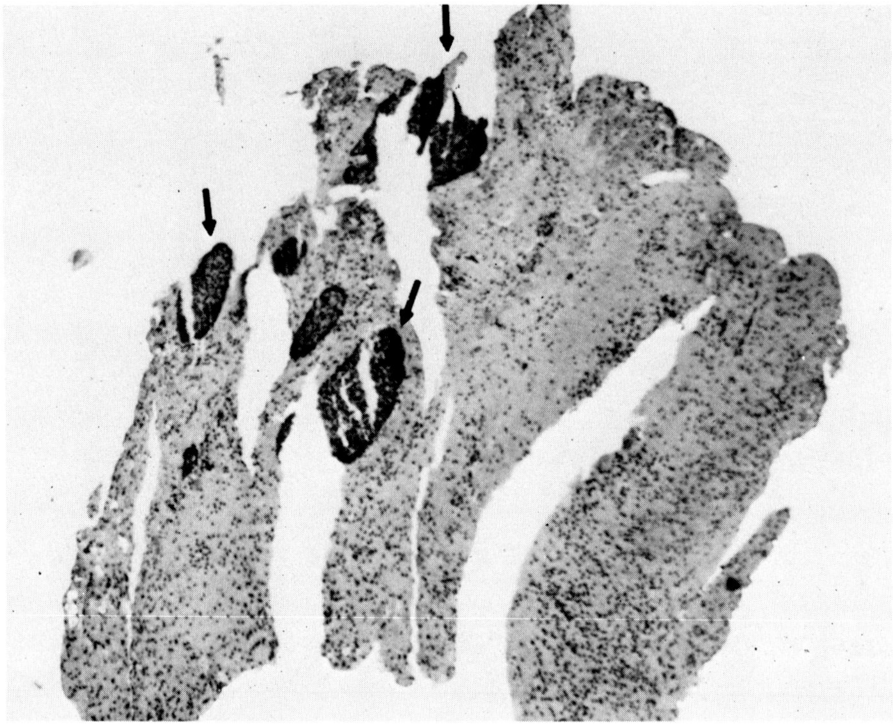

Fig. 16-8. Nicholas D. Histology of tissue from posterior edge of chiasm grossly indistinguishable from remainder of chiasm. H&E stain—only astrocytes with small epithelial nests (arrows).

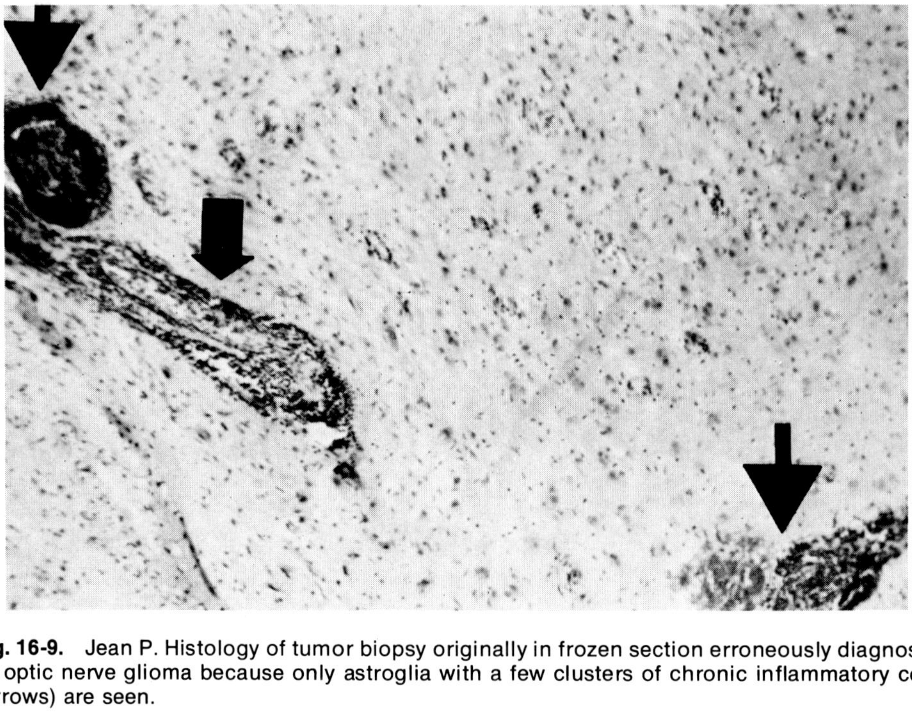

Fig. 16-9. Jean P. Histology of tumor biopsy originally in frozen section erroneously diagnosed as optic nerve glioma because only astroglia with a few clusters of chronic inflammatory cells (arrows) are seen.

midline where it was abutting on the cavity of the third ventricle. Once a clearcut posterosuperior end of tumor was felt, its center was removed and the cleavage plane followed by easing wall of tumor toward the midline from all the way around. Her three quadrant defects in the visual field of each eye and her visual acuity promptly returned to normal. She has had no evidence of recurrence 12 years later. In a second patient the pathologist was promptly able to diagnose a craniopharyngioma from a small biopsy, and the cleavage plane was found in the same way.

I have shown, however, to my entire dissatisfaction that it is possible to remove some hypothalamus along with the gliotic tumor boundary. Figure 16-10 shows this in a patient's biopsy (James D) taken at a second operation 14 years after the first one and 9 years after we had known of his tumor recurrence. The patient had abandoned both medical and further surgical treatment until his condition became desperate. At reoperation the boundary tissue between tumor and hypothalamus was obviously more tenacious than anything I have ever encountered before. Because of a wound infection, the patient did not survive the postoperative period, but the hypothalamic trauma may well have played a role in the fatal outcome. Van der Bergh and Brucher[6] have made several observations of both types; ie., in their Case 1 at postmortem they noted in several places a plane of cleavage between the perineoplastic spongioblastic gliosis and the actual hypothalamic nervous tissue. Contrariwise, in their Case

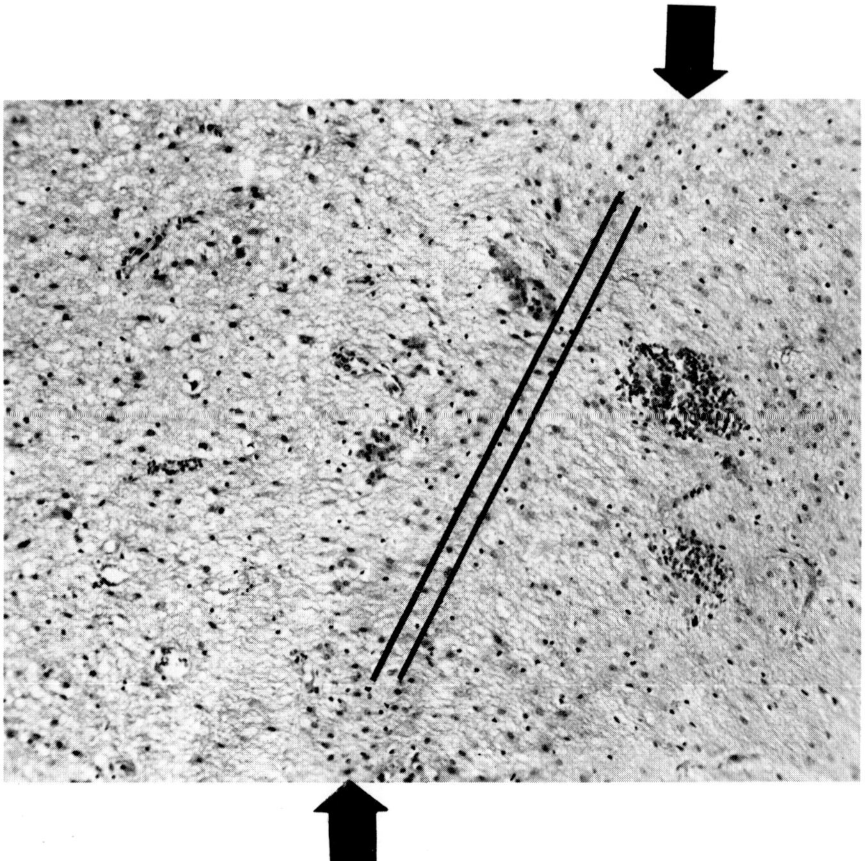

Fig. 16-10. James D. Histology of tissue biopsy, ×130. Hypothalamus is present along with glial reaction in this, tenaciously adherent recurrent tumor of long standing. To the left of the lines joining the arrows is hypothalamus; to the right of that line lies dense astroglia.

5 at postmortem, the dense spongioblastic gliosis with tumor tongues contained as well some normal looking neurons and some atrophic ones with vacuolar degeneration.

Another patient in whom the tumor grew for many years and became firmly adherent to adjoining brain was Anna M, who was treated with 3,000 rads of radiation to her presumed third ventricular pinealoma in 1949. She did well until 1972 when her increasing mental confusion was treated by ventriculoatrial shunt of her grossly dilated lateral ventricles. Finally, over a year later, when she was in a state of useless dementia and the center of her brain was a mass of solid tumor, I made a forlorn effort to remove her craniopharyngioma. The central part of the lesion came away fairly readily, leaving a tenacious glial rind whose separation from brain I had to abandon. The operation served no useful purpose.

However, in all 22 of my other patients in whom tumor could apparently be eased away essentially totally from the surrounding third ventricular wall, the operative specimen shows only gliosis with or without epithelial nests and without neurones. In particular, in 10 of these 22 patients in whose operative specimens I directed Dr. Richardson's attention to a worrying gross appearance to some of the tissue, he saw nothing containing neurons. However, the gliosis elicited by these tumors appears to be an increscence into ventricle, not a part of functional brain, and largely separable from it by gentle dissection. I have no evidence that gliomas of the visual pathways, ectopic pinealomas or any other anterior third ventricular tumor excite this specific, apparently surgically helpful, form of gliosis.

Suggestions Regarding Operative Management

Matson and I independently concluded that these tumors should all be approached via the subfrontal route. Their most tenacious attachments, in my experience, are to the chiasm and adjoining optic tracts, pituitary stalk, and neighboring hypothalamus, or to the medial aspects of the internal carotid, posterior communicating, or anterior choroidal arteries. Only the subfrontal route permits a good view of all of these areas. In particular, since the neoplasm and much of its accompanying special gliosis can almost always be safely drawn downward and forward out of the third ventricle, the two superior approaches *via corpus callosum* or lateral ventricle lose their special advantage of a good view of the walls of the third ventricle. However, these tumors may send a tongue down into the cerebellopontine angle oftener than I had realized two decades ago. As already pointed out, such extension may require a suboccipital craniectomy, or if the tongue is less extensive, a supratentorial lateral approach. Either elevation of the temporal lobe or division of arachnoid at the horizontal limb of the Sylvian fissure and depression of temporal lobe may achieve the necessary exposure. Malis[9] has presented an excellent description of this exposure.

It is important to select the appropriate side from which to work. I favor working from the side of the worse vision and the larger mass of tumor. Figure 16-11 illustrates a little larger tumor to the left of the midline in the CT scan in a patient whose vision was down to finger counting and that only in the upper nasal quadrant of the right eye. As Figure 16-12 shows, this tumor had to be approached from the left since it lay mainly lateral to the left optic nerve, displacing it over against the right optic nerve and pushing the internal carotid downward. The dislocation of the usual normal structures and the frequent presence of unusual arteries require unrelenting maintenance of orientation. After the tumor was removed largely via the space lateral to optic nerve and chiasm, the pituitary stalk appears to run diagonally behind the dorsum sellae with the right posterior communicating artery just to its right (Fig. 16-13). One tongue of the tumor was drawn anterosuperiorly out of the cerebellopontine angle. A sizable unnamed artery lies ventral to the anterior end of the left internal carotid. From it came one of the main feeding arteries to the tumor capsule, an unusually long one. One seeks to find nutrient arteries to the inferior surface of the optic nerves and to save them separate from tumor capsule. In this patient the tumor was located superior to the left anterior and

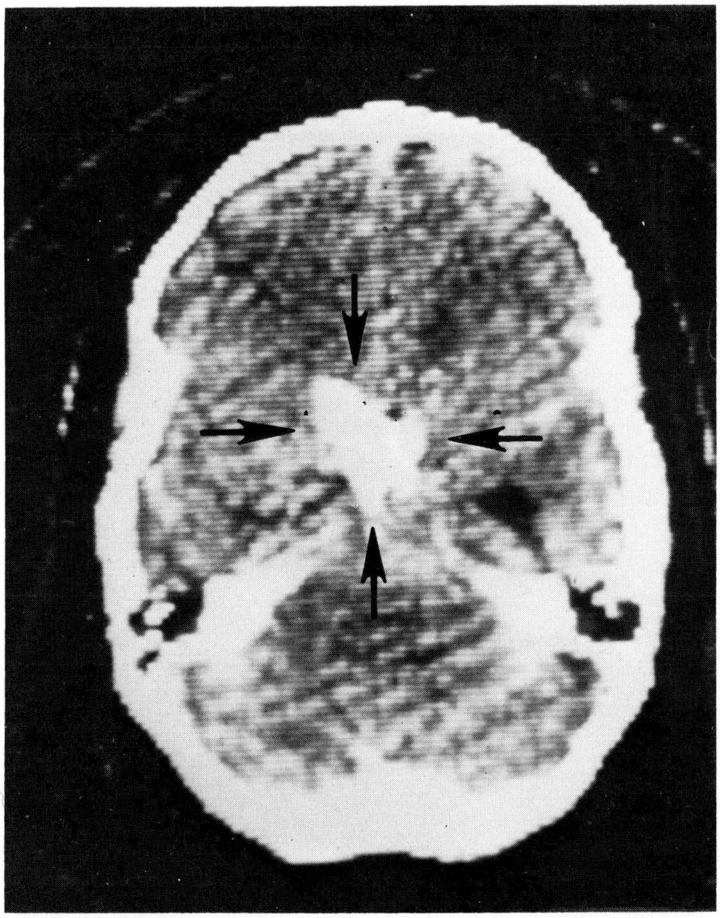

Fig. 16-11. Charles W. CT (EMI) scan. Low horizontal cut shows abnormal parasellar dense calcification of tumor (arrows) not much more to left than to right of midline.

middle cerebral arteries, pushing their perforating branches posteriorly. The tumor, although adherent to these vessels, could be slowly freed from them with no oozing from any of them. The extreme zigzag course of the left optic tract is probably correlated with no recovery of vision related to it despite the resumption of a nearly normal appearance of the optic nerves once the tumor was out.

The tumors in 23 of my 37 patients lay mainly in the third ventricle and in them removal was from between the two optic tracts through the lamina terminalis. Often they pushed the chiasm forward almost to the tuberculum sellae. Especially in the three completely solid tumors, there was initially almost no space to work between the anterior cerebral artery behind and the posterior edge of the chiasm in front. This space gradually increased as the center of the tumor was removed. I sought to avoid piecemeal removal of any of the capsule. This may become tenuous, and it is important to have as much of it as possible on which to exert gentle traction as one seeks to bring tumor downward and forward out of the back of the third ventricle. Use of the double binocular microscope, affording a chance for a second surgeon to bring at least one of his hands into play, has been an advance in technique, as Dr. Kjellberg and I demonstrated to our satisfaction in this situation several years ago. Those tumors largely in the third ventricle often erode through its anterior and/or anterolateral floor,

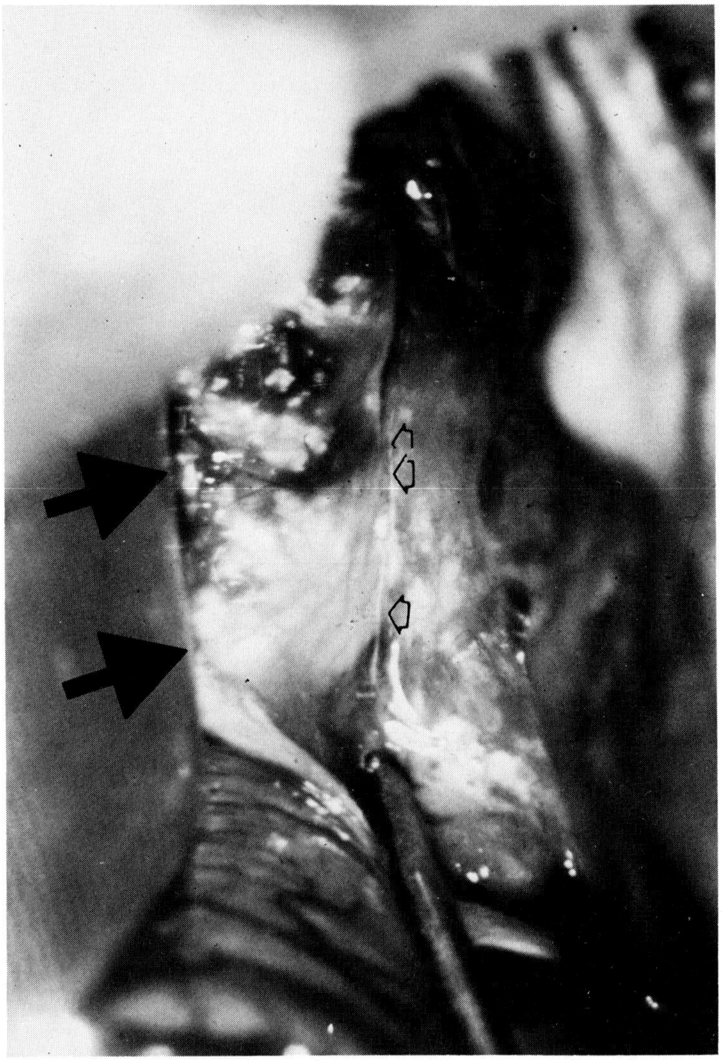

Fig. 16-12. Charles W. Operative photograph. After elevation of left frontal lobe to expose left optic nerve and tumor. Suction tip points to lateral edge of posterior part of grossly elongated left optic nerve. Extreme displacement to right of left optic nerve by tumor (open arrows indicate lateral edge of nerve). Retraction on medial edge of temporal lobe exposes tumor beyond tips of closed arrows.

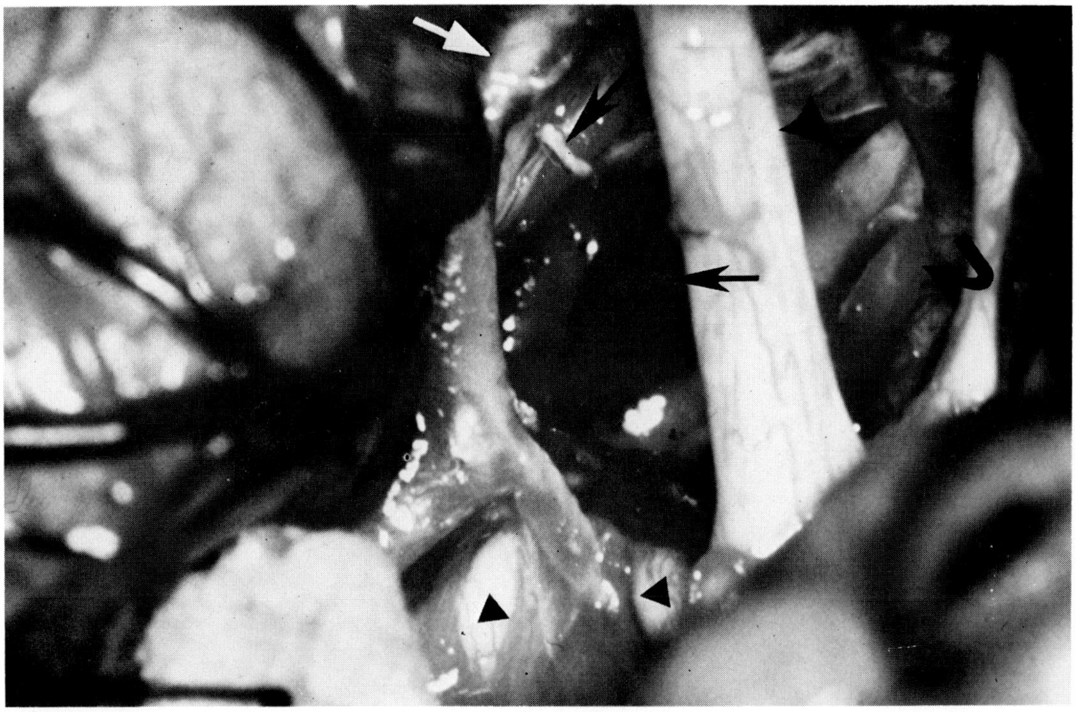

Fig. 16-13. Charles W. Same view as Figure **16-12** after removal of tumor, which extended inferoposteriorly into left cerebellopontine angle (arrow on left optic nerve points to black void of the empty angle). Proceeding clockwise from this arrow, ▶ to right of left optic nerve points to intact pituitary stalk; curving arrow on right optic nerve points to origin of right posterior communicating and anterior choroidal arteries from right internal carotid. Closed triangles lie on zigzag left optic tract which had been displaced by tumor, so as to move straight lateral to the chiasm about 1 cm, then angle sharply backward. The right closed triangle lies just to the right of left anterior cerebral artery crossing the optic tract. The left closed triangle lies between perforating branches running backward from anterior and middle cerebral arteries. The largest arrow at top left points to anterior end of left internal carotid artery. The smaller arrow below and to the right of thispoints to the largest feeding artery to the capsule electrocoagulated and divided several mm from its origin from a large anomalous artery running inferomedial and parallel to the anterior end of the left internal carotid. The shaft of the arrow lies on that anomalous artery.

and I have found it advantageous to push them backward from the suprasellar area under the chiasm or from medial to the carotid artery under the optic tract as shown in Figures 16-14 in one patient and Figure 16-15 in another. In the latter patient, the bloodstained hypothalamic floor seen after the tumor was out proved consistent with useful hypothalamic function. Via the hole in the anterior third ventricle floor made by tumor in such a case, one sees after its removal the basilar artery and its main upper branches through the intact arachnoid over the prepontine and cerebellopontine angle cisterns. The same vessels may be seen from in front of the chiasm when this has been pushed far back by tumor. The arachnoid appears to form a barrier preventing adherence of tumor to the important structures near to it in these cisterns and permitting its forward withdrawal with relative impunity.

Unusual directions of growth were taken by one tumor (Fig. 16-16) which engulfed the right internal carotid and proximal anterior, middle, and posterior cerebral arteries, following the latter two vessels out into the Sylvian fissure and back around the cerebral peduncle. Those vessels were lying free in air after Dr. John Tew and I spent the day picking out neoplasm, birdseed bites at a time. An atypical slight arachnoidal thickening enclosed the optic nerve, chiasm, and proximal optic tracts in this patient.

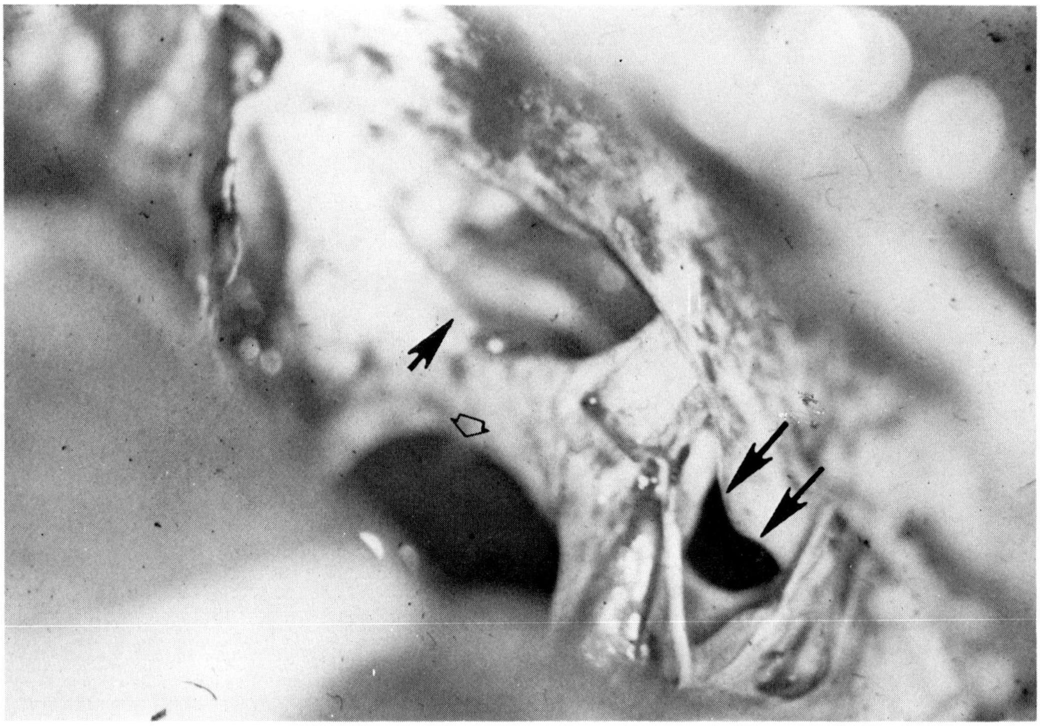

Fig. 16-14. Nancy C. Operative photo after tumor removal via subfrontal approach to show empty spaces anterior to the chiasm (left solid arrow) and lateral to right optic tract and right internal carotid artery (double solid arrows) beneath which tumor was pushed for removal behind the chiasm and between the two optic tracts (open arrow).

The pink posterior communicating and anterior choroidal arteries may make little ridges in the pink wall of the capsule and obviously should not be grasped. Indeed every effort is made to avoid starting up any arterial bleeding of even minimal degree. In 2 patients I started bleeding, which was readily controlled by application of Oxycel. In one of them, a whole succession of tiny holes in one anterior cerebral artery and the opposite internal carotid were made because the adherent tumor capsule was apparently supplied directly therefrom. In the other patient I placed divergent retractors in such fashion as to cause a slight tear at the angle of origin of anterior cerebral from internal carotid, obviously a maneuver to avoid. The ease of stopping the bleeding led me to push on with extirpation. Both patients, at first doing well after operation, died of spreading thrombosis in the basal arteries. In 3 later patients in whom such bleeding occurred, the operation was stopped forthwith to allow time for endothelium to cover the opening. In 2, the operation was successfully completed at a second stage some weeks later, but the third died postoperatively from hemorrhage at the operative site. An additional abrupt death occurred from a tiny hemorrhage into the hypothalamic floor on postoperative day 14. A premonitory moderate subarachnoid hemorrhage had occurred in her on the fourth postoperative day, from which she was recovering and which led to determination of normal blood coagulation mechanisms. Doing well, she suddenly expired without another subarachnoid hemorrhage. No tumor was identified in the hypothalamus, but if I left behind tissue of the type seen in part of the operative specimen from an another patient, showing many blood vessels in the midst of the gliosis, it might have caused the tiny fatal bleed. The result has led me to ease out all I dare of the periphery of tumor.

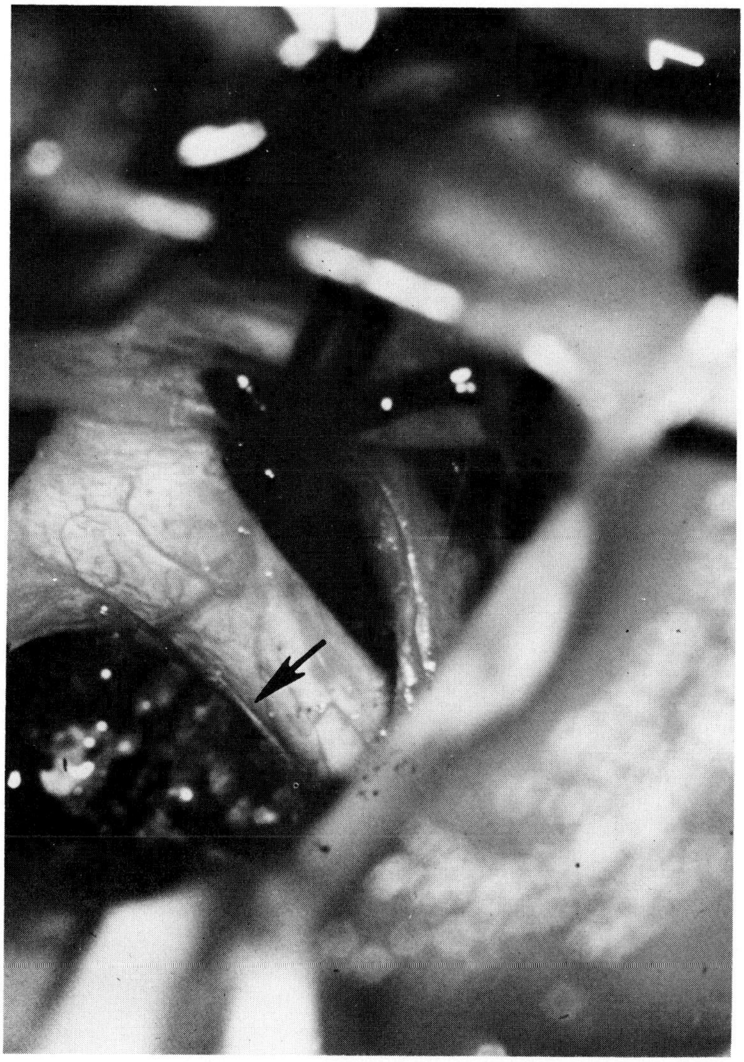

Fig. 16-15. Scott S. Operative photo. Similar general view as for Figure **16-14**; glistening tumor remnants in third ventricle behind chiasm and to left of right optic tract on which arrow lies pointing to tumor. To right of right optic tract lies empty space medial to right internal carotid previously occupied by lateral wall of hypothalamus plus tumor. By *pushing this medially, the lateral wall of hypothalamus was kept intact and tumor all removed medial to tract, via the safest opening available for an intrathird ventricular tumor–ie., that provided by removal of ultrathin, functionless lamina terminalis.*

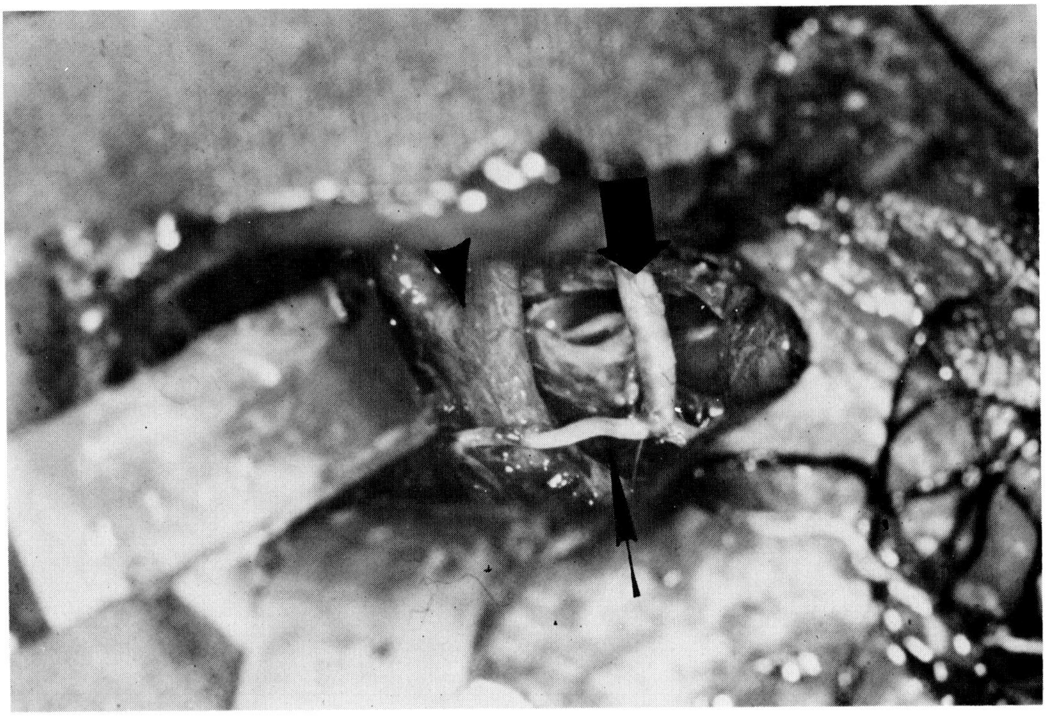

Fig. 16-16. Kevin A. Operative photo after right subfrontal removal of tumor which had engulfed right internal carotid and proximal anterior, middle, and posterior cerebral and posterior communicating arteries. Right internal carotid displaced markedly to right (upper right arrow); horizontal part of anterior cerebral remarkably free of any branches (lower right arrow), apparently because of early embryonic development of congenital nests around it; visual pathways enclosed in unusually thick arachnoid (upper left arrow between right and left optic nerves).

In only 6 patients was I able to keep the pituitary stalk intact; in several I had to cut it as it splayed out into tumor; in others, I did not see it either because it was presumably engulfed in tumor lying in front of and within the third ventricle or lying beneath a broad fixed chiasm. In one patient a huge stalk proved to be invaded by a central cord of neoplasm and was excised.

An important point already stressed by many surgeons is the need to line the working area with cottonoid so that irritative fluid and solid debris in the cyst will not set up a chemical meningitis. Patrick's case[10] of a spontaneous rupture of such a cyst is especially instructive. At the height of the reaction, the cerebrospinal fluid (CSF) total protein was 7.5 g/100 ml, the white cell count 23,700/mm^3, and the pressure $>$ 300 mm H_2O. Every time a new locule of cyst is entered, its contents should be thoroughly sucked and irrigated out before one works on the solid tumor again. The mica-like crystals come to the top of the fluid and irrigation should continue until not a one is visible. Inadequate attention to this may have led to the need for a postoperative ventriculoatrial shunt after 5 of my 44 operations. (The cottonoid strips were removed to facilitate orientation in the operative photographs).

All of these tumors were removed with the aid of magnifying loupes, the operating microscope, or both. As special instruments I have found long, tiny shafted, delicate alligator-type scissors, toothed and smooth forceps, and tiny cup rongeurs useful, especially when three hands are manipulating them in the small field. The surgeon must learn to use reflections from a mirror to look and work beneath the chiasm, hypothalamic floor, and *tuberculum sellae* for tumor remnants.

Postoperative Management

The need for assiduous attention to water and electrolyte balance and to hormonal requirements has received full discussion elsewhere and need not be repeated. Rapid deterioration in the patient's condition may be associated either with hyperosmolarity usually with hypernatremia, or hypo-osmolarity and hyponatremia. A similar clinical picture is present in each type of disorder. Clearly the treatment differs in the two situations. It is imperative that the neurosurgeon have skilled associates, neurosurgical or otherwise, who are constantly on call to manage such problems if he himself is not promptly available.

An avoidable cause of death after one of our reoperations deserves mention. Four hours after the wound was closed, the patient's systolic blood pressure rose from 140 to 220 mm Hg, remained at 230 to 190 levels for 13 hours, and then spontaneously subsided to its preoperative 150/90 level. But probably during this period, oozing began intradurally at his craniotomy site. By his second postoperative day, increasing stupor led to evacuation of the hematoma, but this 63-year-old man did not survive the two operations. Now with constant monitoring of blood pressure, as soon as this rises to 160 to 170 mm Hg, a slow intravenous infusion of sodium nitroprusside is started to maintain the pressure in the normotensive range while active investigation of the cause of that rise proceeds.

It is not superfluous to repeat that for the majority of these patients with varying degrees of hypothalamo-hypophyseal deficits they and their relatives must be aware of their particular vulnerabilities. They must themselves increase their doses of glucocorticosteroid upon any added stress of mild illness or injury, and they must have a physician skilled in the management of their deficits whom they consult at once on minimal provocation.

In our patients the most common annoying postoperative problem is their need to wage an even more relentless battle against the tendency to gain weight than the average over-nourished American. I describe to them in vivid terms 2 patients who lost this battle to the extent that a jejunoileostomy was required by one and extreme corpulence contributed eventually to death in the other. A Danish drug, a resin, containing as the active agent the sympathomimetic drug, phentermine, and marketed in this country as Ionamin has proven helpful in decreasing the incessant appetite for food. A 30-mg capsule each morning usually suffices for an adult. One highly intelligent patient has pointed out to me that when she is very thirsty and needing another dose of pitressin, she may combine unnecessary eating with the necessary drinking of fluids. I pass on to other patients the word that they must satisfy thirst only with water or other noncaloric fluids.

The capacity of some of the tumors to recur even after radical or presumed total excision makes it advisable to restudy the patients at 1- to 2-year intervals for this possibility by CT scanning and polytomograms of the sellar region. The former study has higher sensitivity for tiny bits of calcification in the suprasellar and retrosellar area than do tomograms. However, Figure 16-17 illustrates the special value of sellar polytomography for calcification within the sella near its bony borders. The CT scan could not distinguish the craniopharyngioma calcification from the bony shadows of the anterior clinoid process in Figure 16-17A and from the sellar floor in Figure 16-17B.

Results

Mortality of Virtually Total Removal

Radical operations were done in those 37 of my patients who had a reasonable chance for a productive life; there were 19 children 16 years or under and 18 adults. The lone exception was the deteriorated dement with a known tumor for 30 years mentioned earlier. I did the initial radical operation in 30 of these patients, with a postoperative death in 2. I thought I had left definite tumor remnants behind in 5 of the 28 survivors. On 4 of the 5 I have operated for

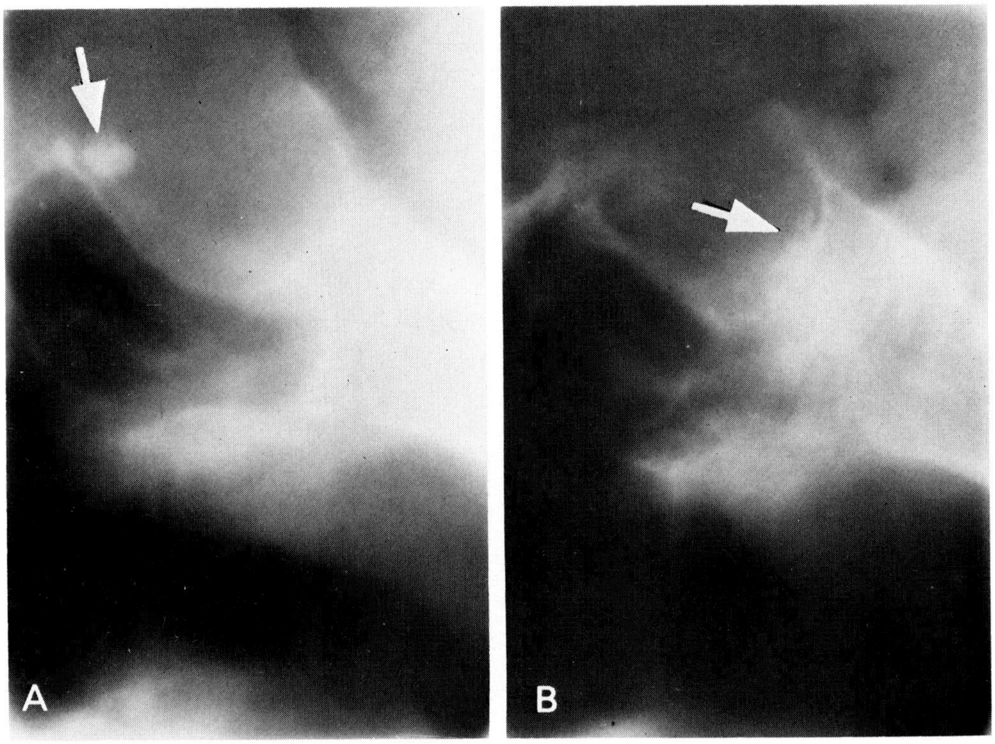

Fig. 16-17. Roger Q. **A.** Tomographic cut to right of midline shows spheroidal calcification independent of normal bony structures (arrow). **B.** Tomographic cut to left of midline shows an additional shell of calcification in tumor lying above the line of the sellar floor (arrow).

recurrences after 8 months, (John G already described), 2½ years, 10 years, and 14 years. Only 1 of these 4 is still living. The fifth died of a myocradial infarct 21 years later. A more conservative operation will not necessarily suffice in the older age group. A tiny remnant beneath the chiasm in a 61-year-old man had regrown to cause near blindness by 2½ years; my colleague, Dr. Ojemann, had the same state develop within 7 weeks in a 69-year-old woman after he had emptied her cyst and removed a generous portion of its wall. In 4 other patients, I suspect I may have left tumor at one point under chiasm or in third ventricle. None of these has clinical, CT scan, or polytomographic evidence of recurrence 8, 10, and 11 years later in the 3 children and 8 years later in the adult. However, 2 children in whom I thought my removal was total have required reoperation 4 and 6 years later; both have died, 1 in the postoperative period and 1 from the late effects of hypothalamic injury.

Of the 7 patients in whom I did a secondary radical operation, 4 are living and 2 died postoperatively. The seventh in this group is lost to followup.

Quality of Survival and Causes of Death

The status of the 26 known to be living is on the whole encouraging. I have used the same classification as Katz[2] did for evaluating the quality of survival in Matson's patients. "Excellent": normal independent functioning; "Good": functioning well despite deficiency; "Fair": functional but dependent; "Poor": nonfunctional. As in Katz' series, our endocrine consultants, Drs. Crawford, Fields, and Kliman, have with the exception of one patient been able to manage the endocrine and metabolic problems so that the quality of survival has been

Table 16-1. Comparison between Results in the Matson (Ma) and Sweet (Sw) Series of Those Still Alive after Surgical Removal

	Primary total excision		No. patients reoperated, presumed total excision		Partial excision	
	Ma	Sw	Ma	Sw	Ma	Sw
Excellent	9	16	1		2	
Good	6	4	1	1	2	1*
Fair	7	1	1	2	1	
Poor			1			
Totals	22	21	4	3	5	1

*At reoperation.

determined by the neurological, primarily the general mental status. Thus we have classified a patient who has dropped from "A–B" student to the "C–D" level as "good." The one metabolic exception is a lad whose hyperphagia could be managed only by jejunoileostomy, but who has in addition now developed Huntington's chorea (Table 16-1).

Results in the two series are summarized in the two tables. The quality of survival as shown in Table 16-1 is remarkably similar. In Table 16-2, the causes of mortality are compared. Matson's total early postoperative mortality is much lower, 10% compared with my 17%. However 9 of his patients died later of hypothalamo-hypophyseal dysfunction, compared with 1 of mine. In particular, persistent hyperosmolarity, usually with hypernatremia, was present in all 9. Katz also notes elevated intracranial pressure in some of their 5 later deaths—a problem we handled by ventriculoatrial shunt. Although 9 of his radical primary excisions have been operated for recurrence to only 5 of mine, his series terminated in 1968 and I have done 9 of my 30 such patients since that time, so the recurrence rates are not validly comparable. The major point evident in both series is the much better chance of long survival after primary than after secondary radical excision (Table 16-2).

None of the patients in either of these two series has been treated by radiation after our radical removal. The subsequent section will summarize the views of others on these topics.

Table 16-2. Operative and Postoperative Mortality, Matson (Ma) and Sweet (Sw) Series

	Radical primary excision			Reoperation	
	Ma	Sw		Ma	Sw
Total No. of patients	34	30		24	12
Postoperative death	0	2		6	5
Later death from hypothalamic, hypophyseal dysfunction	3	0		9	1
Later death from nonneural or nonmetabolic cause	0	2*		2	1
Reoperated for recurrence	9	5			
Still living without recurrence	22	21	Still living	7	4
			Lost to followup		1

*Myocardial infarct after 21 years in an adult; pneumonia after 3 years in a child.

Discussion

Objections to Aggressive Surgery

Olivecrona reported in 1967[11] that in his 107 personal cases only 46% of 25 cases had a "useful survival" after radical removal and 21% of 53 cases had a "useful survival" after partial removal. Hence he favored giving radiation therapy a trial—either by an external source or by stereotactic puncture of and instillation into the cyst of a β-emitting isotope or both. However, study of the detailed tables of Svolos[12] on the same series of cases reveals that the follow-up was carried out in January 1961, that the last operation was in December 1958, and that only 32 of the patients were operated on after 1951. Hence, about three-fourths of the series was carried out in the precortisone days.

However, other discouraging reports on the advisability of radical removal in the post-cortisone era include: (a) Kerr[13]—seven postoperative deaths after radical removals in 16 of 17 patients. Of the 9 survivors, the tumor was thought to be completely removed in 7. (b) Bartlett[14]—only 6 radical removals carried out in 72 patients since about 1948; 2 of these died two decades later of proved recurrence. Of the whole group, only 43% are still alive or survived more than 10 years. He concluded that the problems created by these tumors and attempts at radical excision are so formidable that they should be treated at a few special centers. (c) Hoff and Patterson[15]—a radical removal of tumor at first operation in 4 and at a second operation in only 2 more patients out of a total of 51 during the last 35 years. (d) Kahn et al.[16]—"As a result of our experience over the years we have become less radical in our operations upon children." The long-term survival rate in his 28 children was only 50% and, more importantly, only 21% could be classified as having a good to excellent result. "Eventually severe seizure disorders or organic brain syndrome, total blindness, obesity, marked endocrine dysfunction and lack of general physical and mental maturation" featured the poor quality of survival. This longer followup has led Kahn[17] to modify his earlier optimism regarding radical surgery. (e) Rougerie after a personal experience of 100 craniopharyngiomas has sentiments similar to those of Kahn. (f) Nakagawa and Tsuru[18] did total removals in 5 cases and subtotal removals in 18 of 26 cases after 1958, with an operative and hospital mortality of 27% and 46%, respectively. (g) A tentative attitude toward radical surgery in the postcortisone era is that of Michelsen et al.[19] Their mortality after primary procedures is only 7%. However, the surgeon thought he had achieved total removal in only 11 (34%) of 32 children and 12 (23%) of 52 adults. Moreover, 5 of the 11 children have since shown recurrent or remaining tumor. These authors recommend radical removal "when the operative conditions are ideal."

Evidence Regarding Radiation Therapy

Pari passu with waning enthusiam for radical surgery has appeared an increasing intimation of the efficacy of radiation therapy. Leddy and Marshall,[20] among the first to draw attention to this, gave convincing details of 10 patients who were benefited by tumor doses usually in the range of 1,000 to 2,500 rads by the then available dosimetry. A greater percentage of their patients were still living more than 5 years after operation, if they had received roentgen therapy in addition (5 of 6 such patients), than if they had had operation only (16 of 35 patients). Microscopic examinations months or years after these modest doses revealed no radiation effect on the tumor in cases in whom obvious clinical improvement had occurred. The authors agree with Carpenter and colleagues,[21] who had suggested as the basis for the improvement in their 4 cases that the radiation inhibited the formation of cystic fluid.

Kramer and colleagues[22,23] have used intensive photon radiation from external sources for a longer period than any other group. The 1975 paper gives us a full long-term followup. In

Kramer's first series treated from 1952-1954, heavy radiation with 2 Mev x-rays was given following surgical biopsy and cyst evacuation to 10 patients. The 6 children received 5,000 to 6,550 rads in 37 to 57 days, respectively. All 6 were living 19 to 20 years later, were working fulltime, and there was no evidence of damage from the radiation in any of them. The 4 adults were given 5,600 to 7,000 rads in 29 to 51 days. One survives and is well 20 years later; the other 3 died of unrelated disease 2, 10, and 14 years later. These excellent results were not maintained in a second series of 33 patients treated between 1958 and 1971. Two of the 12 children in this second group died of persistent tumor; 10 are still alive, and only one of these has marked failure to grow. Only 13 of the 21 adults had survived. Although 2 of the 8 deaths were from unrelated diseases, 3 patients died after a second operation undertaken because the patient's condition worsened during or just after the course of radiation. Three more died—one with areas of necrosis possibly related to radiation, another with a huge area of radiation necrosis but no residual tumor, and the third with both residual tumor and areas of necrosis. Bloom and Harmer[24] agree with Kramer et al. in favoring a combination of a conservative cyst evacuation and biopsy only followed by radical irradiation. They are assessing results of treatment in a series of 100 patients of all ages with primary or recurrent craniopharyngioma. The 5- and 10-year survival rates for cases treated as they recommend were 85% and 72%, respectively. Over 90% of the patients were in good general health with no serious neurologic or mental disability at 2 years; vision was at least useful in 82%. Of 12 patients treated on a 6 mev linear accelerator over 5 years ago, 11 were still alive and well.

Hoff and Patterson[15] have also presented evidence that partial removal of the tumor with radiation therapy is better than the same type of operation alone. Ten-year followups revealed a 63% recurrence rate in the 24 patients in whom radiation was added, whereas 85% of 17 patients who were not radiated had shown recurrence. However, Matson and Crigler[1] comment that all but 1 of the 11 patients sent to them for recurrence after an operation elsewhere had also had radiation therapy. The crucial data regarding the detailed parameters of that therapy are given in neither of the last two publications.

Sharma et al.[25] have treated 21 patients by "limited surgery" and 5,000 to 5,500 rads over *circa* 1 month from a Theratron-60 unit. In a followup on 18 patients—from 2 to 7 years later in 11 of them—none had yet shown brain damage or other clinical deterioration and all are alive and well (the remaining three patients were lost to followup).

In a little contrast to these encouraging reports, Backlund[26] cites five publications that describe radiation necrosis disasters at the "radical" dose levels. He and Leksell have for nearly 10 years been developing a regime of a more localized radiation involving the stereotaxic injection of colloidal, β-emitting ^{90}Y into the cystic part of the tumor and stereotaxicly directed focused multiportal gamma-irradiation from ^{60}Co to the solid parts of the tumor. A personal communication from Dr. Backlund, dated October 8, 1975, summarizes his highly gratifying data from a followup just completed in 34 primary cases treated in the last 10 years; there were only two deaths and two "partially disabled." It will be instructive to compare the long-term results of this logical approach as well as those of less focused radiation with those of radical surgery. If radiation is to be used, the combination of β-emitting ^{90}Y into the cyst plus sharply focused protons or photons to the solid tumor is clearly the most controllable technique. The value of high resolution CT scans to demonstrate cystic portions of the tumor plus the use of radiopaque contrast material intravenously to sharpen the definition of solid parts of the tumor in the CT scan has been seen in our own cases and was beautifully demonstrated, during a recent trip to Stockholm, by Leksell and Backlund. These encouraging results from radiation are consonant with the observations of Rubin and Casanett[27] of the "fairly high" radiosensitivity of skin and oropharyngeal epithelium.

Rarely the tumors have or develop so vicious an invasive tendency that at that point no therapy can succeed. Thus, in Iyer's[28] 3-month-old baby, the tumor had critically invaded and replaced not only hypothalamic but also midbrain tegmental structures. Grover and

Rorke's[29] patient had "a 95% removal" of his solid tumor at age 5 followed by 6,100 rads of ^{60}Co radiation at age 12. When he died at age 17, there was almost no residual normal structure inthe left caudate nucleus, thalamus, midbrain, or pons. These areas and the basal subarachnoid space were filled with tumor.

Summary and Conclusions

There is evidence, from this publication and those of Matson and colleagues, that a determined effort at total excision of these tumors as the initial therapy is a tenable course of action. The main bases for this concept are: (a) the dense gliosis characteristically intervening between these epithelial tumors and normal brain constitutes a margin of safety for the surgeon at least for the first several years such tumors are growing in the third ventricle; (b) improved early diagnosis and better operative instruments, magnification, lighting, and technique are decreasing operative morbidity and mortality; and (c) new knowledge and new replacement therapy are reducing the burden of metabolic and endocrine defects.

Competing with this is the concept that rotationally delivered or even more precise focused high-energy photons and intracavitary β-radiation have lower morbidity and mortality. The detailed and long-term data on which to draw conclusions are not yet available. My medical colleagues and I are preparing case-by-case tables with all of the relevant facts to supply one component of the total picture.

Acknowledgement

It is a pleasure to express appreciation to the Neuro-Research Foundation for the support of these studies.

REFERENCES

1. Matson DD, Crigler JF, Jr: Management of craniopharyngioma in childhood. *J Neurosurg 30*:377-390, 1969
2. Katz EL: Late results of radical excision of craniopharyngiomas in children. *J Neurosurg 42*:86-90, 1975
3. Bailey P, Buchanan DN, Bucy PC: *Intracranial Tumors of Infancy and Childhood.* The University of Chicago Press, Chicago, Illinois, 1939
4. Grcevic N, Yates PO: Rosenthal fibers in tumors of the central nervous system. *J Pathol 73*:467-472, 1957
5. Zulch KJ: *Brain Tumors. Their Biology and Pathology.* Second edition. Springer, New York, 1965, pp 228-233
6. van der Bergh R, Brucher JM: L'abord transventriculaire dans les craniopharyngiomes du troisieme ventricule. *Neurochirurgie 16*:51-65, 1970
7. Ghatak NR, Hirano A, Zimmerman HM: Ultrastructure of craniopharyngioma. *Cancer 27*:1465-1475, 1971
8. Timperley WR: Histochemistry of Rathke pouch tumours. *J Neurol Neurosurg Psychiatr 31*:589-595, 1968
9. Malis LI: The transnasal and transpterional approach to lesions of the clivus. Presented at the Congress of Neurological Surgeons Meeting, Atlanta, Georgia, October 1975
10. Patrick BS, Smith RR, Bailey TO: Aseptic meningitis due to spontaneous rupture of craniopharyngioma cyst. Case report. *J Neurosurg 41*:387-390, 1974
11. Olivecrona H: The craniopharyngiomas, *Handbuch der Neurochirurgie*, vol 4, Part 4. Edited by H. Olivecrona, W Tonnis. Springer, Berlin, 1967, pp 269-279
12. Svolos DG: Craniopharyngiomas. A study based on 108 verified cases (of Olivecrona). *Acta Chir Scand Suppl: 403*:1-44, 1969
13. Kerr AS: Craniopharyngiomata. *J Neurol Neurosurg Psychiatr 31*:646, 1968
14. Bartlett JR: Craniopharyngiomas—a summary of 85 cases. *J Neurol Neurosurg Psychiatr 34*:37-41, 1971
15. Hoff JT, Patterson RH: Craniopharyngiomas in children and adults. *J Neurosurg 36*:299-302, 1972
16. Kahn EA, Gosch HH, Seegar JF, et al.: Forty-five years experience with the craniopharyngiomas. *Surg Neurol 1*:5-12, 1973

17. Kahn EA: Some physiologic implications of craniopharyngiomas. *Neurology 9*:82-90, 1959
18. Nakagawa Y, Tsuru M: Postoperative course of craniopharyngioma. *Brain Nerve (Tokyo) 23*:993-1002, 1971
19. Michelson WJ, Mount LA, Renaudin J: Craniopharyngiomas. A thirty-nine year survey. *Acta Neurol Lat Am 18*:100-106, 1972
20. Leddy ET, Marshall TM: Roentgen therapy of pituitary adamantinomas (craniopharyngiomas). *Radiology 56*:384-393, 1951
21. Carpenter RC, Chamberlin GW, Frazier CH: The treatment of hypophysial stalk tumors by evacuation and irradiation. *Am J Roentgenol Rad Thera Nucl Med 38*:162-177, 1937
22. Kramer S: Radiation therapy in the management of craniopharyngiomas. *Neurochirurgie 21*: Suppl 2:204-223, 1975
23. Kramer S, Southard M, Mansfield CM: Radiotherapy in the management of craniopharyngioma: further experiences and late results. *Am J Roentgenol Rad Thera Nucl Med 103*:44-52, 1968
24. Bloom HJG, Harmer CL: Craniopharyngiomas. *Br Med J 2*:288-289, 1972
25. Sharma U, Tandon PN, Saxene KK, et al: Craniopharyngiomas treated by a combination of surgery and radiotherapy. *Clin Radiol 25*:13-17, 1974
26. Backlund EO: Studies on craniopharyngiomas. III. Stereotactic treatment with intracystic yttrium-90. *Acta Chir Scand 139*:237-247, 1973
27. Rubin P, Casanett GW: *Clinical Radiation Pathology*, vol 1 and 2. WB Saunders, Philadelphia, 1968
28. Iyer CGS: Case report of an adamantinoma present at birth. *J Neurosurg 9*:221-228, 1952
29. Grover WD, Rorke LB: Invasive craniopharyngioma. *J Neurol Neurosurg Psychiatr 31*:580-582, 1968

CHAPTER 17

The Transbasal Approach to Tumors Invading the Base of the Skull

Patrick J. Derome

BECAUSE THEY ARE LOCATED in a *frontier area* between the skull and the face (no man's land for different specialties), lesions that invade the base of the skull, particularly the middle areas, were treated by neurosurgeons, ENT and ophthalmologic surgeons, and plastic surgeons. Often, it was impossible to remove the mass completely. In addition many patients were not offered further treatment after a single biopsy through a narrow anterior approach and gradually became blind, before the base of the skull was massively invaded and all cranial nerves involved.

Although it is perfectly acceptable not to remove certain malignant tumors, a benign tumor should always be removed. And, many of the tumors that invade the base of the skull are benign. Admittedly, tumors in the region of the ethmoid, sphenoid, or clivus present many problems and are extremely difficult to remove. Close collaboration between neurosurgeon and plastic surgeon was required. Today the entire procedure can be completed by the neurosurgeon alone, using the transbasal approach.

Tessier[1] developed this approach 12 years ago for craniofacial abnormalities and used it to reduce his first cases of hypertelorism and craniofacial dystosis. It was then adapted for the surgical removal of basal tumors.[2]

Goals of the Transbasal Approach

The first goal is to remove the tumor completely. Some of these are located on the midline, but most extend laterally toward the orbital walls, the lesser and greater sphenoidal wings, and the middle fossa. The second goal is to free the cranial nerves and open the optic foramina, the sphenoidal fissures, and even the foramen rotundum and foramen ovale, areas that cannot be reached through narrow anterior approaches. If the anterior and, possibly, the middle fossae are to be seen, an anterior subdural and extradural approach is required. Anosmia, which very often is present before the procedure, is the only side effect. An anterior approach that can be combined with the intracranial to remove certain tumors of the clivus will be discussed later.

12 Hameau des Pinsons, La Ceffe, St. Cloud, France

Hazards of the Transbasal Approach

The most important complication is the possible communication between the subarachnoid spaces and the upper air-filled cavities of the face (Fig. 17-1A and B). Resection of the ethmoidosphenoidal mass widely opens the frontal and sphenoidal sinuses and the ethmoidal cells. The floor of the nasal fossae and the pharyngeal or cavum mucosae can be reached through the cranial approach. Meningeal tears and dural defects occur frequently. Well-known, possible complications are pneumatoceles or cerebrospinal fluid leaks, ascending infections, and meningitis.

The three structures superimposed between the intradural spaces and the air-filled cavities of the face are: the dura, the bone involved by the tumor, and the rhinopharyngeal mucosal plane. These structures must be repaired carefully to prevent the above-mentioned complications. The dura must be closed tightly and strengthened with a pericranial or dermal graft, depending on the size of the defect. The base of the skull must be reconstructed with bone autografts to eliminate a medial dead space, which may cause later meningoceles or encephaloceles and postoperative extradural hematomas or infections (Fig. 17-2A and B). The mucosal plane is preserved as much as possible, since it sustains and feeds the lower aspect of bone grafts. When these dicta are rigidly applied, the transbasal approach is a benign procedure.

Preoperative Organization

Prophylactic antibiotic therapy is administered routinely for 2 days before the procedure, during the operation, and for 1 week postoperatively. The frontal lobe must be well retracted so that the base of the skull is readily exposed. All of the methods are used simultaneously, ie., assisted ventilation with negative pressure, Mannitol, and continuous intraoperative lumbar drainage. Because the procedure is a very long one (10 to 12 hours and sometimes longer), the anesthesiologist must maintain normothermia, strict biologic control, and avoid hyponatremia. Blood losses must be carefully replaced and strict hemostasis

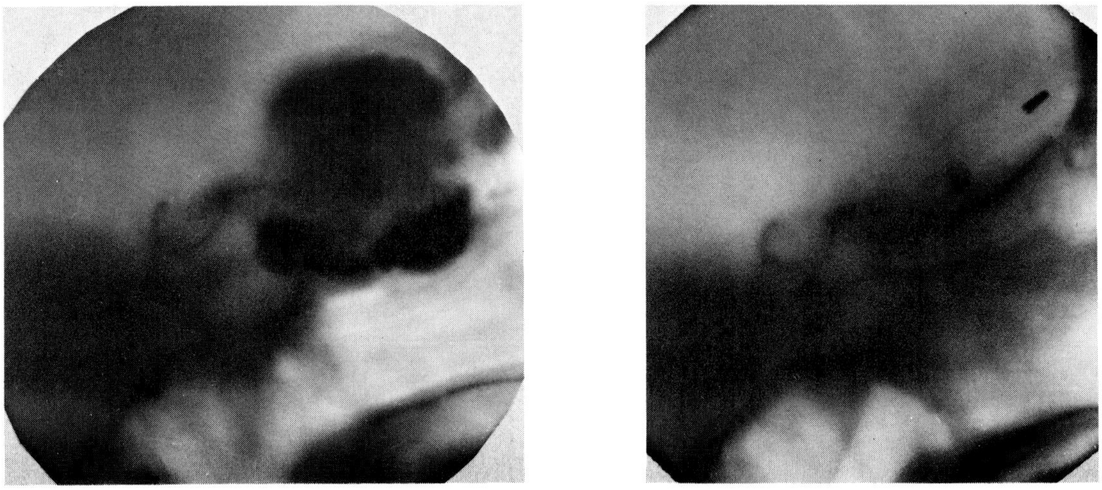

Fig. 17-1. A and **B.** Resection of an ethmoidosphenoidal tumor (osteoma ?) widely opens the upper air-filled cavities of the face.

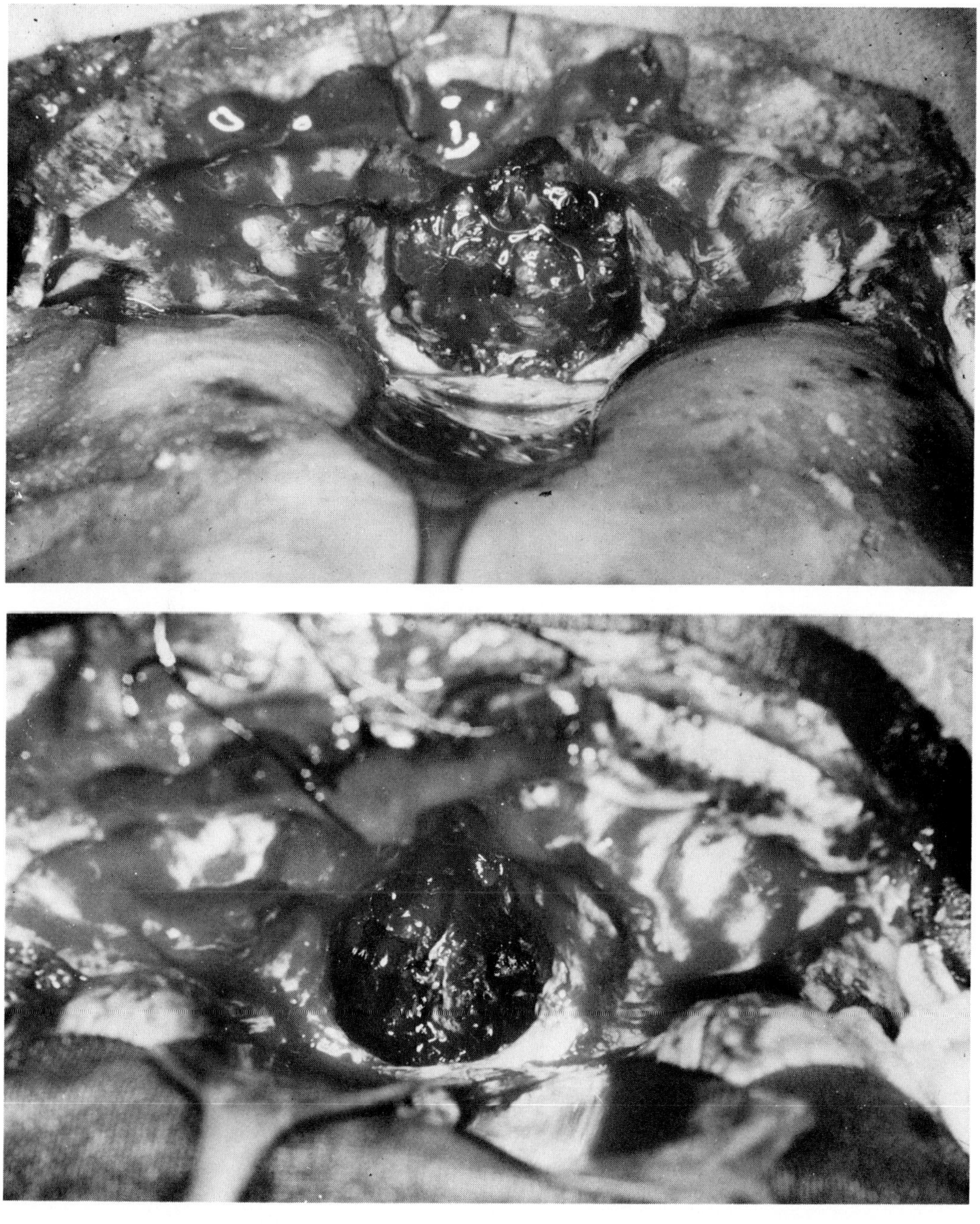

Fig. 17-2. **A.** (top) Intraoperative view of an ethmoidosphenoidal chordoma responsible for extradural compression of both optic nerves. The orbital roofs are partially removed. **B.** (bottom) After removal: large dead space reaches the nasal fossae and deeper aspect of the pharyngeal mucosae. Note the free optic nerves.

applied at each step. If the tumor has a tendency to bleed, special techniques, such as ligating the external carotid artery or preoperative embolization may be used.

The patient is placed in the dorsal decubitus position, without fixing the head, so that all aspects of the procedure (rotation and declivity) can be modified intraoperatively.

Preserving the Mucosal Plane

To preserve the rhinopharyngeal mucosae, they are dissected first through a rhinoseptal approach, as in the first steps of the classic transsphenoidal access to sellar tumors, ie., incise under the upper lip, resect the inferior nasal spine, and separate the mucosae up to the rostrum. The dissector is then pushed backwards and the mucosae of the choanae are separated as much as possible from the vomer and the inferior aspect of the body of the sphenoid. Two tents are introduced, both for protection and as deep landmarks, before the tumor is attacked from above (Fig. 17-3). At the end of the procedure nasal packing is used to reapply the mucosae to the cancellous bone grafts used to repair the base of the skull and the sphenoethmoid (Fig. 17-4).

Exposing the Base of the Skull

A temporo-temporal incision just behind the hairline, is used. The pericranial incision follows both temporal crests laterally to the coronal sutures and is then folded upwards. If it is necessary to proceed more laterally, the entire temporal muscle is dissected from the temporal fossa and from the retromalar area to the zygomatic process.

The bone flap is usually a bifrontal free flap; its inferior margin is strictly supraorbital, without regard for the frontal sinuses. If these sinuses are wide, their posterior walls and mucosae are removed and their ostia closed with bone grafts.

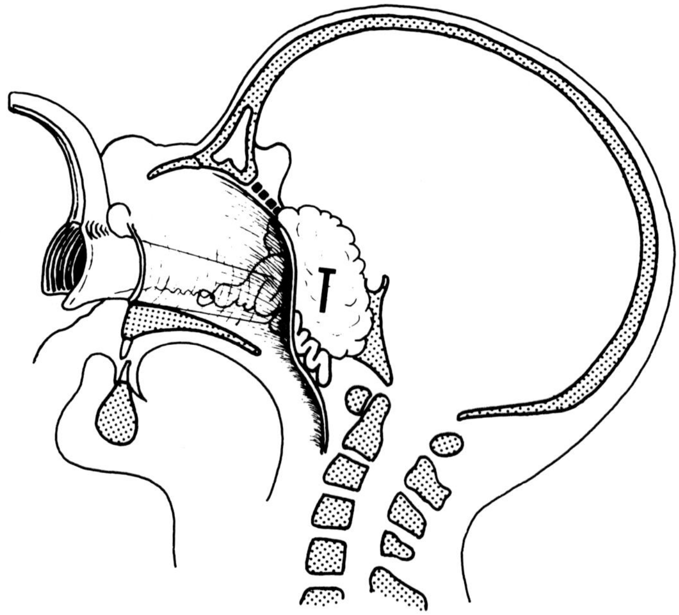

Fig. 17-3. Rhinoseptal approach permits the surgeon to preserve the rhinopharyngeal mucosae. A packing is introduced both for protection and as deep landmarks.

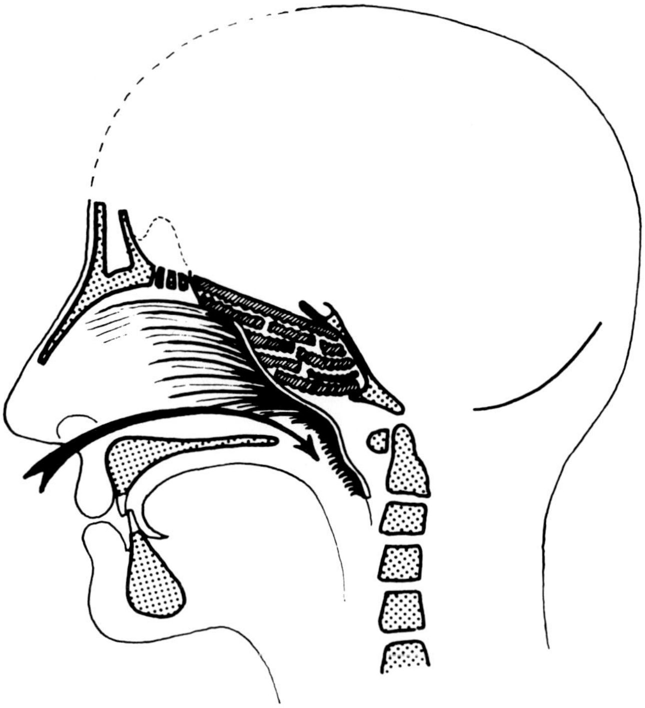

Fig. 17-4. The mucosae are reapplied close to the ethmoido-sphenoidal mass, reconstructed with bone autografts.

After the subfrontal dura is dissected, the anterior fossa is exposed. This dissection is fairly easy, except for the area of both olfactory grooves (sometimes it is possible to avoid meningeal tears by a primary resection of the crista galli apophysis and by cutting the olfactory nerves one by one). The dissection must reach the posterior limits of the anterior fossa: the posterior edge of the lesser sphenoidal wings, the tuberculum sellae, and the base of the anterior clinoid processes. A partially invaded dura or a tumor growing through the meningea into the intradural spaces may cause some problems. The subfrontal and intracerebral parts of the tumor are removed through a classic intradural approach before the subfrontal dura around the basal insertion of the tumor, is dessected.

Meningeal Repair

The dura is closed before the base is resected and the upper air-filled cavities are opened. There are three possibilities:

1. The dura is preserved and there are only a few meningeal tears, generally located in the area of the olfactory grooves. The tears can be sutured with very fine sutures but it would be better to strengthen the dura on the midline with other material (Fig. 17-5).
2. There is a true dural defect. This must be closed with a dural substitute more than twice the size of the defect. This substitute is sutured to the dura at the most remote margins of the anterior fossa (Fig. 17-6).
3. The defect is exceptionally large and the posterior dura in front of the optochiasmatic cistern has disappeared (Fig. 17-7A, B, and C). It is impossible to posteriorly suture the dural substitute, which is folded as a leaf in a book. When it is impossible to achieve an

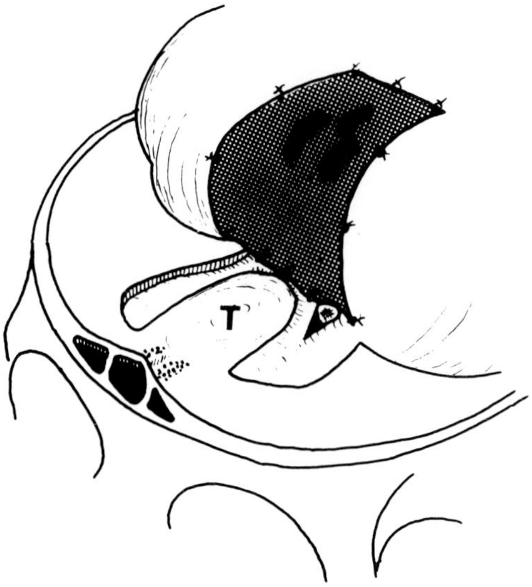

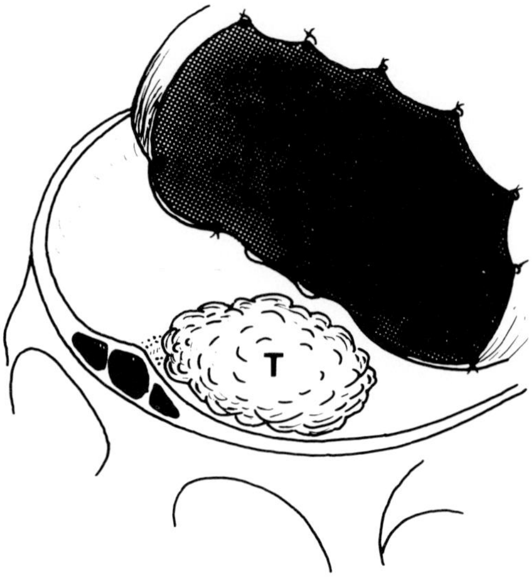

Fig. 17-5. (left) Strengthening the subfrontal dura on the midline with a pericranial graft. T = Tumor.

Fig. 17-6. (right) Dural defect closed with a large graft. Note suture at remote edges of the anterior fossa. T = basal insertion of tumor.

immediate tight closure, the basal part of the tumor is resected in a second stage, 3 or 4 months after the meninges are repaired.

The choice of dural substitute depends on many factors. The material must be thick enough and tight enough to prevent leaks and ascending infection, supple enough to permit brain reexpansion, and it must be revascularized rapidly for quick adherence and to feed bone grafts used to reconstruct the base of the skull. In our experience, rather than prosthetic materials, lyophilized dura, or fascia lata, a pericranial or dermal autograft is preferable.

The pericranial autograft has the same properties as the periosteum. For a thicker material and to preserve the anterior pericranium (covering the bifrontal free flap at the end of the procedure), the graft is taken from the biparietal area through the same scalp incision (Fig. 17-8). If necessary, the size of the sample can be as large as the entire subfrontal dura. This type of pericranial graft is used in almost all cases. Its periostic face lies toward the basal reconstruction.

The dermal autograft is excellent, provided epidermal implants are avoided. It is taken from the abdominal area, using a Padgett's dermatome. A thick dermoepidermal graft (1 to 1.2 mm thick) is cut from the subumbilical area. The graft stuck on the dermatome is recut on the drum to obtain a purely dermal graft (0.5 to 0.6 mm thick). The epidermal part is folded backward and sutured (Fig. 17-9). This substitute is used (a) when the dural defect is large (over 6 cm in diameter), and (b) when the optochiasmatic cistern is opened at the posterior margin of the anterior fossa. The *epidermal* face of the graft is placed on the skull base (the deeper face of the graft close to the frontal lobes).

It must be emphasized that subsequent steps in the procedure depend on the quality of dural repair. In contrast to the anterior approach the transbasal approach makes this repair easier, even with a clival dural defect (Fig. 17-10).

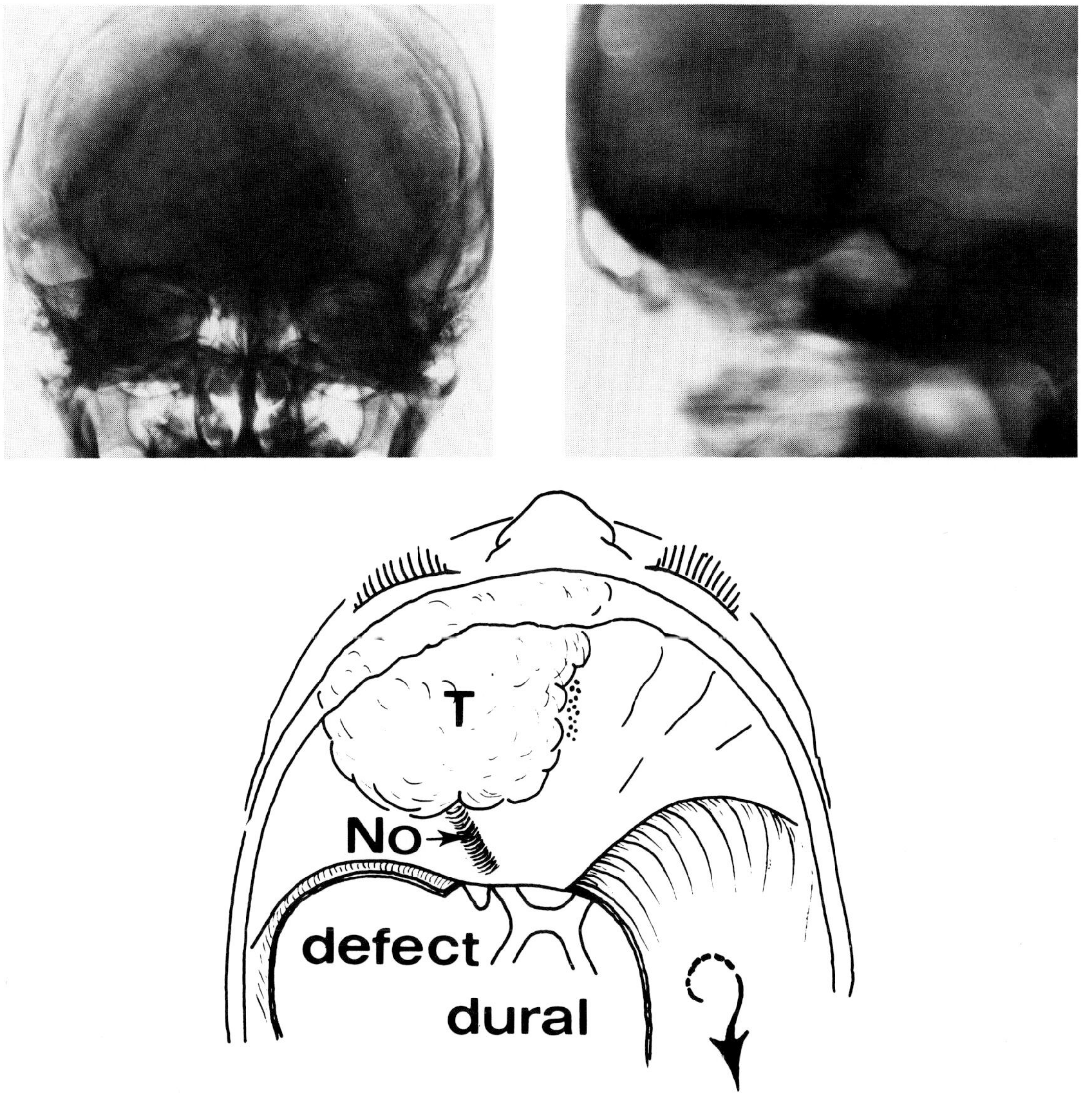

Fig. 17-7. Ossifying fibroma with a large intracranial extension. T = basal insertion of the tumor, No. = extradural part of the left optic nerve. After the intracranial part is removed, the optochiasmatic cistern is opened widely. In this case a dermal graft becomes necessary, because it is more adhesive.

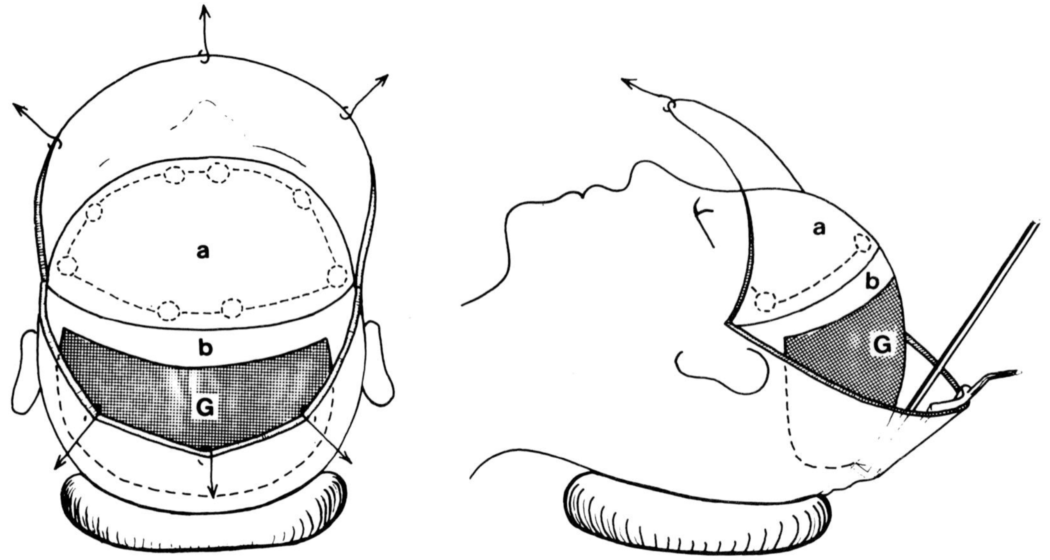

Fig. 17-8. Extracting a pericranial graft. a = anterior pericranium, G = graft, b = pericranial band preserved to allow a suture at the end of the procedure.

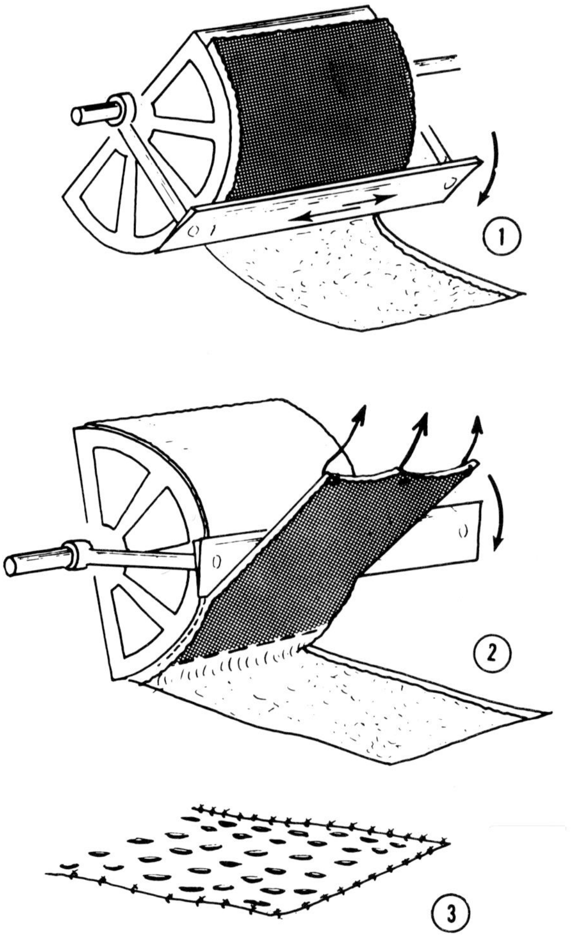

Fig. 17-9. Taking a dermal graft from the abdominal area.

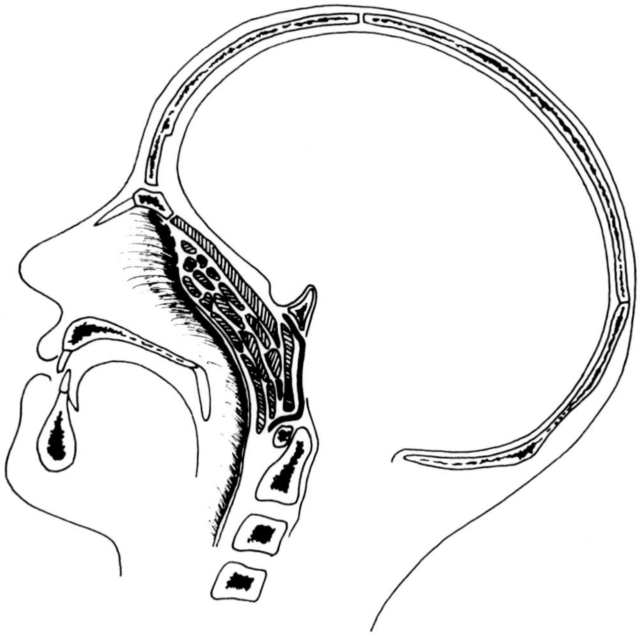

Fig. 17-10. Repair of a clival dural defect. The graft is applied by bone reconstruction.

Removal of the Basal Tumor

The difficulties encountered vary according to the location, extension, and consistency of the tumor. All types of rongeurs and drills can be used to remove pathologic bone.

Tumors in the ethmoidal area can be removed easily because there are no structures in the vicinity that can be injured. The neurosurgeon quickly reaches the nasal fossae where the turbinates, the septum, and septal mucosae are identified and preserved, if they are not invaded by tumor.

In the sphenoidal area the first step is to locate both optic nerves (Fig. 17-11A and B). Therefore partial resection of the orbital roofs is the first step after the periorbitum has been separated through an orbital approach. For this reason, the frontal bone is scraped to the upper margin of the orbits. When the supraorbital fissures are closed, resection of their lower rim helps to preserve the supraorbital vessels and nerves. The optic canals are then opened and the extradural part of the optic nerves identified. The tumor is attacked between the nerves on the jugum plate (Fig. 17-12A). After intratumoral resection, the margins of bone are progressively removed. The medial walls of both orbits and the entire body of the sphenoid are then resected to the packing introduced through the rhinoseptal approach to preserve the pharyngeal and cavum mucosae (Fig. 17-12B). The medial rim of the sphenoidal fissure can be opened from the midline (Fig. 17-13), and it is possible to reach the foramen rotundum and the vidian canal in the root of the pterygoid process.

Laterally, if the tumor involves the lesser and greater sphenoidal wings, resection of the orbital roof is extended to the temporal dura so that the lesser wing and the upper margin of the sphenoidal fissure disappear. Working between the sphenoidal fissure and the optic foramen, the anterior clinoid process is progressively removed. This resection must be done very carefully, step by step, because of the proximity of the internal carotid artery and the insertion of the small circumference of the tentorium, just below the dura. Resection of the

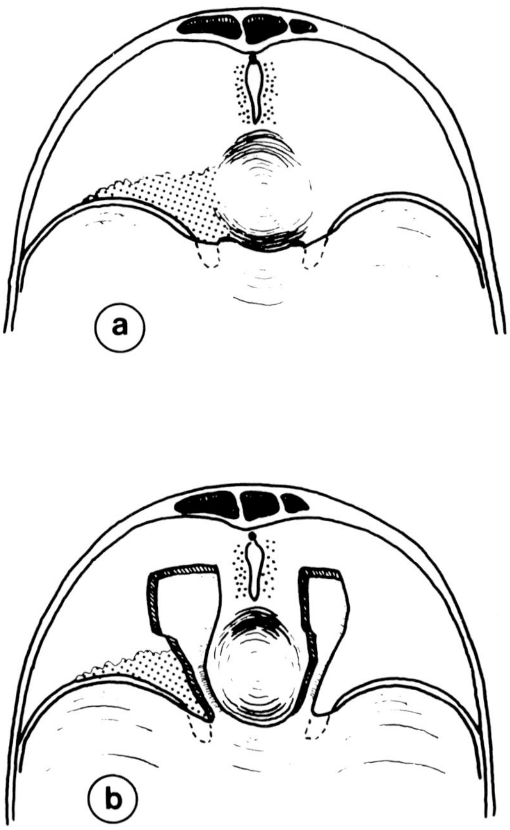

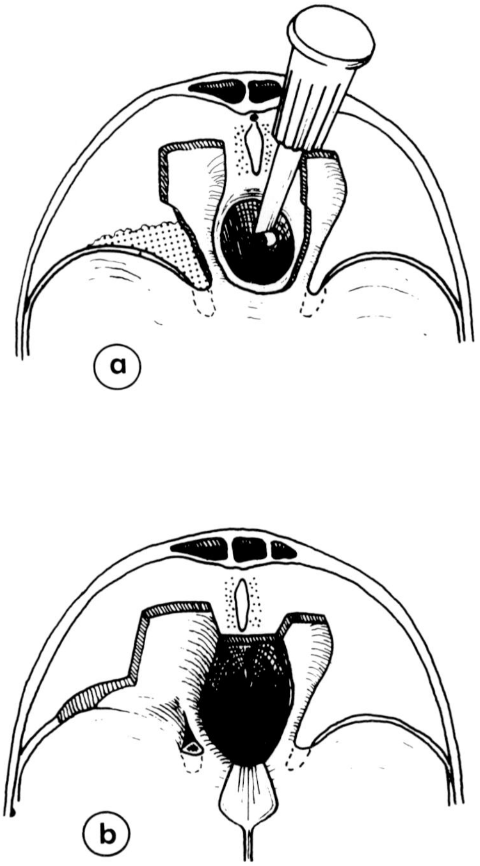

Fig. 17-11. (left) **(A)** = Fibrous dysplasia involving the sphenoidal body and the left lesser wing. **(B)** = Opening the optic canals.

Fig. 17-12. (right) **(A)** = Intratumoral resection between the optic nerves. **(B)** = Total removal of the sphenoid body leading to the pharyngeal mucosae. Opening of the left sphenoidal fissure and resection of the left anterior clinoid process.

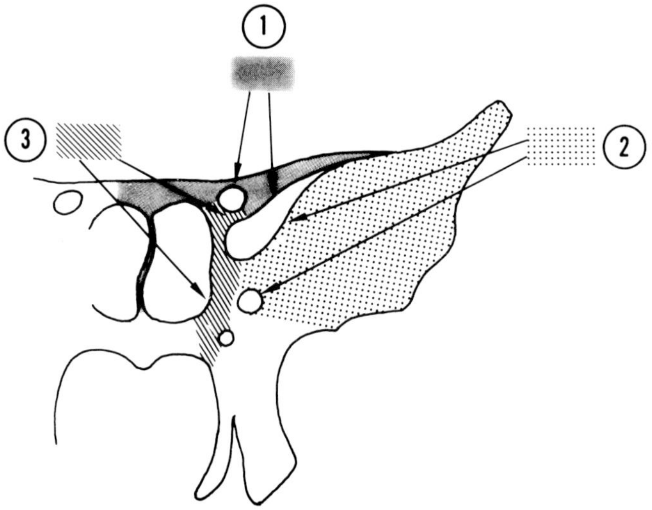

Fig. 17-13. 1 = Vertical attack, 2 = medial attack, 3 = lateral attack.

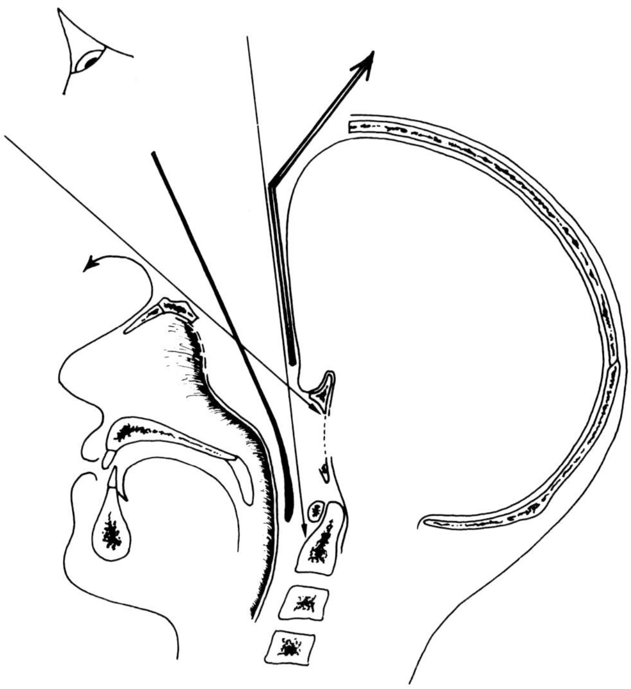

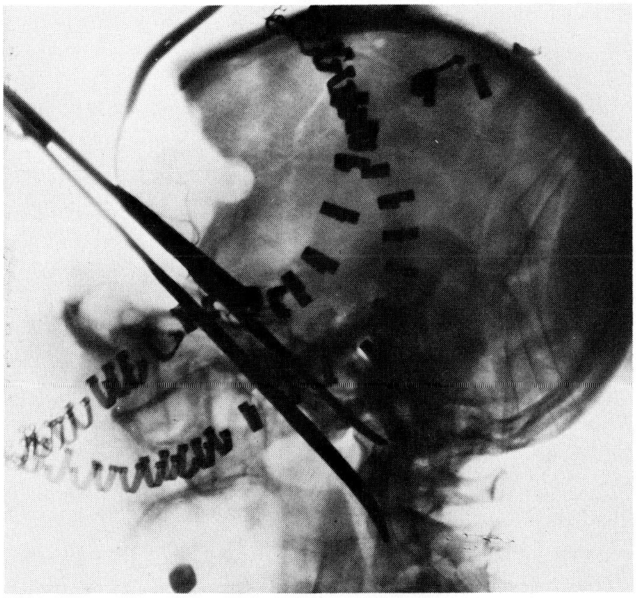

Fig. 17-14. A. (top) Through the transbasal approach, it is possible to reach the clivus, the anterior arch of the atlas, and the body of C1 and C2. Notice the preservation of the pharyngeal mucosae. **B.** (bottom) Intraoperative radiography. The tips of the instruments are located on the anterior margin of foramen magnum and body of C2.

greater wing, between the periorbitum and the temporal dura, is now easy and opens the inferior margin of the sphenoidal fissure, leading toward the floor of the middle fossa, the foramen rotundum, and the foramen ovale (Fig. 17-13). At the end of this procedure all upper cranial nerves are free.

Posteriorly it is now possible to reach the clivus after the tuberculum sellar area and the vertical part of the sellar floor have been removed. Some bleeding may occur in this area because the dura of the sella is extremely vascular. However this bleeding is generally not significant.

Proceeding downwards, the clivus is removed and the clival dura dissected to the anterior margin of the foramen magnum, which is opened. If dissection of the pharyngeal mucosa follows, the surgeon is able to reach the precervical space, the anterior arch of the atlas, and even the body of C2 and C3 (Fig. 17-14A and B). The base of the skull, after this wide dissection, looks much different than usual: the bony tissue has disappeared, the soft tissues of the orbits are attached only to the frontal and temporal dura by the optic nerves and sphenoidal fissures, and between them there is a large dead space bounded by the rhinopharyngeal mucosae.

Repair of the Base of the Skull

This reconstruction is necessary for three reasons: (a) in the midline, because of the dead space and risk of later meningoceles and encephaloceles; (b) laterally, in the orbital area to avoid postoperative enophthalmia, pulsatility, or desaxation of the eyeball; and (c) in the frontal area, for cosmetic reasons, if the orbito-frontal band and supraorbital margins are involved and therefore removed.

Maxillofacial and plastic surgeons have taught us that the best material to use to close air-filled cavities of the face, which have been opened widely and are generally septic, is bone autograft. The grafts are taken from the iliac bone, where it is possible to get a large specimen, during the same procedure. The advantage of an iliac extraction is that it also provides cancellous rather than cortical grafts. If the specimens are not sufficient, which is often the case in children, one, two, or even three rib grafts can also be taken. The rib must be split to get a cancellous face, which is applied close to the upper air-filled cavities and rhinopharyngeal mucosae (Fig. 17-15A, B, and C). After the medial walls and the roofs of the orbits are repaired with two single grafts or one modeled graft, the dead space is packed with cancellous bone. A final cortical graft is used to close the ethmoido-sphenoidal area. It is implanted between the nasion and the clivus, beneath the horizontal portion of the sellar floor. If the clivus has also been removed, the graft is applied close to a vertical graft, fitted between the floor of the sella and the anterior margin of the foramen magnum or the anterior arch of the atlas. Optic nerves must remain completely free. Bone dust is finally packed intracranially to give a tight closure. (Figures 17-16 through 17-19 illustrate the principles of this reconstruction.) If necessary, the supraorbital margins are reconstructed with iliac graft or with one single-modeled split rib graft wired to both orbital processes of the malar bone. Generally, removal of the greater sphenoidal wing and anterior half of the middle fossa does not need repair.

Closure

Clips are placed medially on the subfrontal dura, which has been strengthened by the pericranial graft. They are landmarks that can be used to follow postoperative brain reexpansion radiographically. The bifrontal free flap is replaced with dural suspensions. If the tumor also invaded a part of the flap, the pathologic bone is resected and a cranioplasty performed

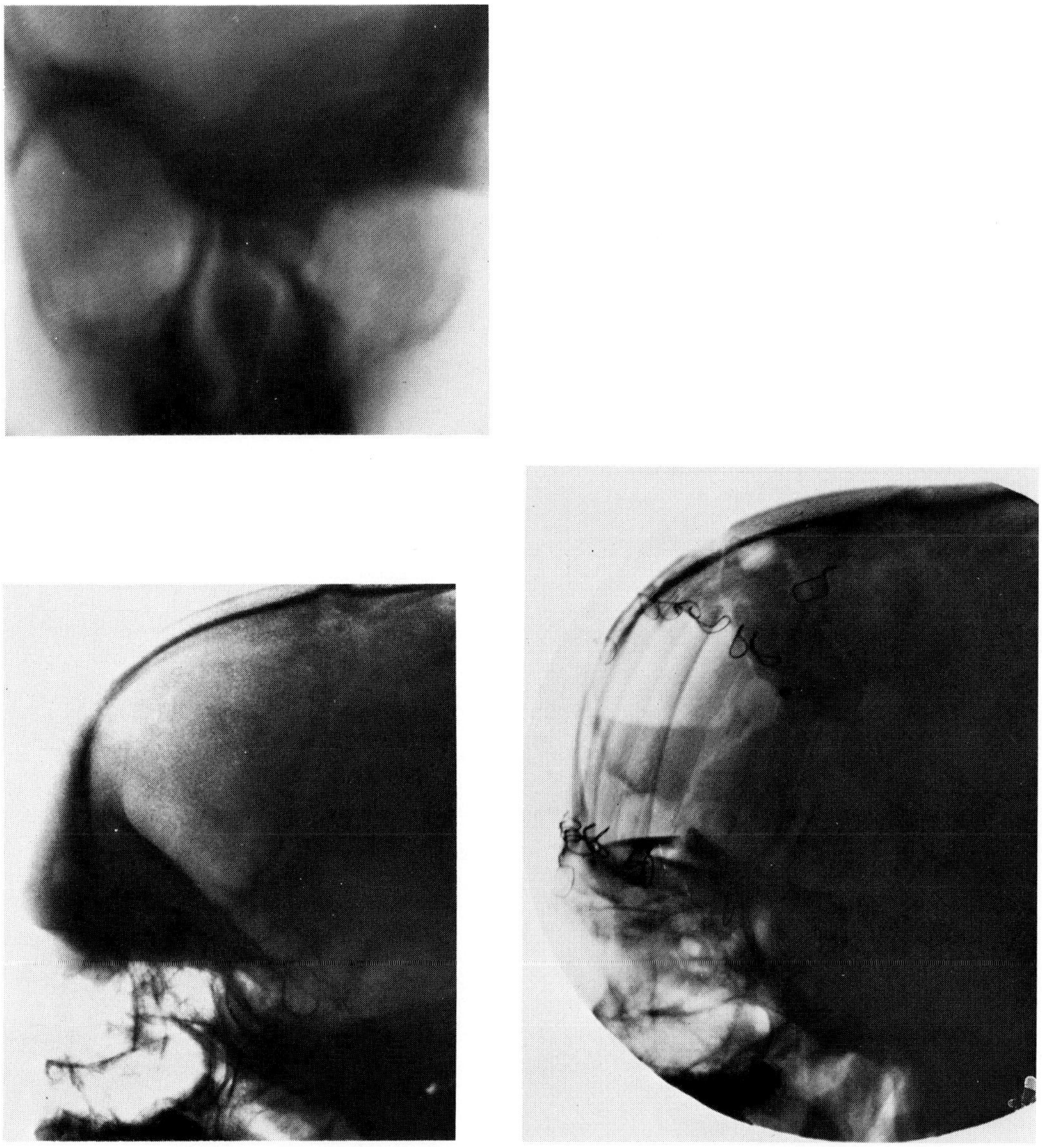

Fig. 17-15. **A.** and **B.** (left) Fibrous dysplasia in an 8-year-old child. **C.** (right) Frontal, orbital, and basal reconstruction with split-rib autografts.

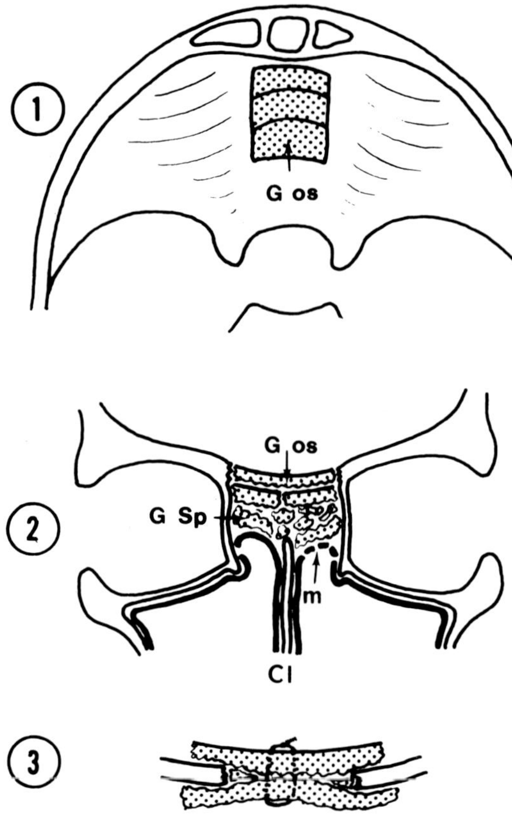

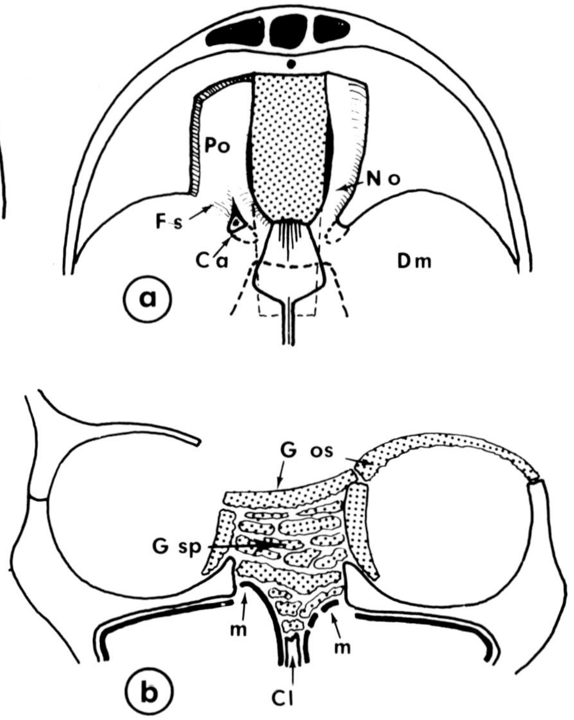

Fig. 17-16. (left) Ethmoidal reconstruction. 1 = Endocranial view of the anterior floor. G os = split rib grafts. 2 = Frontal section. G sp = cancellous bone grafts, m = mucosae, Cl = nasal septum. 3. = "Stud-like" technique insuring the closure of a defect when the bone is thin.

Fig. 17-17. (right) Ethmoidosphenoidal reconstruction. **(A)** = Endocranial view. PO = periorbitum, No = optic nerve, Fs = sphenoidal fissure. Ca = anterior clinoid process, Dm. = dura. **(B)** = Frontal section. G os = cortical bone grafts, G sp. = cancellous bone grafts, m = mucosae, Cl = nasal septum. Simultaneous repair of an orbit roof.

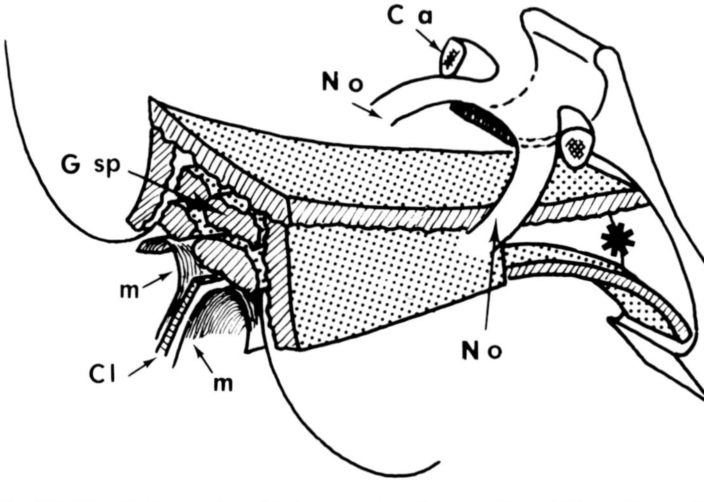

Fig. 17-18. Sphenoethmoidal reconstruction on the midline. (Same legends as for preceding drawings). Between the new medial orbital walls and the large upper graft impacted below the sellar floor, the dead space is packed with cancellous bone grafts. Notice the freedom of both optic nerves. (Abbreviations same as in **Figs. 17-16, and 17-17.)**

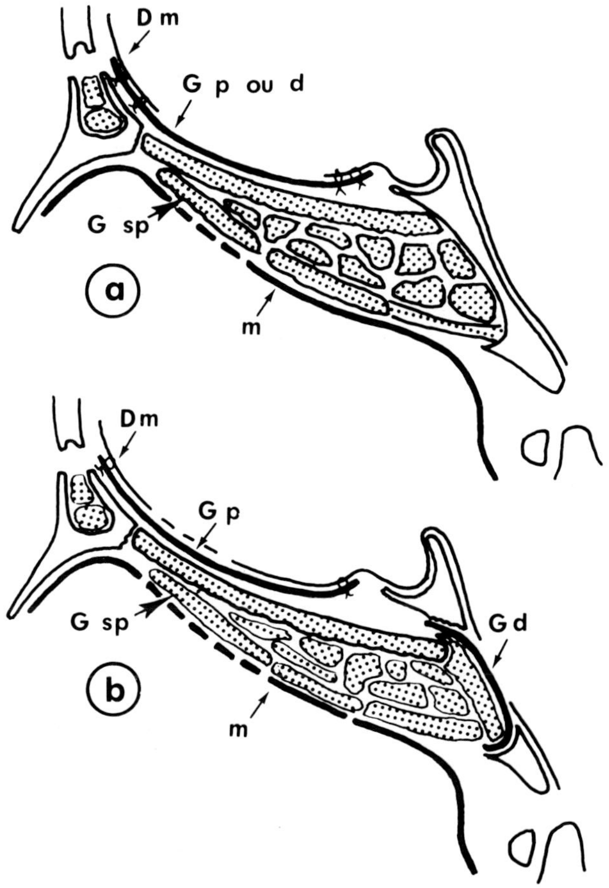

Fig. 17-19. Sagittal section of the reconstruction. **A.** The upper graft is impacted between the nasion and the remnants of the clivus. **B.** If the clivus is removed the posterior edge of the upper graft is impacted close to a graft fitted between the floor of the sella and the anterior margin of the foramen magnum, or the anterior arch of atlas. (Abbreviations same as in Figs. **17-16** and **17-17**.)

at the same stage. Again, a bone autograft is preferred to prosthetic material. (The possible need for such reconstruction must be anticipated when grafts are being taken.) The anterior pericranium is turned down to cover the bifrontal free flap. Before the scalp is sutured, two drains are placed, one extradurally in the subfrontal area and the other in the parietal area where the pericranial graft was extracted.

In the presence of preoperative exophthalmia, the eyelids may be closed temporarily with a silk suture and the eyes included in the dressing to avoid postoperative edema of soft orbital tissues. Lumbar drainage is removed at the end of the procedure.

Limits of the Transbasal Approach and Combination of Several Approaches

Only the subfrontal approach provides the exposure required for extensive removal of tumors invading the base of the skull. The entire anterior fossa and the largest part of the middle fossa can be resected. It is possible to free the vessels and nerves that pass through

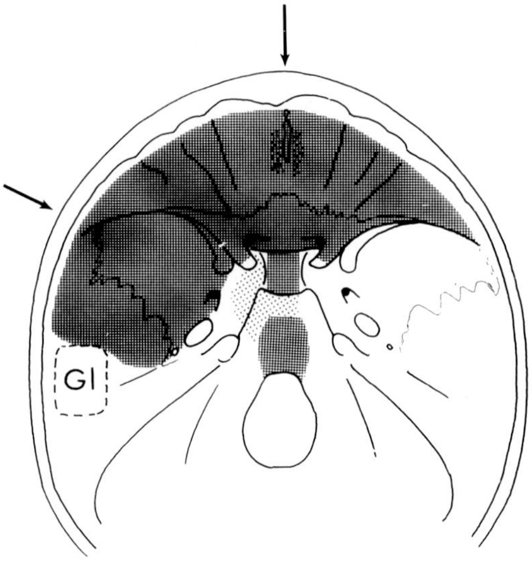

Fig. 17-20. Limits of basal resection through a bifrontal approach.

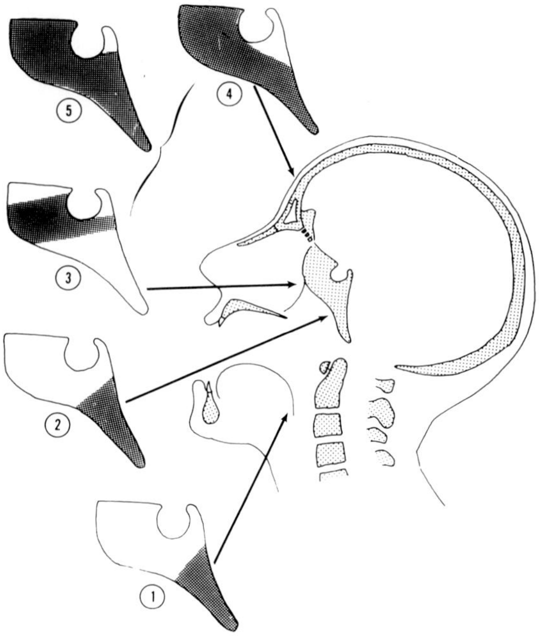

Fig. 17-21. Limits of sphenoidal and clival resection through anterior approaches. 1 = Transcervical approach, 2 = transoral approach, 3 = rhinoseptal approach, 4 = transbasal approach, 5 = association of transbasal and rhinoseptal approach.

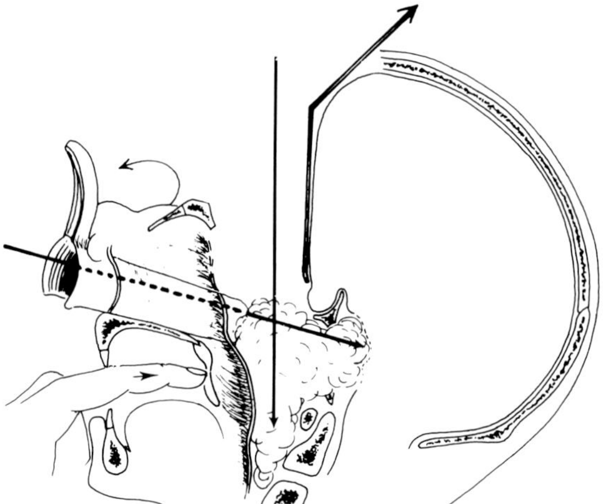

Fig. 17-22. Combination of several approaches during the same procedure (transbasal, rhinoseptal, and "pseudotransoral" approaches.

the optic canals, the sphenoidal fissures, the foramen rotundum and the foramen ovale (Fig. 17-20). The posterior limit is the petrous bone, which can be reached through a posterolateral approach, but its removal is not consistent with conservative surgery because the seventh and eighth nerves are destroyed. Resection of a pathologic skull base in front of the petrous bone preserves all upper cranial nerves, except the olfactory tracts.

Bone resection does not present problems. These occur only when soft tissues are involved, as with meningiomas. In the orbital area it is often possible to overlap the limits of the tumor by careful intraorbital dissection under the microscope. When the cavernous sinus is invaded, overlapping is generally impossible. And, except for rare encapsulated tumors, such as chondromas, the usual invasive and adhesive characteristics of the lesion make its complete removal impossible.

Possibilities for removing the clivus through different anterior approaches are summarized in Figure 17-21. The transcervical[3] and transoral approaches provide access only to its lower half. The rhinoseptal route is convenient to gain access to the sella, but it is narrow, lateral structures are not visible, and only the upper part of the clivus can be resected. Except for the subsellar area, which is hidden by the bulging sellar dura, the body of the clivus and sphenoid can be resected most extensively by the transbasal approach. To preserve the rhinopharyngeal mucosae, a rhinoseptal approach can be used in the same procedure. Thus both approaches can be combined, adding the advantages of each to remove the clivus almost completely, except for the dorsum sellae, which can be reached only intradurally.

The approach to a clival tumor depends on its nature, consistency, level of insertion, main expansion, and its location relative to the dura of the clivus. Some tumors can be removed through a single anterior approach. But, in a few cases the transbasal approach has certain advantages. These are:

1. Tight closure of the dura is possible if there is any risk that the subarachnoidal spaces will have to be opened.
2. The procedure can be combined with a rhinoseptal or *pseudotransoral* (introducing a finger in the mouth to push an anteriorly bulging tumor backward) approach for tumor removal (Fig. 17-22).
3. It is possible to add an intradural approach (subtemporal or through the posterior fossa) without risk of leaks, 2 to 3 months after the anterior part has been removed and the base of the skull reconstructed.

Indications for the Transbasal Approach

A transbasal approach is not required to gain access to all tumors at the base of the skull. Its use depends on the exact anatomic location of the lesion. However, the transbasal approach should be used each time it is likely to increase chances for total removal. The following table summarizes those cases in which this approach seemed to be absolutely necessary (Table 17-1).

Diagnosis of a tumor invading the base of the skull does not routinely lead to the same concept of treatment. The choice between complete removal, decompressive procedures, or radiotherapy without surgery must be based on the histology and extent of the lesion. For example, it is illogical to resect the base widely if an invasive malignant tumor involves the cavernous sinus. These factors must be determined by the preoperative examination.

Arteriography, phlebography, and sometimes pneumoencephalography show upward extension toward the intradural spaces and cavernous sinus. Radiography, tomography, gammagraphy, and, more recently, the computed tomography (CT) scan provide the most complete information about the nature and extent of bone invasion. However the nature of the lesion may be very difficult to diagnose, in which case rhinoseptal biopsy is suggested.

Table 17-1. Cases in which Transbasal Approach Used with Simultaneous Reconstruction (to November 1976)

Tumor	No. of patients
Meningiomas	18
Fibrous dysplasia	18
Chordomas	5
Olfactory placod tumors	5
Ossifying fibroma	2
Osteoma (?)	1
Chondromas	1
Hemangiopericytoma (?)	1
Sarcoma	2
Total	53

Biopsy will prevent errors; some invasive adenomas and sphenoidal mucoceles are often confused, clinically and radiologically, with a destructive chordoma.

Lesions involving the base of the skull may be divided into three groups: (a) tumors of intracranial origin, such as meningiomas; (b) true bone tumors; and (c) tumors of rhinopharyngeal origin, which generally are malignant.

Meningiomas

Meningiomas invade the base of the skull in three different ways: (a) sometimes the anterior fossa is ruptured at its weakest point, the ethmoidal area and cribiforme plates, as with intranasal extension of olfactory meningiomas[2,4-9] in which there is no true bone invasion. (b) With an en plaque meningioma,[2,5,10] the dural tumor is less important than hyperostosis, which is not a single reaction but a true tumoral infiltration of bone. The hyperostosis is responsible for the entire clinical syndrome and compression of the optic nerve into the optic canal. The dural plaque as well as the bone must be removed to avoid recurrence. The pterional location is not an indication for the transbasal approach. This approach is necessary and useful, however, when the lesion overlaps the optic canal and involves the sphenoidal area medially. (c) A bone reaction may be found close to the basal insertion of some en masse meningiomas.[11] The pathologic features of such a reaction are difficult to confirm, but it may be a true invasion, causing the basal malignancy to recur several years after the intracranial part has been removed. The basal invasion of a meningioma must be removed along with the intradural mass in one or two stages, depending on the size of the dural defect and the duration of the intracranial procedure.

True Bone Tumors

Bone tumors include many types of lesions.[11,12] Some are malignant and usually inoperable, such as sarcomas or metastasis. Many are benign, such as osteomas, osteoblastomas, hemangiomas, ossifying fibromas,[2,13] or fibrous dysplasia.[2,8,14] Although fibrous dysplasia is not a tumor, it may be considered one clinically and is sometimes responsible for visual disturbances. It is very difficult to predict the evolution of this type of lesion, which is often found in young patients, but progressive fibrous dysplasias with rapid visual loss are not uncommon (Fig. 17-23).

Our experience suggests that preventive surgery is required if the fibrous dysplasia is progressive or the area of the optic foramen is involved. Also, there are bone tumors that are difficult to classify because their pathologic potential is doubtful, even though some are malignant. Their malignancy, however, is localized probably because it is impossible to remove them completely. Examples of these tumors are giant cell tumors,[4] chondromas,[6] and

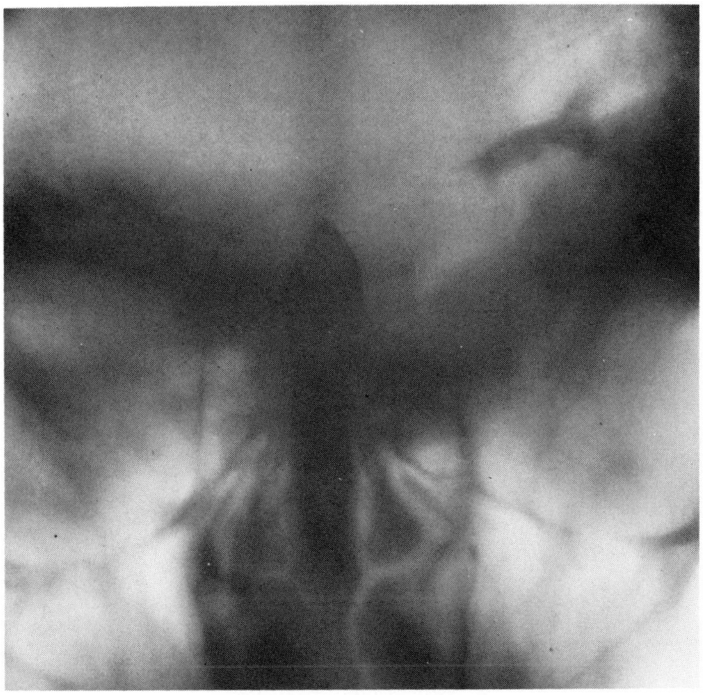

Fig. 17-23. Fibrous dysplasia responsible for visual loss. **A.** Preoperative tomography: invasion of the entire anterior fossa.

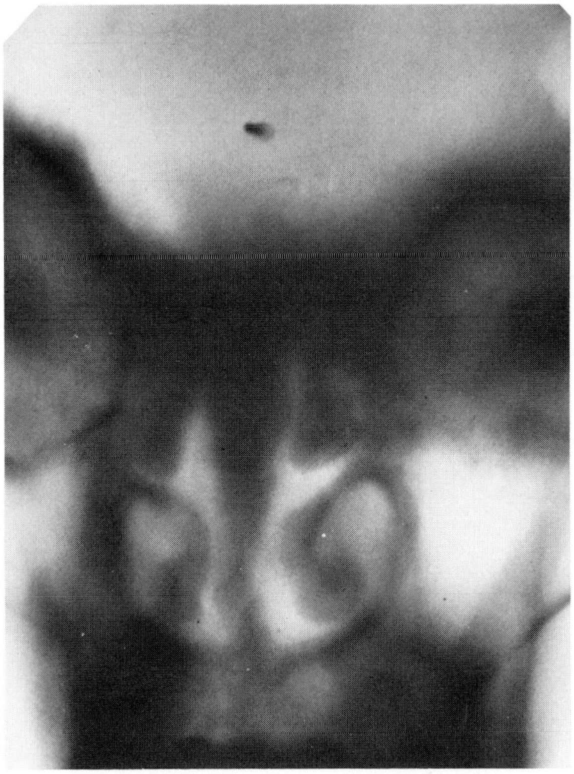

Fig. 17-23. B. Postoperative tomography 15 days after the procedure. Reconstruction of both orbits and the sphenoethmoidal mass.

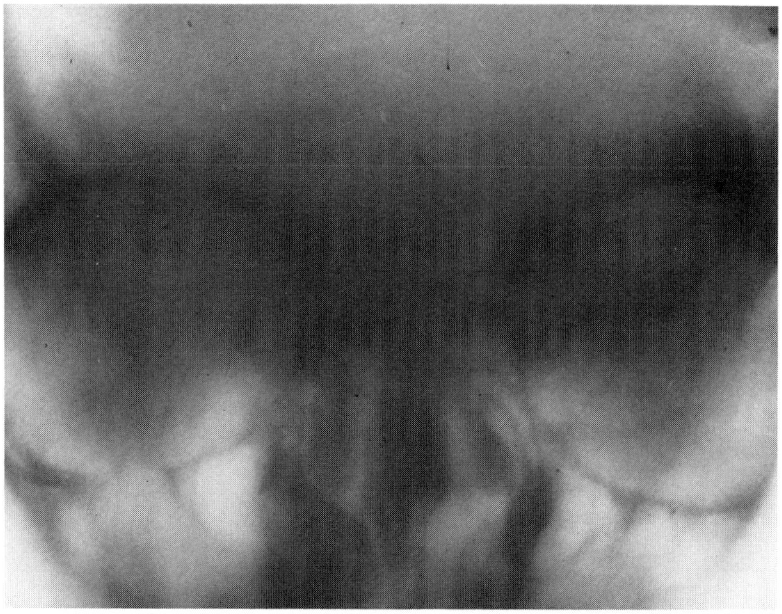

Fig. 17-23. **C.** Postoperative tomography, 2 years after the procedure. Normal aspect of the skull base.

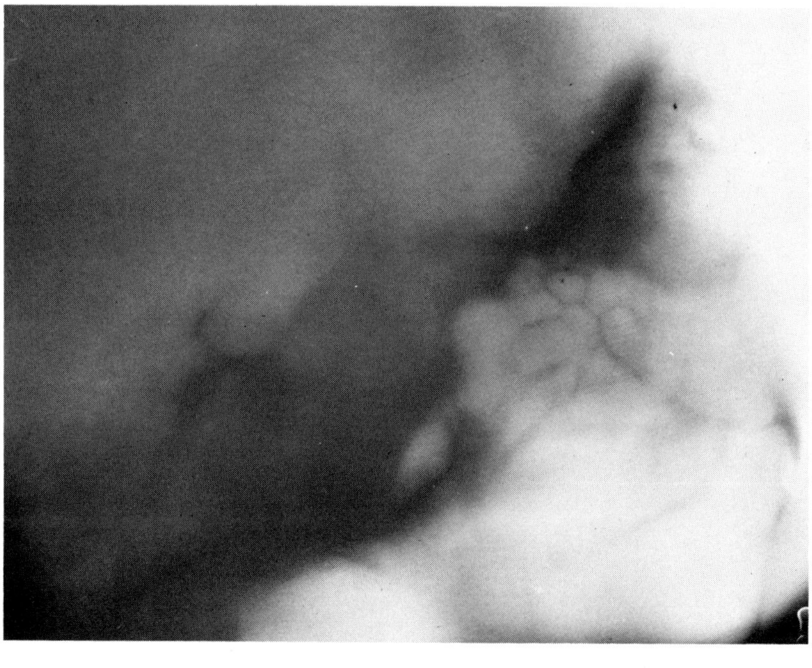

Fig. 17-23. **D.** Preoperative sagittal tomography.

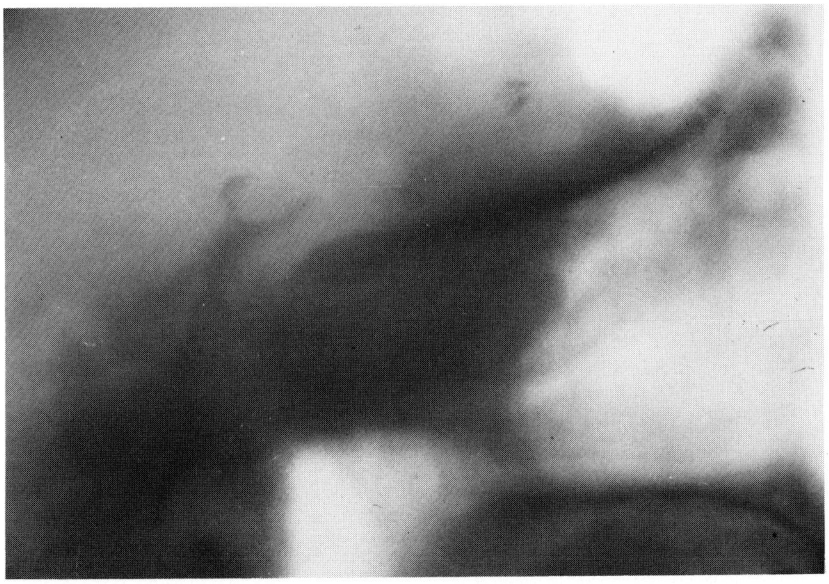

Fig. 17-23. E. Postoperative sagittal tomography, 15 days after the procedure. Notice the large upper graft covering the sphenoidal reconstruction.

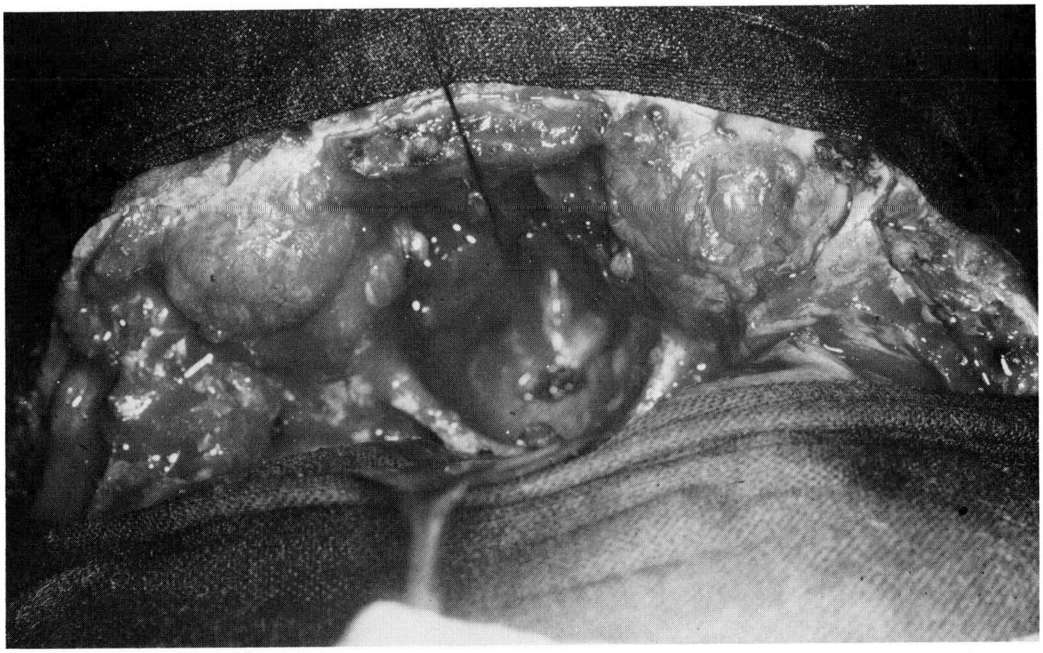

Fig. 17-23. F. Intraoperative view of the removal of the entire anterior fossa. The upper orbital margins, roofs and medial orbital walls, ethmoid, sphenoidal body, lesser wings and anterior clinoid processes are resected. Medially, this resection leads to the nasal fossae and pharyngeal mucosae. Both optic nerves are totally free and the sphenoidal fissures are opened.

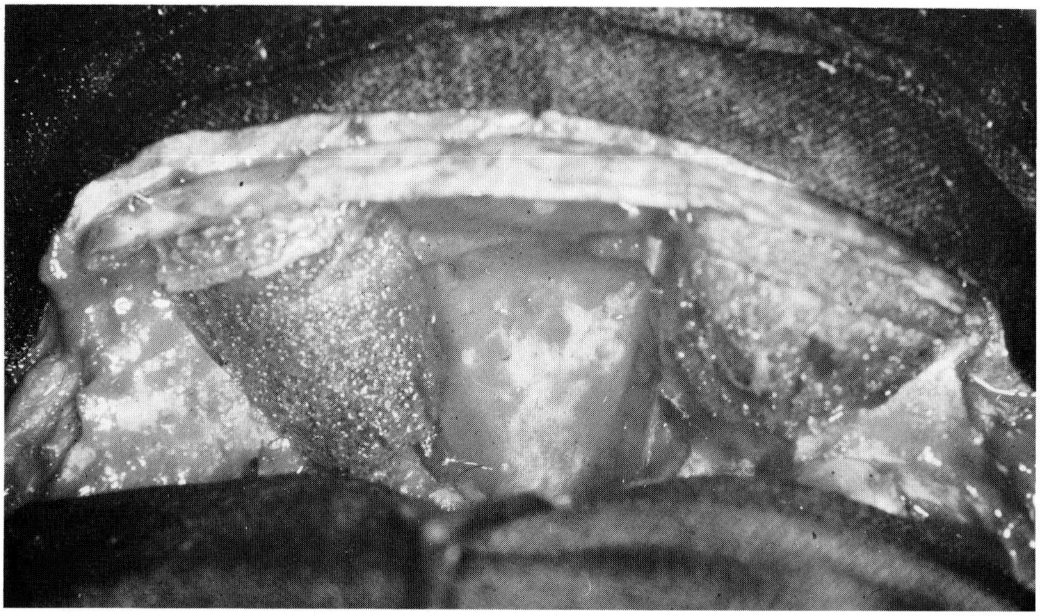

Fig. 17-23. **G.** Intraoperative view of the reconstruction. Both upper orbital margins are repaired with a single-wired split-rib graft. Note the large medial upper graft between the reconstruction of both orbits.

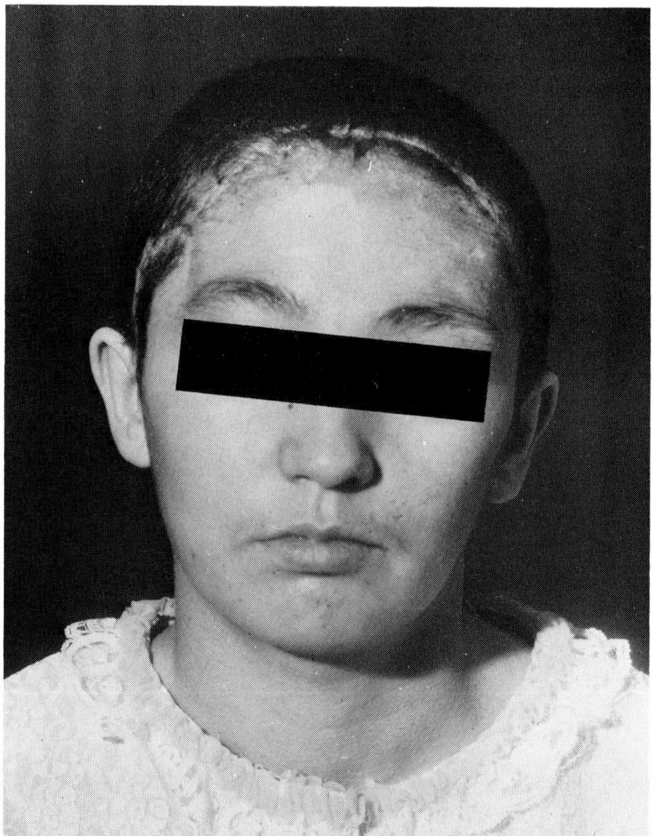

Fig. 17-23. **H.** Patient after 15 postoperative days, with a good cosmetic result and normal vision.

chordomas.[2,7] Surgery is certainly advised for chondromas because radiotherapy is ineffective. These tumors are more or less encapsulated and they probably can be removed almost completely, even when they develop within the cavernous sinus. With chordomas, the decision lies between surgery with or without radiotherapy, radioactive implantation, or radiotherapy alone. Because the transbasal approach increases the possibility that tumor in the clival area can be removed, surgery, in my opinion, is warranted. Even if the tumor cannot be removed completely, the effectiveness of postoperative radiotherapy improves when pathologic remnants have been reduced to a minimum. The combination of the most complete removal and radiotherapy gives the patient the best chance for long-term survival without recurrence.

Tumors of Rhinopharyngeal Origin

Among the rhinopharyngeal tumors that involve the base of the skull, very few are benign, ie., benign olfactory placod tumors[11] (esthesioneurocytomas) or nasopharyngeal fibromas. These tumors generally are malignant carcinomas or epitheliomas and the neurosurgeon's approach to each may vary. If the tumor extends toward the anterior fossa, the intracranial approach is suggested. But, extensive resection of the base of the skull is only indicated when it is possible to widely overlap the area of the tumor, as in surgery for carcinoma.[1,3,13,16] Extensive removal in these cases is more important than reconstruction. Unfortunately when this type of patient is seen by the neurosurgeon, it is often too late to remove all tumorous tissue completely. These patients must be seen very early in the course of tumor development and to do so close cooperation between neurosurgical, ENT, and maxillofacial teams is required.

REFERENCES

1. Tessier P, Guiot G, Derome P: Orbital hypertelorism. II. Definite treatment of orbital hypertelorism by craniofacial or by extracranial osteotomies. *Scand. Plast. Reconstr Surg 7*:39-58, 1973
2. Derome P, Akerman M, Anquez L, et al: Les tumeurs spheno-ethmoidales, Possibilites d'exerese et de reparation chirurgicales. Rapport de la Societe de Neurochirurgie de Langue Francaise. *Neurochirurgie 15*:Suppl 1:1-164, 1972
3. Stevenson GC, Stoney RJ, Perkins RK, et al: A transcervical, transclival approach to the ventral surface of the brainstem for removal of a clivus chordoma. *J Neurosurg 24*:544-551, 1966
4. Geissinger JD, Siqueira EB, Ross ER: Giant cell tumors of the sphenoid bone. *J Neurosurg 32*:665-770, 1970
5. Guiot G, Derome P: A propos des méningiomes en plaques du pterion. Le traitement chirurgical des meningiomes osseux hyperestosants. *Ann Chir 20*:C1109-C1127, 1966
6. Lehrer HZ: Ossifying fibroma of the orbital roof: Its distinction from blistering or intraosseus meningioma. *Arch Neurol 20*:536-541, 1969
7. Krayenbuhl H, Yasargil MG: Cranial chordomas. *Prog Neurol 6*:380-434, 1975
8. Liechtenstein L, Jaffe HL: Fibrous dysplasia of bone. A condition affecting one, several or many bones, the graver of which may represent abnormal pigmentation of skin, premature sexual development, hyperthyroidism, or still other extraskeletal abnormalities. *Arch Pathol 33*:777-816, 1942
9. Pertuiset B, Beciric T: La voie intracranienne dans l'exerese du prolongement nasal des meningiomes olfactifs. *Press Med 63*:1863-1865, 1958
10. Castellano F, Guidetti B, Olivecrona H: Pterional meningiomas en plaques. *J Neurosurg 9*:188-196, 1952
11. Dahlin D: *Bone Tumors*. Charles C Thomas, Springfield, Illinois, 1964
12. Reynaud J, Courson B: A propos des osteodysplasies et osteopathies fibreuses craniofaciales et de leur traitement. *Ann Chir Plast 15*:312-317, 1970
13. Scott M, Peale AR, Croissant PD: Intracranial midline anterior fossae ossifying fibroma invading orbits, paranasal sinuses, and right maxillary antrum. *J Neurosurg 34*:827-831, 1971
14. Plewes JL, Jacobson I: Familial frontonasal dermoid cysts. Report of four cases. *J Neurosurg 34*:683-686, 1971
15. Saunders WH, Miglets A: Surgical techniques for eradicating far advanced carcinoma of the orbital-ethmoid and maxillary aréas. *Trans Am Acad Ophthalmol Otolaryngol 7*:426-431, 1967
16. Van Buren JM, Ommaya AK, Ketcham AS: Ten years' experience with radical combined craniofacial resection of malignant tumors of the paranasal sinuses. *J Neurosurg 28*:341-350, 1968

CHAPTER 18

Transcallosal Approach to Third Ventricular Tumors

Bennett M. Stein

Introduction

TUMORS WITHIN THE THIRD ventricle are strategically located so as to make them extremely difficult to expose and remove.[1] Although they can be reached by a number of routes, it is difficult to expose the region widely. At the very least such surgery requires an operating microscope and microsurgical instruments.

The tumors may arise from structures surrounding the third ventricle, such as the hypothalamus and thalamus, or from within the third ventricle, originating from the ependyma or the paraphysis. Craniopharyngiomas, when they arise from the median eminence, may grow almost entirely within the third ventricle.[2] Tumor histology varies greatly and rivals the pineal region for a gamut of pathology.[3-6] The more common lesions encountered include: astrocytomas of all grades, ependymomas, craniopharyngiomas, colloid and ependymal cysts, choroid plexus papillomas, and other rare lesions. It is important to realize that a wide variety of tumors occur in this region and attempts should be made to accurately diagnose the type of tumor prior to operative intervention. The dorsal part of the tumor is related to the velum interpositum, which contains the internal cerebral veins and choroid plexus. The tumors often reach the foramen of Monro and may enlarge it or grow through it into the lateral ventricles. They are related to the lamina terminalis anteriorly, to portions of the hypothalamus inferiorly, and to the thalamus laterally.

The anatomic location, size, and possible nature of the tumor have a bearing on the choice of approach to be used to expose the third ventricle. Lesions that impinge upon or enlarge the foramen of Monro may be approached most easily from a transcallosal route. It appears that even though the tumor may arise in the chiasmatic or suprasellar area, if it is large enough to reach the foramen of Monro, it will have so thinned-out the hypothalamic region that it can be approached directly by a transventricular route.

Surgical Approaches to the Third Ventricular Region

For tumors that fill the third ventricle and encroach upon the lateral ventricles, a number of surgical approaches have been used. A transfrontal route requires a frontal craniotomy, usually on the right side, with incision into cortical and subcortical tissue, until the epen-

Department of Neurosurgery, Tufts-New England Medical Center, Boston, Massachusetts 02111 dymal surface of the right lateral ventricle is reached. At this point an enlarged foramen of Monro usually permits access to the third ventricle. The interhemispheric, parafalx or transcallosal approach was used by Dandy[7] and others. The advantages of the transcallosal approach to the third ventricle are numerous. The retraction, rather than incision of the right hemisphere, provides an easy route and brain tissue is not sacrificed; sacrifice of an occasional cortical vein as it enters the sagittal sinus has not resulted in significant neurologic deficit, arteries on the surface of the corpus callosum may be easily mobilized and spared, while small veins that run directly on the corpus callosum are of no significance and may be sectioned.

The greatest advantage of the transcallosal exposure is that it permits entry into either or both lateral ventricles and provides direct access to deep regions of the third ventricle, through the foramen of Monro. The surgeon is not encumbered by entering the lateral ventricle at an angle that limits his view of the deep recesses of the third ventricle, especially the optic recesses. In a dilated ventricular system, the exposure is virtually bloodless.

Preoperative Evaluation

The most informative radiographic procedures are those that outline the extent of the tumor. These include contrast ventriculography either with air or pantopaque and, more recently, the computerized tomography (CT) scan. Although arteriography may be valuable for demonstrating the vascularity of the tumor, giving some indication as to its pathology, it rarely outlines the tumor sufficiently to disclose its exact relationship to the foramen of Monro and other third ventricular structures. Because the surgical approach depends upon the size and exact position of the tumor, it is important to outline the extent of the tumor, and particularly, its relationship to the foramen of Monro. If the tumor lies deep within the third ventricle, or is basically a suprasellar tumor indenting the third ventricle and not large enough to reach the foramen of Monro, it is better approached from a subfrontal or translamina terminalis route. If the surgeon can be certain that the tumor impinges upon the foramen of Monro or goes through it, then a transventricular approach, especially the transcallosal, is appropriate (Fig. 18-1). The CT scan often supplants ventriculography, thereby shortening the operative procedure and the morbidity of the diagnostic workup.

Details of the Operative Approach to the Third Ventricle

The patient is positioned in the recumbent supine position, with the head flexed so that the junction of the coronal and sagittal sutures is parallel to the horizontal. Care is taken so that an air embolism can be diagnosed and treated appropriately. This requires placement of a central venous catheter and doppler monitoring. Generally, the patient's head is best held flexed by a pin-type head holder so that there will be no change in position during the operative procedure. The angle of the head in the flexed position should be memorized by the surgeon. Also, it is essential that the head is not tilted so that a direct perpendicular approach can be carried out. If the patient's position varies, and the operating surgeon is not aware of the changes, entry into the lateral ventricular system may be rostral or caudal to the foramen of Monro or the ventricle opposite to the intended one may be entered. A horseshoe incision is made, with its base toward the zygoma and the free portion extending from the right to just over the midline on the left (Fig. 18-2). A free bone flap is elevated, making the superior margin just to the left of the midline so that the sagittal sinus is exposed. The anteroposterior position of the flap is situated so that two-thirds will be anterior to the coronal suture and one-third posterior. Mannitol or spinal drainage may be used, depending on the degree of obstruction within the ventricular system. The dura is then opened in a U-shaped fashion, with its base along the sagittal sinus. It is important to make the cuts directly to the edge of

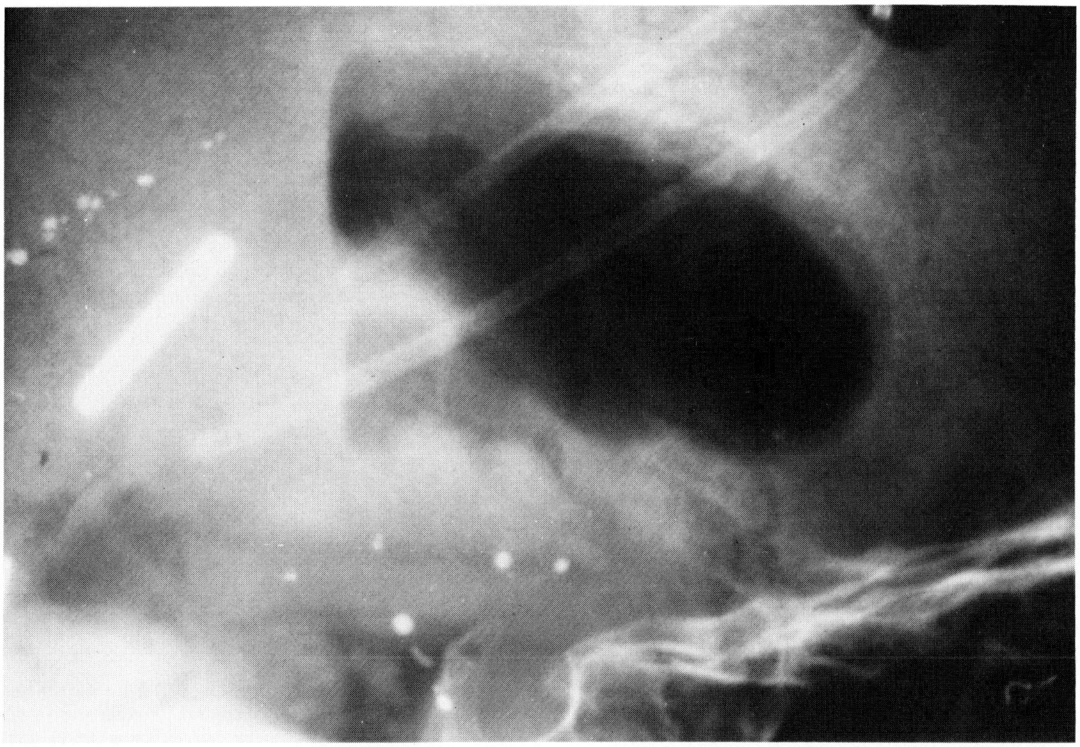

Fig. 18-1. Hanging head ventriculogram showing a dilated foramen of Monro due to a third-ventricular craniopharyngioma. The irregular surface of the tumor may be appreciated by the air within the third ventricle.

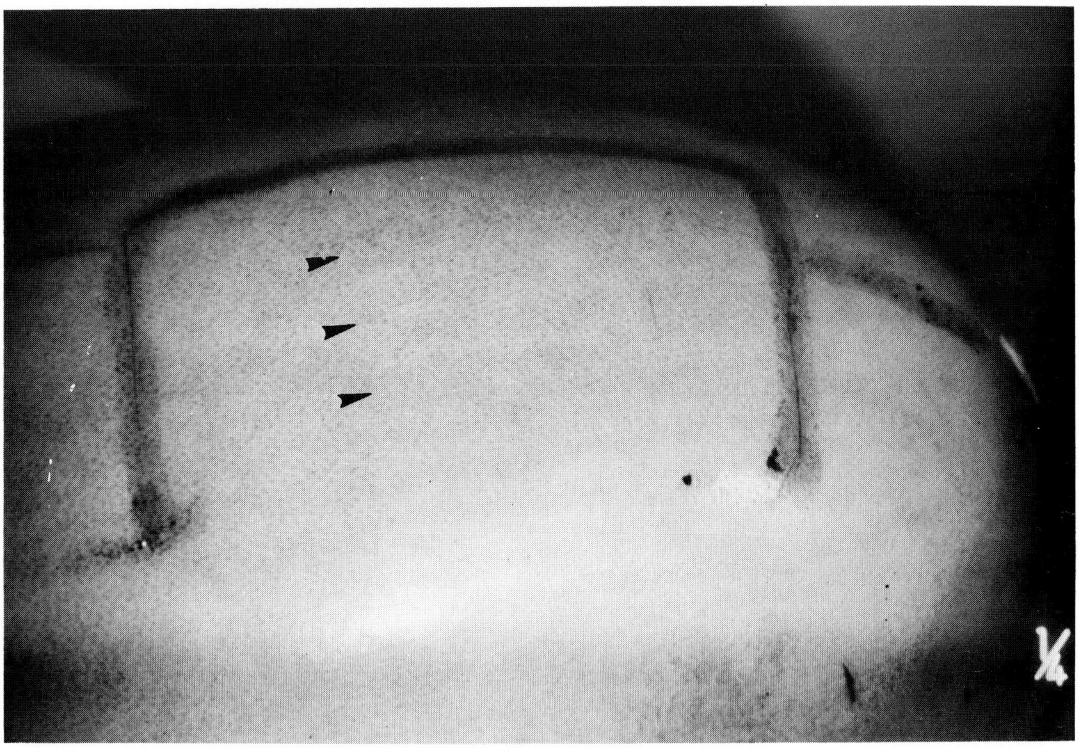

Fig. 18-2. Outline of right paramedian craniotomy flap. Arrow indicates position of the coronal suture.

the sinus so that the dural flap may be reflected strongly to the left side and the falx visualized. A number of modest-sized cortical veins, entering the sagittal sinus, are generally encountered. Some of these can be dissected a considerable distance so that they are displaced out of the operative area. Others may have to be sacrificed, which has not resulted in neurologic deficit. When the medial margin of the hemisphere is free, gentle retraction is applied to separate it from the falx (Fig. 18-3). If tension exists, the right lateral ventricle may be tapped with a ventricular needle and cerebrospinal fluid evacuated to facilitate retraction of the hemisphere. When the interhemispheric fissure is entered, the cingulate gyrus may be confused with the corpus callosum (Fig. 18-4). The gyrii of the right and left cingulate region are often adherent to each other and may be displaced to the left or right of the midline, making a direct approach to the corpus callosum somewhat difficult. This situation should be recognized immediately, otherwise a great deal of difficulty will be encountered and the brain injured. The cingulate gyrus is more vascular than the dorsal surface of the corpus callosum, which is very white and relatively avascular. This is a small point, but if it is not recognized,

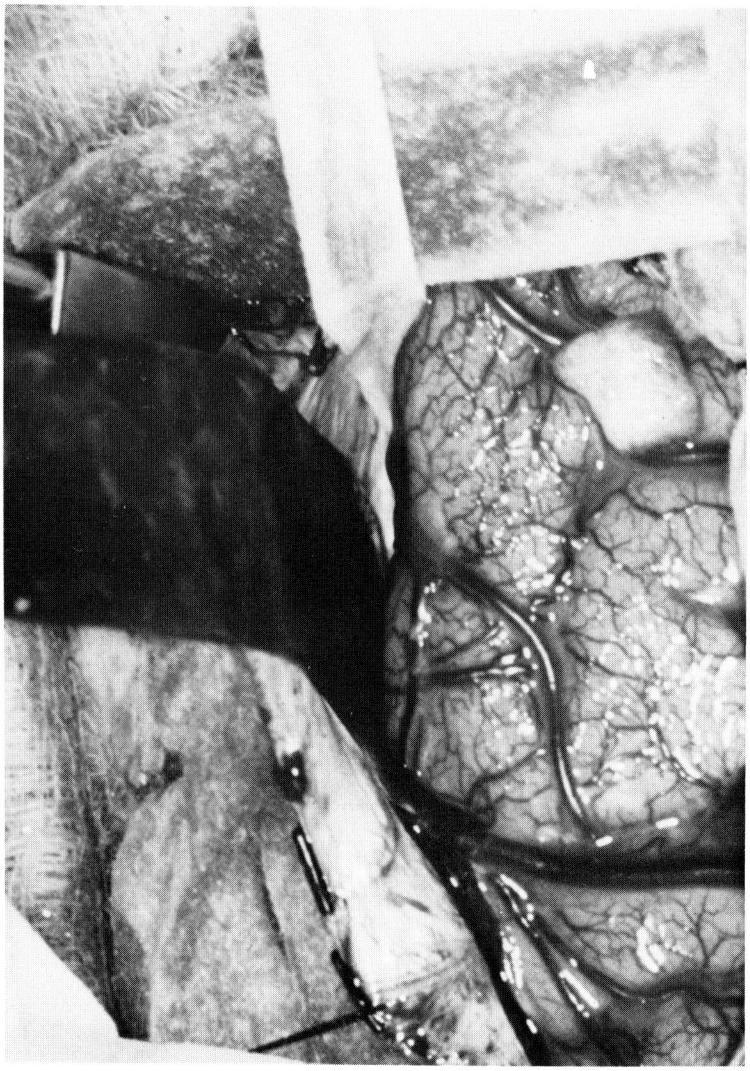

Fig. 18-3. Initial exposure of interhemispheric fissure. Retractor is on the falx.

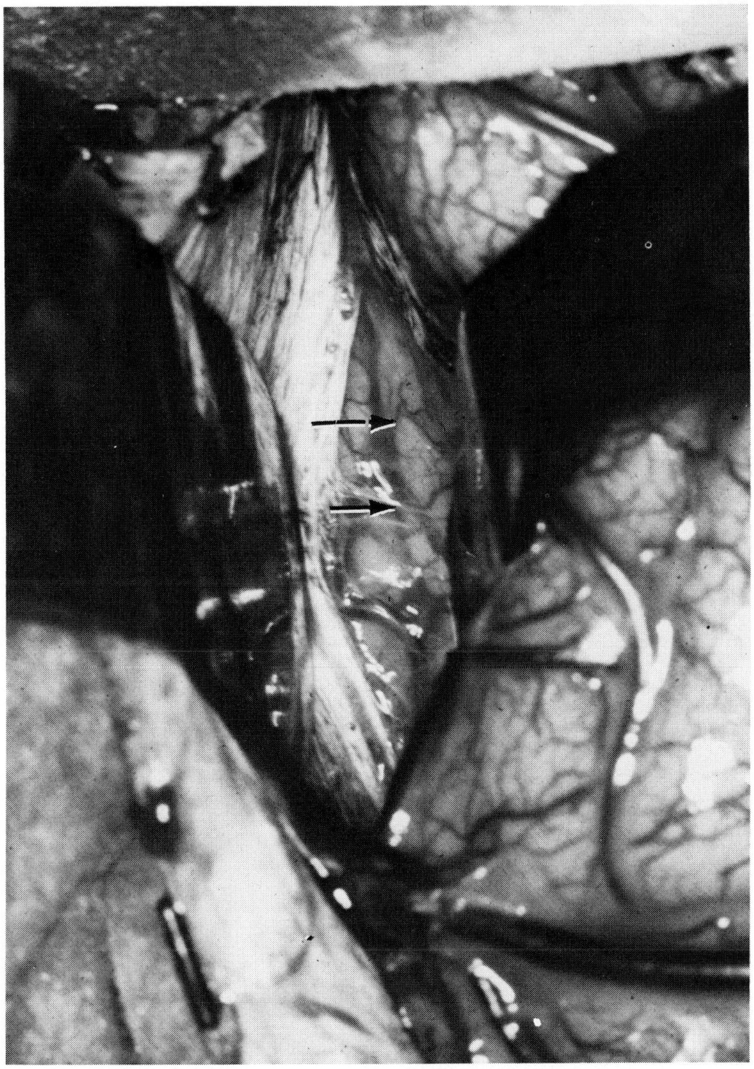

Fig. 18-4. Exposure of cingulate gyrus (arrows). Compare texture with that of corpus callosum **(Fig. 18-5).**

subsequent difficulty will be encountered in the exposure. The dissection is carried to the corpus callosum where the main trunks of the anterior cerebral artery or the pericallosal arteries will be encountered. A brief appraisal of the situation will indicate that both arteries may be displaced either to the left or right without sacrificing all but one or two small branches to the cingulate gyrus. Having displaced the arteries appropriately, the dorsal surface of the corpus callosum, upon which a number of small veins run, is encountered (Fig. 18-5). These veins are cauterized to facilitate section of corpus callosum. The falx is held sharply toward the left by a self-retaining retractor, whereas the brain is held in position, usually covered by cellophane or cottonoid, by a second self-retaining retractor. An anteroposterior section of the corpus callosum, amounting to approximately 3.0 cm is sufficient exposure. The measurement, of course, depends upon the age of the patient and the relative size of the corpus callosum.

The pial margin of the corpus callosum is cauterized and an incision made with cautery, suction, and a blunt dissector. The thickness of the corpus callosum varies, according to the

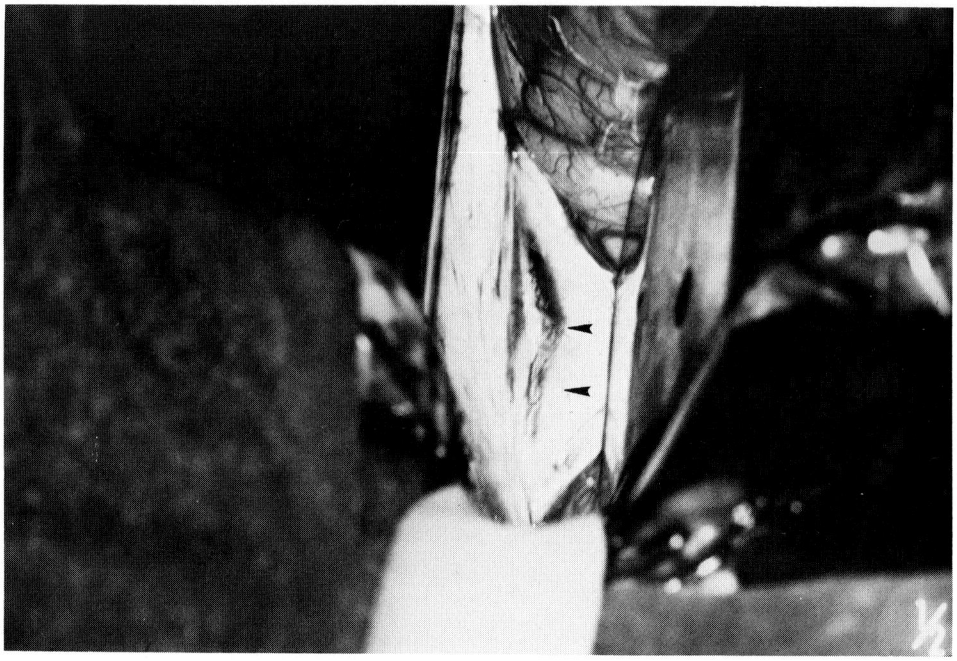

Fig. 18-5. Exposure of corpus callosum (arrows).

degree of ventricular expansion and the age of the patient. There is minimal vascularity within the corpus callosum, whereas veins may be encountered on the ependymal surface. These are easily recognized and cauterized. When the ependymal margin is reached, the anatomy will become apparent, since the color of the tissue changes. Some of the corpus callosum may require suctioning in order to afford adequate exposure into either the left or right lateral ventricle.

It is often difficult, at first, to determine whether the exposure has been made into the left or right lateral ventricle. The surgeon should immediately look for landmarks, which include: (a) the septal vein of the septum pellucidum, (b) the choroid plexus which terminates in the region of the foramen of Monro, and (c) the thalamostriate vein. With a small amount of effort, these landmarks may be identified and at this point one can be certain as to the laterality of the ventricle, which has been opened. The self-retaining retractors are then extended deeper to retract the sectioned corpus callosum, affording an excellent view of the lateral ventricle and foramen of Monro region (Fig. 18-6). If the preoperative diagnosis has been accurate, the foramen of Monro will generally be dilated and the tumor is easily visible, either within or just below the foramen of Monro (Fig. 18-7).

To facilitate removal of the tumor, or surgery within the third ventricle, it is often necessary to open the foramen of Monro. To do so an incision is made anteriorly through one of the fornices. To extend the incision posteriorly would result in injury and hemorrhage from the choroid plexus or the internal cerebral vein and its tributaries. The anterior opening of the foramen of Monro is relatively avascular and section of one fornix is not considered to produce a neurologic deficit. Care should be taken, however, not to section both fornices or damage the septal region. With the exposure enlarged, the tumor may be biopsied or removed by microsurgical techniques, using the operating microscope, tumor forceps, cautery, and various suctions. A 250- or 275-mm objective on the microscope is generally appropriate. Care must be taken not to injure any of the ependymal surfaces and to keep bleeding to a minimum, since blood would permeate the ventricular system and perhaps cause secondary

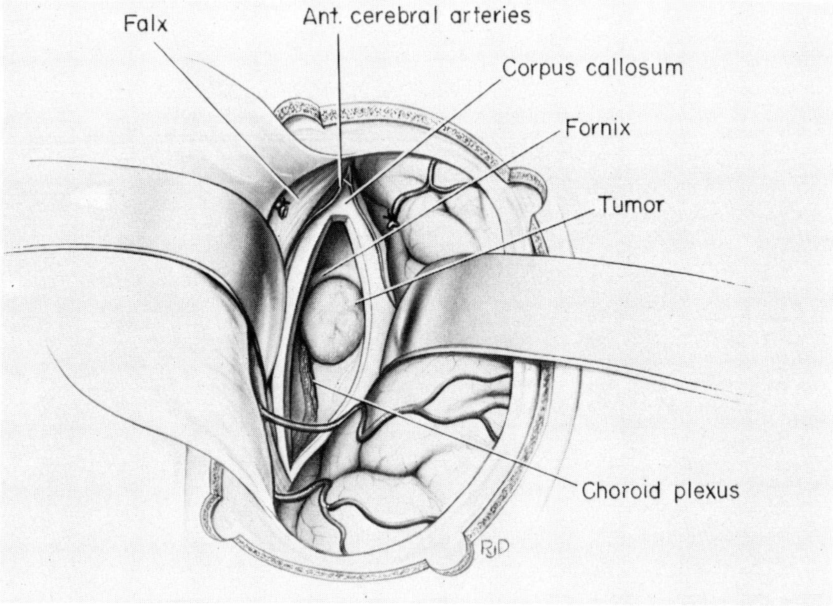

Fig. 18-6. Drawing of intraventricular exposure.

obstruction where there otherwise would be an open ventricular system following operative resection of the tumor.

When work on the tumor is completed, hemostasis must be accurate and no bleeding left within the ventricular system. Hemostatic agents such as Gelfoam, are not utilized, since they may work free and occlude the aqueduct or other portions of the ventricular system.

The major problem encountered in closure is collapse of the lateral ventricular system after the hydrocephalus has been relieved. There appears to be no way to satisfactorily close the corpus callosum so that postoperatively cerebrospinal fluid will undoubtedly leak into the interhemispheric region and, possibly, subdurally. Attempts have been made to inflate the ventricular system by placing a small Foley catheter into the opening in the corpus callosum, the balloon occluding it and the catheter being removed when dural closure has been completed. However, this is temporary at best and has not been very satisfactory. Generally, collapse of the ventricular system, especially on the operative side, is ignored. Since hydrocephalus has been controlled, either by decompression or secondary shunt, the hemisphere, after a period of time, appears to assume a more normal configuration and position. Occasionally, difficulty has been encountered due to subdural hygromas. The closure of the craniotomy is routine.

If a shunt is to be employed because of residual tumor or persistent obstruction of the ventricular system, the ventricular end of the shunt tubing may be placed, at the primary operative procedure, into the appropriate lateral ventricle. If the obstruction remains in the region of the foramen of Monro, an opening is made through the septum pellucidum so that shunting one ventricle will decompress both. This maneuver insures that both lateral ventricles will be decompressed and that the tubing will be accurately located within the ventricular system. The shunt tubing is then brought out through the opening in the corpus callosum through the interhemispheric fissure and extended subcutaneously, exiting through a stab wound in the posterior scalp region. Subsequently, it may be connected into a shunt system by removing some of the subcutaneous portion and attaching it to appropriate distal tubing.

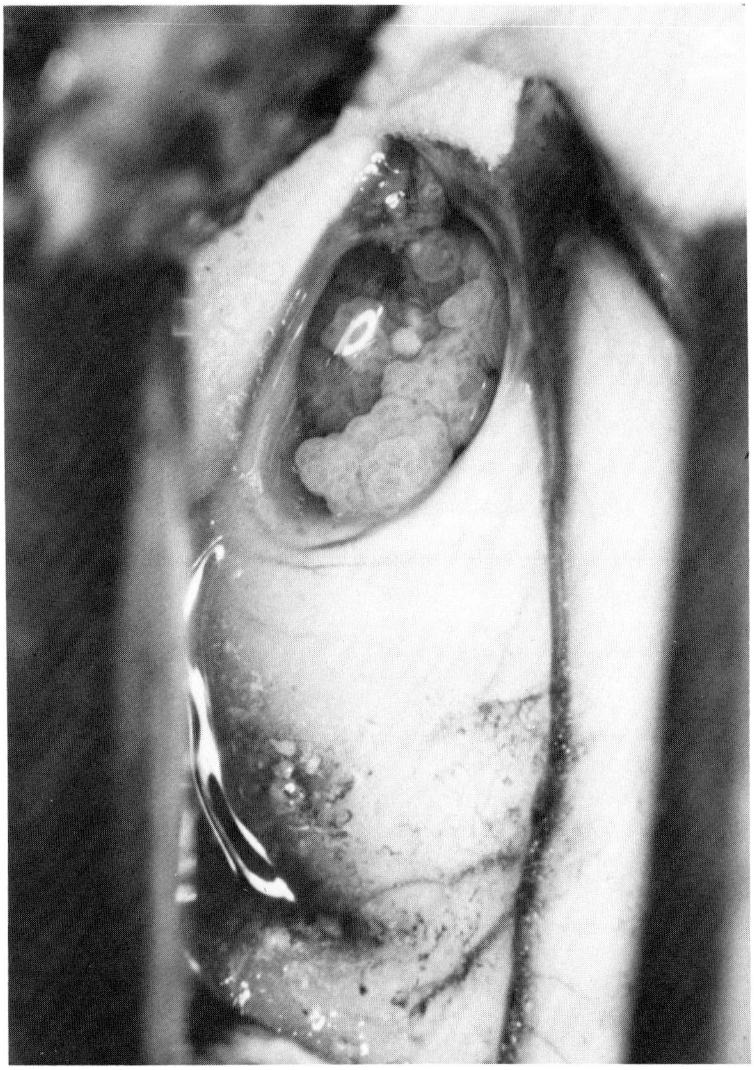

Fig. 18-7. Magnified view of foramen Monro with papillary appearance of a craniopharyngioma within the third ventricle.

Summary

In this personal series 15 transcallosal approaches have been used for lesions within the third ventricle, both in children and in adults (Table 18-1). The vast majority of tumors were infiltrating astrocytomas, presumably of the thalamic region, which are noncystic. Therefore the tumor usually could not be radically removed. In 6 of the 15 cases, however, benign pathology, including craniopharyngioma, colloid cyst, and a cystic teratomatous tumor of the third ventricle were encountered and could be largely or totally removed. In cases in which only a biopsy or subtotal resection was done, important data as to tumor type helped to plan subsequent therapy. There was no mortality nor significant morbidity in this series. The procedure is, therefore, deemed safe and in the author's opinion, allows the best visualization of the third ventricle for lesions that arise primarily within that region and extend to the level of the foramen of Monro, no matter what their nature.

Table 18-1. Transcallosal Approach

Case	Pathology	Technique
1	Astrocytoma	BX and RT
2	Astrocytoma	BX and RT
3	Astrocytoma	BX and RT
4	Astrocytoma	BX and RT
5	Astrocytoma	BX and RT
6	Astrocytoma	BX and RT
7	Astrocytoma	BX and RT
8	Glioblastoma	BX and RT
9	Glioblastoma	BX and RT
10	Craniopharyngioma	Resection
11	Craniopharyngioma	Resection and RT
12	Colloid cyst	Resection
13	Lipoma	Resection
14	Cystic atypical teratoma	Resection and RT
15	Organizing hematoma	Removal

BX = Biopsy
RT = Radiation therapy

REFERENCES

1. Matson DD: *Neurosurgery of Infancy and Childhood.* Charles C Thomas, Springfield, 1969
2. Van den Bergh R, Brucher JM: L'abord transventriculaire dans les cranio-pharyngiomes du troisieme ventricle. Aspects neuro-chirurgicaux et neuro-pathologiques. *Neurochirurgie 16*:51-65, 1970
3. Buchsbaum HW, Colton RP: Anterior third ventricular ventricular cysts in infancy. Case report. *J Neurosurg 26*:264-266, 1925
4. Cassinari V, Bernasconi V: Tumori della parte anteriore del terzo ventricolo. *Acta Neurochir 11*:236-271, 1963
5. Lakke JPWF: Report on 16 intraventricular brain tumors: A clinical study. *Eur Neurol 2*:158-174, 1969
6. Pecker J, Ferrand B, Javalet A: Tumeurs du troisieme ventricule. *Neurochirurgie 12*:7-136, 1966
7. Dandy WE: *Benign Tumors in the Third Ventricle of the Brain: Diagnosis and Treatment.* Charles C Thomas, Springfield, 1933

CHAPTER 19

Supracerebellar Approach for Pineal Region Neoplasms

Bennett M. Stein

Introduction

INCLUDED FOR DISCUSSION IN this chapter are the tumors arising from the pineal gland and from the environs of the pineal region that may involve primarily the posterior third ventricle and the quadrigeminal region. These tumors lie in the central-most portion of the brain and are difficult to expose because of their distance from various cranial points used in the initial opening. The fact that they often involve the deep venous system of the brain adds to the hazard of the operation. In most instances, however, the veins tend to be displaced dorsally and either lie over the dorsal surface of the tumor or within its dorsal portion. The arteries close to or involved in the tumor are generally of small caliber and insignificant in nature. These include the posterior choroidal arteries, branches of the quadrigeminal arteries, and the posterior cerebral arteries.

Although the number of patients who have tumors in this region is relatively small, the fact that the tumors represent a wide variation in histology and have been a challenge to expose surgically has led to a comparatively voluminous literature on these particular tumors. Cushing[1] indicated the difficulty with surgical treatment of pineal tumors by stating "personally, I have never succeeded in exposing a pineal tumor sufficiently well to justify an attempt to remove it." Others[2,3] also emphasized the high mortality following operation on pineal tumors. However, Dandy[4] despite the high operative mortality, continued to advocate surgical exposure and removal of these tumors. More recently, Suzuki[5] reported a large series of pineal tumors in which total or near total removals were effected without overwhelming morbidity or mortality.

The well-recognized fact that a wide variety of tumors may occur in this region and that approximately 25% of them are encapsulated and benign, lends further justification to the surgical approach to tumors of this region with an attempt to remove those that are encapsulated and can be dissected free of surrounding brain tissue. With more invasive tumors, exact histologic identification results in enlightened therapeutic management, since the atypical teratomatous type has a tendency to spread widely throughout the central nervous system. In such instances radiation of the entire neuraxis may be justifiable. On the other hand astrocytomas and ependymomas tend to invade locally and may best be treated by high-dose local radiation and supplemental chemotherapy.

Department of Neurosurgery, Tufts-New England Medical Center, Boston, Massachusetts 02111

Classic Surgical Techniques

Dandy was a master at approaching deep-seated brain tumors and was particularly interested in pineal region tumors. He advocated an interhemispheral approach with section of the posterior portion of the corpus callosum to gain access to the pineal region. This required sacrificing a number of parietal cortical veins and retracting a large portion of the parietal hemisphere, usually the right. In the region of the pineal difficulties were encountered in dissecting through or around the deep venous system, and many of the fatalities appeared to arise from uncontrolled deep vein thrombosis and edema of the diencephalic region. VanWagenen[6] advocated an approach through the right lateral ventricle, which is almost always dilated when tumors compromise or obstruct the aqueductal region. Exposure of the tumor still involved dissection of the deep venous system, since the approach was primarily dorsal to the tumor. In addition it had the disadvantage of a transcortical incision and possible hemispheral collapse when the ventricle was opened. Poppen[7] advocated an approach under the occipital lobe, in which bridging veins were sacrified, a large portion of the hemisphere retracted, and the free edge of the tentorium sectioned to expose the deep venous plexus in a more favorable attitude relative to the underlying tumor. Krause,[8] in 1926, reported 3 cases, each a different variety of tumor in the pineal or quadrigeminal region, which he approached through the posterior fossa, over the cerebellar hemispheres, and under the tentorium. The advantages of this approach are (a) it avoids injury to the deep venous system and (b) the tumor is approached directly. This approach to the tumor appeared to be very reasonable and certainly afforded an exposure similar to that of the supratentorial approaches.[9]

Diagnosis

Clinical Features

The classic symptomatology of Parinaud's syndrome is not always encountered in cases of pineal tumor or, at best, variations of this syndrome may be encountered. More likely are signs of raised intracranial pressure and ataxia due to compromise of the aqueduct and compression of the superior cerebellar peduncle in the midbrain. Precocious puberty occurs in a select group of males and only in 10% of the patients. A similar incidence of diabetes insipidus is encountered. In the latter syndrome, it has been suggested that its presence indicates seeding of the tumor into the hypothalamic region.

Radiographic Findings

Air- or positive-contrast ventriculography outlines, to best advantage, the location of the tumor in the posterior third ventricular region and gives some indication as to its eccentricity, as opposed to a purely midline position. When air is secondarily instilled through the lumbar route, evaluation of the quadrigeminal cistern region and the aqueduct may also help to define the margins of the tumor.

Arteriography has been of less help in defining the exact location of the tumor. If the tumor is highly malignant and therefore hypervascular, the arteriogram may give some indication as to its true nature.

Of great value has been the identification of these tumors by computerized tomography (CT). This scan has not only precisely defined the limits of the tumor, its relationship to the third ventricle, midbrain, and quadrigeminal cisterns, but has also, in some instances, indicated cysts within the tumor. This procedure alone should suffice in diagnosing and planning the operative procedure on such tumors.

On the basis of clinical features and radiographic findings, especially the CT scan, selection of patients for operation can be considered. In most instances operative exposure of tumors of this region is advocated, since the exact pathology must await surgical verification. In certain instances however, when the tumor is eccentric (to one side or the other), we have selected the interhemispheric transcallosal approach, since it can be reached more effectively through one or the other lateral ventricles and generally lies more in relation to the pulvinar of the thalmus than it does to the pineal or posterior third ventricular region. In most cases however, the tumors are central and are best approached through the posterior fossa by the supracerebellar infratentorial technique. If there is evidence of seeding, which has not occurred in this series, then conservative management, with a shunt and radiotherapy, might be considered.

Operative Technique—Posterior Fossa Approach

If the patient has severe intracranial hypertension and marked hydrocephalus, the direct approach to the pineal tumor may be abetted by a preliminary extracranial shunt in order to gradually reduce ventricular size and compensate for the raised intracranial pressure. In most cases however, this is not necessary and a direct approach to the tumor is carried out with or without ventricular drainage during the operation and postoperative period. Unless the patient is under 2 years of age and suffering from a severe degree of hydrocephalus, the sitting position is preferred. The patient's head must be strongly flexed so that the best exposure of the tentorial notch can be achieved, with the greatest comfort to the operating surgeon. In addition to strong flexion of the neck, the patient is tilted somewhat forward, once positioned on the operating table, so that the surgeon actually works over the back of the patient into the posterior fossa. Care is taken to avoid or to recognize an air embolism, using a doppler probe, central venous catheter, and modest positive-pressure ventilation during the opening or when large venous sinuses are exposed.

A long, midline incision is used, extending from C2 high up into the occipital region so that the pericranium and muscle attachments can be elevated to either side without disrupting their continuity. This greatly facilitates closure, since all muscle attachment must be elevated. A wide craniectomy is generally performed, which must extend above the lateral sinuses and torcula in all instances (Fig. 19-1). In the initial series of cases the craniectomy was carried to the foramen magnum and the posterior arch of C1 was removed. In more recent cases we have been doing a limited craniectomy, which involves the superior region of the posterior fossa but does not extend to the foramen magnum. The craniotomy should be wide, laterally as well as superiorly. Adjuvants, such as urea or ventricular drainage, may be used to reduce volume and to facilitate retraction of the cerebellar hemispheres. The opening of the dura is important, for it must be opened bilaterally to the region of the lateral sinus. However these incisions should not be carried too far laterally, since in doing so one is unable to retract the flap of dura adequately in the region of the torcula (Fig. 19-2). Once this is accomplished, the tentorium can be elevated with a self-retaining retractor. The weight of cottonoids or a copper retractor is sufficient to depress the cerebellum (Fig. 19-5).

Gravity helps in this latter maneuver. The operating microscope with a 250- or 275-mm objective has been utilized in all instances. If a greater focal distance is used, the operator is too far from the incisura region and, even with an armrest, finds the position extremely fatiguing. Therefore, the microscope and operator must be relatively close to the field. Some type of armrest is recommended. In addition long instruments will be required because of the distance to the pineal region and beyond; many of these tumors extend well into the third ventricle, some to the region of the foramen of Monro. All bridging veins over the dorsal surface of the cerebellum, including the hemispheres and vermis, may be sacrificed in order

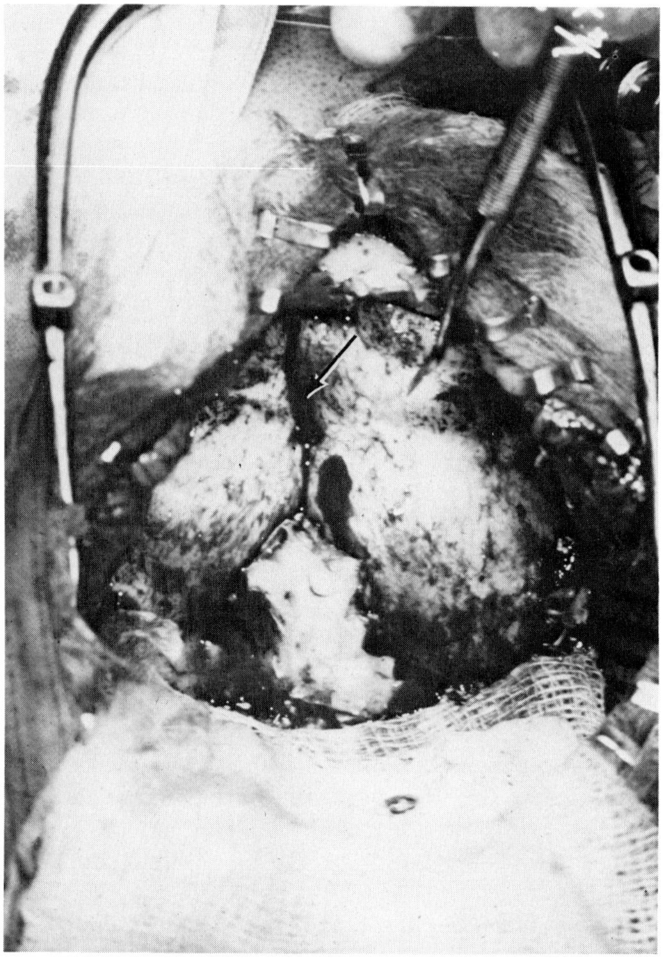

Fig. 19-1. Large suboccipital craniectomy. Arrow and instrument indicate torcula and lateral sinus.

to open the quadrigeminal region and the incisura (Fig. 19-3). The arachnoid, in this region, is almost always thickened and opaque in the presence of tumors, and must be opened by microdissection techniques to expose the surface of the tumor. The great vein of Galen and the internal cerebral veins are generally well above the tumor and are not encountered in these initial maneuvers (Fig. 19-4). Laterally, the medial aspect of the temporal lobe and the veins of Rosenthal may be seen as they course upward toward the confluence of veins in this region. The tumor capsule is then cauterized and opened by sharp dissection. The tumor, depending on its consistency, is removed with tumor forceps, a small loop, suction, and cautery. In general terms, the trajectory of the operation is toward the velum interpositum (Fig. 19-5). This must be considered when attempts are made to remove portions of the tumor in the inferior portion of the third ventricle or directly over the quadrigeminal plate in relation to the anterior lobe of the cerebellum. This is the most difficult aspect to be dealt with; small dental mirrors and angled instruments may be required to effect removal of tumor in this region. The lateral extent of the tumor can be pursued through this particular exposure.

Even with nonresectable tumors, benefit may be accrued through internal decompres-

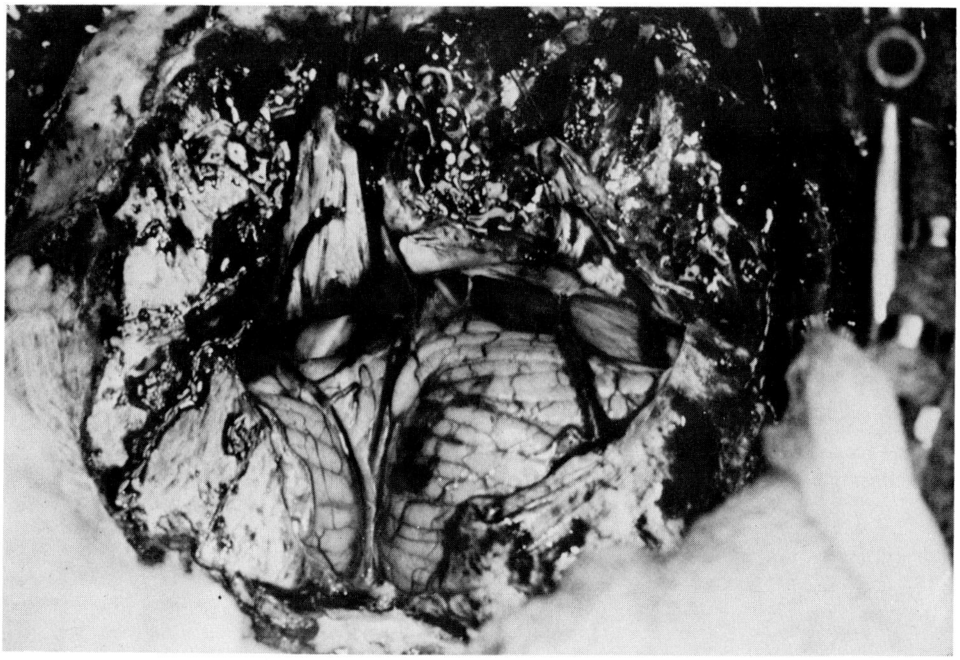

Fig. 19-2. Dural opening. Cerebellum "hangs" on dorsal veins.

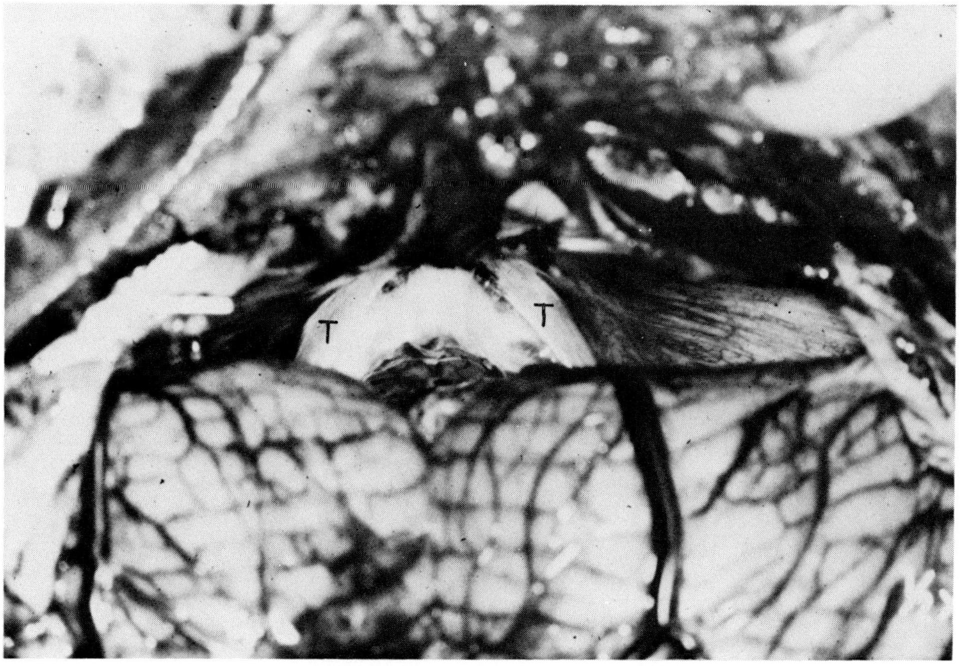

Fig. 19-3. Tentorial incisural exposure. Free edges of tentorium (T).

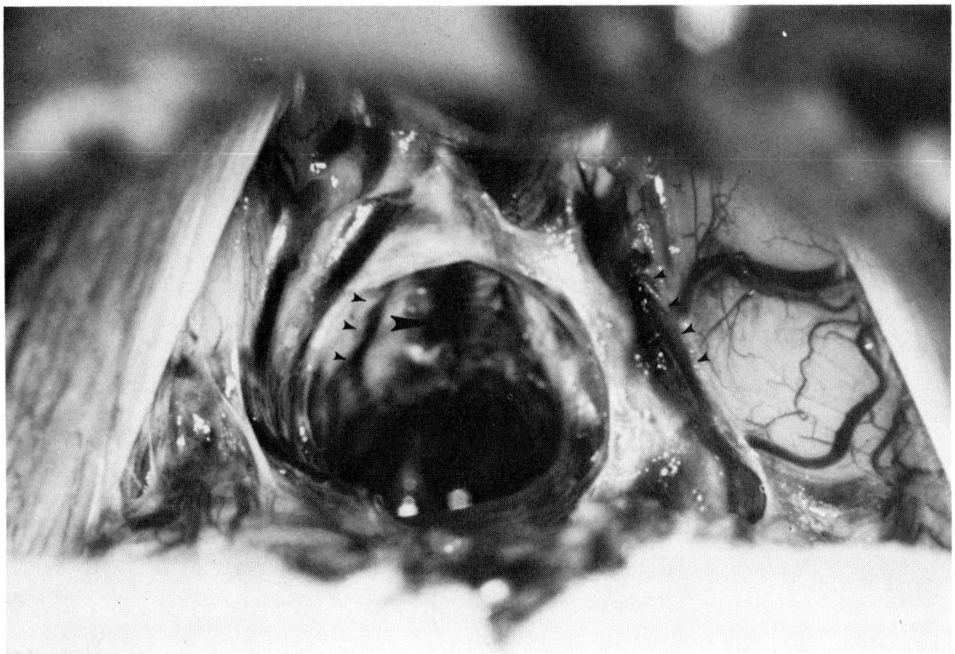

Fig. 19-4. Pineal tumor partially removed revealing veins of Rosenthal (small arrows) and internal cerebral veins (large arrow).

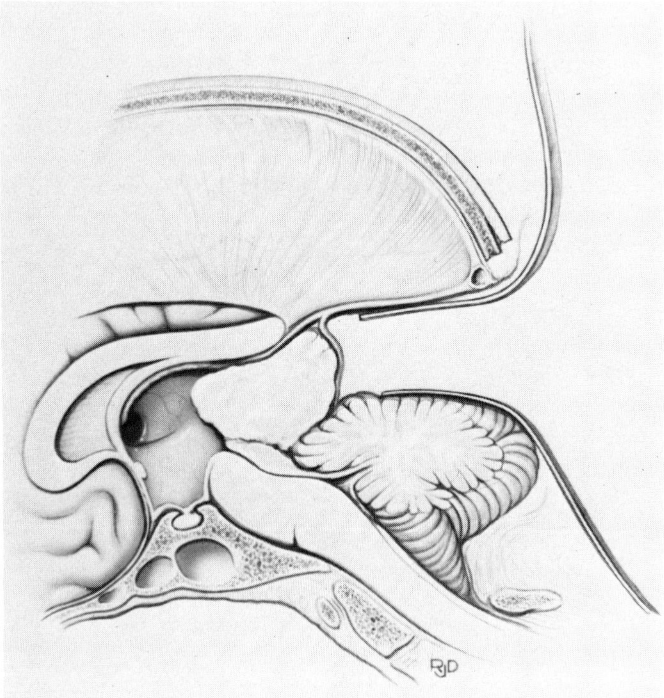

Fig. 19-5. Drawing of exposure.

sion of or an opening through the tumor adequate to expose the posterior third ventricle. This will allow placement of an internal shunt tube from directly within the third ventricle, through the interior of the tumor, and over the cerebellar hemisphere to the region of the cisterna magna. Even in instances in which this tubing occludes, a passageway has been established for cerebrospinal fluid. If the tumor cannot be removed completely or an internal shunt placed, ventricular drainage with subsequent conversion to a shunt may be necessary in the postoperative period.

The dura has generally been left open, but with the smaller openings into the posterior fossa and significant decompression or removal of tumor, the dura may be closed. It would appear that this makes the postoperative course smoother and may limit the degree of posterior fossa postoperative aseptic meningitis.

Summary

To date 17 cases of pineal region tumors have been operated on. These are reviewed in Table 19-1.

It is felt that benefit and useful information was gained in all cases by removing encapsulated or well-defined tumors, and by histologic confirmation in other invasive or nonresectable tumors. In two tumors with large cysts, atypical teratomas were a surprise finding. These tumors are not generally cystic and accordingly, the preoperative diagnosis in these cases was cystic astrocytoma. The difference in longevity of these two types of tumors is obvious and bears upon subsequent therapy. Unfortunately, experience with atypical teratoma tumors has not been favorable in this series; it would appear that radiation has little more than a temporary effect. Approximately 25% of the cases were amenable to total or near total resection, and therefore, would fall into the category of encapsulated, benign tumors.

The operation is generally safe; only 1 death occurred and this was due to delayed hemorrhage in a glioblastoma, 1 week after the primary operative procedure. There has been no significant morbidity in the remaining cases.

Exposure of all tumors in the pineal region is strongly advocated, with confirmation of the histology; removal, if feasible; and, if not, internal decompression or the establishment of an internal shunt from the third ventricle to the cisterna magna third ventricular region.

Table 19-1. Pineal Tumors

No.	Case	Age (yr.)	Diagnosis	Prior treatment	Results
1.	JC	8	Teratoma	——	Normal
2.	MR	24	Cystic astrocytoma	RT	Late death
3.	CG	8 mo	Arachnoid cyst	——	Normal
4.	KL	12	Epidermoid	——	Normal
5.	MS	9	Teratoma	RT	Unchanged
6.	RD	4	Teratoma	——	Improved
7.	RM	5	Atypical teratoma	——	Late death
8.	SA	25	Astrocytoma	——	Improved
9.	EM	10	Astrocytoma	RT	Improved
10.	MD	8	Glioblastoma	——	Died
11.	AO	12	Atypical teratoma	——	Improved
12.	JC	37	Astrocytoma	——	Unchanged
13.	LB	35	Astrocytoma	RT	Unchanged
14.	WJ	16	Atypical teratoma	——	Improved
15.	JP	43	Atypical teratoma	RT	Improved
16.	TA	18	Atypical teratoma	——	Improved
17.	TM	22	Colloid cyst	RT	Unchanged

RT = Radiation therapy

REFERENCES

1. Cushing H: *Intracranial Tumors: Notes Upon a Series of Two-Thousand Verified Cases with Surgical-Mortality pertaining thereto.* Charles C Thomas, Springfield, Ill, 1932, p 64
2. Cummins FM, Taveras JM, Schlesinger EB: Treatment of gliomas of the third ventricle and pinealomas: with special reference to the value of radiotherapy. *Neurology 10*:1031-1036, 1960
3. Horrax G, Daniels JT: The conservative treatment of pineal tumors. *Surg Clin North Am 22*:649-652, 1942
4. Dandy WE: Operative experience in cases of pineal tumors. *Surg Gynecol Obstet 33*:113-119, 1921
5. Suzuki J, Iwabuchi T: Surgical removal of pineal tumors (pinealomas and teratomas): experience in a series of 19 cases. *J Neurosurg 23*:565-571, 1965
6. Van Wagenen WP: A surgical approach for the removal of certain pineal tumors: report of a case. *Surg Gynecol Obstet 53*:216-220, 1931
7. Poppen JL: The right occipital approach to a pinealoma. *J Neurosurg 25*:706-710, 1966
8. Krause F: Operative freilegung der vierhugel, mebst Beobachtungen uber hirndruck and dekompression. *Zbl Chir 53*:2812-2819, 1926
9. Stein BM: The infratentorial supracerebellar approach to pineal lesions. *J Neurosurg 35*:197-202, 1971

CHAPTER 20

Occult Spinal Dysraphic States

Paul H. Chapman

THE TERM SPINA BIFIDA is generally understood to connote a wide variety of congenital pathologic conditions of the spine. Such pathologically dissimilar entities as myelomeningocele, dermoid sinus with or without tumor, spinal lipoma, tethered filum terminale, and diastematomyelia have been variously included under the heading of spina bifida.[1] The common denominator is as implied a congenital defect in the posterior elements of one or more vertebral segments. Such a grouping on the basis of a single pathologic feature has, however, led to some confusion regarding the relationship between these various conditions with regard to clinical presentation, course, and treatment. The major difficulty results from a juxtaposition of myelomeningocele (or meningocele, spina bifida cystica, spina bifida aperta, myeloschisis, etc.) with so-called *spina bifida occulta* and its associated conditions. Myelomeningocele, with its attendant problems, is a common and widely recognized entity. In such cases there is characteristically a dorsal protrusion of more or less severely malformed spinal cord elements and their coverings between the bifid bony elements to present on the surface of the back. Neurologic deficits in the lower extremities are often severe, with associated loss of bladder or bowel control. These deficits are present at birth and are usually unchanging. The Arnold-Chiari malformation of cerebellum and brain stem is usually present, as are lesser deformities of the forebrain. Progressive hydrocephalus is not unusual.

There is, on the other hand, a group of congenital lesions of the spinal canal and its overlying tissues, more common in its caudal portion, which involves the spinal cord to produce progressive neurologic deficits, usually in early life. Because spinal bifida is associated with these lesions, they are often discussed under the designation spina bifida occulta. Use of the term *spinal dysraphism,* to designate them as a group, has also been increasing.[2-5] Pathologically, these lesions are not associated with Arnold-Chiari malformation, hydrocephalus, or other cerebral anomaly. Also, the degree of spinal cord dysplasia is relatively minor compared with that found in the typical case of myelomeningocele. Likewise, the dysplasia of overlying tissues, in particular skin, is usually of a minor sort, although extremely valuable in suggesting the presence of underlying difficulty. This entity typically causes progressive neurologic deterioration, whether of bladder, bowel, or lower extremity sensorimotor function. Initially the deficits are often minor and may or may not occur in the context of preexisting fixed deformities of the lower extremities, such as talipes or unequal size of feet or legs. Finally, approximately two-thirds of the patients are female, whereas in the case of myelomeningocele there is no clear sex predilection.

Neurosurgical Service, Massachusetts General Hospital, and the Harvard Medical School, Boston, Massachusetts 02114

Pathology

The intraspinal pathology of spinal dysraphism is quite diverse. However, certain common features underly this diversity. In most cases, the congenital abnormality, whatever it might be, exerts an immobilizing influence on the spinal cord, usually at its distal extremity. Occasionally, expanding lesions, such as intraspinal dermoids or lipomas, produce neurologic symptomatology by direct compresssion of adjacent spinal cord or nerve roots. Even in these cases, however, the presence of an ancillary immobilizing influence must be considered. In conjunction with this immobilization, the conus medullaris is found to lie at an abnormally low level within the spinal canal. This is demonstrable either at operation or by myelography and constitutes an important feature in diagnosis. During fetal development, there is gradual relative ascent of the conus within the spinal canal due to the disparate rate of longitudinal growth of the spinal cord and spine.[6,7] At 17 weeks' gestation, the spinal cord ends opposite the L4 vertebral level. At term, the mean level of termination is at the lower border of L2. Several months postnatally it has reached the level of the L1-2 interspace. There is no further ascent. As a general rule, therefore, if the conus terminates at the level of L3 or below after 5 to 6 months of age, it can be considered abnormally low lying.

In spinal dysraphism, the conus is not only low lying but also tends to be situated posteriorly within the spinal canal (Fig. 20-6). With caudal fixation of the conus, the lumbosacral lordosis tends to bring it into a posterior position. Another factor may be actual fixation of the conus to the posterior dura by a thickened filum, lipomatous mass, or fibrous bands, as will be discussed.

Aside from these general considerations, the spinal pathology usually assumes one of several forms. An understanding of the pathologic anatomy of these lesions is necessary for their proper recognition in surgical management. Intraspinal lipoma is a common pathologic entity (Fig. 20-1A). Emery and Lendon[8] have studied its various forms in detail. The lipomatous mass is usually situated in the caudal extremity of the spinal canal and is coextensive with conus medullaris. The connection with the conus may be a stalk-like fibrolipomatous structure. On the other hand, the lipoma may gradually merge with the conus in such a way that there is extensive intermingling of fatty and neural tissues at a rather indistinct interface. This obviously can cause some difficulty when attempting surgical removal of the lipoma and generally precludes its total excision. The caudal portion of the fatty mass may be fixed at the end of the spinal canal, being entirely intraspinal, or it may extend through a dural defect posteriorly and present as a subcutaneous mass.

A simpler type of abnormality is the short, thickened filum terminale (Fig. 20-2A). The filum terminale is normally a threadlike structure. It represents a nonneural continuation of the conus medullaris. The filum inserts at the distal end of the dural sac and generally contains a microscopic continuation of the central canal of the spinal cord. In its abnormal state the filum is thickened to a diameter of 3 to 5 mm. It is shorter than normal by virtue of the low position of the conus and lies posteriorly within the dural sac, often in contact with the posterior dura. A lipoma in continuity may be present, particularly at the point of distal insertion of the filum. The thickened filum may insert posteriorly in the dura, proximal to the termination of the dural sac. Microscopically the abnormal filum is collagenous, with a centrally placed core of ependymal cells representing the remnant of the central canal. There may be small islands of fatty tissue within the collagenous substrate.

Fibrous bands may occasionally be found. These arise from the inferiorly placed conus and insert on the dura posteriorly, laterally, or, occasionally, anteriorly. Such bands may continue through the dura to end in relation to overlying bony elements or within subcutaneous tissue. At times, these have the appearance of aberrant nerve roots, although stimulation reveals no motor function.

Diastematomyelia is a common form of spinal dysraphism. The pathology consists of a bony or fibrocartilaginous spur that traverses the spinal canal in an anteroposterior direction

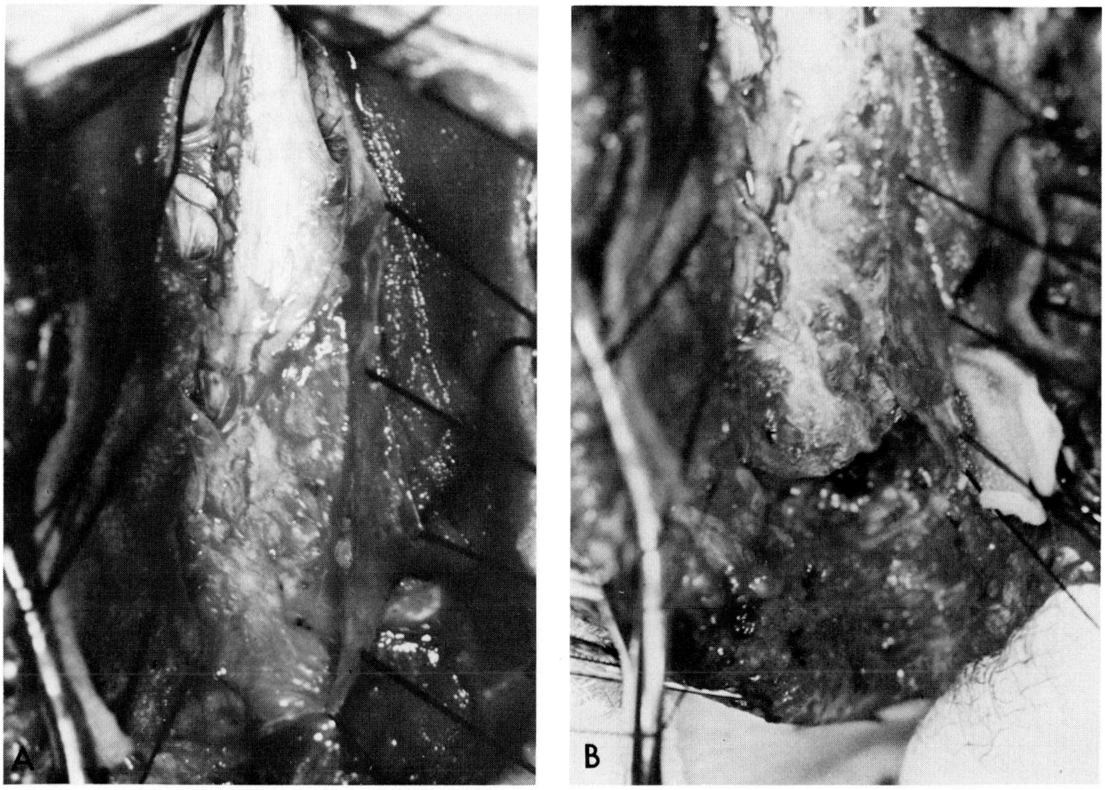

Fig. 20-1 **A.** Intradural lipoma confluent with the conus medullaris. Note the horizontal direction of exiting nerve roots. **B.** Closer view of the lipoma shown in Figure 20-1A following subtotal resection. Operation resulted in improved bladder function.

in the midline. It is attached anteriorly to the vertebral body and posteriorly to the arch of bone constituting the back of the spinal canal. The spur may incompletely span the canal, in which case it might be based either anteriorly or posteriorly. Abnormalities such as small or hemivertebrae, disc space narrowing, fusion of anterior or posterior elements, or transverse widening of the canal generally occur at that level. The spur characteristically divides the spinal canal in a midsagittal direction, thus effectively skewering the divided cord, the halves of which rejoin above and below the spur. The spur may occur at any point along the thoraco-lumbar spine but is most common in the lower thoracic or upper lumbar area.

Dermal sinus, with or without a related intraspinal dermoid tumor, is found in association with occult spina bifida. The tumor is often situated partially within the substance of the spinal cord, particularly in the region of the conus. In such cases, it cannot be totally extirpated. Microscopically, these tumors consist of dermal elements, including appendages such as hair follicles, with hair and sweat, and apocrine glands. Occasionally epidermoid tumors occur as well.

Although these various lesions have been described as discrete entities, the pathology is often more complex than such a description would indicate. There is a tendency for more than one type of lesion to occur in a single case (Fig. 20-3). Thus, one occasionally finds a short thick filum, fibrous bands, or intraspinal lipoma in the context of diastematomyelia. Alternately lipoma, tethering bands, and a thickened filum may occur in varying combinations. Finally, the lesions encountered are not strictly limited to those just described. Lesions such as occult meningocele and hydromyelia have also been observed either singly or in

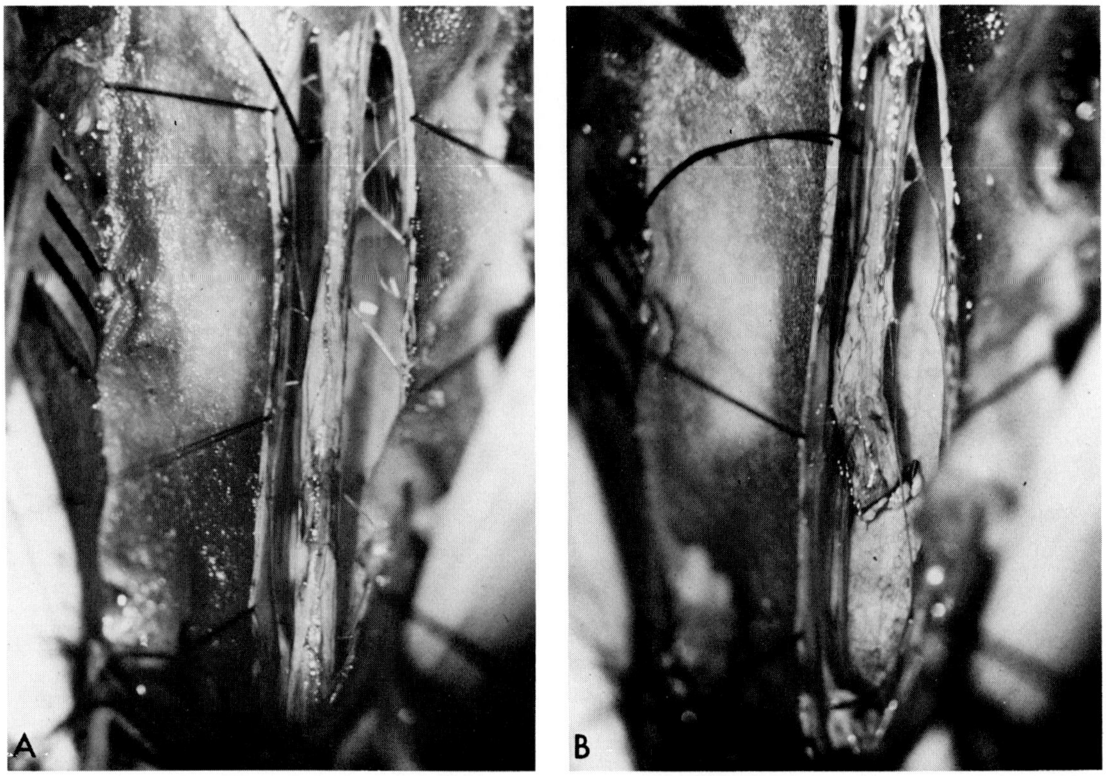

Fig. 20-2 A. Thick filum terminale with low conus medullaris (top). **20-2 B.** Filum shown in Figure 20-2A following division. Note the distance between the divided ends of the filum and the more vertical direction of the nerve roots, indicating upward migration of the conus and proximal filum after division of the filum.

combination with the more common lesions. Despite the occasional lesion associated with Arnold-Chiari malformation, this hindbrain deformity has not generally been found in cases of spinal dysraphism, where it has been specifically sought.[9]

The mechanism by which these diverse pathologic conditions produce neurologic impairment is unclear. Except when a mass lesion or fibrous bands exert obvious pressure on neural elements, the common denominator appears to be the immobilizing effect of the lesion on the distal spinal cord and, possibly, nerve roots (Fig. 20-2B). It has been suggested that this prevents normal ascent with growth of the spinal cord in the canal, and that the traction thus exerted results in progressive neurologic deficits. Since there is no appreciable ascent of the spinal cord after several months of age, this does not provide a good explanation for disabilities appearing beyond that age, as so often occurs. Such an explanation might be invoked, on the other hand, to explain deficits and deformities present at the time of birth. The normal degree of mobility of distal spinal cord elements in response to changes in position is unclear. Some mobility can be demonstrated at myelography, although this alone has not provided a clear differentiation between normal and pathologic conditions. It is possible that immobilization of neural elements prevents normal protective accommodative movements in response to changes in position during activity. The possibility of vascular insult, as a result of cord immobility, has also been considered.[10]

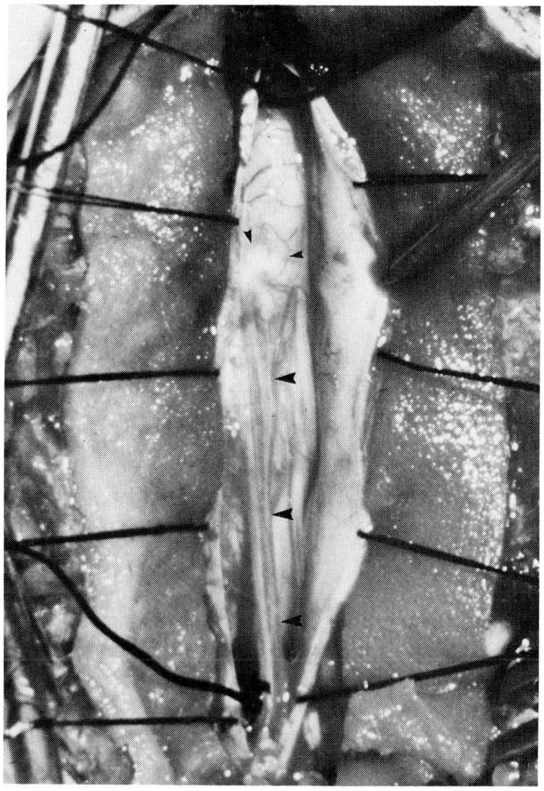

Fig. 20-3. Fibrous bands (large arrows, lower) attaching to conus posteriorly in the region of an associated small intramedullary dermoid tumor (small arrows, upper). No sinus tract was demonstrated pathologically.

Spine Abnormalities

The presence of spina bifida occulta is, as the name implies, an important feature in the diagnosis of this condition. Some confusion may arise in that a substantial proportion of the normal population harbors an occult spina bifida without intraspinal pathology. When spina bifida is a normal variant, the split element is generally at S1 and occasionally at L5. The degree of bifida has its highest incidence in early life and is more common in males. Its incidence appears to vary with different racial groups.[14] In symptomatic spina bifida occulta associated with spinal dysraphism, spinal segments other than L5 and S1 are usually involved, often multiply, and the degree of diastasis is more pronounced. Although spina bifida may be the only demonstrable bony abnormality, other defects do occur. Examples of these were enumerated briefly in the discussion of diastematomyelia. Although there is a general geographic relationship between the site of bony abnormality and the underlying intraspinal lesion, this is not exact. The two lesions may be separated by several segmental levels. This fact assumes importance in properly recognizing the site of intraspinal pathology at surgical exploration. It also emphasizes the need for careful preoperative myelographic evaluation.

Skin Abnormality

Cutaneous stigmata are often, though not invariably, present and may provide a valuable clue to the problem. These abnormalities usually occur in the mid or lower back in the midline and, like the bony deformity, may not correspond to the segmental level of the intraspinal lesion (Fig. 20-7). The nature of the skin lesion varies. It may consist of a circumscribed area of hyperpigmentation or capillary hemangioma. The latter is quite common as a normal variant over the inferior occipital area and is of no concern there. If such a lesion is found in the midline thoracic or lumbar region, unseen difficulties should be anticipated. There may be a hairy patch of skin, either with or without associated abnormal skin pigmentation. Hair growth can be extremely luxuriant, constituting what is aptly called a *fawn's tail*. A subcutaneous lipoma may be present. As indicated previously, such fatty masses are often coextensive with intraspinal lipomas.

A midline skin pore is common in association with intraspinal dermoid tumors. It represents the opening of a sinus tract that extends inward to attach to the tumor. This tract is directed rostrally so that the skin pore lies caudal to the level of the tumor. It is important to distinguish between a true dermal sinus pore and a simple pilonidal or postanal dimple. The latter, which lies more inferiorly, usually at the tip of the coccyx, is of no consequence in the present context.

Clinical Presentation

About two-thirds of patients with spinal dysraphism are females. Although symptoms may arise at any age, most occur initially in the pediatric group. In most cases the presenting problem reflects neurologic impairment of the lower extremities or of bladder function. Gait disturbance is most common and may represent simple weakness or postural deformity of one or both lower extremities, particularly distally. Equinus deformities are common. In addition there may be shortening of the involved foot or leg and/or wasting of the extremity. Orthopedic deformities are present at birth in some instances. Further neurologic impairment may then be superimposed on this preexisting disability. In this context it may be difficult to detect progressive functional impairment early, especially in younger children. The problem might manifest itself only as repeated failure of orthopedic corrections, for instance. A significant percentage of patients present initially with urinary incontinence, which can be minor or severe. This problem may only become apparent when the child is well past the usual age of training, despite its presence from infancy. Finally, a number of cases come to medical attention because parents are concerned about the skin lesion, particularly subcutaneous lipomata or hairy patches.

Although the foregoing covers the principal modes of presentation, occasionally other problems prompt initial concern. Impaired sensation in the lower extremities can result in trophic ulceration of the involved part. Septic meningitis, especially recurrent or due to an unusual organism, should elicit careful examination for the presence of a dermal sinus tract. Back pain, although uncommon, may be the chief concern. This pain is characteristically exacerbated by movement or exercise and the child limits his activity, even though he may not complain specifically about it.

Diagnostic Assessment and Indications for Surgery

The initial assessment of these children requires a careful history and examination designed to detect what might be minor degrees of neurologic impairment. In any suspected case plain x-rays of the spine should be obtained to corroborate the diagnosis. In any patient with documented neurologic deterioration, the next step should be myelography preparatory to surgery. Also, any case of dermal sinus, regardless of neurologic status, should be handled similarly. In the latter instance the high incidence of associated intraspinal tumor or potential communication with the subarachnoid space, with attendent risk of meningitis, demands surgical intervention. An element of controversy arises regarding the proper management of patients with clinical and radiologic stigmata of spinal dysraphism but without evidence of deterioration or neurologic deficit. In spinal lipoma delayed neurologic deterioration is well documented, both in childhood[15-17] and in adult[18] life. Because of such cases the opinion has been expressed[3] that the presence of a lumbosacral lipoma per se is an indication for surgery in anticipation of future neurologic difficulty. This opinion is shared by Till,[4] who further feels that any child with clinical and radiologic stigmata of spinal dysraphism should undergo myelography, regardless of neurologic status. If the myelogram is abnormal, showing either a specific lesion or low conus, then surgical exploration is warranted. This view represents an extension of the concept of prophylactic surgery for all patients with spinal dysraphism. It is based on the observation that neurologic deficits that occur, even under close followup, cannot predictably be reversed by subsequent surgery. Implied is the fact that surgery, when properly executed, has a sufficiently low risk to warrant such action. Finally Till[19] has reviewed his own extensive experience with regard to the question of prophylactic surgery.

Myelography

Because of the diverse and often complex intraspinal pathology associated with spinal dysraphism, it is important to gain maximum information from myelography prior to surgical exploration. To do so requires a technique that clearly defines structures within the caudal spinal canal. Iophendylate (Pantopaque, Lafeyette Pharmaceutical, Inc.), introduced by the lumbar route, has frequently been used[10,20] but has several disadvantages. Because it is a dense contrast medium, structures, such as fibrous bands, tracts, or a thickened filum may be poorly visualized. The level of termination of the conus may not be apparent. The position of the conus is important. A low lying conus represents a more or less constant pathologic concomitant of spinal dysraphism and may be the only abnormality found on myelography. Puncturing the spinal canal in an area where displaced neural tissue may be situated logically presents the risk of injury to these structures (Fig. 20-4). Finally it may be difficult to enter the subarachnoid space, especially if a lipoma is present. Introducing the contrast by cisternal tap[9] presents problems with retrieving the substance.

An alternative is air myelography[4] (Figs. 20-5 through 20-8). The gas is introduced by cisternal or lateral cervical puncture, with the anesthetized patient positioned 20° head down. During the incremental introduction of air, enough spinal fluid is removed to give a final positive pressure of about 200 mm of water in the lower lumbar canal. This distends the lumbar subarachnoid space for better visualization. Tomographic views are taken in the lateral and anteroposterior supine projections. It may be useful to have the patient's lower spine moderately flexed when lateral views are taken. This brings the conus forward in the canal so that its posterior as well as its anterior profile can be seen. After the study, it is advisable to keep the patient in a head-down position for 24 hours, if the air is not removed. The usefulness of oxygen as opposed to air is limited by its rate of disappearance after introduction. Recently we have begun to replace the air with artificial cerebrospinal fluid at the end of the procedure. This is achieved by introducing a lumbar needle, once the pathologic anatomy has been defined. This technique, suggested by Thibaut,[21] has been quite useful in avoiding problems associated with residual air.

Finally a water-soluble contrast agent, such as metrizamide, may, in the future, prove superior to either immiscible positive contrast or gas myelography in studies of dysraphic states. At present, however, experience with the technique in this country is limited.

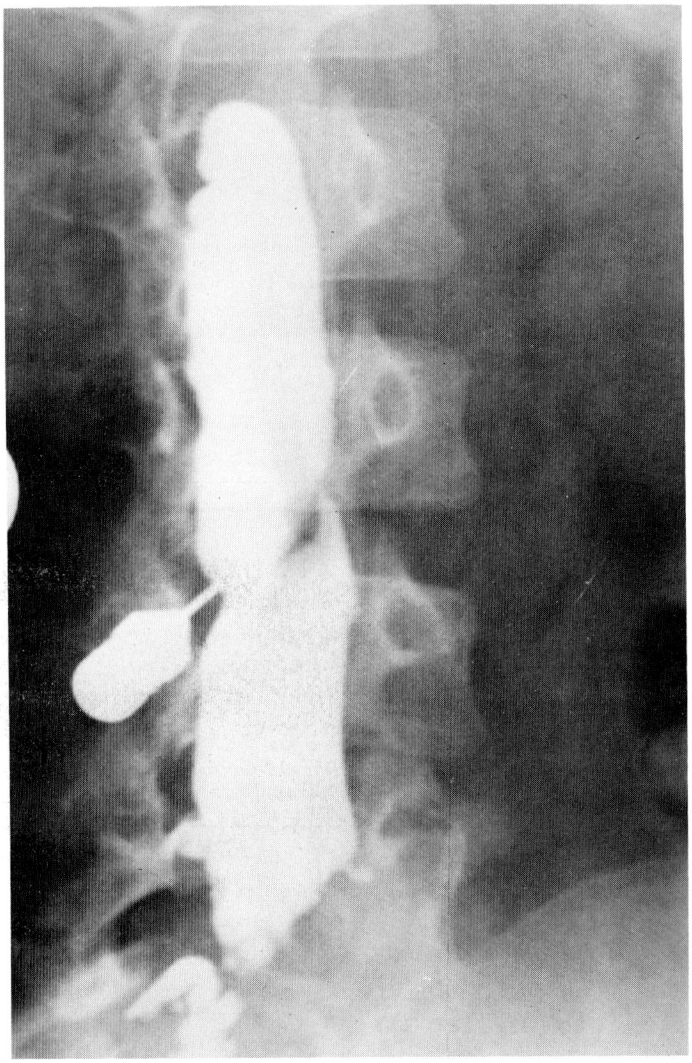

Fig. 20-4. Iophendylate myelogram. Contrast was introduced by L3-4 spinal puncture. The needle tip is shown impinging on an elongated spinal cord. No neurologic deficit resulted.

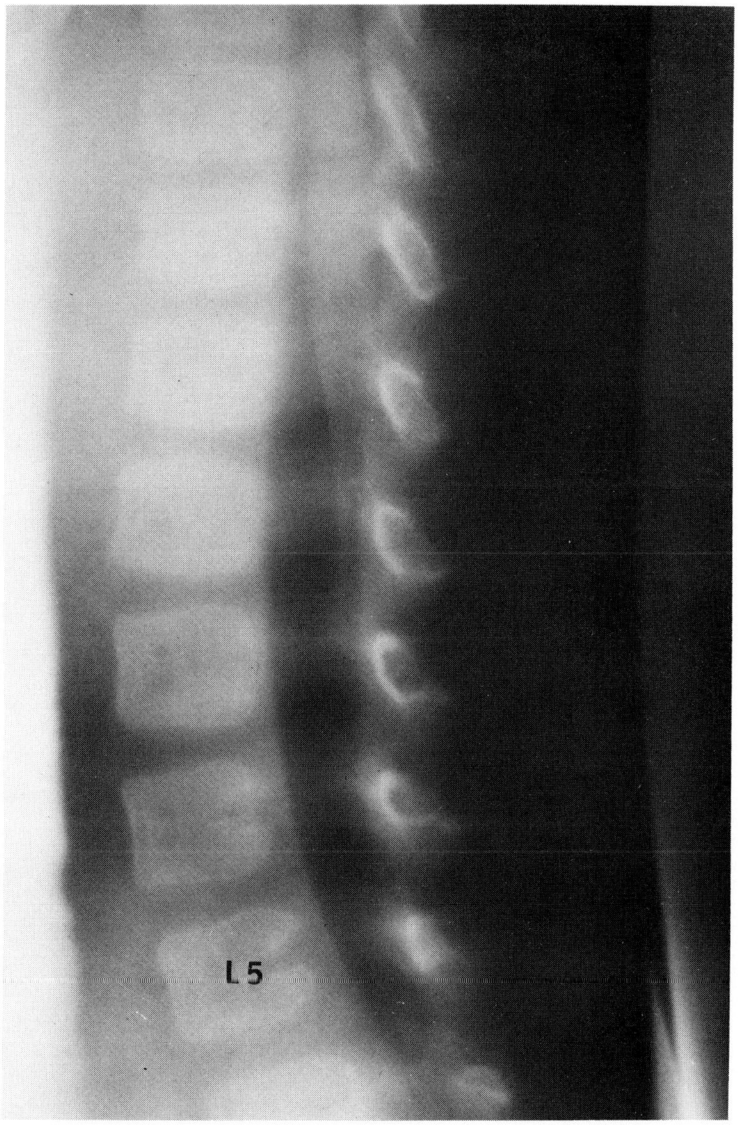

Fig. 20-5. Lumbar, air myelogram, lateral view, showing normal level of termination of the conus.

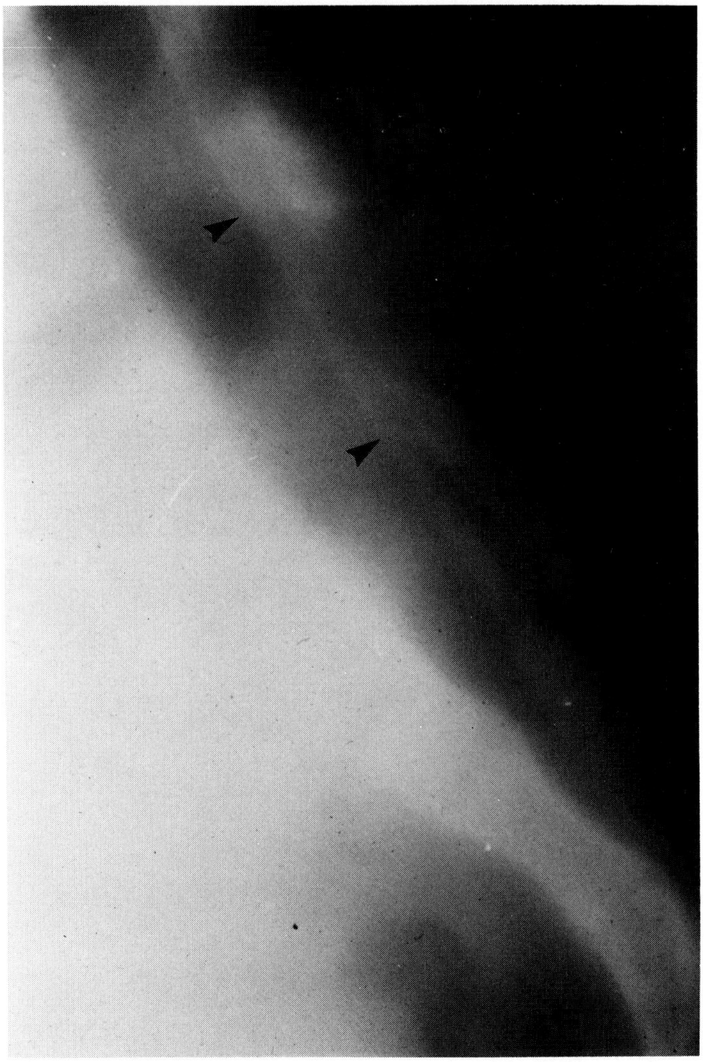

Fig. 20-6. Elongated, attenuated conus (arrows) terminating in a distal intraspinal lipoma. Note the posterior position of spinal cord within the spinal canal. Operative findings are shown in Figure 20-1.

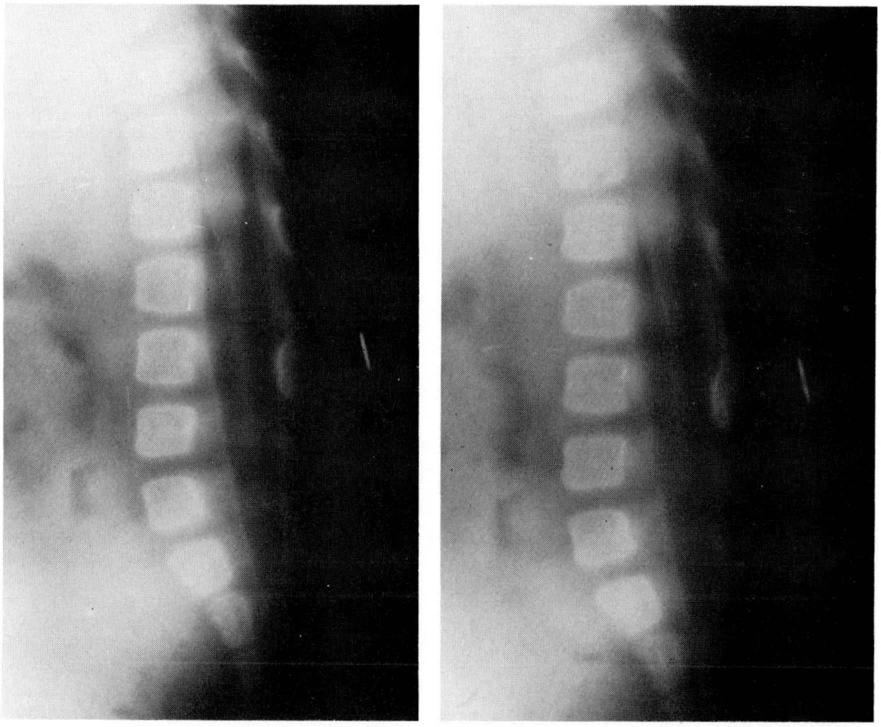

Fig. 20-7. Intramedullary dermoid tumor of the conus. The lead marker shows the site of the skin abnormality, a capillary hemangioma. Operative findings are shown in Figure 20-3.

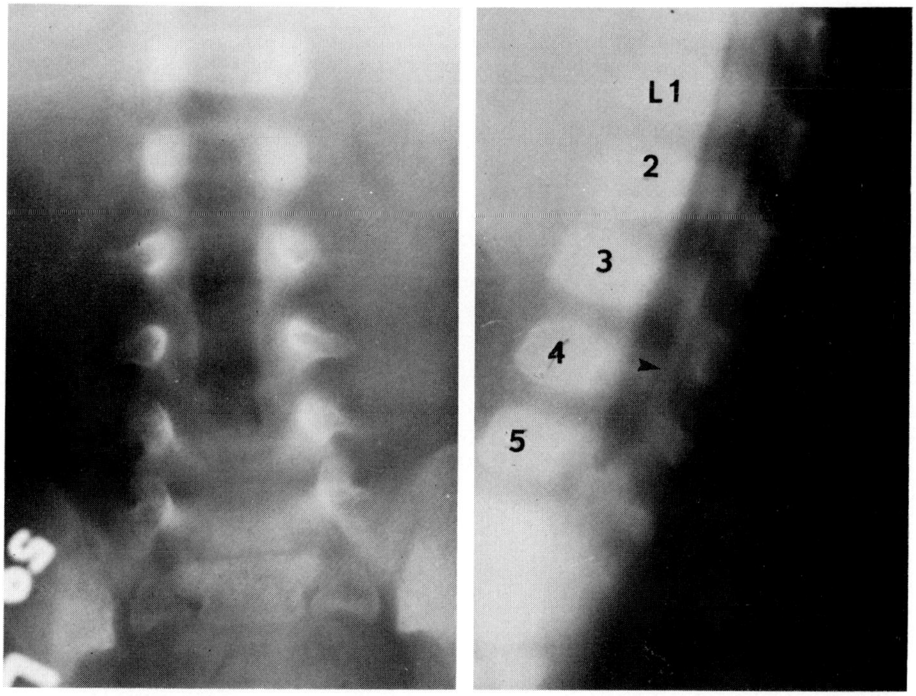

Fig. 20-8. Dermoid tumor of distal spinal canal. Note the associated low conus and thick filum (arrow) proximal to the tumor.

Surgery

Technique

Successful surgery of spinal dysraphism depends on detailed knowledge of the pathologic anatomy that will be encountered, especially when lesions are complex or multiple. This is predicated on gaining maximum information from preoperative myelography, as discussed. Diastematomyelia may be associated with a thick filum, which, if overlooked, can lead to further functional deterioration even though the bony spur has been successfully dealt with. The principle of surgery is usually to relieve the mechanical constraint the intraspinal lesion exerts on conus or nerve roots. This may involve merely dividing a thickened filum or tethering bands. In diastematomyelia the midline bony or fibrocartilagenous septum is excised. Intraspinal lipoma represents a special problem, since its interface with neural tissue is often complex and indistinct, and nerve roots of the cauda equina may traverse the substance of the lipoma (Fig. 20-1A). In these cases as much of the fatty mass is removed as is safely possible, leaving the remnant of tumor that mingles with nerve elements (Fig. 20-1B). If a fibrous stalk joins lipoma to conus, this stalk can be transected, taking care to leave more proximal neural tissues undisturbed. Again the purpose of surgery is to relieve the restraining influence the lipoma exerts on the distal spinal cord. Complete excision is rarely possible and is not necessary to achieve the desired result. Dermoid tumors, along with their associated dermal sinus tracts, should be excised in toto where possible in view of their propensity to recur. As in the case of lipomas however, they are often intimately associated with the conus (Fig. 20-3), making attempts at total excision inadvisable. In some instances it may be worthwhile to marsupialize a large tumor cavity to overlying dura to facilitate reexploration if the tumor recurs.

For more formidable lesions, microsurgical techniques are useful. These include bipolar coagulation. The nerve stimulator can help to identify motor nerve elements within a complex anomaly. Manometric monitoring of urinary bladder tone during stimulation, using an indwelling catheter, is a useful adjunct. Cerebrospinal fluid leak is the single most common complication of surgery. For this reason, careful attention should be given to achieving a watertight dural closure. Caudal dura is not infrequently deficient, particularly in association with lipomas. A fascial graft may therefore be necessary. Because it is difficult to obtain a truly watertight closure with synthetic dural substitutes, these should not be used.

Results and Followup

Most authors report some cases of improved sphincter or sensorimotor function after operation. As a rule however surgery should not be undertaken in anticipation of achieving neurologic improvement. Rather it should be performed to prevent further deterioration. As stated previously the rationale for prophylactic surgery rests, in part, upon this fact. It also implies that surgery should not be delayed once any degree of progressive impairment of sphincter or limb function is recognized in patients chosen for followup without initial myelography. Finally occasional instances of delayed postoperative deterioration in function have been reported. The deterioration may be due to a previously undetected lesion, such as a thickened filum accompanying a treated diastematomyelia. Such cases warrant reinvestigation.

Conclusion

In summary, successful management of the patient with spinal dysraphism demands proper regard for the underlying problem. This requires, in the first instance, recognition of the true nature of difficulties, which, at first glance, may appear to be orthopedic, urologic, or cosmetic in origin. Early attention to lesions that will cause progressive deficits is vital. Finally, the surgeon dealing with these lesions must respect their often complex nature and the technical difficulties implied with surgery. In such cases a thorough understanding of the pathologic anatomy, aided by appropriate preoperative studies, will be helpful.

REFERENCES

1. Ingraham FD: *Spina Bifida and Cranium Bifidum.* Harvard University Press, Cambridge, 1944
2. James CCM, Lassman LP: Spinal dysraphism. An orthopedic syndrome in children accompanying occult forms. *Arch Dis Child 35*:315-327, 1960
3. James CCM, Lassman LP: *Spinal Dysraphism. Spina Bifida Occulta.* Butterworths, London, 1972
4. Till K: Spinal dysraphism. A study of congenital malformations of the lower back. *J Bone Joint Surg 51B*:415-422, 1969
5. Anderson FM: Occult spinal dysraphism: A series of 73 cases. *Pediatrics 55*:826-835, 1975
6. Reimann AF, Anson BJ: Vertebral level of termination of the spinal cord with report of a case of sacral cord. *Anat Rec 88*:127-138, 1944
7. Barson AJ: Vertebral level of termination of spinal cord during normal and abnormal development. *J Anat 106*:489-497, 1969
8. Emery JL, Lendon RG: Lipoma of the cauda equina and other fatty tumors related to neurospinal dysraphism. *Dev Med Child Neurol (Suppl) 20*:62-70, 1969
9. Gryspeerdt GL: Myelographic assessment of occult forms of spinal dysraphism. *Acta Radiol* [*Diagn*] *1*:702-717, 1963
10. Fitz CR, Harwood-Nash DC: The tethered conus. *Am J Roentgenol Rad Ther Nucl Med 125*:515-523, 1975
11. Fawcitt J: Some radiological aspects of congenital anomalies of the spine in childhood and infancy. *Proc R Soc Med 52*:331-333, 1959
12. Lorber J, Levick K: Spina bifida cystica. Incidence of spina bifida occulta in parents and in controls. *Arch Dis Child 42*:171-173, 1967
13. Manley CB, Frech RS: Urinary tract infections in girls: Prevalence of spina bifida occulta. *J Urol 103*:348-352, 1970
14. Sutow WW, Pryde AW: Incidence of spina bifida occulta in relation to age. *Am J Dis Child 91*:211-217, 1956
15. Swanson HS, Barnett JC Jr: Intradural lipomas in children. *Pediatrics 29*:911-926, 1962
16. Dubowitz V, Lorber J, Zachary RB: Lipoma of the cauda equina. *Arch Dis Child 40*:207-213, 1965
17. Yashon D, Beatty RA: Tethering of the conus medullaris within the sacrum. *J Neurol Neurosurg Psychiatry 29*:244-250, 1966
18. Loeser JD, Lewin RJ: Lumbosacral lipoma in the adult. Case report. *J Neurosurg 29*:405-409, 1968
19. Till K: Occult spinal dysraphism. The value of prophylactic surgical treatment, *Recent Progress in Neurological Surgery.* Excerpta Medica ICS 320, Amsterdam, 1973, pp 61-66
20. Gold LHA, Kieffer SA, Peterson HO: Lipomatous invasion of the spinal cord associated with spinal dysraphism: myelographic evaluation. *Am J Roentgenol Rad Ther Nucl Med 107*:479-485, 1969
21. Thibaut A: Myélographie gazeuse sélective totale. Une amélioration technique. *Acta Radiol (Diagn)9*:754-758, 1969

CHAPTER 21

Microsurgery of Arnold-Chiari Malformation and Hydromyelia in Adults

Albert L. Rhoton, Jr.

HYDROMYELIA, A CONDITION IN which the central canal of the spinal cord communicates with the fourth ventricle and is distended by cerebrospinal fluid, often accompanies Arnold-Chiari malformation in the adult. Unfortunately, a painless, slowly progressive cord deficit caused by hydromyelia suggests a degenerative disease. The first manifestation is often a loss of pain and temperature sensation with tactile preservation in the cervical dermatomes because the cord destruction in hydromyelia often begins around the central canal of the cervical cord. The cavity then extends into the anterior horn, destroying anterior horn cells and causing atrophy and weakness in the involved segments. These deficits caused by a lesion beginning in the central portion of the spinal canal suggest a diagnosis of syringomyelia. Syringomyelia is classified in Merritt's neurology textbook[1] as a degenerative process for which "There is no satisfactory treatment." The location of the lesion has led to the constellation of typical neurologic findings being referred to as a central cord syndrome and the association of these deficits with syringomyelia has led to the name *syringomyelic cord syndrome*.

Evaluation of the initial patients in this series led the author to conclude that Gardner's mechanical concept of a pressure distention origin of syringomyelia cord syndrome is correct,[2,3] and provided the rationale for the treatment outlined here. Unfortunately most of these patients had a previous diagnosis of untreatable degenerative disease and severe deficits had developed in some prior to treatment.

The common association of bulbar symptoms with the syringomyelic cord syndrome has often led to a diagnosis of syringobulbia. This experience has led the author to conclude that this bulbar dysfunction is not caused by a rostral bulbar extension of the syringomyelic degenerative process but by the Arnold-Chiari malformation.

Division of Neurological Surgery, University of Florida Health Center, Gainesville, Florida

Clinical Material

Clinical Material

Fifteen adults, age 19 to 64 years, having surgery by the author provided the basis for this review.[4] Eleven patients had an Arnold-Chiari malformation with hydromyelia and 4 had Arnold-Chiari malformation only. No patient had a prior history of myelomeningocele. All patients with hydromyelia had signs and symptoms referable to it. Of 11 patients with hydromyelia, 4 also had bulbar signs and symptoms. Seven patients with both Arnold-Chiari malformation and hydromyelia had symptoms referable only to the hydromyelia. The 4 patients with Arnold-Chiari malformation without hydromyelia presented with a combination of progressive bulbar and cerebellar signs.

With hydromyelia sensory loss usually preceded lower motor neuron signs. The deficits in this series ranged in severity from a minimal subjective sensory loss to a widespread sensory loss with quadraparesis with marked atrophy of all extremities. Four patients with hydromyelia followed without surgery after initial diagnosis because their deficits were minimal, worsened and had surgery within 1 year of the initial diagnosis. The patients with symptoms due to the Arnold-Chiari malformation had a combination of upper and lower motor neuron signs in the bulbar musculature, gait difficulties due to cerebellar and long tract involvement, and some nystagmus. A 24-year-old man with Arnold-Chiari without hydromyelia was admitted with severe respiratory stridor caused by bilateral vocal cord paralysis of sudden onset. Bertrand[5] describes the mechanism for sudden onset or change of symptoms with this condition.

No adult in this series had hydrocephalus or evidence of increased intracranial pressure even though defective ventricular drainage is thought to be important in development of the hydromyelia.

Radiologic Findings

These patients with spinal cord deficits had Pantopaque myelograms through the foramen magnum in the supine and prone position (Figs. 21-1 and 21-2). The supine myelogram outlined the Arnold-Chiari malformation in all cases; the prone study was frequently normal. Spinal cord deficits were assumed to be caused by hydromyelia, even if the cord size was normal or only minimally enlarged, if the deficit was typical of a central cord lesion and the Pantopaque myelogram done in the supine position showed the Arnold-Chiari malformation.

The radiologic diagnosis was somewhat more difficult to obtain if the patient had Arnold-Chiari but not hydromyelia. These adults, because of the brain stem findings, often had posterior fossa angiography or pneumoencephalography initially. The diagnosis of Arnold-Chiari malformation was suspected in several patients after angiography because of the low descent of the caudal loop of the posterior inferior cerebellar artery (Fig. 21-3A). After angiography, these patients often had pneumoencephalography rather than ventriculography because there was no evidence of increased intracranial pressure. The ventricles frequently did not fill at pneumoencephalography and subsequently a ventriculogram was done and showed the typical caudal displacement of the fourth ventricle (Fig. 21-1D). No patient had significant hydrocephalus even though dense scar over the foramen of Magendie frequently prevented filling of the fourth ventricle at pneumoencephalography and supine Pantopaque myelography.

Operative Findings

All patients had a suboccipital craniectomy and upper cervical laminectomy. All dissection after the bone removal was done using the 3-40X magnification provided by the surgical microscope (Figs. 21-3, 21-4, and 21-5).

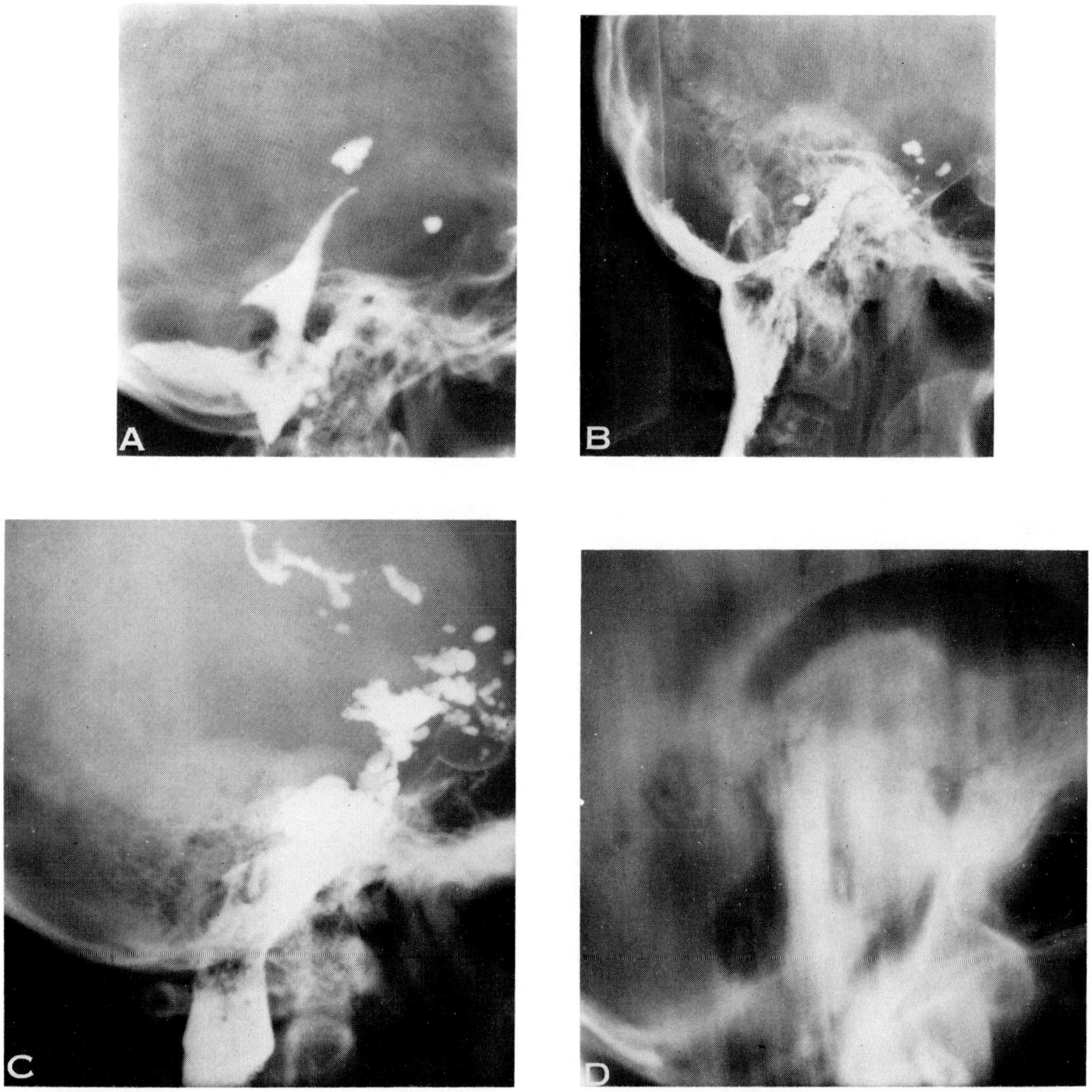

Fig. 21-1. Myeolography and pneumoencephalography in Arnold-Chiari malformation. **A.** Normal lateral view of Pantopaque study with patient in supine position. Pantopaque fills cisterna magna and fourth ventricle to the level of the aqueduct. **B.** Pantopaque myelogram done in supine position outlines tonsilar herniation with Arnold-Chiari malformation. **C.** Pantopaque study of foramen magnum in supine position showing Arnold-Chiari malformation. No Pantopaque passes into the cisterna magna above level of foramen magnum. At surgery, dense adhesions in area of cisterna magna bound the medulla and cerebellum to dura. **D.** Lateral view of ventriculogram showing blunting of lower margin of caudally displaced fourth ventricle with Arnold-Chiari malformation. (Reproduced by permission from Rhoton AL: Microsurgery of Arnold-Chiari malformation in adults with and without hydromyelia. *J. Neurosurg 45*:473-483, 1976)

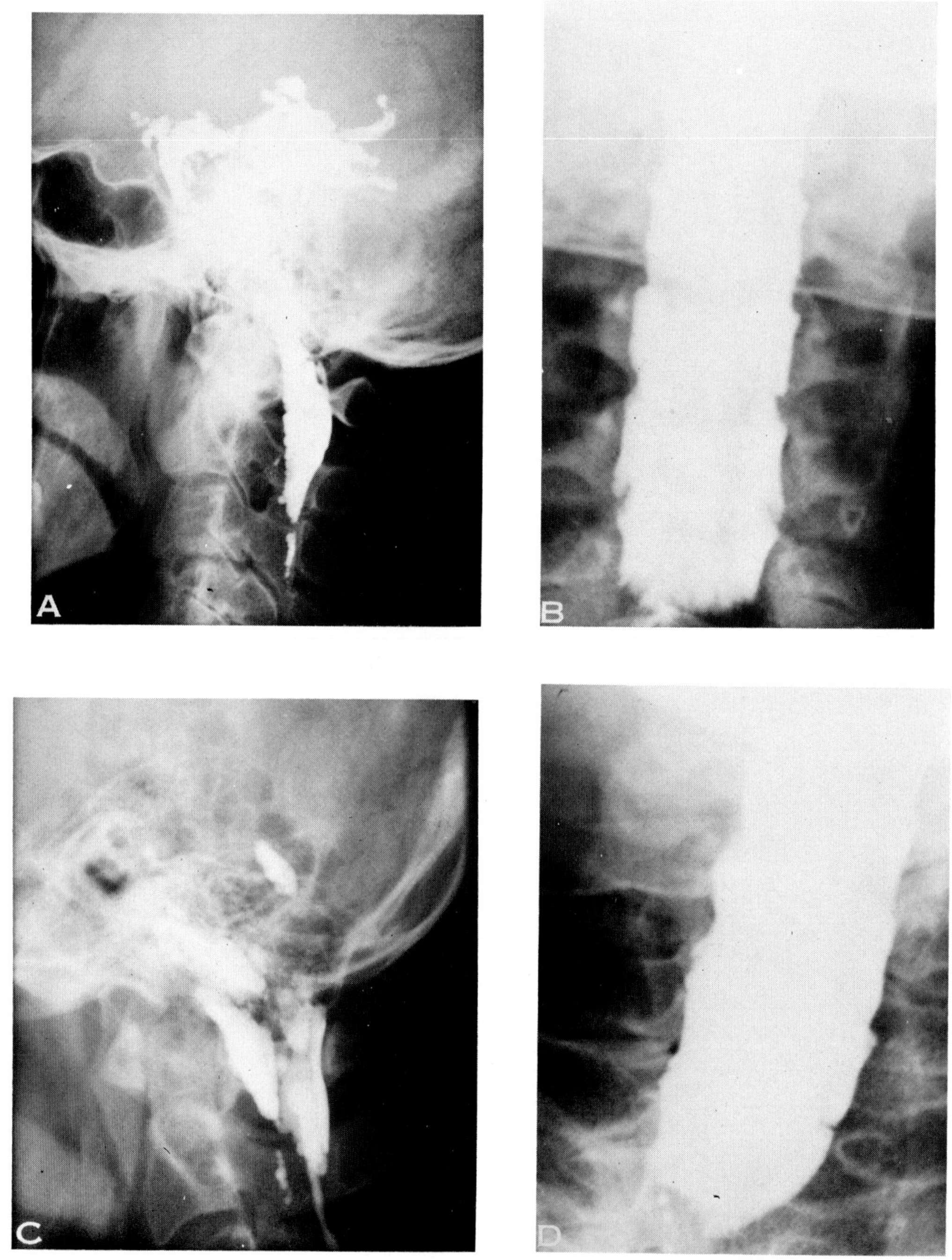

Fig. 21-2. **A** and **B** are from the one patient and **C** and **D** are from another patient. Both patients had previous myelograms to define the cause of progressive central cord deficits which were reported to be normal. The myelograms (**B** and **D**) show no striking abnormalities in the cervical regions. A diagnosis of degenerative disease had been made because cord size appeared normal on previous myelograms. Lateral view of the Pantopaque study of the foramen magnum in the supine position in both patients (**A** and **C**) shows the obstruction to filling of the cisterna magna. The findings from supine Pantopaque myelography lead to a diagnosis of Arnold-Chiari malformation with hydromyelia. (Reproduced by permission from Rhoton AL: Microsurgery of Arnold-Chiari malformation in adults with and without hydromyelia. *J. Neurosurg, 45*:473-483, 1976)

The hydromyelic cords in the upper cervical area varied from those that had a normal surface appearance to those having an almost transparent covering over the fluid cavity. The thinnest part of the cord was the dorsal root entry zone between the lateral and dorsal columns. The thickness of the cord covering the cavity at the dorsal root entry zone varied from no thicker than a layer of arachnoid to 4 mm. The posterior columns were relatively preserved in comparison to the remainder of the cord even with far advanced cord destruction.

The cerebellar tonsils and fourth ventricle were displaced caudally into the foramen magnum or upper cervical area. The caudal loop of the posterior inferior cerebellar artery often descended to the level of C2, marking the lower margin of the cerebellar tonsils (Fig. 21-3A). The elongated cerebellar tonsils varied in appearance from those normal in color and consistency to those which were white and firm because of scarring and gliosis (Fig. 21-3B). If Pantopaque passed into the area between the cerebellar tonsils and the dura, the cerebellar tonsils were near normal in consistency being covered with only mild arachnoidal adhesions. If no Pantopaque passed into the area between the cerebellar tonsils and the dura, an intense mat of scar which included the dura, arachnoid, cerebellar vermis and tonsils, and dorsal surface of the medulla was found at surgery (Figs. 21-3E, 21-4A, and 21-5A). Intense scarring over the foramen of Magendie was commonly seen with hydromyelia. Those with less scarring were less likely to have hydromyelia.

Typically, there was a kink in the lower medulla at or just below the foramen magnum. In cases having only the Arnold-Chiari malformation without hydromyelia, the caudal margin of the fourth ventricle, the obex, and the upper end of the central canal of the cord lay caudal to the lower margin of the cerebellar tonsil and because of this caudal fourth ventricular extension, the hind brain hernia did not overlap and occlude the central canal (Fig. 21-3D). The fact that the tonsils did not block the central canal of the cord explains the lack of hydromyelia.

Operative Procedures

Prior to surgery, the patients sat for 20 to 30 minutes in the cervical semiflexed position to be used for surgery to make certain that the position would not increase their deficit or cause respiratory problems, as has been reported with the use of the flexed position in Arnold-Chiari malformation.[6] A suboccipital craniectomy and Cl-3 laminectomy was done through a midline incision to decompress the foramen magnum. The surgical microscope was brought in the field after bone removal was complete. The dura was opened in the midline over the cervical cord and above this the incision was U-shaped with the lower margins of the U encompassing the mat of scar tissue often attached to the upper cord and lower medulla (Figs. 21-3E, 21-4A, and 21-5A). If a plaque of arachnoid and dura was densely adherent to the dorsal medulla and cord, it was left attached because an attempt to disconnect this might injure the dorsal surface of the medulla cord. The degree of adherence of dura to cord and medulla could usually be predicted from the myelogram. If no Pantopaque passed posterior to the cord and cerebellar tonsils at the foramen magnum, the dura was usually matted to the cord. If Pantopaque passed freely, although slowly, between the arachnoid and cerebellar tonsils, the meninges were usually easily separated from the tonsils. If the foramen of Magendie was blocked, its lower part was opened in the midline, care being taken to make certain that the dissection was far enough superior to enter the fluid cavity of the fourth ventricle rather than the cord or medulla (Figs. 21-4A, 21-4B, and 21-5A). After the fourth ventricle was opened, a Silastic wick was attached to the dura and passed up into the new midline opening (Fig. 21-4B). The opening at the outlet of the fourth ventricle should be large enough that it would not close even if no wick was threaded into it. The wick was used to maintain the patency of the outlet rather than as a conduit for drainage.

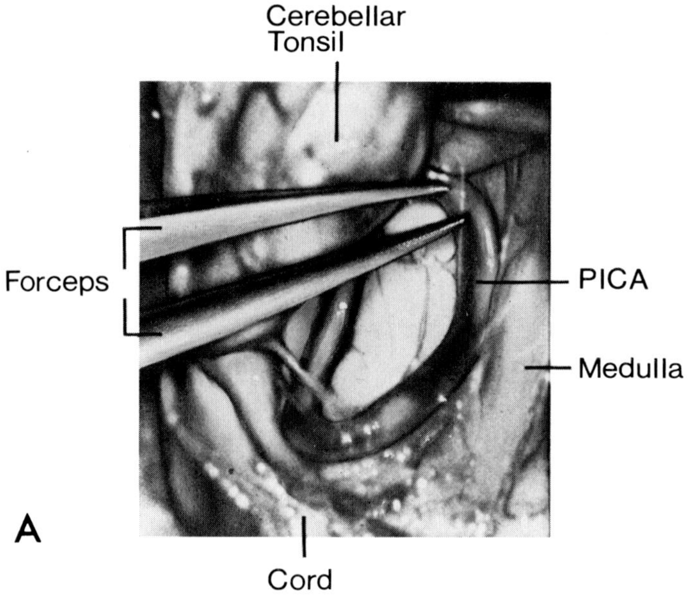

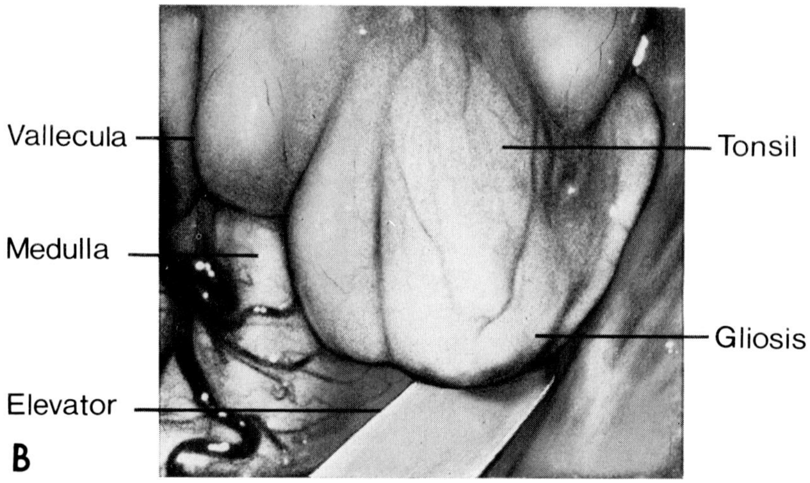

Fig. 21-3. Posterior views of Arnold-Chiari malformations through suboccipital craniectomy. The pictures were taken through surgical microscope at 6X magnification and retouched and labeled to increase clarity. Only B and C are from the same patient. **A.** Caudal loop of the posterior inferior cerebellar artery (PICA) displaced around caudal margin of herniated cerebellar tonsil. Lower margin of tonsil was at C-2. **B.** Lower margin of herniated cerebellar tonsil. Same patient as shown in **Figure 21-1B.** Pale color at tip of left cerebellar tonsil is caused by gliosis in herniated tonsilar tips.

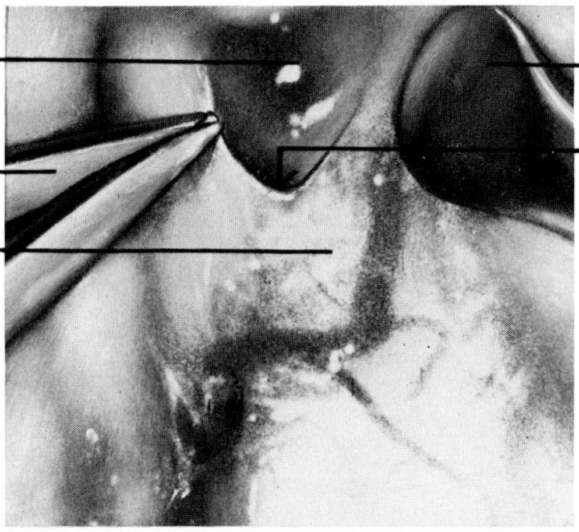

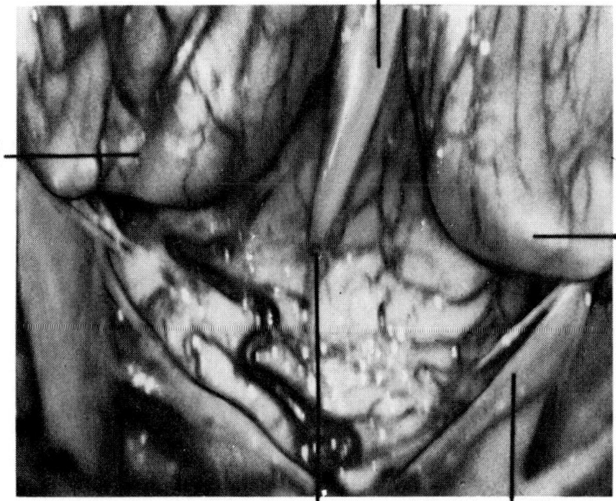

Fig. 21-3. (continued) **C.** Posterior view of fourth ventricle after separation of cerebellar tonsils shown in **B.** There is a small membrane at the lower margin of fourth ventricle which blocks view of upper end of the central canal and which would retain a small muscle plug if it were placed in the central canal. **D.** This patient did not have hydromyelia because the tonsils did not extend far enough caudal to block the central canal. The tonsils were separated to expose the fourth ventricle. The obex lies slightly below the caudal level of the cerebellar tonsils. The elongated, narrow fourth ventricle is seen in the midline.

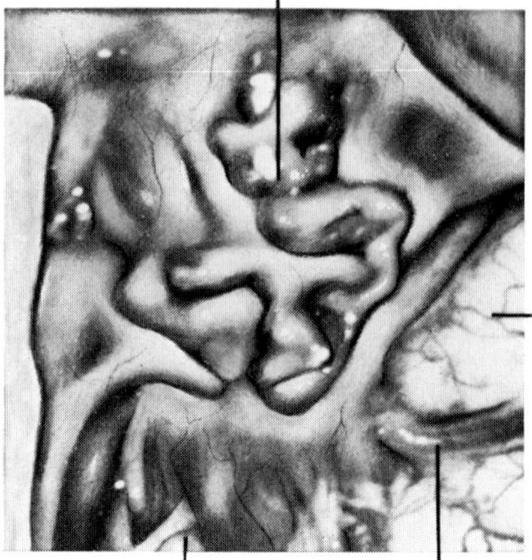

Fig. 21-3. (continued) **E.** Dense mat of scar which includes dura blocks the area of the foramen of Magendie and is adherent to surface of medulla. The caudal loop of PICA enters the scar. (Reproduced by permission from Rhoton AL: Microsurgery of Arnold-Chiari malformation in adults with and without hydromyelia. *J. Neurosurg, 45*:473-483, 1976)

The hydromyelia was drained by incising in the dorsal root entry zone between the posterior and lateral columns because that was usually the thinnest area (Figs. 21-4D and 21-5B). A midline myelotomy in such cases could have led to a lower extremity posterior column deficit which was nonexistent prior to surgery, but posterolateral myelotomy near the dorsal root entry zone on the side of the upper extremity with the greatest deficit usually will not increase the already existing deficit in that extremity. A needle was introduced into the cavity at the thinnest area and fluid collected for cell count and protein determinations before incising the cord (Fig. 21-4C). The protein in hydromyelia is normal. An elevated protein or colored fluid suggests a diagnosis of intramedullary tumor. A vertical incision at least 1 cm in length was made into the thinnest area along the dorsal root entry zone and a Silastic wick, anchored to the dura above, was threaded downward into the myelotomy (Fig. 21-4E). Usually the cord was thinnest on the side of the greatest neurologic deficit. The dura was loosely closed utilizing a dural graft, care being taken not to constrict the area.

Only one patient had an increased deficit as a result of surgery, a mild proprioceptive sensory loss in the right thumb, which did not impair the patient in his work requiring a moderate dexterity. Most patients noted some subjective improvement in sensory and motor deficit but the neurologic signs remained about the same as prior to surgery.

Discussion

Barnett et al. agree that a hydromyelic cavity is the most likely cause of a spontaneously appearing central cord syndrome, although they refer to the condition not as *hydromyelia,* but as *communicating syringomyelia.*[7] The author prefers to refer to the dynamic cord pathology associated with Arnold-Chiari malformation as hydromyelia, as proposed by Gardner,[2,3] rather than as communicating syringomyelia because of the traditional association of the term *syringomyelia* with an untreatable degenerative disease. Merritt's neurology textbook classifies syringomyelia as a degenerative process.[1]

Of 19 cases of central cord syndrome seen by this author, in which there was no prior history of spinal trauma, 11 were caused by hydromyelia associated with Arnold-Chiari malformation and 8 by intramedullary tumor. The fact that most syringomyelic cord syndromes are caused by treatable conditions means that an active investigational attitude should be adopted so that early cases of this disorder are recognized and treated because patients beyond a certain stage of disability have little likelihood of useful recovery. A number of patients in this series initially diagnosed as having untreatable degenerative disease because myelographic cord size was normal, progressed and developed crippling deficits prior to surgery. Four patients in whom the correct diagnosis was made, but surgery was deferred because the central cord deficit was mild, progressed and required surgery within 1 year of diagnosis.

Spinal cord size on Pantopaque myelography may be normal even in the presence of a hydromyelia causing a marked cord deficit. The diagnosis can be established in the presence of a normal cord size by myelography in the supine position. The presence of a central cord syndrome and tonsilar herniation on Pantopaque myelography establishes the diagnosis of Arnold-Chiari malformation with hydromyelia.

On myelography, hydromyelia commonly produces a less striking picture of cord enlargement than does an intramedullary tumor (Fig. 21-6). Intramedullary tumor, even when diagnosed early, often causes striking cord enlargement and frequently is associated with an almost complete block. The enlargement with hydromyelia is diffuse over many segments and that with a tumor is more localized.

The author recommends that Arnold-Chiari malformation and hydromyelia be treated with a suboccipital craniectomy and upper cervical laminectomy to decompress the malformation at the foramen magnum. In addition, an outlet for the fourth ventricle should be established if it is blocked and if there is a hydromyelic cavity it should be drained. The increased accuracy of dissection obtained by the use of surgical magnification facilitates dissection through the scar over the fourth ventricle, inspection of the lower fourth ventricle, identification of the proper area to incise the cord, and the final incision into the spinal cord.

The cord should be incised longitudinally in the posterolateral cord at the dorsal root entry zone because this is the thinnest area. The natural dissection of the cavity along the dorsal root entry zone also leads to a proprioceptive deficit in the upper extremities, hence, incision here will not aggravate the patient's deficit. The posterolateral myelotomy used in hydromyelia is different from the midline myelotomy between the gracile fasciculi made to expose and remove an intramedullary tumor. An incision approximately 1 cm long is made to drain a hydromyelia.

Percutaneous needling of the hydromyelia cavity has been advocated as a possible mode of therapy,[8] however, aspiration of fluid at surgery is followed by rapid refilling of the hydromyelic cavity from the ventricular system and it seems unlikely that a needle tract would remain patent. In hydromyelia, the longitudinal opening into the cord should be long enough that there is no tendency for spontaneous closure.

Gardner initially recommended treatment consisting of decompression at the foramen magnum and plugging of the upper end of the patent central canal at the area of the obex with a small piece of muscle.[2,3] There is often a membrane stretched across the fourth ventricle just posterior to the patent central canal which would help retain a pledget of muscle (Fig. 21-3C), however, the author favors incision between the posterior and lateral columns to drain the hydromyelia rather than risk damage to the hypoglossal and vagal nuclei which are near the obex.

Recently Gardner et al.[9] have advocated a procedure called terminal ventriculostomy. The terminal ventricle is a dilated portion of the central canal extending below the tip of the

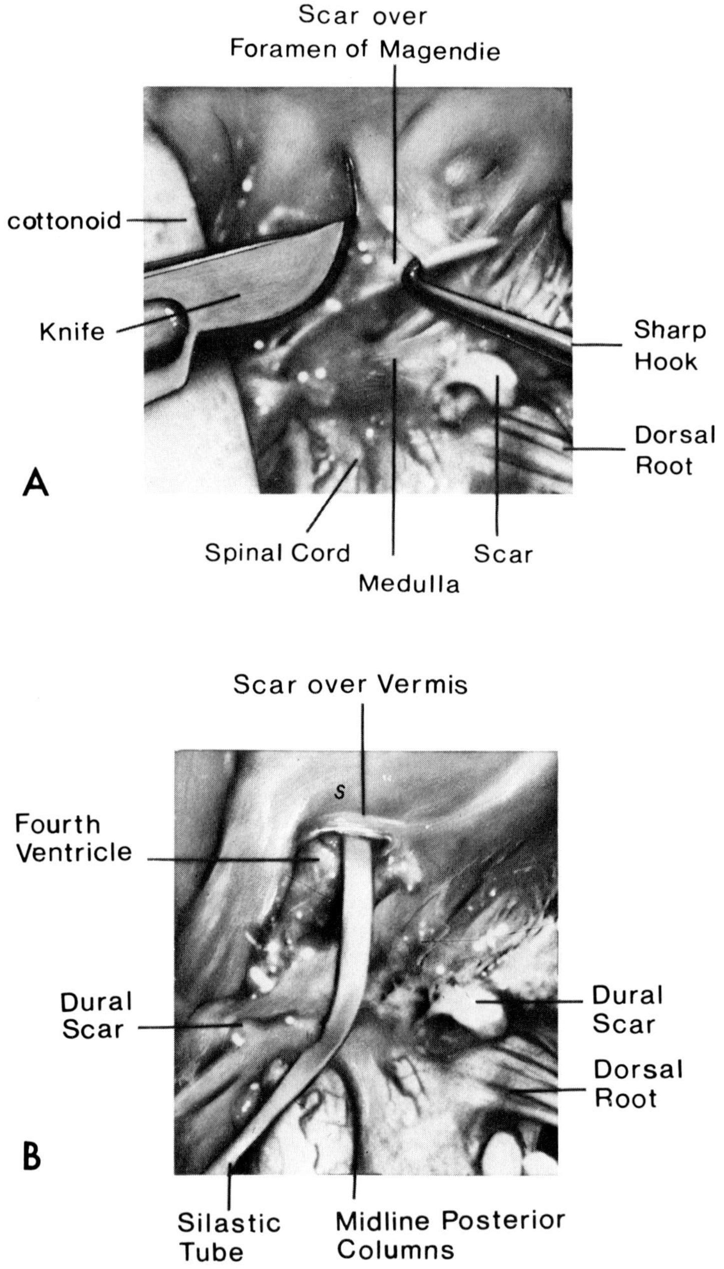

Fig. 21-4. Posterior views of Arnold-Chiari malformation and hydromyelia through a suboccipital craniectomy and C1-3 laminectomy. Pictures taken at 6X magnification through surgical microscopes and retouched for clarity. All pictures are from the same patient. **A.** Incision of dense mat of scar over the foramen of Magendie. **B.** Opening into fourth ventricle is completed and a Silastic tube anchored to dura below is threaded rostrally.

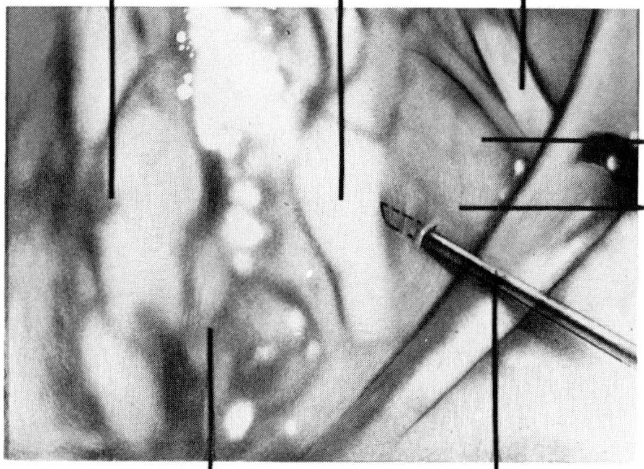

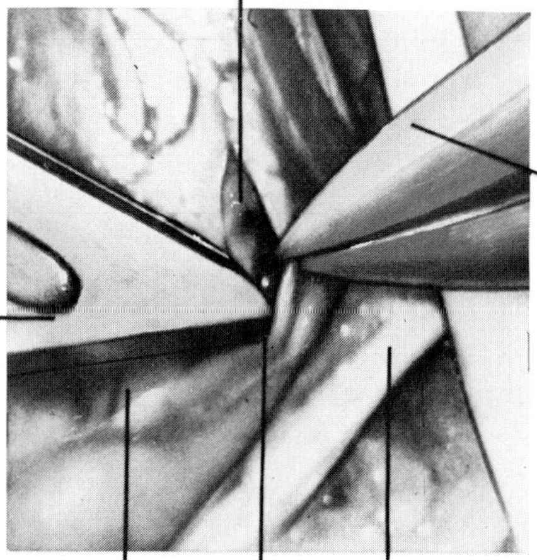

Fig. 21-4. (continued) **C.** A needle is introduced into the right half of the spinal cord lateral to the posterior column near the C-3 dorsal root entry zone. Clear fluid was obtained. The cord was so thin in this area that the needle tip could be seen through the bulging surface. **D.** One cm in length incision made in dorsal root entry zone using No. 11 knife blade. Cord thinner than the dura.

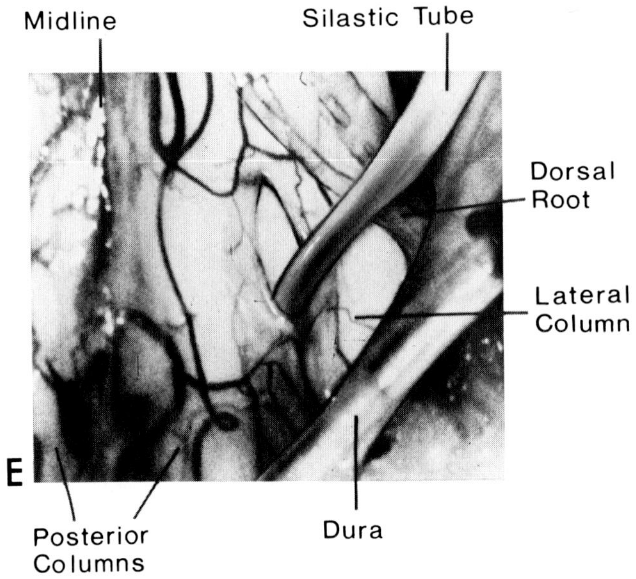

Fig. 21-4. (continued) **E.** Silastic wick attached to the dura above led downward into the hydromyelic cavity. (Reproduced by permission from Rhoton AL: Microsurgery of Arnold-Chiari malformation in adults with and without hydromyelia. *J. Neurosurg, 45*:473-483, 1976)

conus medullaris into the filum terminale. A laminectomy is done over the caudal limit of the fluid sac and the filum is opened. This procedure does not decompress the malformation at the foramen magnum but may prove satisfactory if only hydromyelic symptoms are present.

Cerebrospinal fluid (CSF) shunting from the lateral ventricle to the atrium or peritoneum has been recommended.[10] However, the adults in this series, even those with marked hydromyelia deficits, have no significant ventricular dilatation and the small ventricles make shunting difficult. In addition, CSF pressure had been normal in our adult cases. Even if shunts were done, there remains a hydrostatic fluid column from the ventricles acting on the cord when the patient is in the upright position. Shunting would be indicated if the ventricles were large or intracranial pressure was increased.

The finding of normal sized ventricles in these patients had led the author to conclude that intracavitary pressure too low to dilate the ventricles may cause progressive cord destruction by distention. A recent case in an infant supports this concept. This child had hydrocephalus after birth which required shunting, the shunt became infected, was removed, and not replaced because head and ventricular size remained normal. The child then developed a progressive, severe lower motor neuron deficit in the arms. Repeat contrast studies showed normal sized ventricles but positive contrast ventriculography showed a hugely dilated cervical cord (Fig. 21-7).

Summary

Microsurgical exploration of 15 adults with Arnold-Chiari malformation with and without hydromyelia using 3 to 40X magnification has led to the following conclusions.

Hydromyelia, associated with Arnold-Chiari malformation, is a progressive mechanical disorder which causes spinal cord deficits by pressure distention of the cord. Arnold-Chiari

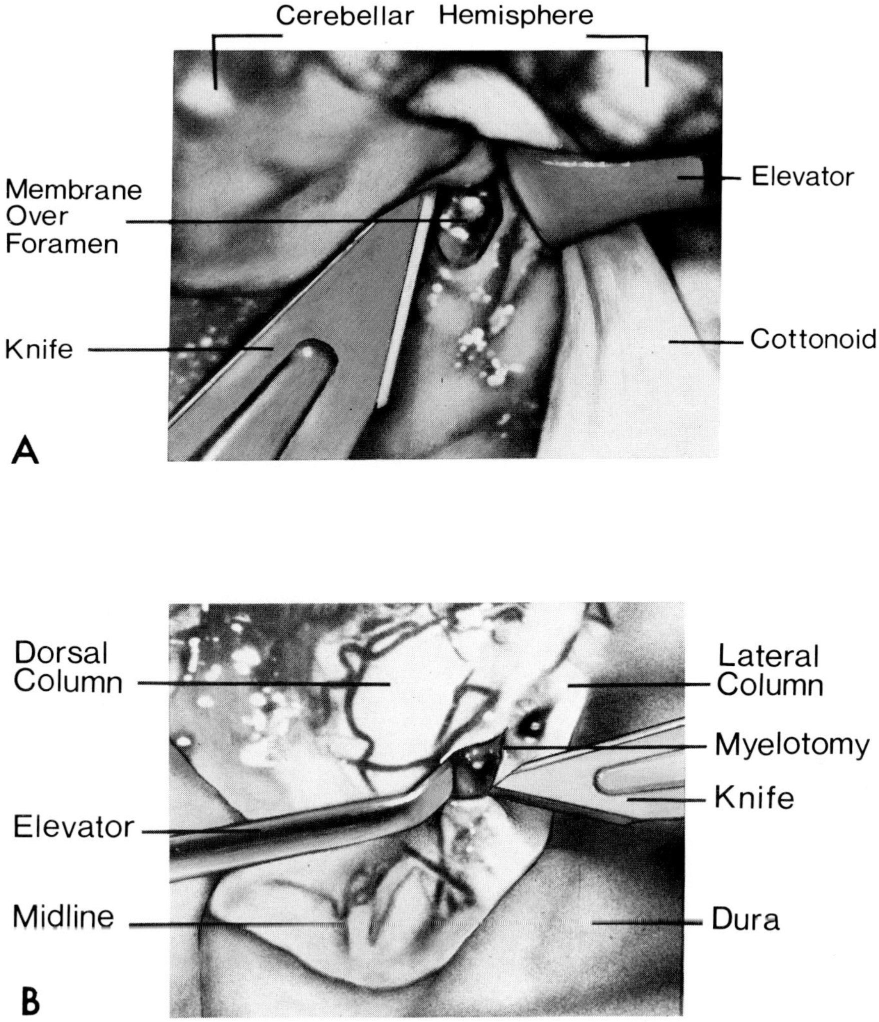

Fig. 21-5. **A.** View through suboccipital craniectomy of membrane occluding foramen of Magendie. A hydromyelia was also present and is shown in **B.** The occluding membrane was incised with a No. 11 blade. **B.** The cord was incised at C3 dorsal root entry zone. The covering over the hydromyelic cavity was only as thick as a layer of dura. A Silastic wick was left in both the fourth ventricle and cord. (Reproduced by permission from Rhoton AL: Microsurgery of Arnold-Chiari malformation in adults with and without hydromyelia. *J. Neurosurg, 45*:473-483, 1976)

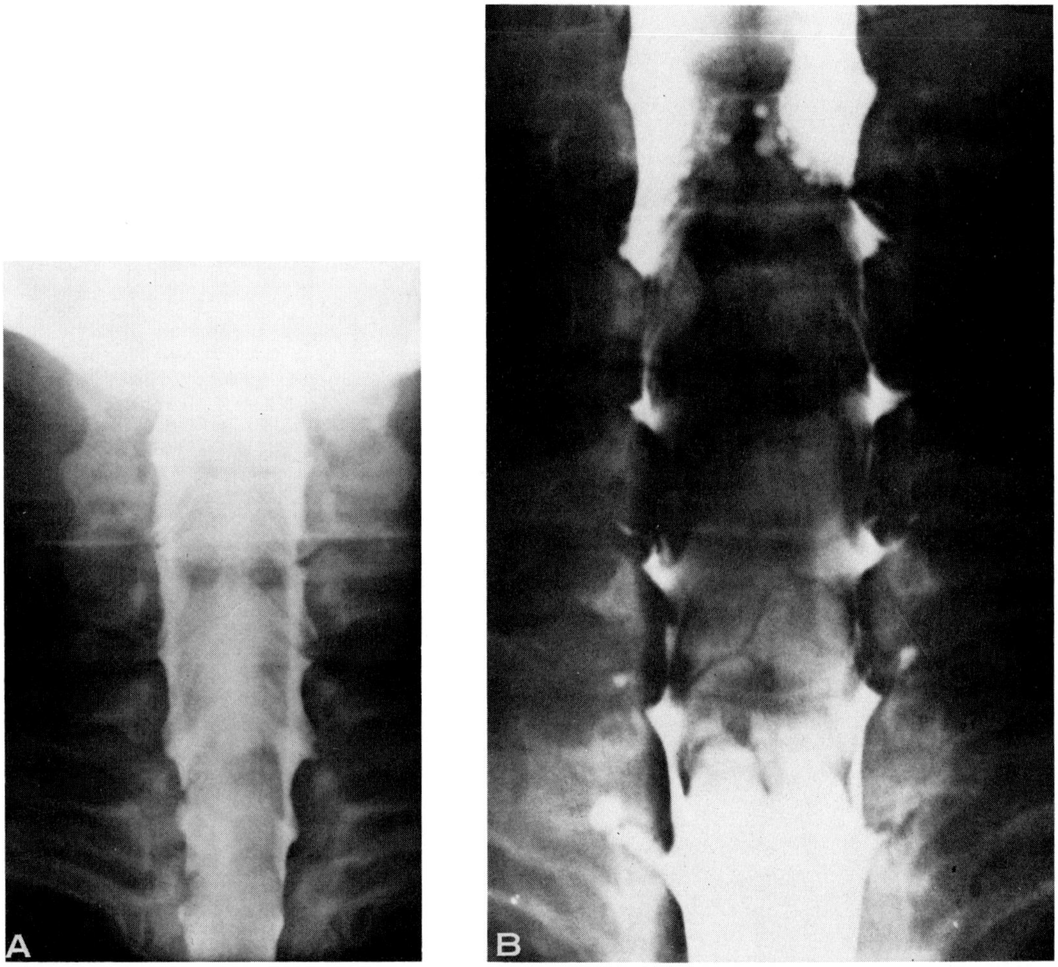

Fig. 21-6. **A.** Pantopaque study of cervical region showing dilatation of cord associated with a far advanced hydromyelic deficit. Even in the advanced stages of a hydromyelia, the myelographic picture is not as striking as with the obstruction due to an intramedullary tumor. **B.** Pantopaque study showing an intramedullary tumor. The hydromyelia presents a more diffuse enlargement; the tumor enlargement is more localized. (Reproduced by permission from Rhoton AL: Microsurgery of Arnold-Chiari malformation in adults with and without hydromyelia. *J. Neurosurg, 45*:473-483, 1976)

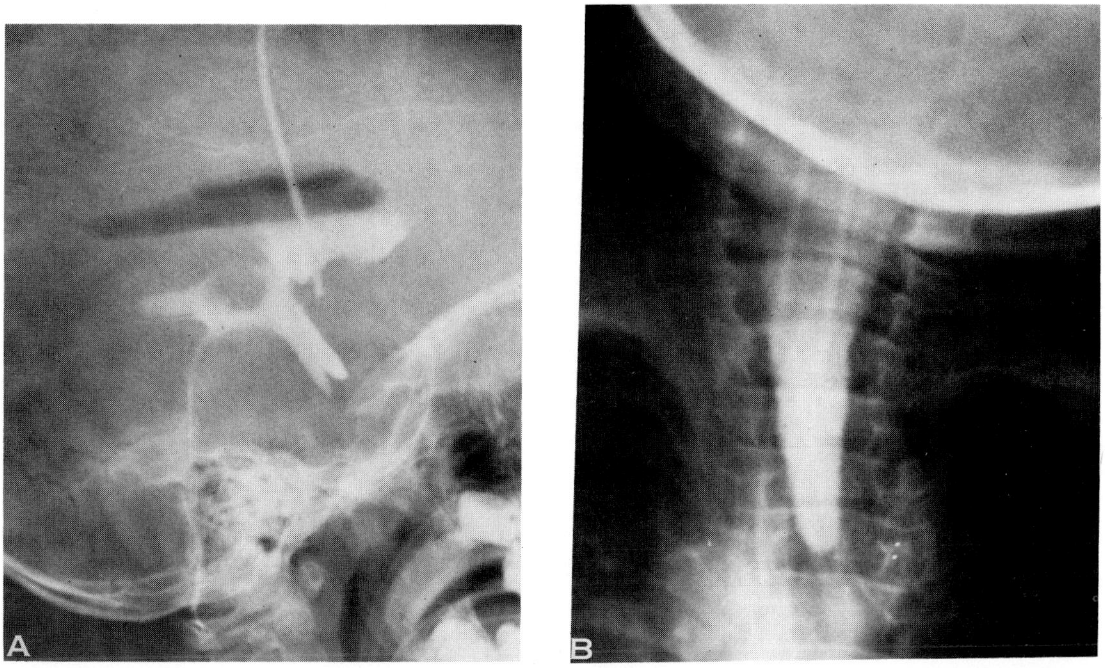

Fig. 21-7. **A.** Lateral view of positive contrast ventriculogram from infant previously treated with a shunt for hydrocephalus. Shunt removed because of infection. This study was done because of a progressive low motor neuron deficit in the arms after shunt removal. Lateral ventriculogram shows normal sized ventricles. **B.** Contrast media enters a large cavity in the cervical cord which communicates with ventricles. (Reproduced by permission from Rhoton AL: Microsurgery of Arnold-Chiari malformation in adults with and without hydromyelia. *J. Neurosurg, 45*:473-483, 1976)

malformation causes slowly or suddenly progressive bulbar dysfunction by impaction of the malformation in the foramen magnum. Decompression of both can be achieved by a suboccipital craniectomy, upper cervical laminectomy, establishing an outlet from the fourth ventricle, and opening the distended cord in the thinnest exposed area which is usually along the dorsal root entry zone. The diagnosis of hydromyelia as a cause of central cord deficit can be made, even if myelographic cord size is normal, if Pantopaque myelography in the supine position shows the Arnold-Chiari malformation. Syringomyelia, traditionally considered a degenerative disease, is a less common cause of a spontaneous appearing, slowly progressive central cord deficit than either hydromyelia or intramedullary tumor. The common association of bulbar symptoms with the syringomyelic cord syndrome has often led to a diagnosis of syringobulbia; however, this bulbar dysfunction is most commonly caused by an Arnold-Chiari malformation and is best treated by decompression.

Acknowledgment

This work was supported in part by NIH Grant No. NS 10978-02.

REFERENCES

1. Merritt HH: *A Textbook of Neurology.* Lea and Febiger, Philadelphia, 1973, p 513
2. Gardner WJ: Rupture of the neural tube. *Clin Neurosurg 15*:57-59, 1968
3. Gardner WJ, Angel J: The mechanism of syringomyelia and its surgical correction. *Clin Neurosurg 6*:131-140, 1959

4. Rhoton, AL: Microsurgery of Arnold-Chiari malformation in adults with and without hydromyelia. *J Neurosurg,* in press.
5. Bertrand G: Dynamic factors in the evolution of syringomyelia and syringobulbia. *Clin Neurosurg* *20*:322-333, 1973
6. Mullan S, Raimondi A: Respiratory hazards of the surgical treatment of the Arnold-Chiari malformations. *J Neurosurg 19*:675-678, 1962
7. Barnett, HJM, Foster JB, Hudgson P: *Syringomyelia.* WB Saunders, London, 1973, p 121
8. Schlesinger ER, Tenner MS, Michelsen WJ: Percutaneous spinal cord puncture in the analysis and treatment of hydromyelia. Presented at the Annual Meeting of the American Association of Neurological Surgeons, Houston, 1971
9. Gardner WJ, Steinberg M, Bell H, et al: Terminal ventriculostomy in the treatment of syringomyelia. Presented at the Annual Meeting of the American Association of Neurological Surgeons, Miami Beach, 1975
10. Conway LW: Hydrodynamic studies in syringomyelia. *J Neurosurg 27*:501-514, 1967

CHAPTER 22

Approaches to the Cervical Spine C1-T1

Robert A. Robinson

THERE ARE THREE SURGICAL approaches to the cervical spine:

1. The posterior approach
2. The anterior and anterolateral approaches
3. The lateral approach

The posterior approach to the spine is the oldest. Paul of Aegina (700AD),[1] after warning of the danger, advised that if the spines were broken, fragments should be removed by an incision through the skin and the wound sutured. As early as 1549 Ambrose Paré,[2] the redoubtable French army surgeon, operated, through a posterior incision, for depressed splinters of bone impinging on the spinal cord and nerve roots. Therefore I shall first consider the posterior approach to the cervical spine, since it is the oldest.

Exposure of Posterior Elements of the Cervical Spine

The posterior exposure necessary to perform a variety of procedures is the same.[3-12] It is performed with the patient in the prone, lateral, or sitting position. In general adjustable, but secure, fixation of the patient's head, with resulting control of the cervical spine during the surgical procedure, is mandatory. Proper positioning of the patient for surgery requires that (a) the cervical spine be maintained in optimum position for the procedure to be undertaken; (b) the head should be fixed so that gross motion of the cervical spine during the operative procedure is not allowed but the position of the neck can be adjusted, (c) pressure on the eyes is prevented during the procedure, and (d) adequate ventilatory exchange and cardiac function are monitored throughout the procedure.

The Halo-cast was developed in 1959.[5] If the skeletal stability of a neck has been compromised by poliomyelitis, dysplasia (such as a deficient odontoid), infection, tumor, or injury, it can be stabilized for surgery in such a device, or by skull tong traction on a Stryker frame, or, occasionally, in a full-length plaster bed. These external devices are applied before anterior, lateral, and posterior spine surgery to avoid damage, by unguarded motion, to the

Department of Orthopaedic Surgery, The Johns Hopkins University, School of Medicine and the Johns Hopkins Hospital, Baltimore, Maryland 21205

spinal cord, vertebral arteries, and nerve roots, since spinal instability is markedly increased under anesthesia.

The skin overlying the occipital portion of the skull, the posterior portion of the neck, shoulders, and upper back is included in the prepared operative field. If a bone graft is to be used, the relevant skin area is also prepped and draped. A midline incision over the cervical spine, with "Y" extensions superiorly, if needed, is made overlying the palpable tips of the spinous processes.

After the skin incision has been made a dilute solution of saline and adrenalin (usually less than 1:100,000) may be injected into subcutaneous and muscular tissues through which the incision will be carried. If the injection is administered before the skin incision is made, bony landmarks may be obliterated, obscuring the midline. The incision is carried through the subcutaneous tissue until the tips of the spinous processes of the cervical spine are identified. The spinous processes and laminae of the appropriate cervical vertebrae are then exposed subperiosteally.

X-ray control should be used to confirm cervical spine vertebral levels during surgery. Very often the posterior spinous process of C3 is completely hidden under that of C2 and the posterior spinous processes of C7 and T1 can be confused.

If the posterior arch of the first cervical vertebra is to be exposed, the posterior elements of the second cervical vertebra are first exposed subperiosteally, the occipital portion of the skull exposed, and dissection carried into the midline between these two structures until the posterior tubercle of the arch of the first cervical vertebra is identified. Dissection is then carried laterally to each side of the midline for a distance of ½ inch, thus exposing the posterior arch of the first cervical vertebra. Care must be taken not to expose more than 1 inch of the posterior arch of the first cervical vertebra to prevent inadvertent damage to the vertebral artery or surrounding plexus of veins. It must be emphasized that subperiosteal exposure of the posterior elements of the cervical spine must be carried out with a sharp periosteal elevator. At no time should decortication of the posterior elements of the cervical spine be attempted using a mallet with an osteotome or gouge. That is, only manual subperiosteal elevation or decortication should be carried out; a mallet should never be used in the posterior portion of the cervical spine. If the spine appears to be very unstable, a Kocher clamp placed upon the spinous process of the unstable segment may be used to steady it during subperiosteal dissection.

It should be pointed out that the ligamentum flavum runs from the posterior arch of one vertebra to another, except at C1. Normally its attachment to the laminae of C1 is relatively slight and it is continuous from the posterior arch of C2 up to and through the posterior rim of the foramen magnum. However, the sagittal cross section of the posterior arch of C1 is triangular, with its apex pointing toward the spinal canal. Therefore if it appears that attempts to loosen the ligamentum flavum from the arch of C1 may cause pressure on the spinal contents, as, for instance, when trying to loosen it in order to pass a wire loop around the posterior arch of C1, it is my opinion that it would be better to drill holes vertically through the arch of C1 posterior to its anterior leading edge. A wire can be passed through these holes to fix a posterior bone graft between C1 and C2. If the posterior arch of C1 is absent, or its bone quality is poor, as it may be in rheumatoid disease, such C1-2 stabilization procedures should probably be extended upward to the base of the skull and downward to the posterior spinous processes of both C2 and C3.[3,13]

In general the bone need be exposed only subperiostally in the cervical spine in order to create a biologically efficient bed for a bone graft. Some surgeons prefer to roughen the periosteal bone surfaces with a burr preparatory to fusion, but as pointed out some years ago by William Rogers, this is not necessary.

The idea that a wire loop alone will cause an injured cervical motion segment to fuse solidly with bone, without a bone graft, is fallacious. Therefore bone grafts and 12 weeks of postoperative immobilization are advised. In posterior fusions wire is used to stabilize the graft, while in anterior fusions braided silk is now used, if necessary, to stabilize the bone graft instead of wire.[10,14]

Once the posterior part of the cervical spine is exposed and the exact *geography* determined by x-ray, various types of surgery can be carried out. If extensive laminectomies, sometimes including facetectomies, are carried out in a spine that is unstable before surgery, or instability has been created during surgery, then there are surgical methods for reestablishing spinal stability at the same operation through the same posterior cervical spine exposure. When fusion of the cervical spine is *critical,* both an anterior and posterior fusion of the same motion segments are recommended.[8]

Anterolateral Approaches to the Cervical Spine

These approaches became popular shortly after 1950.[15-21] Aseptic surgery, general anesthesia with controlled pressure, gaseous anesthesia with endotracheal intubation, readily available stored blood for transfusions, antibiotics (particularly streptomycin and penicillin), and intraoperative x-ray control had all been developed during the 100 years preceding 1950. In fact, the antituberculous drug, streptomycin, was developed approximately 5 years before that time.

However, as in so many advances in surgery of the spine, there has long been a human desire to help those afflicted with spinal tuberculosis. To directly approach the usual site of tuberculous lesions in the spine, the vertebral bodies had to be approached anteriorly. Therefore, although anterior approaches to the cervical spine were only used by rare surgeons prior to about 1950, nevertheless they were used. According to Verbiest,[22] Boudot,[23] basing his thesis on an operation of Professor Michel, is probably the first to have pointed out the possibility of a retromastoid approach permitting one to expose the transverse cervical apophyses. Chien,[24] Cheyne,[25] Burckhardt[26] and Auffret[27] all drained retropharyngeal abscesses, most of which were probably tuberculous, by an anterolateral approach, either just anterior or posterior to the sternocleidomastoid muscle.

Küttner[22,28] treated aneurysms of vertebral arteries through a lateral approach about 1917.

According to Verbiest,[22] Auffret, in 1986, was the first to use the transbuccal, direct anterior approach to the C2, C3, and C4 vertebral bodies. However, he preferred the anterolateral approach for the transverse processes of C2 through C7 and the bodies of C5, C6, and C7. He stated: "The fact that I originated the direct exposure of the anterior aspect of the first three cervical vertebrae does not totally blind me from recognizing that it is possible when necessary, that is from extreme necessity, to approach these vertebral bodies laterally". He judged that the lateral approach was still full of problems.

Burckhardt[26] preferred to drain retropharangeal abscesses by an approach medial to the sternocleidomastoid muscle and neurovascular bundle.

Lahey[29] used a parasternocleidomastoid approach to marsupialize and eventually remove esophageal diverticulae. (It interests me that Dr. Lahey does not mention the anterior cervical spine which must have been visible to him; obviously his chief interest was anterior to the spine.)

In any event anterior approaches to the cervical spine are at least 100 years old and probably much older. For instance, retropharyngeal abscesses that interfered with breathing may have sometimes drained spontaneously, or may have unreportedly been incised through the back of the throat via the mouth, as long as surgery has been practiced as were peritonsillar abscesses. Recently Fang et al.[30] electively used this direct anterior approach to the cervical spine through the mouth to fuse the lateral masses of C1 and C2.

Anterolateral Exposure from the First Cervical Vertebra to the First or Second Thoracic Vertebra

The technique used for anterolateral exposure of the cervical spine has been described in detail previously.[9,31] As I do it, the patient is supine on an operating table with a radiolucent top. The neck is at first stabilized by 5 lb of traction applied through a head halter. The shoulders are gently pulled caudally, with adhesive tape, and the table then placed in about 5° Trendelenburg position. A cylindrical pneumatic support is placed transversely under the neck, the shoulders are slightly elevated by a folded sheet, and the occiput, after traction is applied, just clears the table. As the cervical spine is exposed, traction is usually increased to 20 lb.

The procedure is often performed through a transverse skin incision, which should be centered over the anterior border of the sternomastoid muscle, and placed over the segment of the spine to be exposed. When the platysma muscle has been exposed, it is grasped between forceps and sharply incised at the lateral limb of the transverse incision, just anterior to the external jugular vein, bluntly separated from the underlying structures, and sharply incised in the line of the skin incision. The underlying sternomastoid muscle is then visible. The anterior border of the sternomastoid muscle must be clearly identified and mobilized throughout the limits of the exposure so that its medial border can be retracted laterally, exposing the middle layer of the cervical fascia. The omohyoid muscle can be seen crossing the field at about the C5-6 level and may be mobilized and retracted inferiorly, superiorly, or transected in its midtendinous segment. The carotid sheath is then identified, and the middle layer of cervical fascia incised just medial and parallel to the carotid sheath, allowing retraction of the carotid sheath and sternomastoid muscle laterally. Usually very little traction is necessary once the esophagus and trachea are retracted medially. However, at first, the neurovascular bundle is retracted slightly and the anterior surface of the cervical spine visualized, as is the esophagus, lying just posterior to the trachea, or in the superior portion of the neck, the larynx. The prevertebral and alar fascias are incised longitudinally in the midline of the neck and retracted medially and laterally. The prevertebral fascias are easily retracted laterally over the underlying anterior longitudinal ligament of the cervical spine. The longus colli muscles may then be elevated sharply from the intervertebral discs and vertebral bodies and retracted laterally. Just before doing this, one should cauterize the vein and artery which emerge on either side of each spinal segment and enter the vertebral body just superior to their point of emergence laterally from under the longus colli muscles. Cauterization helps keep the wound relatively bloodless.

At this point in the exposure a lateral x-ray of the cervical spine can be obtained, placing a needle into a disc for exact localization. However, a very excellent anatomic landmark is the bony promontory on the transverse processes of C6, the *carotid tubercle,* opposite the vertebral body of C6. The intervertebral disc between C5 and 6 vertebral bodies can thus be spotted for placement of the needle.

When many motion segments of the cervical spine from C1-2 through T1-2 are to be exposed anteriorly, a more vertical incision, extending from near the tip of the mastoid process to the suprasternal notch along the anterior border of the underlying sternocleidomastoid muscle, may be used. Through such an incision, different types of anterior and lateral operations can be done on cervical vertebral bodies and intervertebral discs, transverse processes, and vertebral arteries. In general, after the initial exposure is made through the superficial layer of the deep fascia surrounding the sternocleidomastoid muscle, I proceed to the front of the spine at C5-6 and then, layer by fascial layer, proceed upward toward the tip of the mastoid process. Through this incision, I have removed the bulk of a plasma cell myeloma in C2 and replaced it with an inverted clothespin-shaped graft, and drained an acute pyogenic abscess involving the C1 odontoid joint.

More Extensive Exposure of the Cervical Spine Anterolaterally

The exposure, which has just been described, is known to head-neck surgeons as the Lincoln Highway to the neck. In its unmodified form it is usually adequate for disc surgery and draining abscesses, and for the removal and replacement of vertebral bodies. It was extended upward and developed for microsurgery of clivus tumors by Stevenson et al.[34] Verbiest, with modifications of his own, uses the extensive anterolateral approach for his "lateral" approach to the cervical spine.[4]

However, in 1973 and 1975 we presented a description and anatomic drawings of an exposure to the front and side of the cervical spine, which allows visualization of the anterior arch of the first cervical vertebra, anterior structures of the remainder of the cervical spine, and the base of the skull. It was demonstrated to Dr. Lee Riley and myself[32,33] by Dr. Robert Chambers, a head and neck surgeon, and has been used to achieve the exposure necessary to perform excision of lesions of the upper cervical spine and fusion of the first, second, and third vertebral segments.[17]

A tracheotomy must be performed and anesthesia maintained through the tracheotomy. The incision is begun just to the left of the midline in the submandibular area, carried posteriorly to the angle of the mandible, then gently curved lateral to the posterior border of the sternomastoid muscle to the base of the neck, and finally curved anteriorly and inferiorly, crossing the clavicle and ending in the suprasternal space. The incision is developed through the platysma muscle and the skin and muscle flap so outlined is retracted medially to expose the sternomastoid and strap muscles, the pharynx, the thyroid gland, the edge of the mandible, and the submaxillary triangle. The anterior surface of the lower cervical spine is identified by reflecting the sternomastoid muscle and carotid sheath laterally, transecting the omohyoid muscle in its tendinous portion, incising the prevertebral fasciae in the midline, and retracting the prevertebral fasciae, thyroid gland, esophagus, and trachea medially. Development of this plane superiorly however is impeded by the superior thyroid artery, the superior laryngeal neurovascular bundle, the hypoglossal nerve, the stylohyoid muscle, and the digastric muscle. The superior thyroid artery should be ligated and divided, the stylohyoid muscle and digastric muscle divided and reflected, and the superior laryngeal nerve and hypoglossal nerve identified and protected. When this has been done, the larynx and pharynx may be retracted medially, the external carotid artery laterally, and the floor of the submaxillary triangle retracted superiorly, so that the base of the skull and the anterior arch of the first cervical vertebra can be visualized. If further exposure is required, it is provided by excising the submaxillary gland and anterior dislocation of the temporal mandibular joint, which is easily performed manually with the patient anesthetized, permitting rotation of the mandible superiorly and to the right side of the patient. Complete exposure of the anterior arch of the first cervical vertebra, the odontoid process, and both vertebral arteries may now be obtained.

Anterior fusion at C1-3 is accomplished by cutting a trough in the anterior aspect of the second and third vertebral bodies to the level of the posterior cortex of the odontoid process and removing the cancellous bone from the odontoid process with a small curette, converting it into a hollow shell surrounded by cortical bone. A bone graft is then cut from the anterior iliac crest and shaped to the dimensions of the previously constructed trough in the anterior aspects of the vertebral bodies of the second and third cervical vertebrae. The superior end of the bone graft is shaped to resemble a saddle or clothespin, with one protrusion of the *clothespin* being fitted into the odontoid process and the other protrusion cradling the anterior arch of the first cervical vertebra. The distal end is locked into the trough in the bodies of the second and third cervical vertebrae. A loop of heavy, braided silk suture is placed through the caudal portion of the bone graft and through the cortex of the second and third vertebral bodies. The graft is tied into place to prevent anterior displacement of the caudal portion of the bone graft.

Exposure of the Transverse Processes, Pedicles, and Vertebral Artery from the Third through the Seventh Cervical Segments

This is achieved through a skin incision which begins behind the junction of the upper and middle third of the sternocleidomastoid muscle, runs down to the junction of the middle and lower thirds along the posterior border of the sternomastoid muscle and then swings anteriorly to the suprasternal notch.[32] The incision is deepened to the platysma muscle, which is then grasped between forceps at the lateral limb of the incision, bluntly elevated from the underlying structures, and divided in line with the skin incision. The anterior and posterior borders of the sternomastoid muscle must be clearly demonstrated. The deep surface of the sternomastoid muscle is freed from the underlying structures so that it is possible to pass a finger under the sternomastoid muscle, which is then sharply divided and retracted superiorly and inferiorly. The omohyoid muscle, lying deep to the sternomastoid, is divided and retracted in a similar fashion. This brings into view the anterior scalene muscle, the phrenic nerve lying on the anterior surface of the anterior scalene muscle, and the cords of the brachial plexus emerging from under the lateral border of the anterior scalene muscle. The phrenic nerve is mobilized throughout the limits of the incision and may be gently retracted anteriorly. The medial and lateral borders of the anterior scalene muscle are identified and mobilized. Great care must be exercised at this stage of the exposure to prevent damage to the cords of the brachial plexus as they emerge from under the lateral border of the anterior scalene muscle. The brachial plexus must be identified and protected. The anterior scalene muscle is then sharply divided, approximately 1 inch inferior to the site of desired exposure, and the entire superior portion of the muscle is excised. Care must be taken to avoid damage to the vertebral artery as it passes between the bony foramen and the transverse processes of the second through sixth cervical vertebrae, as the slips of origin of the anterior scalene muscle are dissected from the anterior tubercles of the transverse processes. If the pedicles are to be exposed, the vertebral artery should be identified and controlled with tapes placed about it proximal and distal to the site of desired exposure. With sharp dissection, the longus colli muscle is reflected medially and any remaining fibers of the scalene muscle reflected distally and laterally to expose the transverse processes in their entirety as well as the uncovertebral joint, the pedicle, the neural foramen, and the emerging nerve root.

Closure is effected by leaving a drain to the level of the resected portion of the anterior scalene muscle and reapproximating the omohyoid, the sternomastoid, and the platysma muscles. The skin edges should be approximated with fine interrupted sutures, which may be removed on the third postoperative day.

There are also lateral approaches to the cervical spine. One approach was described by Barber.[35] It is a lateral approach to the joint between C1 and C2 by an incision below the mastoid process on either side of the neck. E. Simmons[36] of Toronto will soon report his experience with this lateral approach for fusion of C1 to C2.

Another lateral approach to C2-3 through C6-7 is one reported by Verbiest.[14,22,37] It is really one that involves the deep rather than the superficial (eg., skin incision) approach to the intervertebral foramina of the cervical spine and the posterior aspects of the vertebral bodies through the intervertebral foramina, procedures that can be carried out through the exposures reported by Robinson and Riley [9,33] and by Riley.[32]

Verbiest discusses such lateral transforaminal surgery for a vareity of clinical problems[14,37] through this approach. He specifically discusses the advantages and dangers of direct lateral removal of bony spurs and disc protrusions by mobilizing the vertebral artery from the transverse process of the cervical vertebrae as described by Henry.[38] Part or all of the transverse process were removed, on occasion,[22] and then osseous and discal material protrusions that may be compressing the vascular and neural tissue in the intervertebral foramina and more medially on the anterior and anterolateral face of the spinal canal through the intervertebral foramen, as recommended by Jung.

Remarks

Throughout the writings concerning indications for neck surgery during the past 25 years, there has been some basic disagreement among authors, which I believe is due to a lack of understanding of one outstanding feature of the biology of living bone—its ability to constantly remodel.

In my approach to bony protrusions (actually osseous-cartilaginous protrusions) that irritate vascular and neural tissue when they move (eg., lateral spurs from the edges of vertebral bodies), or neural tissue, it appears to me that two etiologic factors responsible for the development of such osseocartilaginous protrusions or spurs are: (a) a degenerated disc and (b) residual motion at the motion level of that disc.

My attack on the problem is very simple. I remove the degenerated disc (that is, whatever is left of it), and then, with a bone graft, increase the height of the disc cavity to take any buckling out of the posterior longitudinal ligament, and the ligamentum flavum; increase the vertical dimension of the intervertebral foramen, and stop motion.

I try to limit the patient's activity until there is true osseous fusion between the two vertebrae in the motion segment that has had the fusion operation. Once solid bone fusion is achieved, the remodelling process takes over and spurs are resorbed by this process in 9 to 18 months.

Therefore I have seldom used the intraforaminal approaches, used by Jung and by Verbiest,[22] to remove spurs. Neither do I use Cloward's[16] method to remove bone spurs from the edges of vertebral bodies contiguous to a degenerate intervertebral disc. I am more interested in the effect of immobilization of bone spurs by solid osseous interbody fusion and the subsequent effect of the bone remodeling process on those cartilaginous-osseous protrusions called *bone spurs*.

On the other hand, to remove malignant or benign tumors of the cervical spine that constantly compress neural or vascular tissue, any and all combinations of the approaches discussed and listed in the bibliography of this paper are important.

REFERENCES

1. Jung A: Resection de l'articulation unco-vertebrale et ouverture de trou de conjugaison par voie auterieure dons le traitement de la neuralgie cervico brachiale. Technique operatoire. Mem Acad. Chir *89*:361, 1963
2. Walker AE: *A History of Neurological Surgery.* (Facsimile of 1951 Edition) Hafner, New York, 1967, p 366
3. Forsyth HF, Alexander ED, Davis C, et al: The advantages of early spine fusion in the treatment of fracture dislocation of the cervical spine. *J Bone Joint Surg 41A*:17-36, 1959
4. McGraw RW, Rusch RM: Atlanto-axial arthrodesis. *J Bone Joint Surg 55B*:482-489, 1973
5. Perry J, Nickel VL, Downey MD: Total cervical spine fusion for neck paralysis. *J Bone Joint Surg 41A*:37-59, 1959
6. Rogers WA: Treatment of fracture-dislocation of the cervical spine. *J Bone Joint Surg 24*:245-258, 1942
7. Rogers WA: Fractures and dislocations of the cervical spine. *J Bone Joint Surg 39A*:341-376, 1957
8. Robinson RA: Anterior and posterior cervical spine fusions. *Clin Orthop 35*:34-62, 1964
9. Robinson RA, Riley LH: Techniques of exposure and fusion of the cervical spine. *Clin Orthop 109*:78-84, 1975
10. Robinson RA, Southwick WO: Indications and techniques for early stabilization of the neck in some fracture dislocations of the cervical spine. *South Med J 53*:565-579, 1960
11. Scoville WB: Discussion: The anterior approach for removal of ruptured disks. *J Neurosurg 15*:615, 1958
12. Scoville, WB: Types of cervical disk lesions and their surgical approaches. *JAMA 196*:49-481, 1966
13. Robinson RA, Southwick WO: Surgical approaches to the cervical spine: Instruction Course Lectures of the American Academy of Orthopedic Surgeons. Vol. 17. CV Mosby, St Louis, 1960, pp 299-330
14. Verbiest H: Anterolateral operations for fractures and dislocations in the middle and lower parts of the cervical spine. *J Bone Joint Surg 51A*:1489-1531, 1969
15. Bailey RW, Badgley CE: Stabilization of the cervical spine by anterior fusion. *J Bone Joint Surg 42A*:565-594, 1960

16. Cloward RB: The anterior approach for ruptured cervical disks. *J Neurosurg 15*:602-614, 1958
17. Dereymaeker A, Mulier J: Nouvelle cure neurochirurgicale des discopathies cervicales. *Neurochirurgie 2*:233-234, 1956
18. Robinson RA, Smith GW: Antero-lateral cervical disc removal and interbody fusion for the cervical disc syndrome. *Bull Johns Hopkins Hosp 96*:223-224, 1955
19. Robinson RA, Walker AE, Ferlic DC, et al: The results of anterior interbody fusion of the cervical spine. *J Bone Joint Surg 44A*:1569-1587, 1962
20. Smith GW, Robinson RA: The treatment of certain cervical spine disorders by anterior removal of the intervertebral disc and interbody fusion. *J Bone Joint Surg 40A*:607-624, 1958
21. Southwick WO, Robinson RA: Surgical approaches to the vertebral bodies in the cervical and lumbar regions. *J Bone Joint Surg 39A*:631-643, 1957
22. Verbiest H: La chirurgia anterieure et laterale du rachis cervical. Suppl 2, Tome 16, Neuro-Chirurgie. Paris VI e, 120 Boulevard Saint Germaine, Masson et cie, Mai 1970
23. Boudot L: Des resections des apophyses transverses des vertebres. These, Strasbourg, No. 812, 1964
24. Chien J: Retropharyngeal abscess. *Br Med J 2*:255-256, 1877
25. Cheyne WW: Case of retropharyngeal abscess pointing in the pharynx but opened by an incision behind the sternomastoid cure. *Med Times Gaz 2*:254, 1881
26. Burckhardt H: Ueber die eröffnung der retropharyngealen abscesse. Zentralblatt Chir *15*:57-60, 1888
27. Auffret C: Intervention dans les lesions du rachis. *Arch Med Navale 66*:435-450, 1896
28. Küttner H: Die verletzungen und traumatischen aneurysmen der vertebralisgefässe am halse und ihre operative behandlung. *Beit Klin Chir 108*:1-60, 1917
29. Lahey FH: The technique of the two stage operation for Pulsion Oesophageal diverticulum. *Surg Gynecol Obstet 43*:359-365, 1926
30. Fang HSY, Ong GB: Direct anterior approach to the upper cervical spine. *J Bone Joint Surg 44A*:1588-1604, 1962
31. Riley LH: Cervical disc surgery: its role and indications. *Symposium on Disease of the Intervertebral Disc,* Orthopaedic Clinics of North America. WB Saunders, Philadelphia, 1971, pp 443-452
32. Riley LH: Surgical approaches to the anterior structures of the cervical spine. *Clin Orthop 91*:16-20, 1973
33. Robinson RA, Riley LH: Anterior interbody fusion of the cervical spine, chap. 144. *The Craft of Surgery.* Second edition. Little Brown and Co, Boston, 1971, pp 1873-1881
34. Stevenson GC, Stoney RJ, Perkins RK, et al: A transcervical transclival approach to the ventral surface of the brain stem for removal of a clivus chordoma. *J Neurosurg 24*:544-551, 1966
35. Barber: *Extensile Exposure.* Second edition. Williams and Wilkins, Baltimore, 1957, pp 58-66.
36. Simmons EH: Personal Communication, 1975
37. Verbiest, H: A lateral approach to the cervical spine: technique and indications. *J Neurosurg 28*:191-203, 1968
38. Henry AK: *Extensile Exposure.* Second edition. Williams and Wilkins, Baltimore, 1957, pp 58-72

CHAPTER 23

The Anterolateral Approach to the Cervical Spine in the Management of Cervical Spondylosis and Its Complications

Henry H. Schmidek

OVER THE PAST TWO DECADES operations have been devised in which a direct anterior or anterolateral approach has been used to gain access to the spine from the base of the skull to the sacrum. This inventiveness has been particularly apparent with regard to the surgical management of disorders of the cervical spine.[1] In the neck, anterior approaches have undergone constant redevelopment and reassessment so that they could be used to treat cervical disc disease, cervical fractures, tumors, and infections of the body of the vertebrae. At the present time at least a half dozen variations of the anterior approach have been fashioned.[2-8] All allow access to the ventral aspect of the dura, the nerve root sheaths, and the vertebral arteries, and all provide for considerable flexibility in the approach available to remove lesions that impinge on these structures or are associated with spinal instability. Not only do they allow for the removal of extruded cartilage or bony overgrowth, but they can be used with the supine position during surgery and with dissection in avascular planes. Their associated low morbidity has resulted in their widespread acceptance in the treatment of sequelae of cervical spondylosis.

The anterolateral approaches to the cervical spine originated in the desire to help those afflicted with tuberculosis of the spine. To reach the usual site of these lesions the vertebral bodies had to be approached anteriorly. This approach was then applied to the treatment of cervical disc disease associated with radiculopathy and myelopathy. This application began with the reports of Robinson[9-11] and of Cloward[5,6,12] in the 1960s and has become a part of the standard neurosurgical armamentarium. This is easy to understand, since changes associated with cervical spondylosis are situated ventral to neurovascular structures within the spine. With the anterolateral approach, these structures can be directly decompressed.

Department of Neurosurgery, Hahnemann Medical College and Hospital, Philadelphia, Pennsylvania 19102

Surgical Indications

Cervical disc disease often involves several levels of the spine, although it is seen most often at C4-5, C5-6, and C6-7. As the disc degenerates its nucleus is affected first and begins to bulge transversely. The patient may then experience neck and arm pain. The *painful disc syndrome* has been defined as a mechanical pain in the neck, shoulders, and arm, often with subjective numbness in a dermatome. In the early stages of the disc's deterioration, pain may develop when the fibers of the annulus or adjacent structures, such as the anterior and posterior ligaments, become stretched. In these cases standard radiographic studies remain normal but discography may help to identify the particular disc responsible for the patient's symptoms.

Further degeneration leads to cracks and fissures of the disc, which may extend into the joints of Lushka; nuclear material may be extruded into these joints, beneath or through the posterior longitudinal ligament or through the cartilagenous plates into the vertebral bodies. Changes in the cartilage further interfere with nutrition of the disc, contributing to its degeneration. Radiographically the disc space is now narrowed and the spine is slightly shortened. Sliding movements between the vetebrae and alterations in the bone adjacent to the disc develop. The end of the vertebral body mushrooms and expands and bony outgrowths develop around the periphery, due to periosteal activity provoked by the abnormal direction and stresses on lamellar fibers. Osteophytes develop around the lateral margins of the vertebrae.

Surgical decompression is appropriate in cervical radiculopathy with subjective and objective evidence of nerve root compression in which conservative treatment, involving adequate sedation and analgesics, traction, and physical therapy, fails. As mentioned by Scoville et al.,[13] unrelenting symptoms should usually be present for a 3- to 4-week period, although some patients who experience severe pain and neurologic deficit require operation shortly after their symptoms start. Cervical traction often accentuates their discomfort, and inevitably a large disc fragment is found to be responsible for their problem (Fig. 23-1).

Spondylotic Myelopathy

This entity often occurs in patients who have a narrower than normal canal (normal: 17 ± 5 mm with a 6 ft tube → film distance) and in whom osteophytes and ligamentous hypertrophy further compromise the size of the canal.[1] The pathogenesis of the disease remains uncertain. Compression of the cord by disc material or traction of the cord against osteophytes are etiologically important, particularly in the case of an acute myelopathy, eg., associated with traumatic disc protrusion. However in chronic myelopathy the factors of disc degeneration, spur formation, foraminal encroachment, and a congenitally narrow canal are probably potentiated by motion at the involved level. It may be that the motion results in the progression of signs and symptoms.

Studies of the vascular supply of the spinal cord[14] have shown a large radicular artery analogous to Adamkiewicz from C6-7, and in some cases a watershed area may exist in the cord at C4. Zulch has noted, in a few cases, that following a C5-6 fracture dislocation, there may be extensive necrosis from C4 → T4, corresponding to the vascular supply in the cord. Whether or not compromise of this radicular vessel is important in some cases of myelopathy is not known. Acute myelopathy secondary to anterior spinal artery thrombosis is very rare and does not explain the progression seen in chronic myelpathy. It may be that secondary to the spondylotic changes, and the distortion and flattening of the cord, there is distortion of its intrinsic arterioles and the subsequent compromise of the cord's feeding or intrinsic vessels, leading to vascular insufficiency of the cord. It has been suggested, by Robinson,[15] that the stepwise progression of neurologic deficit characteristically seen in certain cases with cervi-

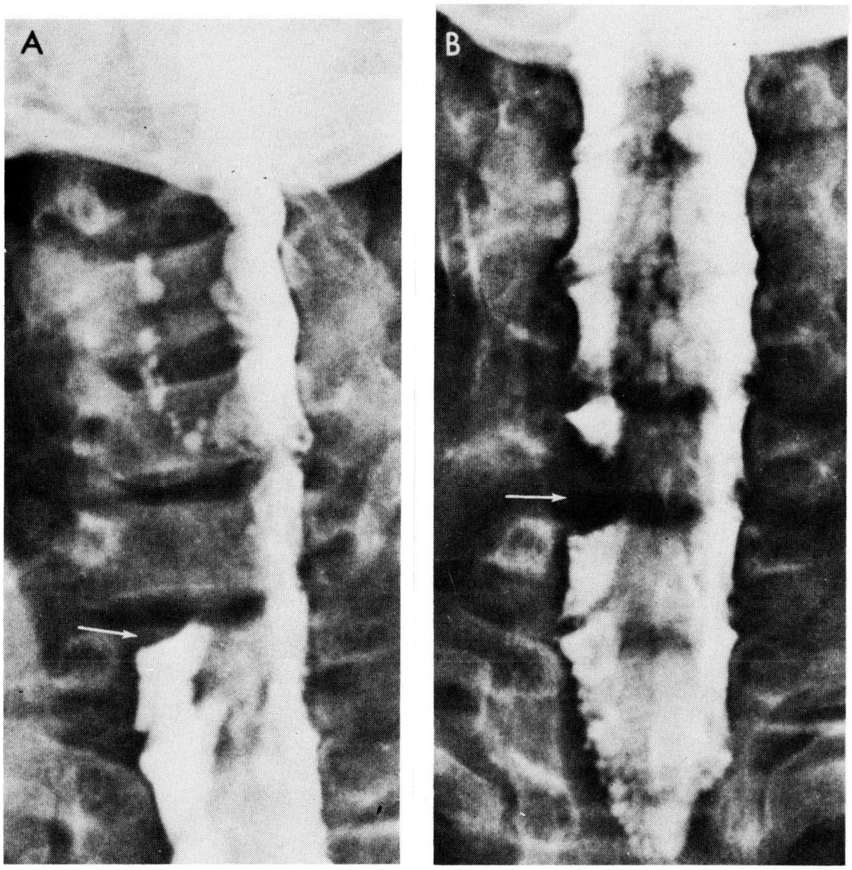

Fig. 23-1. Cervical myelogram showing laterally situated free disc fragment in patient with intractable radiculopathy.

cal spondylotic myelopathy actually represents repeated small infarctions within the cord substance.

Cervical spondylotic myelopathy was identified and characterized as a distinct entity in the classic paper by Clarke and Robinson,[16] who reviewed the case histories of 120 patients with myelopathy and evidence of spinal cord compression on myelography. They noted that although complete remission was never seen, regression occurred in 2. Of their 120 cases, 75% had a series of episodes with progression, 20% were steadily and slowly progressive, and 5% had a rapid onset of findings, with a plateauing prior to further deterioration at a later date. It was also noted that of 22 patients managed nonoperatively, 16 were treated with a neck brace alone. In 8 of the 16 patients, walking, the ability to dress, and radicular signs in the arms improved, strikingly so in 2. Although the remaining patients did not improve, neither did their disease progress.

At a later date Lees and Turner[17] and Balla et al.[18] also attempted to define the natural history of cervical myelopathy. In Lees' series deterioration often ceased after the first few years; other patients experienced remissions lasting for years and then became worse. Progression and recurrence were particularly evident in patients with a congenitally narrow canal. Balla et al.[18] in a series of 123 patients followed for up to 10 years found that without treatment 52% improved, 35% remained unchanged, and 13% became worse.

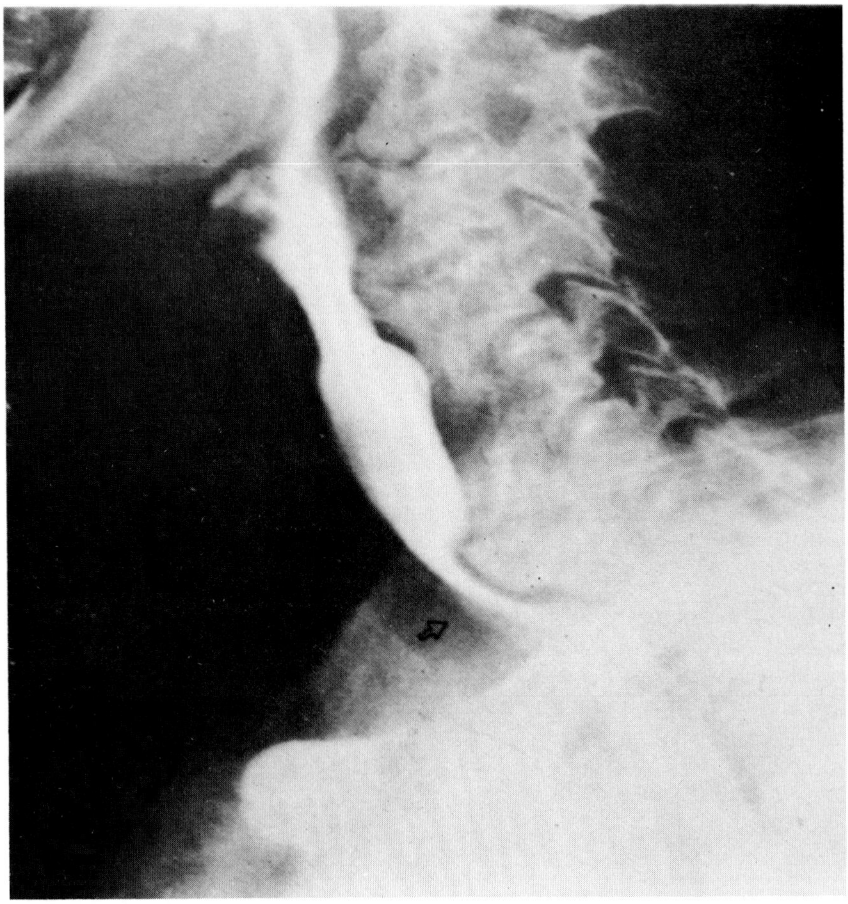

Fig. 23-2. Cervical osteophyte in a patient with dysphagia.

Dysphagia

Compression of the esophagus or hypopharynx by osteophytes has been reported in the literature since 1926. A review, in 1960, reported 36 cases of dysphagia associated with osteophytes.[19] In 1971 Maran and Jacobson[20] reported the tenth case treated surgically. These authors also advocated interbody fusion in addition to excision of the osteophyte to prevent recurrent spur formation at the involved level.[21,22]

Compression of the hypopharynx is not experienced as dysphagia but as a lump in the throat and is seen with osteophyte compression above C6. Cervical osteophytes have been reported along the entire cervical spine, with C5-6 being the most common site. In two-thirds of the cases one level is involved and in the remaining one-third, osteophytes at several levels contribute to the symptoms. Surgical removal of the exostosis is usually not indicated, although with persistent symptomatology the lesion can be excised by the anterolateral approach (Fig. 23-2).

Vertebral Artery Compression

Osteophytes projecting into the vertebral canal or subluxation of adjacent vertebrae has been reported to cause vertebral artery compression. To be clinically significant, this compression must involve the carotid and vertebral arteries to the extent that narrowing of a single vertebral artery impairs blood flow to the brain stem. Hutchinson and Yates[23] have shown that the effect of vertebral artery compression by osteophytes can be enhanced by rotating the head or extending the neck, which may result in giddiness or drop attacks. However, these symptoms may also occur in the absence of head movement. Disease of this kind is exceedingly rare, and in his entire experience Fisher[24] has seen only a single case in which it may have been appropriate to remove an osteophyte that compressed the vertebral artery. This was not done, however, since the patient suffered a major stroke at the time of angiography. To date I have not seen a case in which surgery would have been suggested as useful to relieve these symptoms.

Diagnostic Evaluation

Investigations of cervical spondylosis involve not only standard roentgenograms but flexion and extension views of the spine to obtain evidence of spinal stability. The musculature of the cervical region, the ligamentous structures, especially the ligamentum nuchae and posterior longitudinal ligament, and the bond between vertebral bodies due to the discs, are major factors responsible for the stability of the cervical spine. White et al.[25] (Figs. 23-3 and 23-4) in a recent biomechanical study of adult cadaver spines, have shown that the ligaments normally permit very little motion between vertebrae and that horizontal motions (greater than 3.5 mm) of one vertebral body on another, as seen on plain lateral roentgenograms, indicate instability. If the angulation of one vertebral body with respect to another is 11° greater than the angulation of adjacent vertebrae and the vertebral body is not compressed,

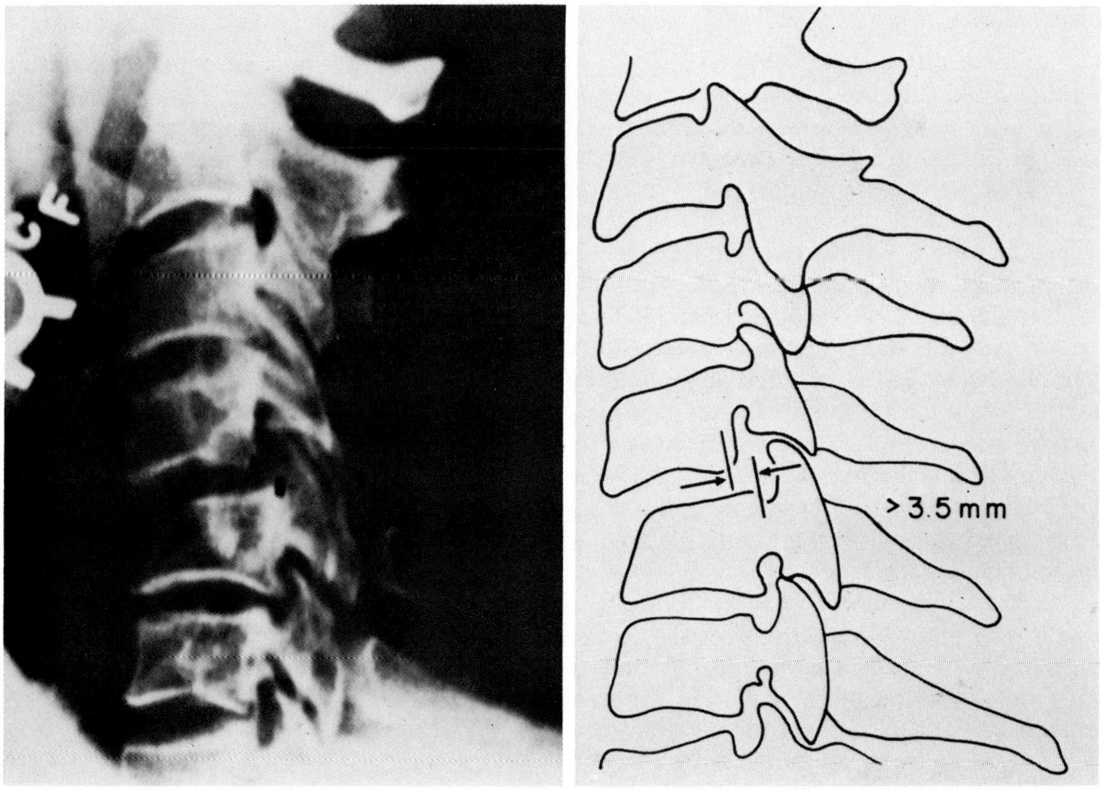

Fig. 23-3.

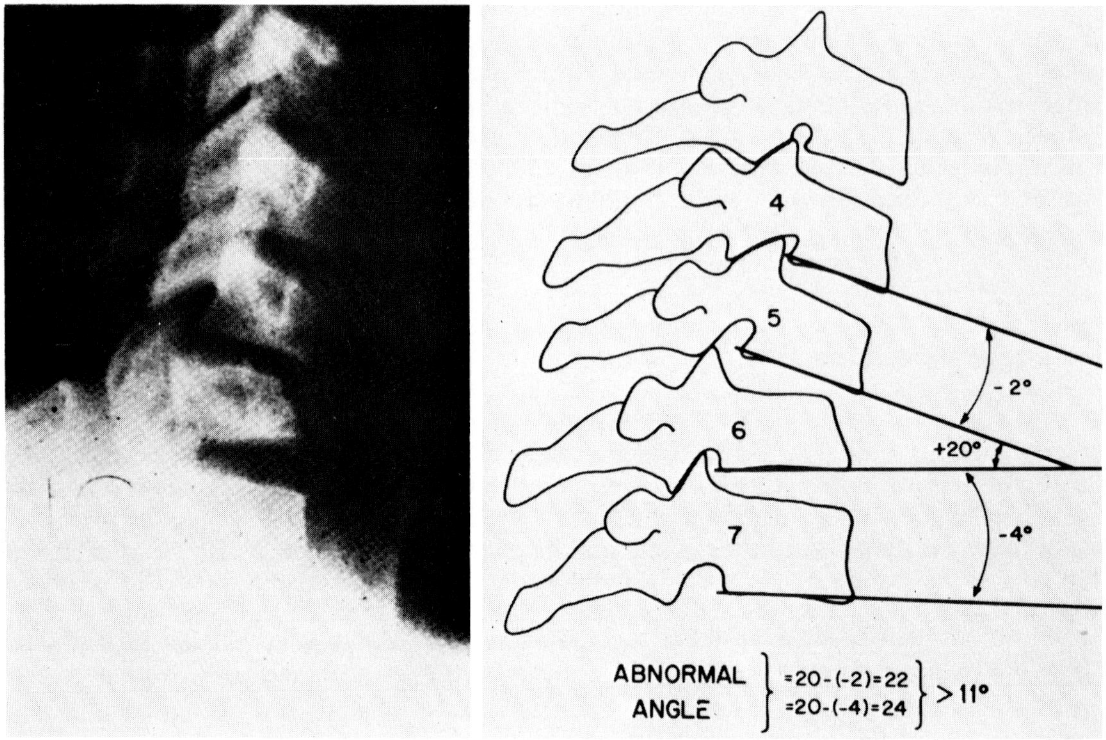

Fig. 23-4.

the spine is relatively unstable. A major number of ligaments must be injured to permit motion exceeding these limits and most spines begin to fail under physiologic loads when these displacements are exceeded. The instability causes the spine to lose its ability to move without further deformity, excessive pain, and potential neurologic worsening.

With rare exception, cervical myelography is performed preoperatively. The neurologic examination alone does not provide all information required preoperatively to plan an appropriate operation. With severe myelopathy a lateral C1-2 puncture is preferable to instilling the dye or air by the lumbar route, since the study will not require hyperextension of the cervical spine, which results in maximal impingement on the cord and has been associated with neurologic worsening following standard myelography. Air myelography is used in patients who may be allergic to the iodine in contrast media and is probably superior to Pantopaque for studies of a myelopathic process. Since air fills both the dorsal and ventral subarachnoid spaces, cord compression, if it exists or is accentuated by neck flexion and extension, is readily detectable. Metrizimide (Squibb), a water-soluble contrast medium, is currently being used abroad, but only experimentally in the United States. This radiopaque agent has an advantage in that dorsal and ventral aspects of the spinal subarachnoid space can be seen during myelography.

Electromyography provides additional *objective* evidence of root compression in patients with relatively minor neurologic findings. It is also important in differentiating root, plexus, peripheral nerve, and muscle disorders, which, in early stages, may mimic cervical radiculopathy. This study may also help to uncover a second problem that may coexist with radiculopathy, eg., carpal tunnel syndrome.

Discography involves injections of saline and local anesthetic into the disc and is used in the patient with painful cervical disc syndrome with a suggestive history, mild objective findings, and otherwise normal radiographs.[25]

Angiography to demonstrate cerebral vasculature is occasionally warranted and should include a survey of both intra- and extracranial vessels for a comprehensive evaluation of cerebral circulation. This should be done in conjunction with head turning to determine whether this maneuver further compromises flow in the vertebral artery and reproduces symptoms.

Computerized tomography of the cervical spine is not yet widely available but preliminary results in bony pathology is very encouraging. This procedure will add another new dimension to investigations of spinal disorders.

Surgical Anatomy

Even though the anterolateral exposure to the cervical spine has been previously described, it is worth reviewing the following anatomic points. The anterior approach is easiest along the anterior margin of the sternomastoid and medial to the carotid sheath (Fig. 23-5). The incision may be centered by noting the hyoid bone at the level of C3, the thyroid cartilage opposite C4, and the cricoid opposite the level of C6 (Fig. 23-6).

Dissection is carried out in avascular planes, passing through the pretracheal fascia first and then the prevertebral fascia. The longus colli muscles, covering the lateral parts of the vertebral body, the vertebral canal, and the transverse processes, can then be seen (Fig. 23-7). These muscles extend from the atlas to the body of T3 and are a major factor in the stability of the cervical spine. There is no muscle covering the anterior aspect of the vertebrae in the midline (Fig. 23-8). The cervical sympathetic chain lies on the longus colli muscles and extends from C2 to T1 (Fig. 23-8). Since a Horner's syndrome will result from damage to sympathetic nerve fibers, it is important to retract the longus colli, starting at its medial edge.

The anterior longitudinal ligament is a strong band that extends from the base of the skull to the sacrum (Fig. 23-9). It is thickest in its midportion, tapers laterally, and is bound to the anterior annulus, functioning to limit the extension of the spine. The posterior longitudinal ligament also extends as a thick band, from the skull to the sacrum, between the posterior annulus and the dura. Since the ligament does not extend laterally over the nerve roots, its normally thick portion, which prevents disc material from extruding into the spinal canal, is absent, permitting disc material to enter the foramen. Functionally this ligament limits flexion of the spine.

Physiologically the ligamentum flavum does not compress the dura or spinal cord; however as elasticity is lost, the ligamentum buckles, compressing the spinal cord.

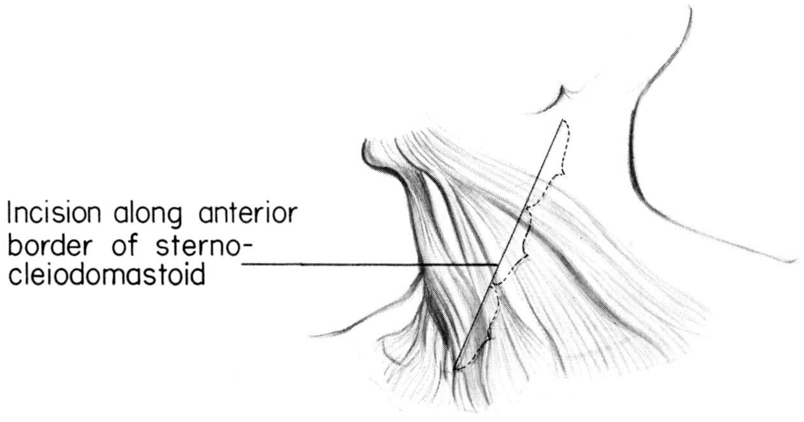

Fig. 23-5.

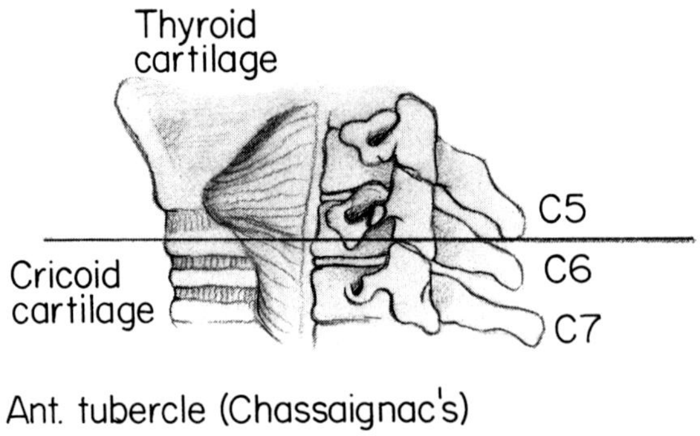

Fig. 23-6.

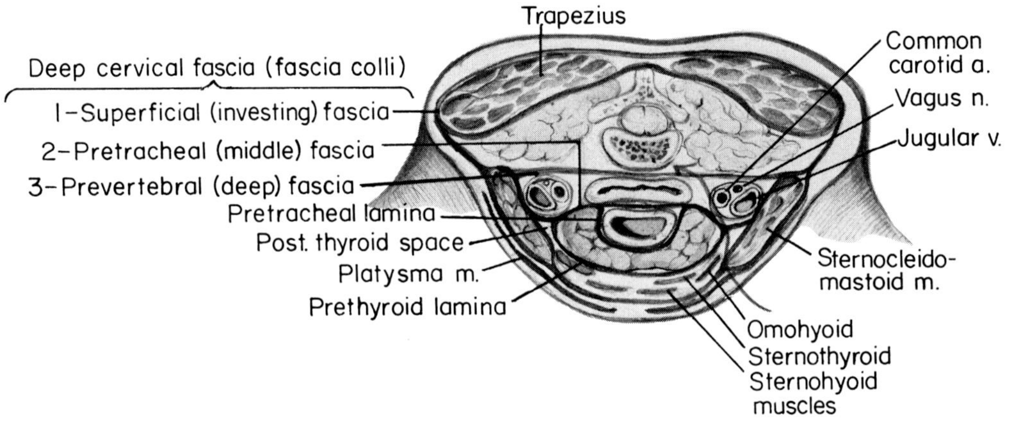

Fig. 23-7. Cross section representation at C5 level of spine indicating fascial planes and avascular surgical approach to the anterior spine.

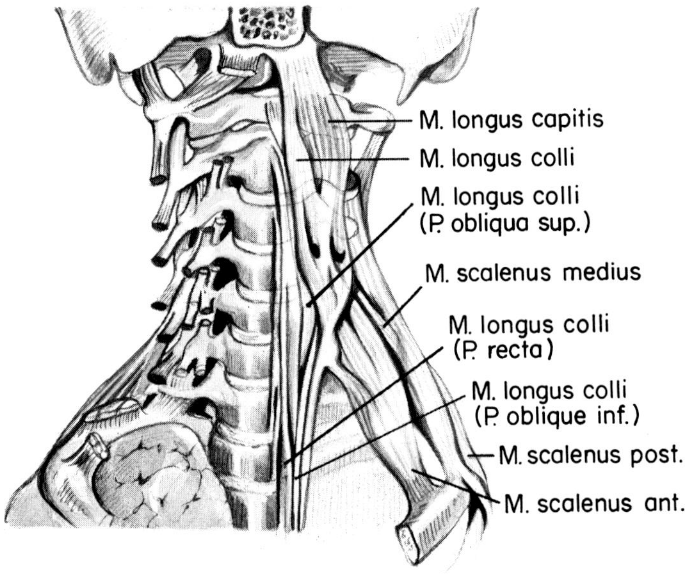

Fig. 23-8. Relationships of anterior cervical musculature to the cervical spine.

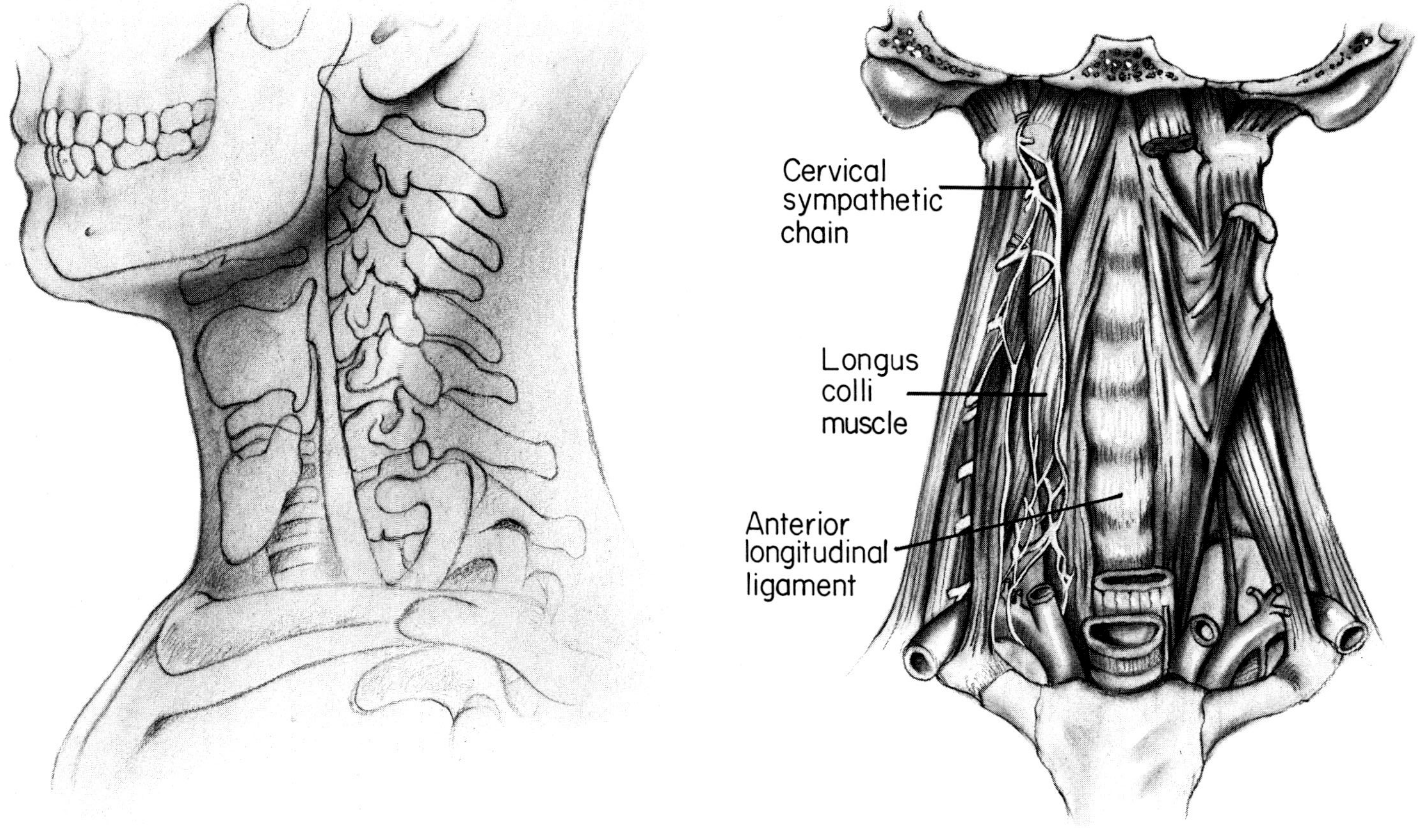

Fig. 23-9. Illustration showing relationship of the cervical sympathetic chain, anterior spine musculature, and anterior longitudinal ligament to the spine.

The left recurrent laryngeal branch of the vagus nerve arises at the level of the aortic arch, loops beneath the arch, and then passes between the trachea and esophagus to reach the larynx. On the right side, the recurrent laryngeal nerve has an inconstant course; it usually descends within the carotid sheath, looping beneath the subclavian artery to reach the larynx between the trachea and esophagus. The nerve may have one of several aberrant courses, leaving the carotid sheath at a higher level. To avoid injury to an aberrant right recurrent laryngeal nerve, it is preferable to operate on the left side of the neck, irrespective of the side of radicular symptoms.

Surgical Procedure

The patient is placed in the supine position on an operating table. Under general anesthesia, the neck may be stabilized by 5 lb of traction applied through a head halter, and is moderately hyperextended by placing a roll beneath the shoulder blades until the occiput just clears the table. The head is turned about 10° to the right. After the patient is draped, the carotid bifurcation is injected with local anesthetic to block the carotid baroreceptor mechanism.

Dissection is then carried out with headlight illumination and magnifying loupes of 3.5 to 4.5X.

Before dissection is started, a lateral cervical scout roentgenogram is taken to insure adequate radiographic technique, and a needle is placed on the spine to localize the interspace to be operated upon.

The procedure is routinely performed through a transverse or longitudinal skin incision on the left side, centered over the anterior border of the sternomastoid muscle and the segment of spine to be exposed (Figs. 23-4 and 23-5). When more than one level is to be operated upon, the vertical incision is most often used, since different types of anterior and lateral operations on cervical vertebral bodies and intervertebral discs, transverse processes, and vertebral arteries can be carried out without undue traction.

When the platysma muscle has been exposed, it is grasped between forceps and incised parallel to the anterior margin of the sternomastoid. The underlying sternomastoid muscle is then visible (Fig. 23-10). The anterior border of the sternomastoid muscle must be clearly identified and mobilized throughout the limits of exposure so that the medial border of the sternomastoid muscle can be retracted laterally to expose the middle layer of the cervical fascia. The omohyoid muscle can be seen crossing the field at about the C5-6 level and may be retracted or transected in its midtendinous segment. The carotid sheath is then identified. An avascular plane is developed through the cervical fascia, medial and parallel to the carotid sheath. The carotid sheath and the sternomastoid muscle are retracted laterally (Fig. 23-11). As this is done, the anterior surface of the cervical spine is seen. The esophagus and trachea are retracted medially. The prevertebral fascia is cauterized with the Malis bipolar cautery and incised longitudinally in the midline of the neck, exposing the underlying anterior longitudinal ligament. The medial aspect of the longus colli muscles are identified and then cauterized for a length corresponding to the discs to be exposed (Fig. 23-12). This helps to keep the wound essentially bloodless. The disc space at the highest level of the field is marked with a fine needle and a cross-table lateral cervical spine roentgenogram is obtained for exact localization. An excellent anatomic landmark is the bony promontory on the transverse processes of C6, the *carotid tubercle*. This is opposite the vertebral body of C6, and the intervertebral disc between C5 and C6 vertebral bodies can thus be spotted for placement of the needle.

After the levels to be operated upon have been established, Cloward blades are placed beneath the previously cauterized medial edges of the longus colli muscles (Fig. 23-13). This is probably the single, most important maneuver in the operation and failure to correctly

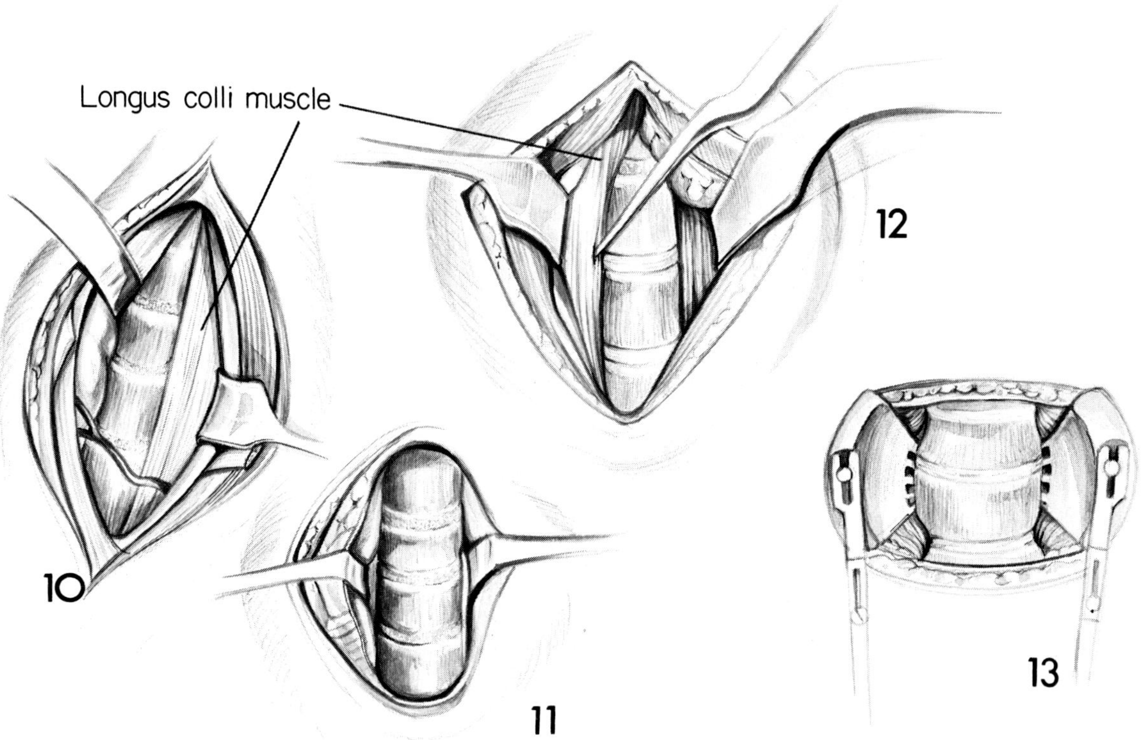

Figs. 23-10 and 11. View of the anterior spine after medial retraction of trachea and esophagus and lateral retraction of the carotid sheath and its contents.
Fig. 23-12. Cauterization of the medial aspects of the longus colli muscles prior to placement of Cloward retractor blades.
Fig. 23-13. Position of Cloward blades beneath longus colli muscles.

position the blades is responsible for many of the reported complications associated with this operation. When the vertical incision is used, it is unnecessary to use the horizontal blades of the Cloward set, also reducing postoperative retraction-related morbidity.

The margins of the disc to be entered are cauterized and the disc incised (Fig. 23-14). It is often necessary to remove the bony spurs, overhanging the disc space, from the upper vertebra before significant amounts of intervertebral disc can be removed. Once the anterior

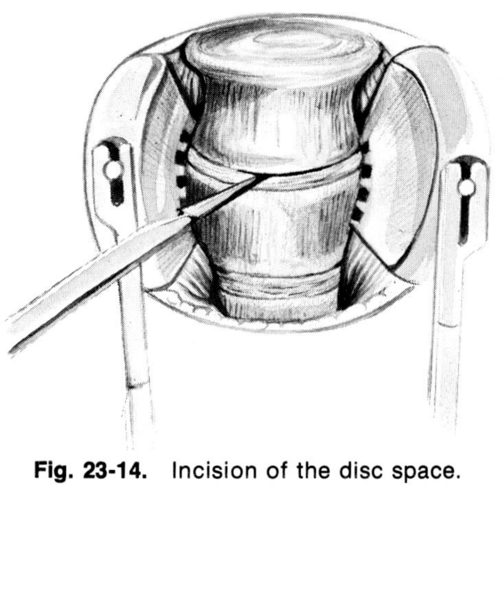

Fig. 23-14. Incision of the disc space.

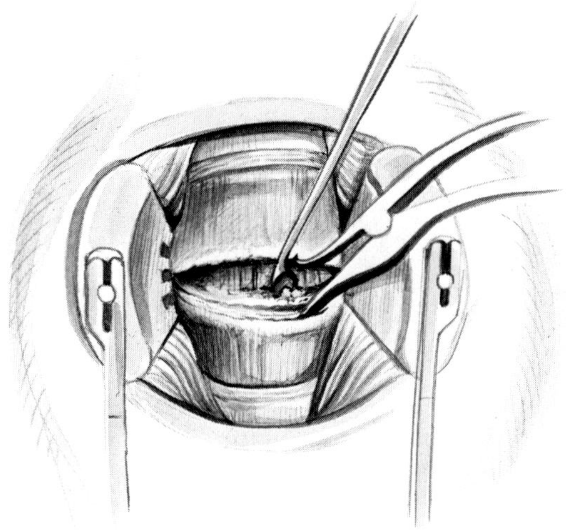

Fig. 23-15. Removal of interspace contents and placement of the intervertebral spreader.

one-half to two-thirds of the disc and the cartilagenous plates have been removed, the disc-space spreader is introduced between the bodies (Fig. 23-15). Dissection to this point is performed under 3.5 to 4.5X loupes. The procedure may then be completed at 6 to 15X magnification, using the microscope.

Under magnification, the remainder of the disc is excised to the posterior longitudinal ligament, which is seen as a structure with glistening yellowish-white vertically aligned fibers (Fig. 23-16A, B, and C). The remaining cartilage and disc is removed with fine curettes. The posterior ligament is removed when there is an otherwise inaccessible large fragment beneath it or in the presence of severe cord compression. The defect can often be seen in the posterior ligament, through which a fragment of disc is extruding. Lateral dissection will expose the uncovertebral joints and the dura, which are no longer covered by the posterior longitudinal ligament (Fig. 23-17A and B).

Using a 20° angled drill, the osteophytes above and below the disc space are carefully removed.

If a fusion is to be performed, a horseshoe-shaped plug of bone with three cortical edges, is taken from the ilium, using a reciprocating saw with blades 8 to 10 mm apart. The graft is countersunk in the disc space and a lateral cervical film taken to check its position (Fig. 23-18). The wound is irrigated and a 1.0-inch Penrose drain is placed above the anterior aspect of the spine, bringing it out through the lower end of the incision. The platysma and skin are closed with fine suture and the drain removed in 12 hours.

Relief following surgery for radiculopathy is apparent to many patients soon after they awaken from anesthesia; codeine suffices. The patient is allowed out of bed within a day, often in a collar fashioned from a towel, and discharged home within 4 to 6 days. The use of a collar is elective. Following surgery for myelopathy, the patient is immobilized in a Philadelphia collar until there is radiographic evidence of bony fusion.

Complications

Tew[26] has recently summarized a combined experience with possible complications of this operation and they appear formidable. In reality, however, the complication rate of the procedure in experienced hands is very modest. The exception lies in the reoperative case in which reexploration of the neck can be extremely difficult. In this group of patients serious problems can and do arise.

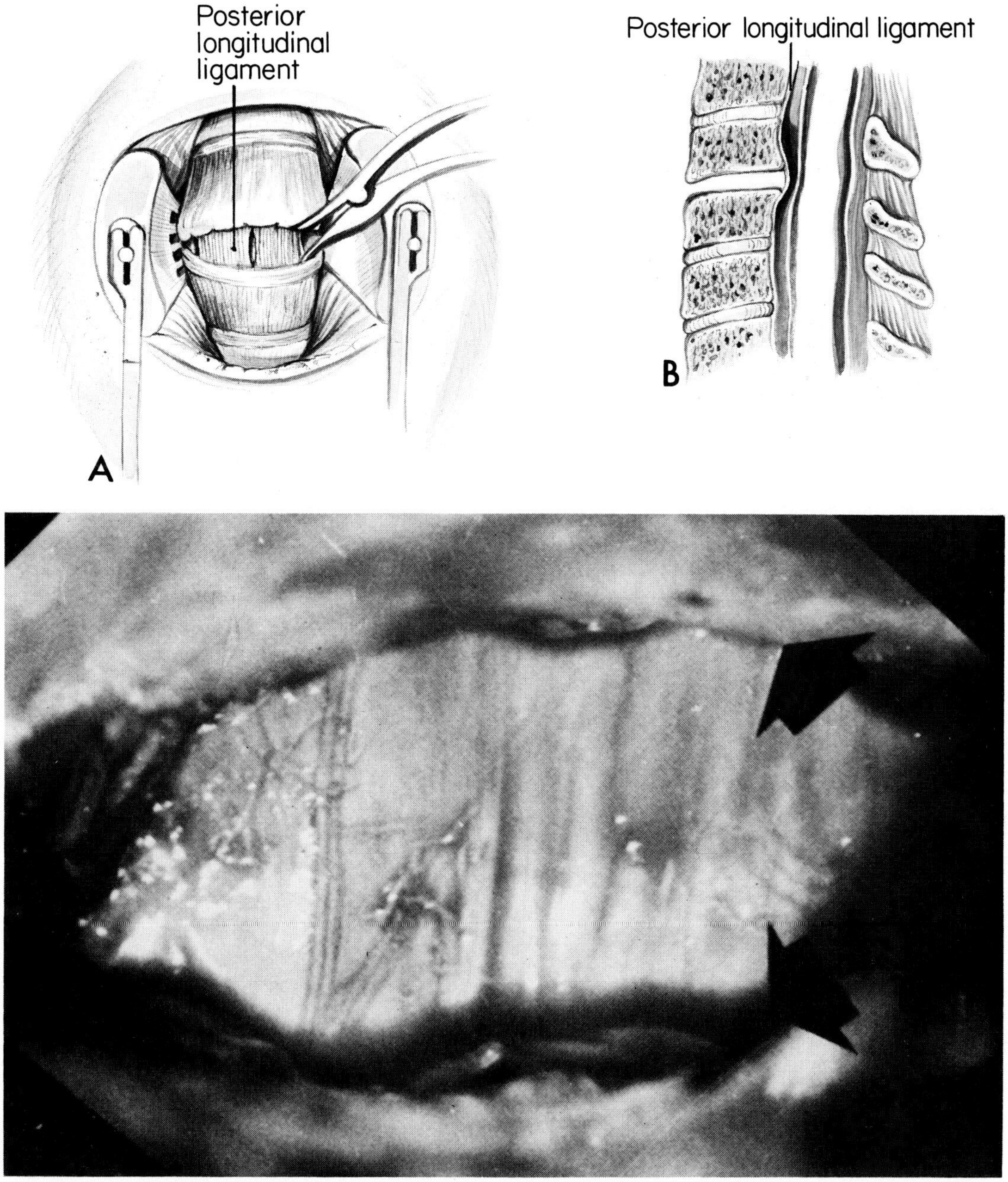

Fig. 23-16. **A.** Appearance of the posterior longitudinal ligament following removal of disc material and cartilaginous plates. **B.** Relationship of the posterior longitudinal ligament to the intervertebral disc and cervical dura. **C.** Appearance of the posterior longitudinal ligament under magnification, as seen through the disc space in the cervical region.

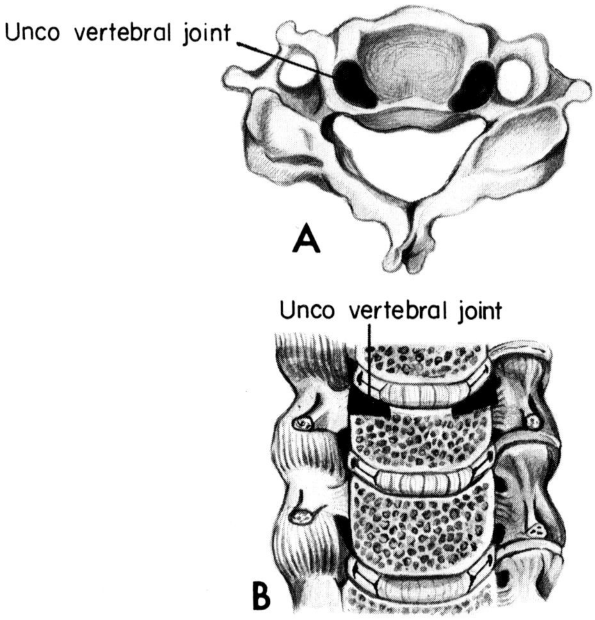

Fig. 23-17. A and B. The uncovertebral joints and their local relationships.

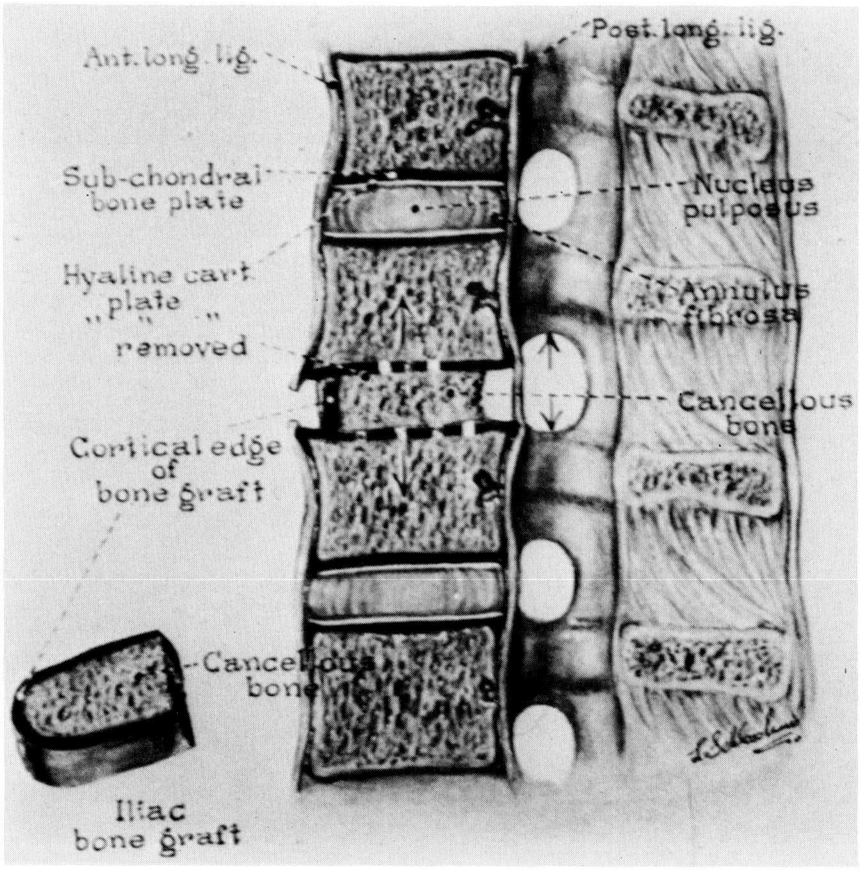

Fig. 23-18. Appearance and positioning of iliac crest bone graft in Smith-Robinson type anterior cervical fusion.

Retraction-related problems are the most common form of postoperative morbidity, and result in laryngeal edema, hoarseness, dysphagia, or a sensation of a lump in the throat.[27] These can be avoided by a generous vertical incision, preferably on the left side; meticulous placement, under magnification, of the blades of the Cloward retractor beneath the medial aspect of the longus colli muscles, a gentle degree of retraction; and a drain placed prevertebrally at the end of the operation. Should these retraction-related problems arise, a short course of steroid therapy has been found useful. Occasionally emergency tracheostomy has been necessary because of upper airway obstruction secondary to extensive retraction on it.

Profuse bleeding from the disc space is unusual but disconcerting when it does occur. The bleeding is due either to injury to the bone as the cartilagenous plates are removed, injury to the vertebral body with the disc-space spreader, or a small dural tear with a cerebrospinal fluid leak, which decompresses epidural veins and can result in profuse venous bleeding. I have seen this bleeding occur during an open cordotomy through the disc space when the dura is opened purposely. In this case the epidural oozing can be very annoying. The vertebral artery is rarely injured.

Esophageal perforation is another retraction-related complication that can be prevented by using the blades properly and which, if recognized, should be repaired immediately. Interrupted nonabsorbable suture is used to repair the rupture and the area drained. Fusion is not performed.

Fusion-related problems are the main reason for the current enthusiasm for anterior discectomy without fusion. Graft extrusion and donor site problems occur in about 2% to 4% of cases, and with the interbody technique fusion failed in 10% of Tew's[26] cases and the incidence of failures was even higher with the Cloward technique. On the other hand significant postoperative discomfort followed discectomy without fusion in 50% to 75% of cases. The discomfort, characterized by a nagging neck, shoulder, and intrascapular pain often lasting several months after surgery but subsiding eventually, is a significant consideration when deciding the merit of this modification of the anterolateral operation in the treatment of spondylosis.

The second consideration is the effect of eliminating the graft on the stability of the cervical spine. Apparently interbody fusion is often unnecessary because spontaneous fusion occurs within 6 months after one-, two-, or three-level disc excision in which the disc, cartilagenous plates, and osteophytes have been removed. The overall results depend on the number of variables responsible for maintaining stability, altered by the spondylotic processes prior to surgery. In a patient with a disc degeneration alone the stability may well be maintained by various muscular and ligamentous structures and the disc can be removed and fusion occur without a graft. However, in patients with advanced spondylosis degenerative changes affect most of the supporting structures of the spine and subluxation is often seen even before surgery. This latter situation, particularly if it is associated with myelopathy and buckling of the ligamentum flavum, would not favor eliminating the graft. The significant degree of angulation seen in up to 20% of the cases in recently reported series according to the criteria discussed earlier, represent spinal instability. This instability may eventually escalate into a series of problems significantly worse than the reticulopathy for which the operation was originally performed.

Results of Anterolateral Disc Excision for Cervical Spondylosis

The results of surgery for cervical radiculopathy have been consistently reported as excellent in many series,[4,6,9,10,13,16,28-34] irrespective of whether an anterior or posterior approach is used to decompress the nerve root. Improvement is seen in over 90% of the cases, an observation I have reconfirmed with my own and with another 350 cases performed by the staff of Massachusetts General Hospital in Boston, which I reviewed. The advantages of the anterior approach for the treatment of this condition have been enumerated, and for these reasons this operation should be standard for the management of cervical radiculopathy due to disc disease at one or many levels.

Radiculopathy associated with evidence of disc degeneration at more than one, two, or three levels may be managed without fusion, following disc excision. This has been our routine practice in these cases for the past 2 years. Following discectomy without fusion, intrascapular, neck, and shoulder pain are considerably more frequent than with fusion, although the complaints usually subside within 6 to 12 weeks. Later secondary fusion may however, be required in some patients with persistent symptoms.

When radiographic findings are extensive and suggest alterations, not only in disc but also of ligamentous and bony structures, then disc excision with coincident removal of the annulus, anterior longitudinal ligament, and, possibly the posterior longitudinal ligament, may potentiate the area's instability.

It has, by now, been repeatedly shown that it is possible to excise the discs from between four contiguous cervical vertebrae, without fusion and without instability.[31,34,35] Fusion fails considerably less often than would be expected theoretically. In the patient with a four-level fusion, it is also remarkable how little actual functional restriction results after five vertebrae are fused.

The results of decompressive surgery for myelopathy associated with cervical spondylosis has also been reviewed several times.[36-42] When cervical spondylosis was first recognized as a cause of myelopathy, it appeared that favorable results should be produced by removing the mechanical impingement. Allen[43] attempted to remove the protrusions extradurally through a posterior laminectomy, with disastrous results. Subsequently posterior laminectomies and foraminotomies were fashioned to allow the cord to migrate away from the spondylotic projections along the anterior aspect of the spine. Collating the various reports, and in my own review of 45 such cases, good to excellent results were obtained in approximately 60% of patients; another 20% became worse immediately after the operation. Long-term followup revealed that none of the patients ever returned completely to normal. Stoops and King[44] reported 42 patients treated by extensive laminectomy without opening the dura. These patients were followed for up to 6 years. Even though 80% were said to show improvement, no prognostic factor could be identified.

Crandall,[26] reporting on his long-term study of 55 patients with cervical myelopathy followed from 2 to 25 years, felt that a history of deficit for less than 1 year was associated with a better prognosis. In contrast a poor outcome is predictable among patients with preoperative sphincteric disturbances shown to be due to the myelopathy. Among these cases, none improved, irrespective of the type of operation.

The debate concerning the appropriate surgical procedure(s) in the management of cervical myelopathy continues. The operative procedure needs to be tailored to the particulars of the case. Posterior cervical laminectomy has a specific indication in patients with prominent dorsal encroachment on the cord due either to bony or ligamentous structures[46] (Figs. 23-19A, B, C, and D). Excessive cervical lordosis may be seen in patients with spondylotic myelopathy; overlapping of the lamina, referred to as *shingling*, may contribute to the myelopathy. Vertebral subluxation may also be seen and may lead to pinching of the cord, from posteriorly, by the laminae and infolded ligamentum flavum.

Inaccessibility to a disc space, eg., C2-3 or C3-4 in some cases, is an indication for posterior decompressive cervical laminectomy, as is a secondary procedure in the presence of neurologic progression, particularly with posterior column signs, and in some cases with widespread bony changes and spontaneous fusions anterior to the spinal cord. I do not believe it should be used routinely in the management of myelopathy. It has been reported in several series that even in the presence of technically faultless surgery up to 20% of cases treated by laminectomy had an increased deficit after surgery. In our experience this is particularly true if the dura is opened and the dentate ligaments sectioned. Also, following laminectomy, cervical instability is a risk, particularly when there has been a generous decompression, both rostrocaudally and laterally.

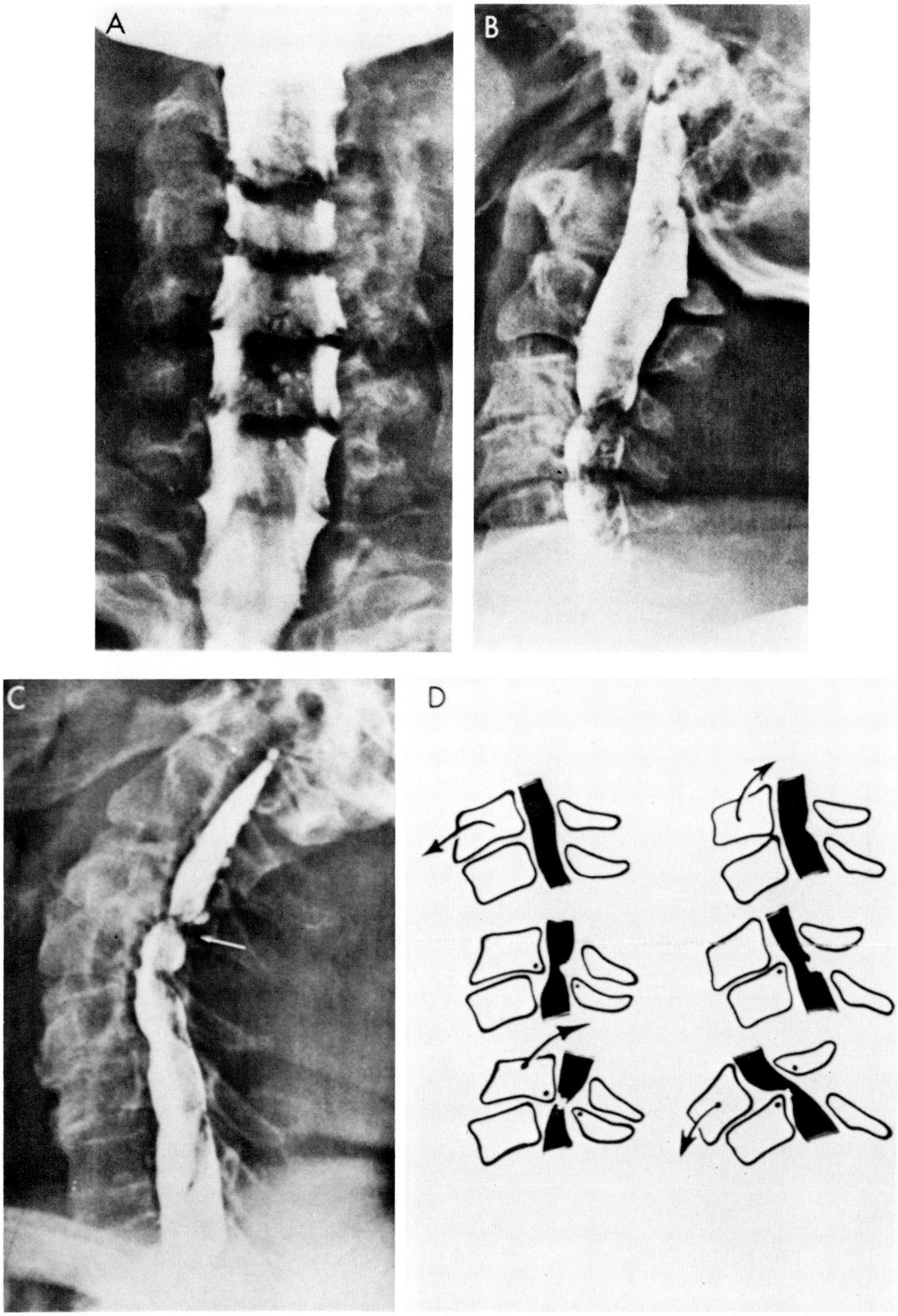

Fig. 23-19. A, B, C, and D. Cervical myelogram showing significant anterior and posterior compression of the spinal cord.

Dereymaeker et al.[47] analyzed two groups of patients with spondylotic myelopathy operated upon either by the anterior or posterior approach and followed for 2 to 6 years. Clinical and radiographic findings showed that of 31 patients with anterior fusion, 20 were improved; of 12 who had laminectomy with excision of the disc, 4 were improved.

Crandall and Batzdorf[38] reported that of 28 cases of myelopathy treated by anterior discectomy and fusion, 71% were improved when posterior projections were removed from the floor of the canal and the involved interspaces stabilized. In no case was the patient made worse by the operation. This experience was reaffirmed in Crandall's latest report,[26] showing that none of his cases treated by the Cloward operation was worse postoperatively but postoperative disability was again increased following decompressive laminectomy. Bohlman[45] has reported his experience with anterior discectomy and interbody arthrodesis in 17 cases of myelopathy. In most no attempt was made to remove the PLL or osteophytes. Cartilagenous plates and disc material were removed, under magnification, up to the posterior longitudinal ligament. In none was neural function lost and of the 17 cases treated, 14 were improved over their preoperative condition. Bone remodeling occurred at the fused levels and the size of the osteophytes decreased with time.

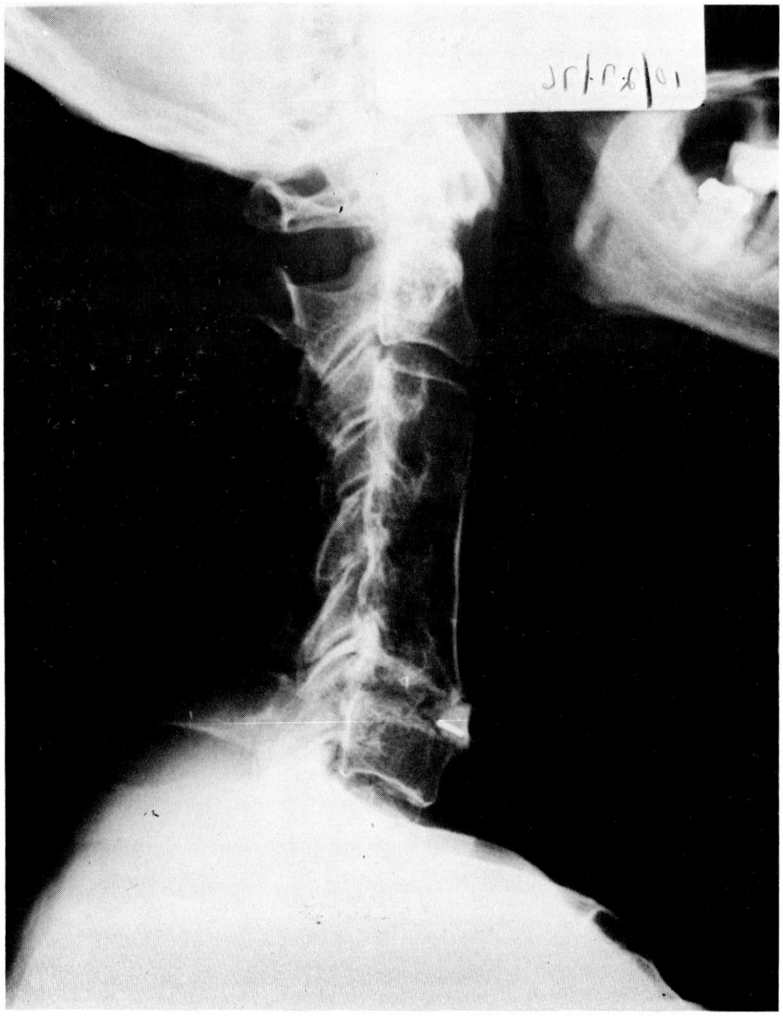

Fig. 23-20. Methyl methacrylate fusion at C6-7.

Based on this experience, and using currently available surgical aids, such as the microscope, the anterior approach has evolved into the operative procedure of choice for cervical spondylotic myelopathy, even if surgery necessitates operation at two to three or four levels, provided major compressive elements are situated anterior to the spinal cord.

Whether the osteophytes require radical removal in this situation is problematic. Should it be possible to do so without substantial risk, this is desirable, although not essential, to achieve a good neurologic result. If a fusion is not performed, increased movement at the operated levels and the possibility that the spinal cord's function will be made worse, are risks.

What of the possibility of producing anterior interbody fusion using methyl-methacrylate alone or in conjunction with bone in the interspace?[48-50] Inherent in this possibility are the theoretical advantages of instantaneous fixation and immobilization of the interspace. When combined with a bone graft, movement at that interspace is minimal, increasing the chances for a successful bony fusion without angulation. The major theoretical disadvantage is infection.

I have used methyl methylacrylate in this fashion in 4 cases, 2 following cordotomy by an anterior approach through the disc space in patients with intractable pain and malignancy. Postoperatively patients were free of pain after neck surgery at C4-5 and could be mobilized the next day. In 2 other cases methylacrylate was used in conjunction with a bone graft. In 1, following resection of the vertebral body, a bone graft was placed between the vertebrae and immobilized with glue. In the last case a fourth-level cervical spine fusion was done anteriorly. To prevent angulation and graft extrusion a bone and methacrylate fusion was performed on this level (Fig. 23-20). This was carried out without difficulty. Postoperatively no movement could be demonstrated at this level and the site has healed well, without angulation or extrusion of the bone graft.

REFERENCES

1. Adams CBT, Logue V: Studies in cervical spondylotic myelopathy. 3. Some functional effects of operations for cervical spondylotic myelopathy. *Brain 94*:587-594, 1971
2. Aronson NI: the management of soft cervical disc protrusions using the Smith-Robinson approach. *Clin Neurosurg 20*:253-258, 1973
3. Bailey RW, Badjley CE: Stabilization of the cervical spine by anterior fusion. *J Bone Joint Surg 42A*:565-594, 1960
4. Bailey RW: *The Cervical Spine*. Lea and Febiger, Philadelphia, 1974
5. Cloward RB: New method of diagnosis and treatment of cervical disc disease. *Clin Neurosurg 8*:93-132, 1962
6. Cloward RB: Lesions of the intervertebral disc and their treatment by interbody fusion methods. *Clin Orthoped 27*:51-77, 1963
7. Smith GW, Robinson RA: The treatment of certain cervical spine disorders by anterior removal of the intervertebral disc and interbody fusion. *J Bone Joint Surg 40A*:607-624, 1958
8. Murphy MB, Bado M: Anterior cervical discectomy without interbody bone graft. *J Neurosurg 37*:71-74, 1972
9. Robinson RA, Smith GW: The treatment of certain cervical spine disorders by anterior removal of the intervertebral disc and interbody fusion. *J Bone Joint Surg 40A*:607, 1958
10. Robinson RA, Walker AE, Ferlick DE: The results of anterior interbody fusion of the cervical spine. *J Bone Joint Surg 44A*:1569-1587, 1962
11. Robinson RA: Anterior and posterior cervical fusions. *Clin Orthop 35*:34-62, 1964
12. Cloward RB: Treatment of acute fractures and fracture-dislocations of the cervical spine by vertebral body fusion. *J Neurosurg 18*:201-209, 1961
13. Scoville WB, Dohrmann AM, Corkill AR: Late results of cervical disc surgery. *J Neurosurg 45*:203-310, 1976
14. Zulch KJ: Personal communications, 1976
15. Robinson RA: Personal communications, 1976
16. Clarke E, Robinson PK: Cervical myelopathy: complication of cervical spondylosis. *Brain 79*:483-510, 1956

17. Lees F, Turner JWA: Natural history and prognosis of cervical spondylosis. *Br Med J 2*:1607-1610, 1963
18. Roth DA: Cervical analgesic discography: a new test for the definitive diagnosis of the painful disc syndrome. *JAMA 235*:1713, 1976
19. Hilding DA, Tachdjian MO: Dysphagia and hypertrophic spurring of the cervical spine. *N Engl J Med 263*:11, 1960
20. Maran A, Jacobson I: Cervical osteophytes presenting with pharyngeal symptoms. *Laryngoscope 81*:412, 1971
21. Facer JA: Osteophytes of the cervical spine causing dysphagia. *Arch Otolaryngol 86*:341, 1967
22. Meeks LW, Renshaw TS: Ankylosing vertebral hyperostosis and dysphagia, *The Cervical Spine*. Edited by RW Bailey. Lea and Febiger Philadelphia, 1974, pp 242-249
23. Hutchinson EC, Yates PO: *Brain 79*:319-[redacted], 1956
24. Fisher CM: Personal communication, 1976
25. White AA, Southwick WO, DePonte RJ: Relief of pain by anterior cervical spine fusion for spondylosis. A report of 65 patients. *J Bone Joint Surg 55A*:525-534, 1973
26. Tew JM, Jr, Mayfield FH: Complications of surgery of the anterior cervical spine. *Clin Neurosurg 23*:424-434, 1976
27. Heeneman H: Vocal cord paralysis following approaches to the anterior cervical spine. *Laryngoscope 83*:17-21, 1973
28. Aronson N, Bagan N, Filtzer DL: Results of using the Smith-Robinson approach for herniated and extruded cervical discs. *J Neurosurg 32*:721-722, 1970
29. Aronson N, Filtzer DL: Treatment concepts of cervical spine disease using the anterior approach, *American Academy of Orthopedic Surgeons Instructional Course Lectures*, vol 21. CV Mosby, St Louis
30. Hirsch C: Cervical disc rupture: diagnosis and therapy. *Acta Orthop Scand 30*:172-186, 1960
31. Martins AN: AC discectomy with/without interbody bone graft. *J Neurosurg 44*:290-295, 1976
32. Riley LH, Jr, Robinson RA, Johnson DA: The results of anterior interbody fusion of the cervical spine. Review of 93 consecutive cases. *J Neurosurg 30*:127-133, 1969
33. Rothman RH, Simeone FA: *The Spine*. WB Saunders, Philadelphia, 1975
34. Robertson JT: Anterior cervical disc removal with and without fusion. Presented at the 33rd Annual Meeting of the American Academy of Neurological Surgery, Lake Tahoe, Nevada, September 29, 1971
35. Hankinson HL, Wilson CB: Use of the operating microscope in anterior cervical discectomy without fusion. *J Neurosurg 43*:452-456, 1975
36. Bishara SN: Treatment of cervical spondylosis with myelopathy. *J Neurol Neurosurg Psychiatr 34*:393-[redacted], 1971
37. Brain WR: Some unsolved problems of cervical spondylosis. *Br Med J 1*:711-773, 1963
38. Brain WR, Northfield DWC, Wilkinson M: Neurological manifestations of cervical spondylosis. *Brain 75*:187, 1952
39. Brain L: Some unsolved problems of cervical spondylosis. *Br Med J 1*: 771-773, 1963
40. Brain L, Wilkinson M: *Cervical spondylosis.* WB Saunders, Philadelphia, 1967
41. Northfield AC: *The Surgery of the Central Nervous System.* Blackwell, Oxford, 1973, pp 711-752
42. Robinson RA, Afeiche N: Cervical spondylotic myelopathy: etiology and treatment concepts, Cervical Spine Research Society. Philadelphia, Pennsylvania, November 19, 1976
43. Symon L, Lavender P: The surgical treatment of cervical spondylotic myelopathy. *Neurology 17*:117-127, 1967
44. Allen KL: Neuropathies caused by bony spurs in the cervical spine with special reference to surgical treatment. *J Neurol Neurosurg Psychiatr 15*:20-36, 1952
45. Stoops WL, King RB: Neural complications of cervical spondylosis: their response to laminectomy and foraminotomy. *J Neurosurg 19*:986-999, 1962
46. Bohlman HH: Cervical spondylosis with moderate to severe myelopathy: treatment of anterior cervical discectomy and fusion. Presented at Cervical Spine Research Society, Philadelphia, Pennsylvania, November 20, 1976
47. Epstein JA, Carras LA, Epsein BS, et al: Myelopathy in cervical spondylosis with vertebral subluxation and hyperlordosis. *J. Neurosurg 32*:421-426, 1970
48. Dereymaeker A, Chosez J-P, Henkes R: Le traitement chirurgical de la discopathie cervicale. Resultats compares de l'abord posterieur (laminectomie) et de l'abord ventral (fusion corporeale)
49. Cleveland D: Interspace reconstruction and spinal stabilization after disc removal. *J Lancet 76*:327-331, 1956
50. Scoville WB, Palmer AH, Samra K: The use of acrylic plastic for vertebral replacement or fixation in metastatic disease of the spine. Technical note. *J Neurosurg 27*:274-279, 1967
51. Hansby WB, Glaser HT: Replacement of spinal intervertebral discs with locally polymensing methyl methacrylate. *J Neurosurg 16*:311-313, 1959

CHAPTER 24

Transthoracic Disc Excision

Frederick A. Simeone Ralph Rashbaum

SYMPTOMATIC HERNIATIONS OF THORACIC intervertebral discs are the rarest, yet most devastating of all disc lesions. They present problems in diagnosis, and historically treatment by ordinary laminectomy has been attended with appalling results. Of Mueller's 4 cases, 3 were paraplegic after surgery.[1] Perot reviewed 91 cases from various sources in 1969.[2] Forty of these patients were not improved by surgery, and 16 were rendered paraplegic as a result of the operation. The results were most unfavorable in *central* disc herniations, particularly with advanced preoperative neurologic deficit. As might be expected, patients with lateral disc herniations and minimal neurologic deficit fared better postoperatively. All patients treated by ordinary laminectomy were characterized by the same discouraging conclusions.[3-9]

In 1960 Hulme[10] treated 4 cases through a lateral (costotransversectomy) approach with encouraging results; 3 were cured and 1 showed improvement. Perot[2], 9 years later, described the transpleural approach through an ordinary thoracotomy incision in 2 patients, both of whom made a complete recovery. During the same year, Ransohoff and coworkers[9] described a similar procedure. These two approaches will be described in detail, with additional comments about the use of the operating microscope when dissection near the spinal cord begins. In most series described thoracic disc herniations represent 0.25% to 0.75% of all symptomatic disc lesions. They are seen between the fourth to twelfth thoracic interspaces, with the gretest percentage between T8 and T11. Patients may present with pain in a radicular distribution, acute or chronic in nature, with laterally placed lesions. Patients with central herniations develop paraparesis, with or without sensory complaints and with an acute or chronic onset. There is nothing characteristic about chronic thoracic disc herniations, which can lead to a clinical distinction among other causes of thoracic spinal cord compression.

On radiologic examination the offending disc is often calcified, though calcification in thoracic disc is sufficiently common that this finding itself normally just increases the suspicion of thoracic disc protrusion. Accurate myelography, particularly with painstaking efforts to achieve optimum lateral views, is absolutely necessary. No operation for thoracic disc herniation should be undertaken without myelograms that clearly outline the lesion; contrast medium may have to be instilled cisternally. When the offending lesion is identified, great pains must be taken to develop criteria for localizing the proper disc intraoperatively. The

Division of Neurosurgery, University of Pennsylvania School of Medicine, and Pennsylvania Hospital, Philadelphia, Pennsylvania

thoracic spine is approached by the alternative routes described below; it is most difficult to find the appropriate level during surgery. Consequently, we will often insert a sterile needle into a spinous process on the morning of surgery (with radiologic control) and retain this marker throughout the operation.

Surgical Technique

Costotransversectomy and Disc Excision

This procedure is carried out under general anesthesia, with a cuffed endotracheal tube in place. The anesthesiologist must be able to inflate the patient's lungs, should the pleural cavity be entered inadvertently.

The patient lies in a modified lateral decubitus position, with 30° elevation from the straight prone, so that the operator may stand opposite the abdomen (Fig. 24-1). A pad is placed in the axilla and below the shoulders. To avoid increased venous pressure the abdomen must be kept free by carefully placed supports under the chest and iliac crest. The uppermost knee is flexed and a pillow placed between the legs. The approach may be made from either side. The choice depending on the presence of lateralizing features in the clinical presentation. If unilateral root pain is the principal symptom, then the interspace should be approached from the same side. With central disc herniations, or in the absence of lateralizing findings, the right-sided approach has been used because, statistically, the important artery of Adamkiewicz usually originates from the left lower intercostal vessels (roughly T8 to L2).

It is essential to localize the lesion at this point, either with a needle previously inserted into the spinous process, as mentioned earlier, or by marking the rib to be removed by injecting indigocarmine subcutaneously onto it.

The skin incision follows a long semilunar course, extending the length of at least three vertebral bodies above and below the disc space in question (Fig. 24-2). The incision extends at least 20 cm laterally from the mid-line at the apex of the curve. Dissection proceeds through the skin and subcutaneous tissue to the deep fascia, which are elevated and retracted medially to the spinous processes (Fig. 24-3). The trapezius muscle can be incised in line with the skin incision and retracted medially. This exposes the erecta spinae mass (semispinalis, longisimus, and iliocostalis muscles), which is reflected medially by stripping the muscles from their attachments. Alternatively, the muscle mass can be transected over the rib to be removed and the muscles retracted in a cephalic and caudal direction, for easier access to the lamina as well as to the rib to be removed. This rib is identified and the intercostal neurovas-

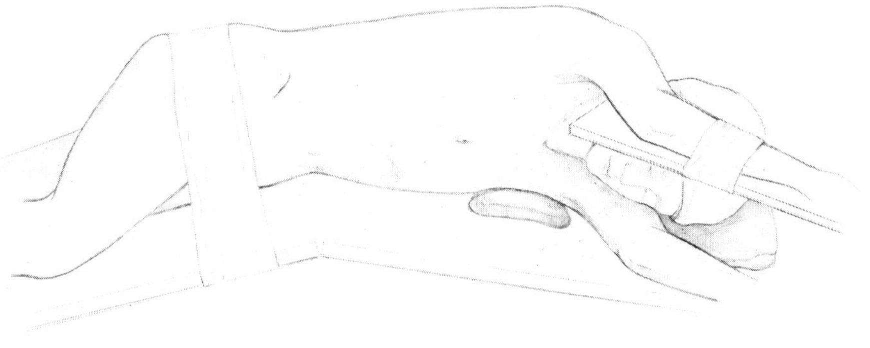

Fig. 24-1.

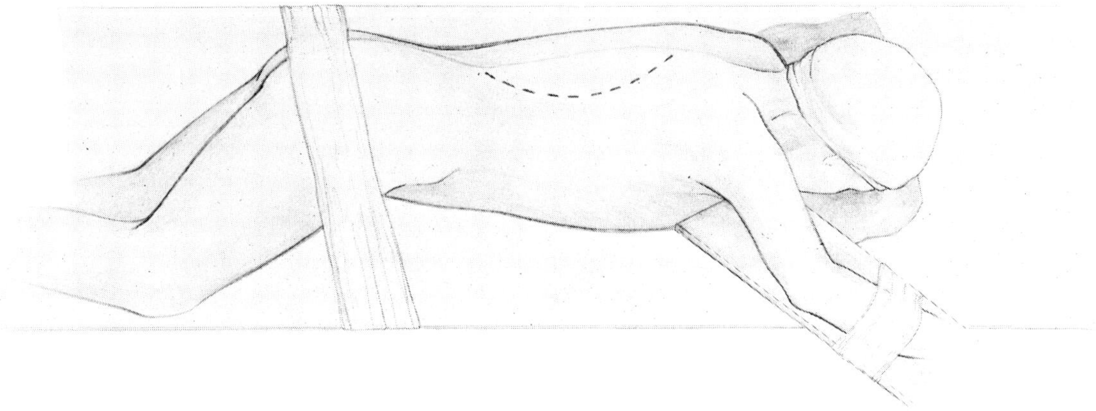

Fig. 24-2.

cular complex is separated from its inferior surface. The periosteum is stripped from the rib, about the width of the incision, with a Doyen separator (Fig. 24-4).

Attention is then directed to the attachment of the rib with the vertebral bodies. The transverse process is removed with a rongeur so that the articulation of the rib head and its costotransverse and capsular ligaments can be identified and sectioned. The rib is cut at the most lateral portion of the incision (approximately 20 cm of rib are removed), and it is disarticulated from the vertebral body (Fig 24-5).

When the rib is removed, the intercostal vein, artery, and nerve can be followed through their entrance into the spinal canal. It is not necessary to sacrifice any of these structures,

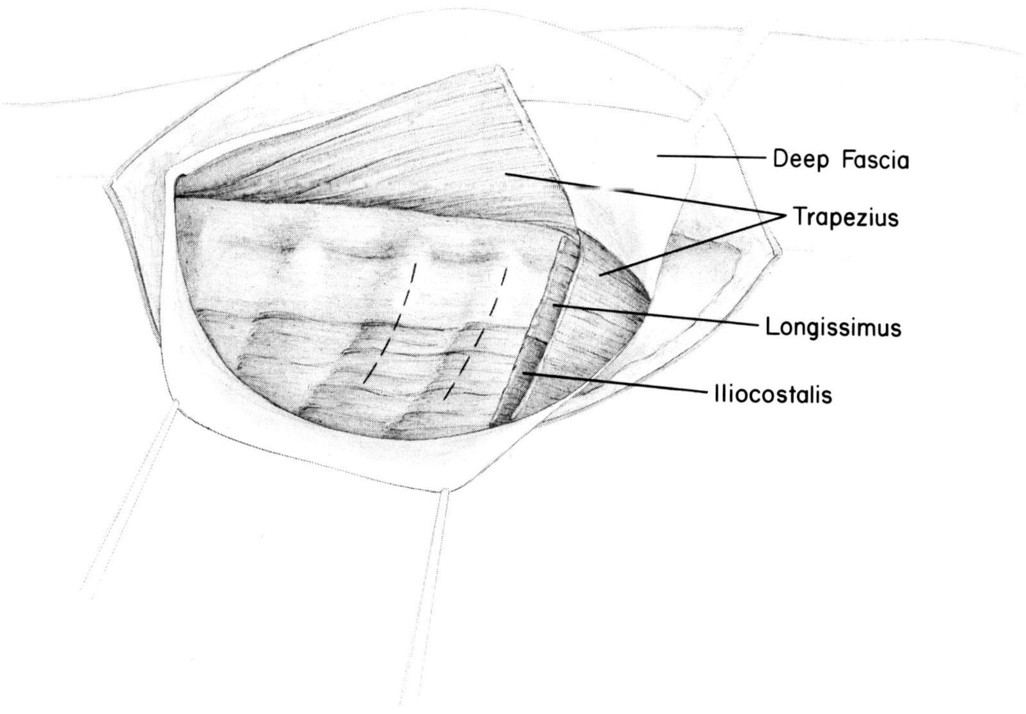

Fig. 24-3.

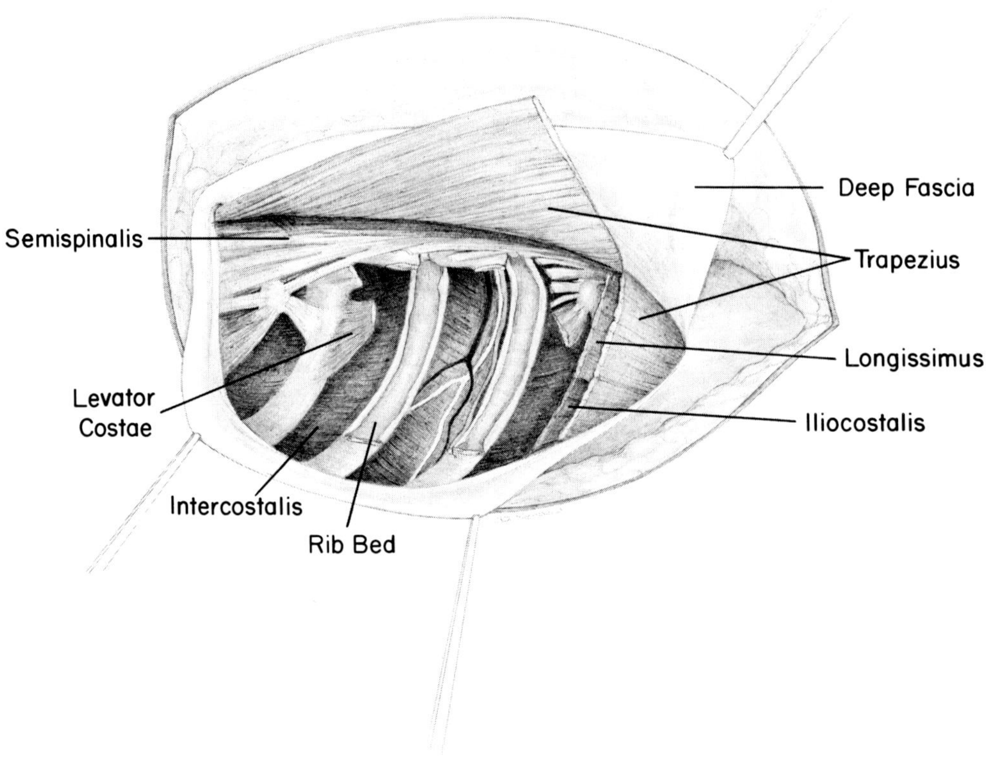

Fig. 24-4.

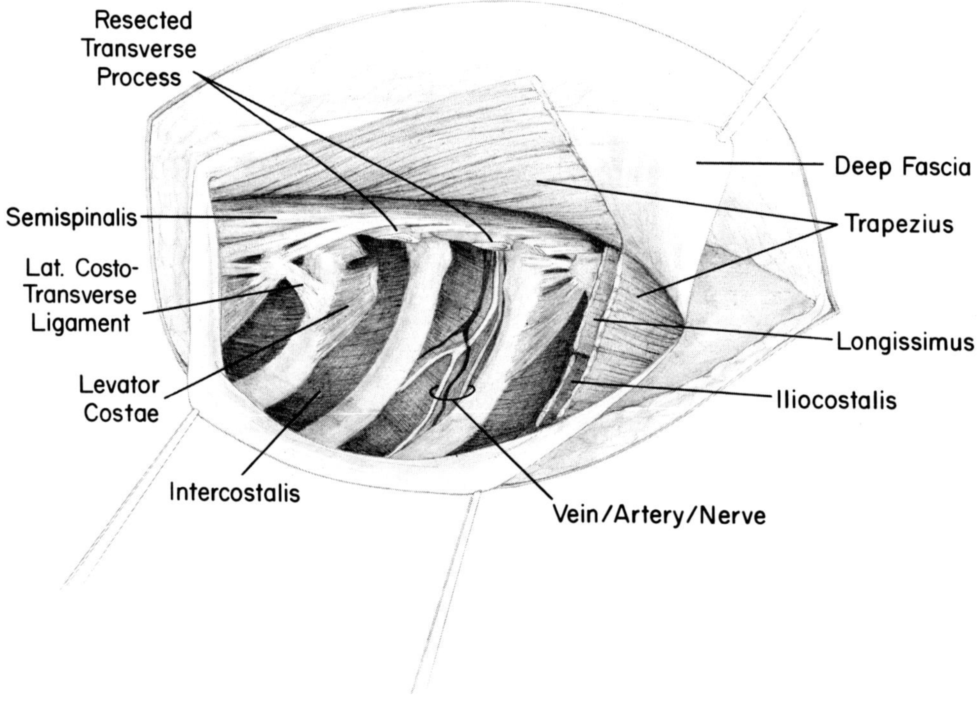

Fig. 24-5.

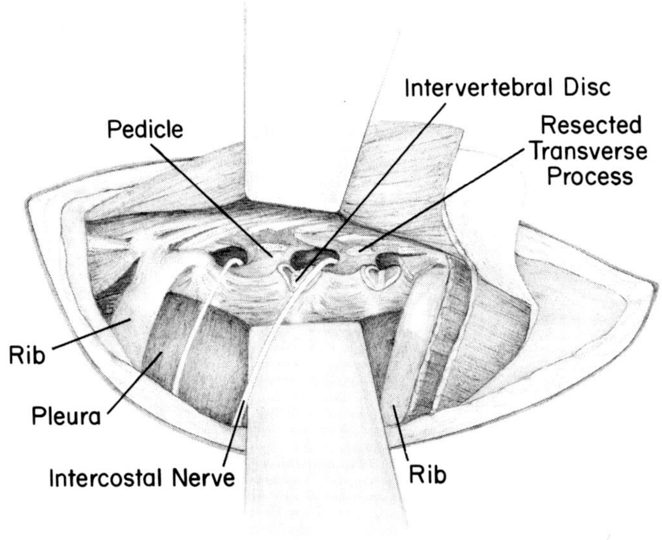

Fig. 24-6.

although the muscular branches of the intercostal artery can be cauterized as needed (Fig. 24-6). The parietal pleura is separated from the ribs, above and below, as well as from the spinal column, and it is depressed with a malleable ribbon or large Deaver retractor. The segmental vessels along the side of the vertebrae are identified. They should not be damaged; but if bleeding develops, it may be controlled by silver clips or coagulation.

The intervertebral foramen is identified by tracing the intracostal nerve medially. The nerve enters the spinal canal between two pedicles. The latter structures are cleaned with a periosteal elevator and then removed piecemeal with a Kerrison rongeur. A high-speed air drill may facilitate removal of the pedicle. If an air drill is used, we also prefer to use an operating microscope at this time, because it provides excellent illumination and magnification of important neural structures underlying the bone to be removed. The microscope is used throughout the rest of the procedure on the vertebra and discs. When the pedicle is removed, the lateral aspect of the dural sac and the intrusion of the disc into the canal can be appreciated (Fig. 24-7). An incision is made into the midportion of the disc space, well away

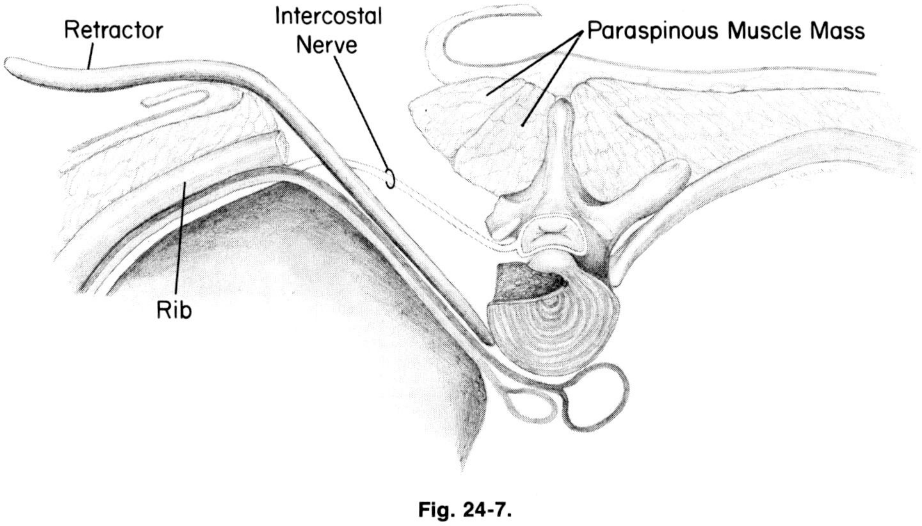

Fig. 24-7.

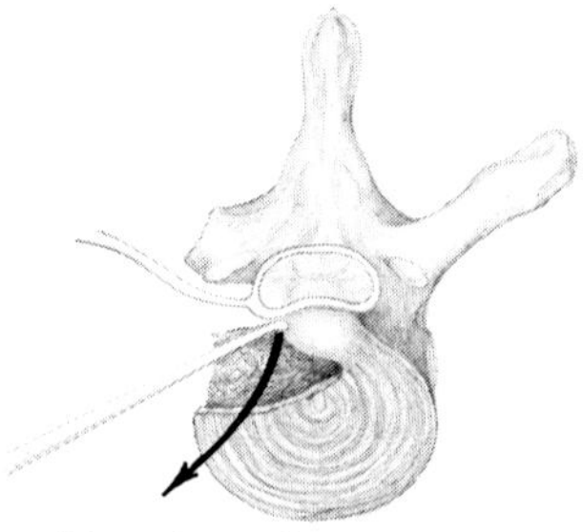

Fig. 24-8.

from the spinal cord, and the space is emptied by curettage and pituitary rongeurs. A small portion of the opposing margins of the vertebral bodies, nearest the spinal canal, can be curetted away to ease access of the disc space (Fig. 24-8). Through this, fragments closer to the dural canal may be separated and pushed into the emptied disc space for later removal. A Penfield dissector can be used to palpate the posterior longitudinal ligament for sequestered disc material. This instrument can also depress the annulus fibrosis into the intervertebral disc space to determine if the spinal canal is really fully decompressed.

The interspace is irrigated thoroughly and meticulous hemostasis is achieved. Through positive pressure ventilation, the pleura is checked for leaks. If it has been violated, an extrapleural chest tube may be placed prior to completion of the closure. The wound is closed in layers. A chest x-ray film taken in the recovery room will help if there are concerns about a pneumothorax.

Transthoracic (Transpleural) Disc Excision

This procedure is considerably more formidable than costotransversectomy, but it provides direct access to the anterior and lateral portions of the disc. A thoracic surgeon is required, at least in the early experience with this approach. The patient's general medical and pulmonary status must be checked preoperatively. A postoperative unit for the management of thoracotomy patients is required. The degree of postoperative pain is greater, as is the possibility of significant intraoperative bleeding.

The operation is carried out under general anesthesia, using a cuffed endotracheal tube. A Carlens tube should be used so that each lung may be ventilated separately if the surgical situation requires this.

The chest is entered through a standard right posterior thoracotomy incision (Fig. 24-9). The right side is chosen because of the fact that the artery of Adamkiewicz usually enters on the left side (80% of cases) and because the heart and great vessels pose a problem through a

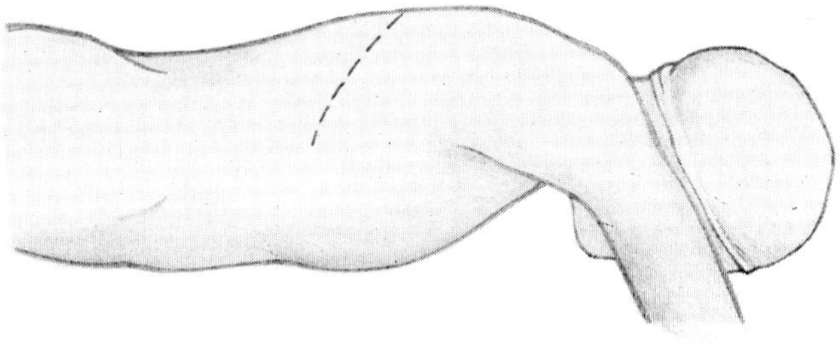

Fig. 24-9.

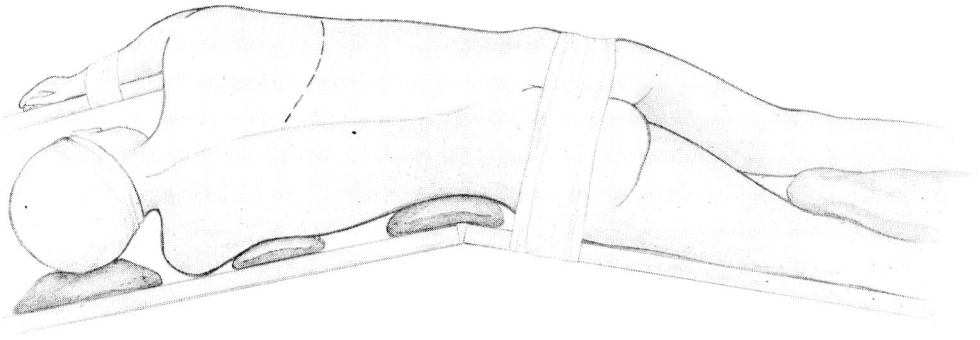

Fig. 24-10.

left transthoracic incision. The patient is positioned in the straight lateral posture, leaning somewhat towards his abdomen so that the chest contents (with the exception of the azygous vein) will gravitate out of the operative field. The surgeon stands on the spinal side of the patient, and a better view is obtained if the patient is tilted slightly towards him (Fig. 24-10). Careful positioning of the patient over the table break or kidney rest will enable the anesthesiologist, at the appropriate time, to laterally flex the thoracic spine thereby opening the interspace. In younger patients, there will be sufficient elasticity of the rib ligaments so that the rib spreader will provide sufficient exposure. If such is not the case, the rib opposite the offending intervertebral disc may be removed (Fig. 24-11). The lateral aspect of the rib is sectioned first, and the head of the rib can be removed through the endothoracic fascia (Fig. 24-12). At least 15 cm of rib, including the rib head, must be removed in order to gain complete exposure to the lateral-most portion of the spinal canal. (Fig. 24-13). Prior to disarticulation of the rib, identification of the intercostal nerve and vessels is important. The vessels should be preserved and the intercostal nerve may be followed to the appropriate intervertebral foramen. A specifically numbered rib will articulate with a posterior-superior margin of the vertebral body whose number it shares, as well as the posterior inferior margin of the next vertebra above. For example, the T8 rib will articulate with the body of T8 and T7, and it will cross the T7-8 interspace.

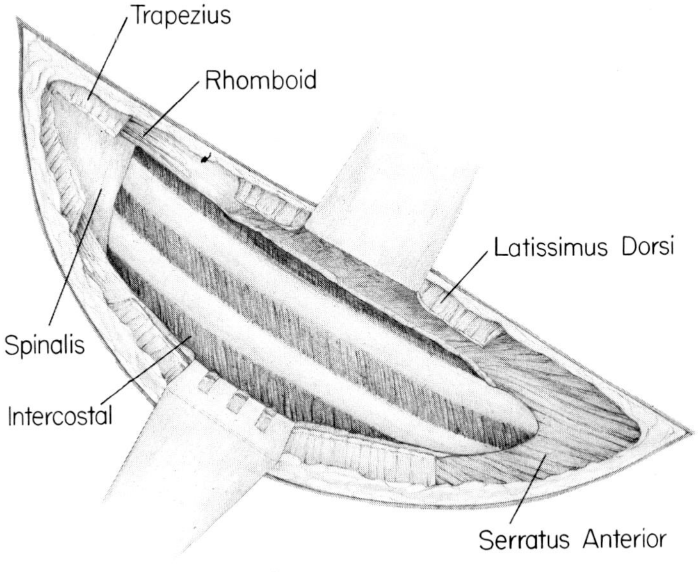

Fig. 24-11.

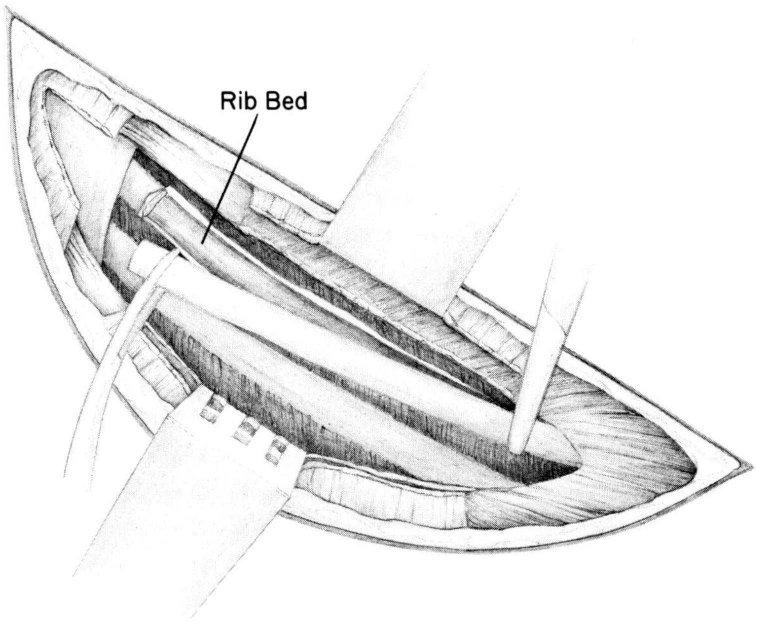

Fig. 24-12.

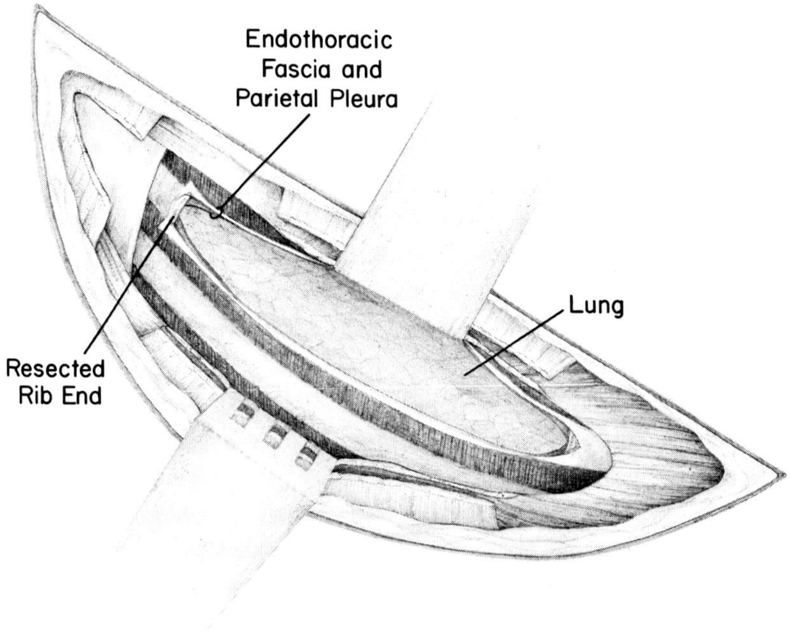

Fig. 24-13.

Attention is now directed to the lateral aspect of the vertebral body above and below the offending disc. A linear incision is made in the parietal pleura extending from the middle of each vertebral body. The incision is extended at its ends, and the pleura is reflected laterally (Fig. 24-14). Careful dissection of the parietal pleura from the vertebral body will expose the intervertebral vessels, as well as the sympathetic chain. It is necessary to ligate the segmental artery and vein above and below the disc lesion to gain adequate exposure. The intercostal nerve is followed to its foramen and gently retracted to expose the pedicles above and below (Fig. 24-15). The Kerrison rongeur or high-speed air drill are used to remove the pedicles so that the dural sac above and below the disc lesion is readily demonstrated. With the use of an operating microscope, disc protrusion into the canal is readily seen. The intervertebral disc is incised anterior two-thirds and its contents are emptied with pituitary rongeurs and curettes. No attempt is made to remove the extruded fragment initially. With flexion of the table or alteration of the kidney rest, the interspace may be opened and a lamina spreader introduced. When the space is emptied, the surgeon may use an air drill to remove a small segment of the vertebral body at the opposing margins (Fig. 24-16). A larger window into the spinal canal made in this fashion will enable disc fragments to be picked away from beneath the dural sac with small curettes. The dura is not retracted, but the floor of the spinal canal is palpated repeatedly with flat instruments (Penfield dissectors) to retrieve sequestered fragments and to ascertain effectiveness of decompression. The annulus fibrosis and its associated ligaments

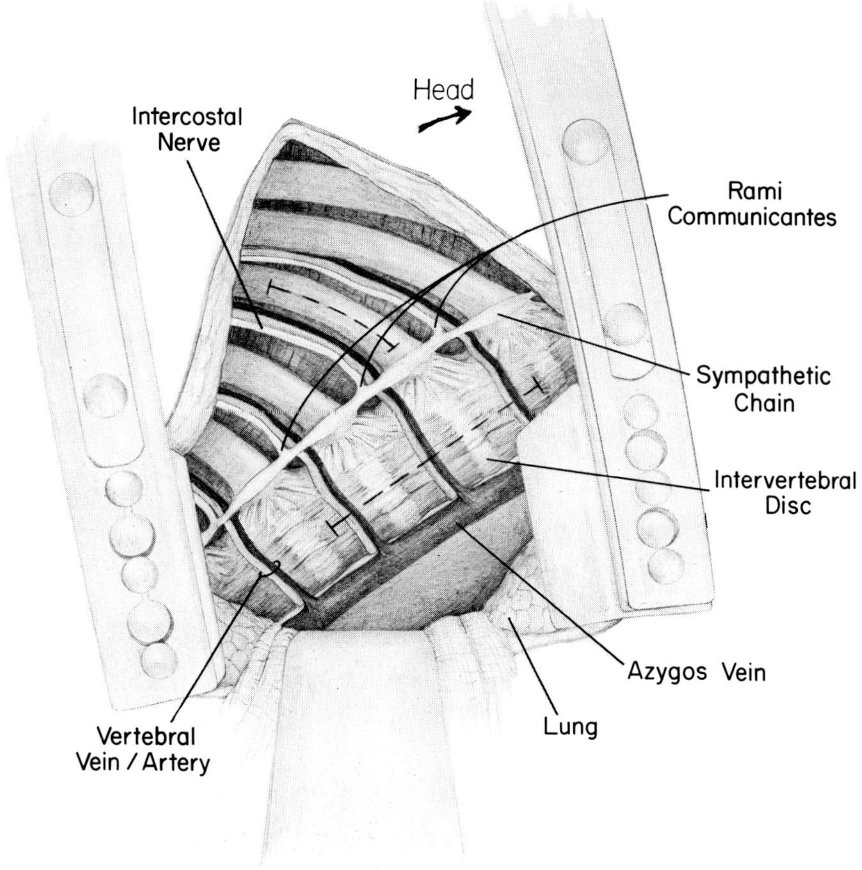

Fig. 24-14.

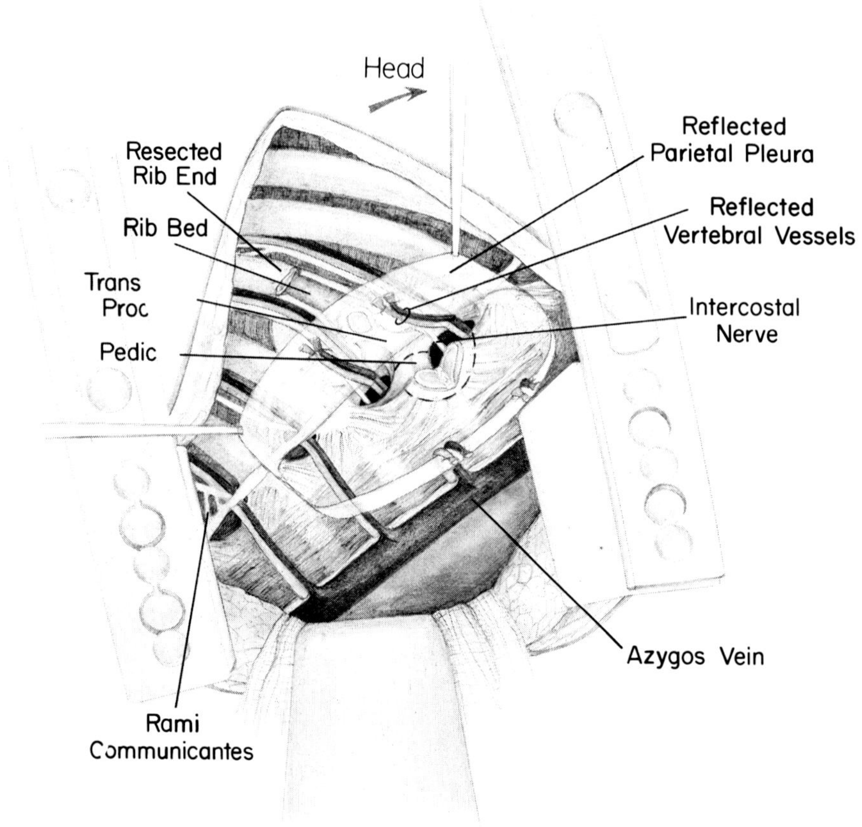

Fig. 24-15.

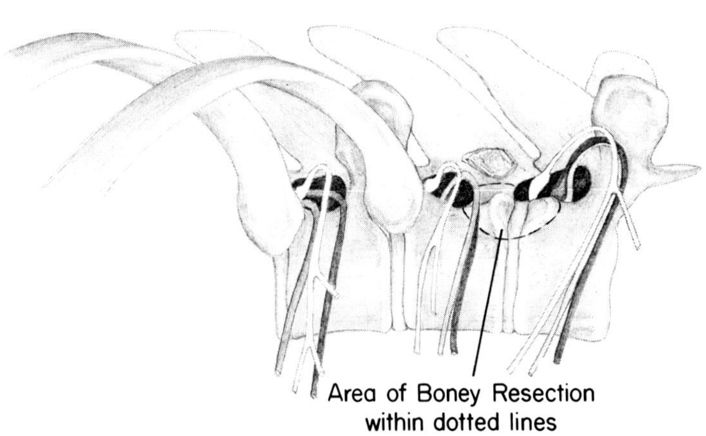

Fig. 24-16.

may be forced into the interspace and subsequently retrieved, and the area is irrigated thoroughly when the operator is confident that the spinal cord has been decompressed.

The parietal pleura may now be sutured over the vertebral bodies with running chromic catgut. Following the placement of an apical dependent chest tube through separate stab wounds, the chest is closed in routine fashion. The chest tubes are subsequently placed to underwater suction drainage, which can be removed when no further air leaks or drainage are present (usually 2 to 4 days). Repeated chest x-rays are used to follow the size of the pneumothorax if one persists during the immediate postoperative period.

Conclusion

Costotransversectomy and the transthoracic approach to thoracic disc herniations have offered patients new hope for cure without great fear of postoperative paraplegia. The costotransversectomy approach is a less formidable operation, and with the operating microscope, provides an adequate exposure to the lateral spinal canal. This approach is probably satisfactory for most symptomatic thoracic disc herniations. Where a more aggressive attack on the anterior surface of the spinal canal is required, transthoracic disc excision provides excellent visualization of the ventral surface of the spinal cord.

REFERENCES

1. Muller R: Prolapse of thoracic intervertebral discs. *Acta Med Scand 139*:99, 1951
2. Perot PL, Munro OD: Transthoracic removal of midline thoracic disc protrusions causing spinal cord compression. *J Neurosurg 31*:452-462, 1969
3. Arseni C, Nash F: Protrusion of thoracic intervertebral discs. *Acta Neurochir 11*:1-33, 1963
4. Logue V: Thoracic intervertebral disc prolapse with spinal cord compression. *J Neurol Neurosurg Psychiat 15*:227-241, 1952
5. Love JG, Schorn VG: Thoracic disc protrusions. *JAMA 191*:627-631, 1965
6. Reeves DL, Brown, HA: Thoracic intervertebral disc protrusion with spinal cord compression. *J Neurosurg 28*:24-28, 1968
7. Svein HJ, Karavitis AL: Multiple protrusions of intervertebral discs in the upper thoracic region: Report of case. *Proc Staff Meet Mayo Clin 29*:375-378, 1954
8. Tovi D, Strang RR: Thoracic intervertebral disc protrusions. *Acta Chir Scand Suppl 267*: 1960
9. Ransohoff J, Spencer F, Siew F, et al: Transthoracic removal of thoracic disc. Report of three cases. *J Neurosurg 31*:459-461, 1969
10. Hulme A: The surgical approach to thoracic intervertebral disc protrusions. *J Neurol Neurosurg Psychiatr 23*:133-137, 1960

CHAPTER 25
Lumbar Disc Excision

Bernard E. Finneson

Caveat Disc Surgeon

The first disc operation is relatively easy. But the repeat operative procedure presents a problem both technically and, even more, in satisfactory outcome. My recommended solution to this problem is to avoid the first operation that is apt to lead to a less than satisfactory result, and create a clinical condition that requires repeat disc surgery.

Patient Selection

The most important single consideration affecting the outcome of lumbar disc surgery is patient selection. What factors help predict if a patient will benefit from surgery? The surgeon who can select a patient who will benefit from surgical intervention has won half the battle before the incision is made. It is perhaps even more important to be able to predict individuals who will not benefit from surgery. The surgeon who operates on this type of patient is handicapped before he starts. A satisfactory clinical result is not likely even with the finest, most meticulous surgical technique. The most that can reasonably be expected is that the patient is not too discernibly worse after surgery. Let me emphasize that the lack of response to nonsurgical treatment is, in itself, not an indication for surgery. All too often the patient with low back pain who is not readily *cured* with nonsurgical management is brought to the operating room under the banner of "we must do something for this poor suffering patient." This *something* is often a variety of new, and sometimes irreversible, surgically produced signs and symptoms, which are superimposed upon the original complaints.

Fallability of the Neurologic Examination

Neurosurgeons, in comparison to their orthopedic colleagues, are perhaps a bit more prone to rely upon the neurologic examination to identify the level of disc protrusion. There are, of course, certain findings, such as severe paraspinal muscle spasm in the lumbar area or poor mobility of the lumbar spine, common to most levels of disc protrusion, which are not considered of localizing value. The classic findings of a diminished or absent Achilles reflex and numbness on the lateral aspect of the foot in the presence of sciatic pain would generally be accepted as an L5-S1 disc protrusion. If the lumbar spine films demonstrate a narrow

Department of Neurosurgery, Hahnemann Medical College and Hospital, Philadelphia, and the Crozer-Chester Medical Center, Chester, Pennsylvania 19013.

L5-S1 disc space, some disc surgeons forego the myelogram and proceed with surgery at the L5-S1 level. In most cases they would be right and a surgically treatable lesion would be found at the L5-S1 level. However, three factors can be responsible for neurologic changes that may mislead the surgeon as to the involved interspace:

1. Location of disc protrusion (Fig. 25-1). The disc fragment may extrude laterally into the foramen so that it compresses the existing root from the interspace above. Such a laterally placed fragment at the L5-S1 foramen may produce an L4-5 syndrome.
2. Neuroanatomic changes (Fig. 25-2). A partially lumbarized first sacral segment, which may be dismissed as of no clinical significance, might be associated with a *postfixed* plexus. In such a situation an L5-S1 disc protrusion may produce great toe weakness and numbness over the dorsum of the foot within the L5 dermatome and might be identified as an L4-5 protrusion on the basis of the neurologic examination.
3. Temporal changes. As the patient grows older, degenerative changes within the discs occur in a progressively cephalad direction. This is well documented by discography, which demonstrates that degenerative changes usually occur first at the L5-S1 level; some years later they advance to the L4-5 interspace, and with advancing age, progressively cephalad. For this reason, an individual over the age of 50, who has severe sciatica associated with an absent Achilles reflex and a narrow L5-S1 disc space, could be suffering from an acute L4-5 lesion. The absent Achilles reflex may be a residual finding from a previously protruded L5-S1 lesion, which has fibrosed and is no longer a source of pain; the acute lesion at L4-5 not having been present long enough to establish definitive neurologic findings.

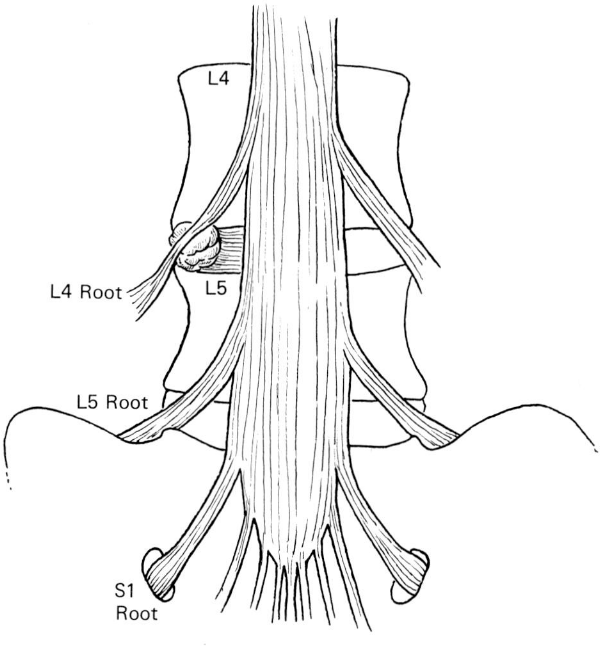

Fig. 25-1. Foraminal root compression syndrome. The laterally situated L4-5 disc protrusion will extend into the intervertebral foramen impinging upon the L4 root and simulate an L3-4 syndrome (Reprinted from Finneson BE: *Low Back Pain*. Philadelphia, Lippincott, 1973, with permission).

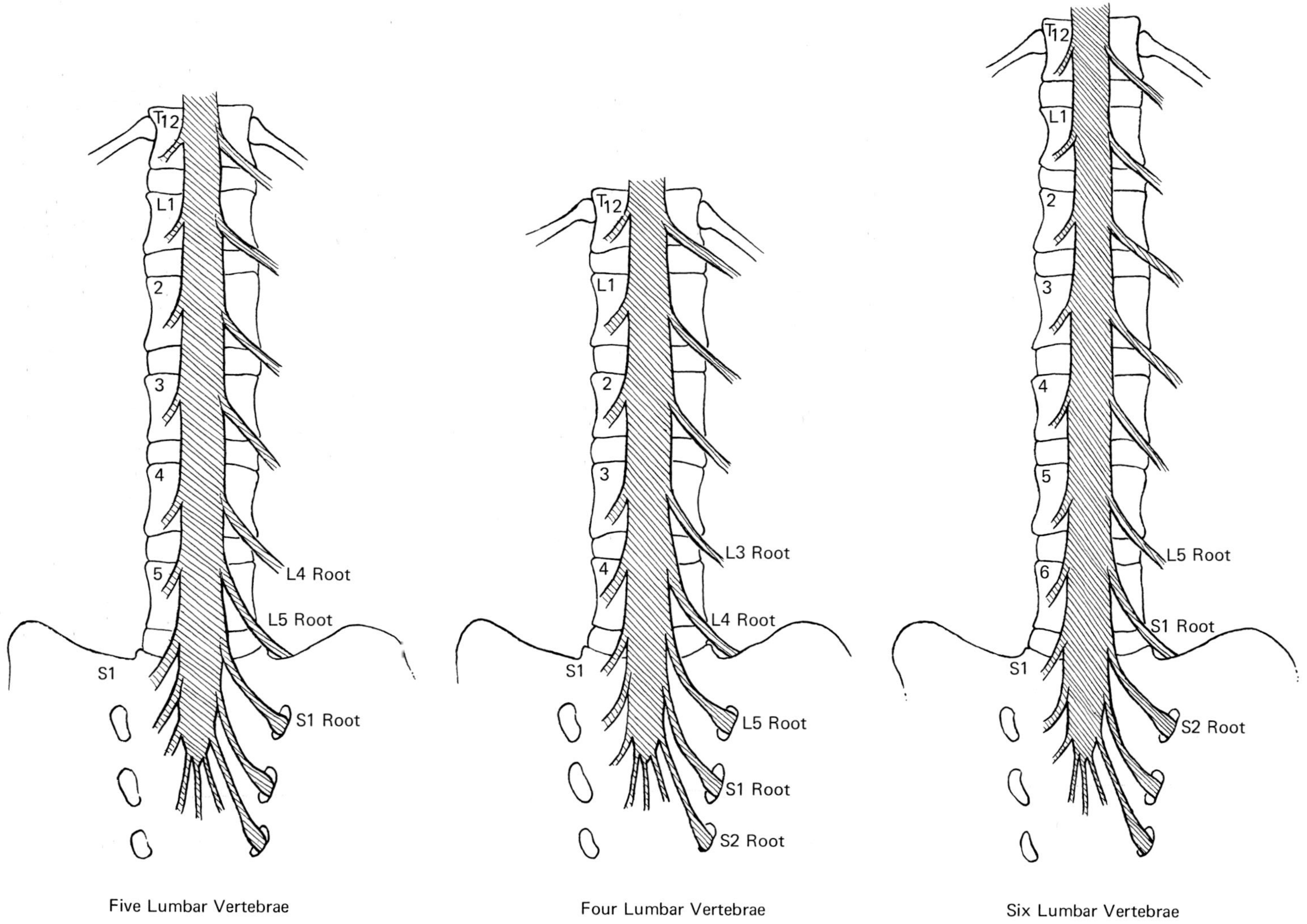

Fig. 25-2. Transitional lumbosacral verteb-al and root function (Reprinted from Finneson BE: *Low Back Pain.* Philadelphia, Lippincott, 1973, with permission).

Myelography

Lumbar myelograms are done on all patients before lumbar disc surgery. These are used principally to confirm clinical localization and to determine if more than one disc herniation is present. They also help to rule out possible lumbar spinal tumors, which can very easily simulate herniated lumbar discs. Although used mainly as a preoperative test, myelography is occasionally performed on patients who have not fared well with an adequate course of conservative management and in whom there is significant uncertainty regarding the nature of their complaints. The myelogram is not infallible and is associated with a significant incidence of both false negatives and false positives. Most false negatives are noted at the L5-S1 level, where there is a large space between the anterior dural edge and the posterior bony spine. This space is less wide above the L5-S1 level, so the incidence of false negatives is much less from L4-5 up. The incidence of false positives is greater in patients over the age of 55, because of the hypertrophic osteoarthritic degenerative changes associated with advancing years.

Predictive Factors

The four most important factors in determining a satisfactory outcome for surgery are:

1. Sciatic pain more severe than the back pain.
2. An abnormal myelogram that correlates with the clinical picture.
3. Positive Lesegue sign.
4. Neurologic deficit.

The crossed Lesegue sign is probably the most specific test for lumbar disc herniation (Fig. 25-3). If all four of the above are present, technically adequate surgery is likely to produce a satisfactory result. If one of them is absent, one should be very satisfied with the accuracy of the other three factors. Surgery considered with only one or two of these positive is likely to be associated with a high incidence of less than satisfactory results. With these factors in mind, there are four indications for surgery:

1. Intractable pain.
2. Progressively worsening neurologic deficit.
3. Intractable recurrence of pain.
4. Cauda equina syndrome.

With the exception of the cauda equina syndrome, each of these indications is relative and will depend on how well the patient tolerates the symptoms, the extent of the neurologic deficit, and the psychologic and sociologic background of the patient.

Choice of Operative Procedure

Once the decision is made that surgery is indicated, the surgeon must determine which operative procedure is most suitable for the patient's particular low back dysfunction.

Is a disc herniation producing a clear single root syndrome? If so, interlaminar disc excision is the procedure of choice.

Is it primarily a stenotic lumbar spinal canal syndrome associated with sciatica produced by foraminal impingement secondary to a bony spur? Attempting to treat this condition with an interlaminar disc excision is often technically difficult and is likely to result in a disappointing clinical result. The operation of choice for a stenotic lumbar spinal canal is decompressive laminectomy. This particular error may lead to permanent nerve root damage from surgery.

If the symptoms are unilateral and the myelographic defect is bilateral, should surgery be

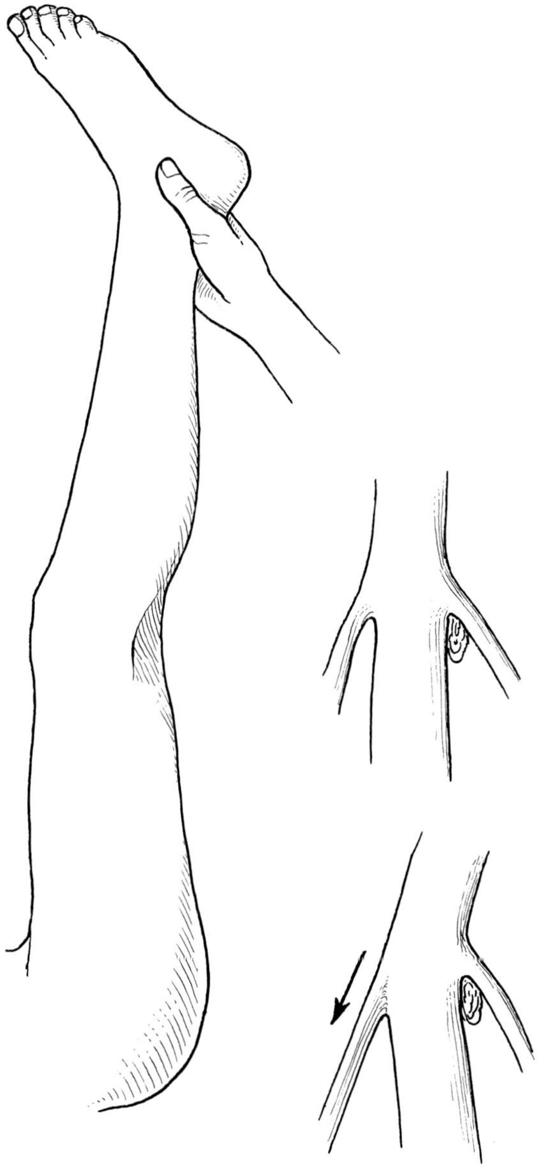

Fig. 25-3. The well leg raising test of Fajerstajn (Reprinted from Finneson BE: *Low Back Pain.* Philadelphia, Lippincott, 1973, with permission).

confined to the side of the pain or should a bilateral interlaminar disc excision be performed? This is often a gray area and may be open to controversy. I prefer to deal with this on an individual case basis rather than generalize, and have gone either way. I will state that as a basic principle I prefer to do the minimal amount of surgery that can adequately relieve symptoms rather than attempt prophylactic surgery of symptoms that have not previously developed. Whichever decision is made in this situation can be wrong. Both sides can be operated on and the patient will wake up with pain in the previously painless leg. Surgery can be confined to the painful side, and in the near or distant future, pain may develop on the nonoperated side.

Should disc excision be followed by a fusion? As director of a low back pain clinic, I have had the opportunity to review many cases of failed back surgery. Our limited experience in this regard seems to point to referral patterns rather than to a medical factor in determining whether disc surgery alone or disc excision followed by fusion is performed. Cases referred by an orthopedic surgeon to a neurosurgeon for disc surgery have the highest incidence of fusions; while the patient who was primarily managed by the neurosurgeon is more likely to have a disc excision alone.

Position

For the unilateral disc excision, many people prefer the lateral position, which was probably first developed by Doctor Thomas Hoen and popularized by Doctor William Scoville. This is the position of choice from the point of view of anesthesia, because it does not hamper respiratory excursions as much as the prone position. The principal surgical advantage is that it allows the abdomen to be relatively free, reducing pressure on the great veins and, in turn, reducing epidural venous distention and bleeding. A third technical advantage is that, in addition to posterior lumbar flexion the surgeon can laterally spread the uppermost interlaminar space by positioning the patient on the table so that the involved disc space is above the flexion break and then flexing the table.

Because of these advantages, I have repeatedly tried to adapt myself to the lateral

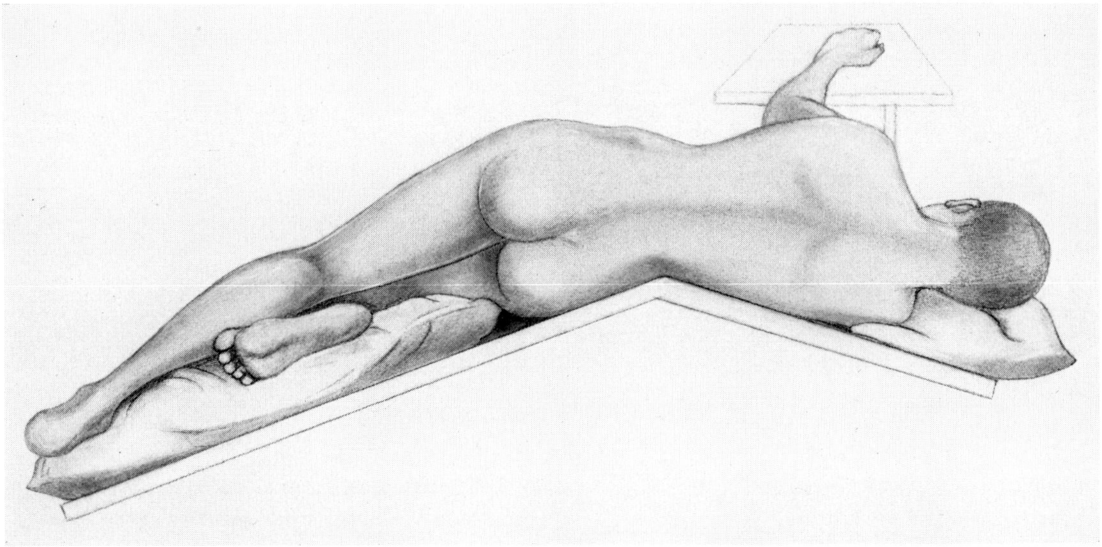

Fig. 25-4. Lateral position for lumbar disc surgery (Reprinted from Finneson BE: *Low Back Pain.* Philadelphia, Lippincott, 1973, with permission).

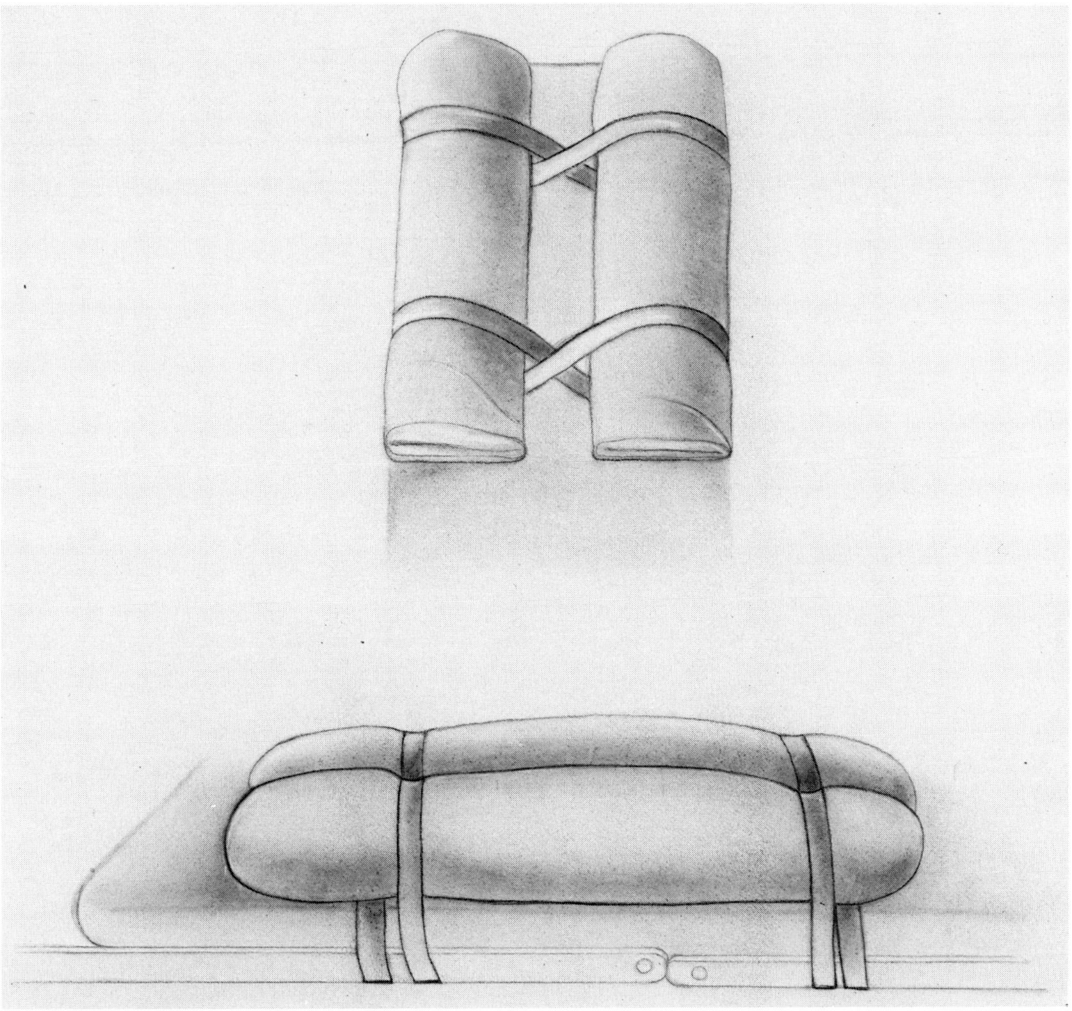

Fig. 25-5. Blanket rolls taped in place (Reprinted from Finneson BE: *Low Back Pain.* Philadelphia, Lippincott, 1973, with permission).

position but have been unsuccessful. Most of the advocates of the lateral position use it only for the unilateral operation and will generally use the prone position for a bilateral procedure. Scoville is one of the few who do all lumbar spinal procedures, unilateral or bilateral, in the lateral position. I still occasionally use it for very obese patients, but each time I do a case in the lateral position, I feel a bit clumsy and am not able to handle tissues as well as I can when the patient is in the prone position, so for reasons of habit I prefer to do lumbar disc surgery in the prone position. I use either a blanket roll (Fig. 25-5), extending from the pelvis to the shoulders, placed well laterally on either side of the table to avoid direct pressure on the midthorax or midabdomen, or the Wilson laminectomy frame, which is placed on the operating table (Fig. 25-6). There are a number of tuck and semituck positions that put much less pressure on the chest and abdomen, and there are strong advocates of these various modifications (Fig. 25-7). Because of the technical problems requiring special equipment and additional operating room personnel to properly carry out these positions, I tend to draw back to the less complex prone position, with the knees moderately flexed by placing a pillow or two beneath the shins. Usually I have the table flexed moderately (Fig. 25-8); but if the patient is a

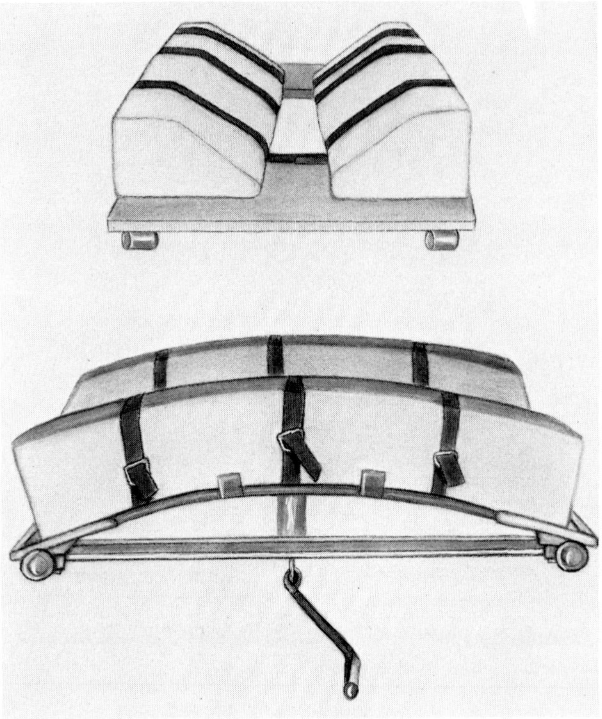

Fig. 25-6. Prone position frame (Reprinted from Finneson BE: *Low Back Pain.* Philadelphia, Lippincott, 1973, with permission).

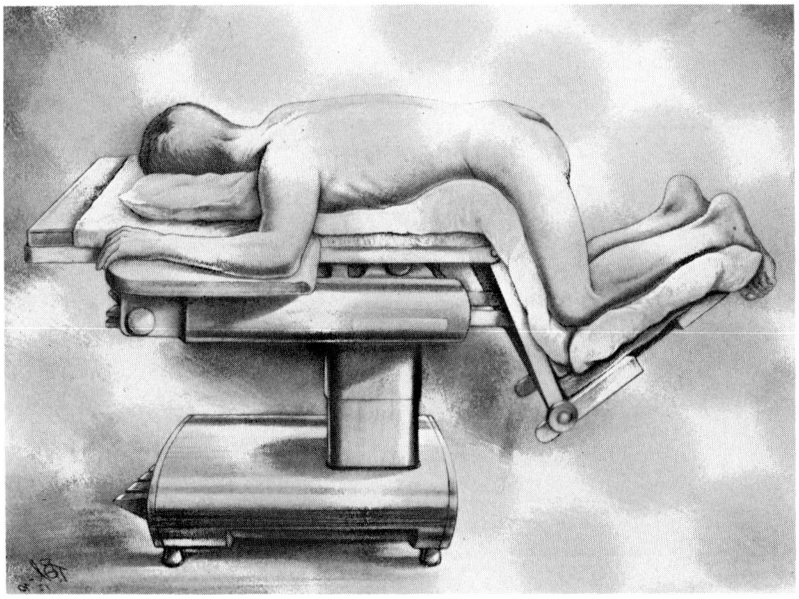

Fig. 25-7. Modified prone position (Reprinted from Finneson BE: *Low Back Pain.* Philadelphia, Lippincott, 1973, with permission).

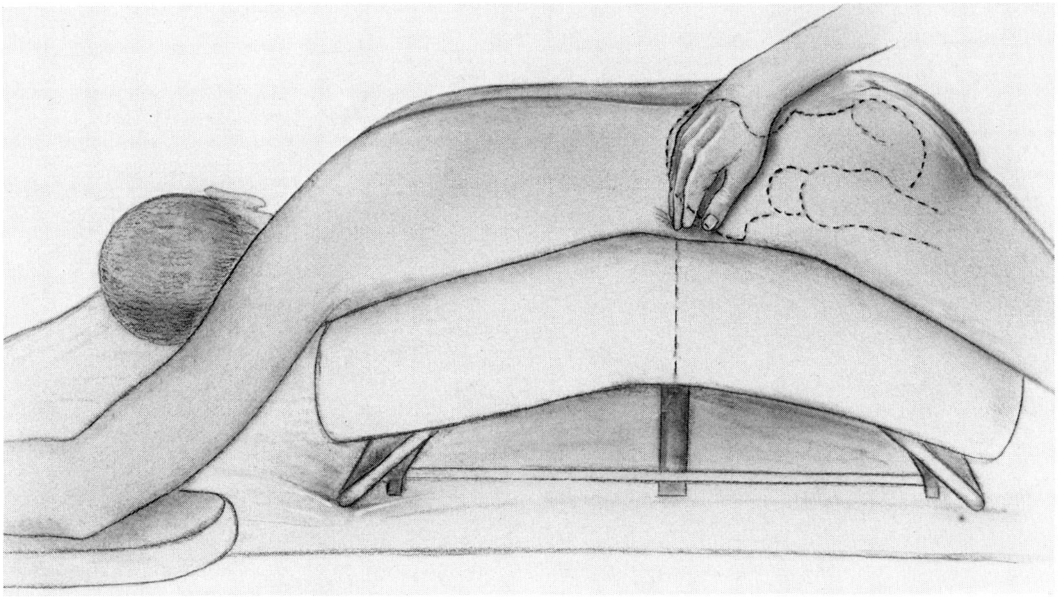

Fig. 25-8. Flexion "break" in table or frame at level of iliac crest (Reprinted from Finneson BE: *Low Back Pain.* Philadelphia, Lippincott, 1973, with permission).

bit obese or if upon removing the yellow ligament, the epidural veins seem a bit more distended than usual, the table is unflexed and surgery is carried out in the unflexed position. Flexion will increase abdominal pressure, causing increased venous pressure and increased venous bleeding.

Incisions

For many years my routine incision extended over approximately three spinous processes as an aid to interspace localization and to improve illumination with the ends of the incision, permitting overhead lighting to *funnel in*. I considered the short incision an *ego trip* on the part of the surgeon. I presently believe that the short incision is beneficial to the patient's postoperative recovery. There is no question that the patients feel immeasurably better in the immediate postoperative interval with the short-incision operation, compared to a large-incision operation. Of greater importance is the fact that the long incision, which extends over several spinous processes, produces a band of scar extending from the skin attaching to the spinous processes and laminae, along the extent of this incision. This scar tissue is not as supple as nonscarred muscle and fascia. This lack of elasticity and suppleness is not conducive to a nicely distributed lumbar curvature after wound healing occurs, and this nonsupple lumbar spine makes the patient more vulnerable to recurrent low back dysfunction in the future. When making a small incision, precise localization of this incision is crucial.

If the patient has recently had a lumbar myelogram, the surgeon can utilize the lumbar puncture needle mark as a cutaneous point of reference and then can count down to the appropriate interspace. When the myelogram is positive and surgery is deferred, the myelogram lumbar puncture needle site can be used as a reference to the appropriate interspace, which is then identified by a small dot tattooed into the skin to permanently mark the site of the involved interspace. This is done by placing a small drop of India ink on the skin and tapping

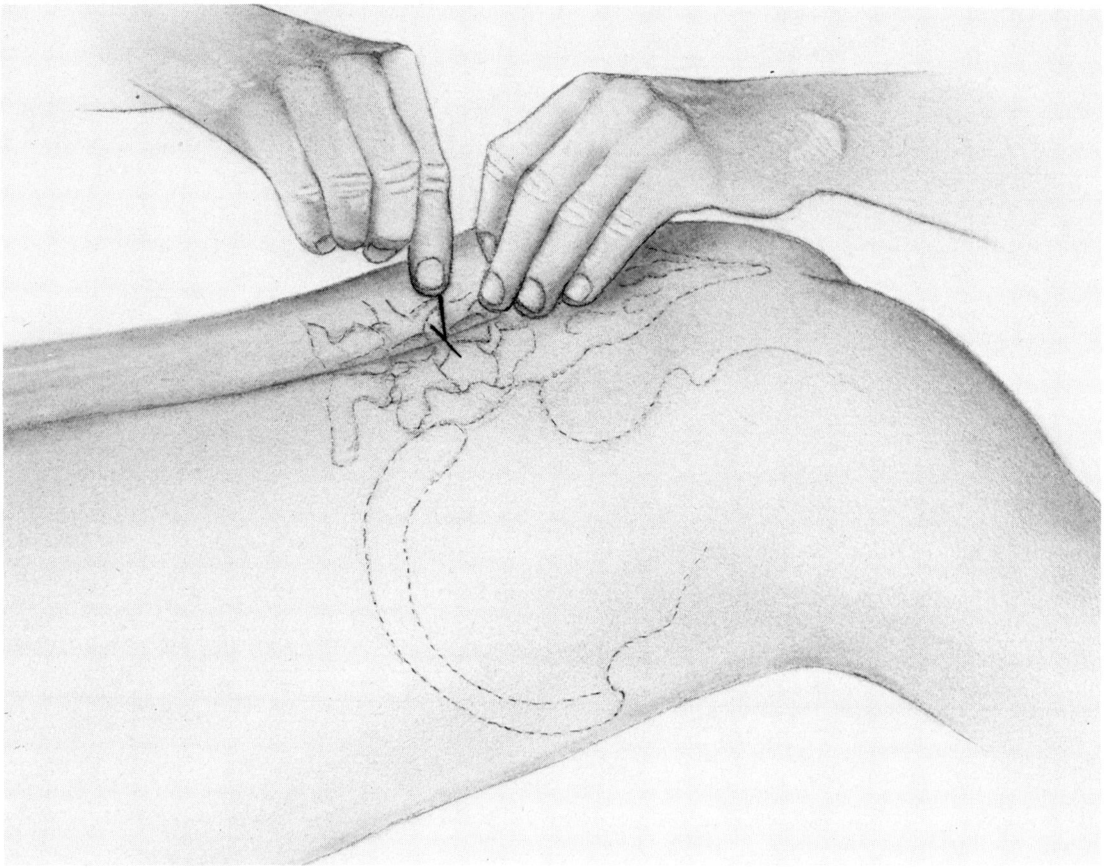

Fig. 25-9. The skin is scratched at the "involved" interspinous space (Reprinted from Finneson BE: *Low Back Pain.* Philadelphia, Lippincott, 1973, with permission).

the skin with a 25-gauge hypodermic needle through this drop of India ink. When using the small incision, fiberoptic lighting and magnification are a necessity. The fiberoptic lighting and operating telescopes or the operating microscope are of great advantage. For many years I carried out lumbar disc surgery without magnification or special lighting and tended to label those individuals using such appliances as gadgeteers. I presently use a Malis fiberoptic headlight and 2½ and 4½ power operating telescopes. These instruments aid greatly in assuring delicate handling of tissue and help precent nerve root damage. I consider them an integral and essential aid to the surgery.

Technique of Surgery

The subperiosteal muscle can be dissected by a variety of methods. I prefer to use a periosteal elevator pressed against the edge of the spinous process and cut directly against the spine, preserving the posterior spinous ligament or supraspinal ligament, a strong fibrous cord that extends without interruption along the tips of the spinous processes from C7 to end at the median sacral crest. Between the spinous processes, it is continuous with the interspinal ligaments. I believe it is valuable to preserve this structure in an effort to avoid weakening the involved spinal ligament unnecessarily. To prevent excessive scarring, I use a scalpel rather than a cutting cautery to incise the fascia. The muscles are best stripped from the

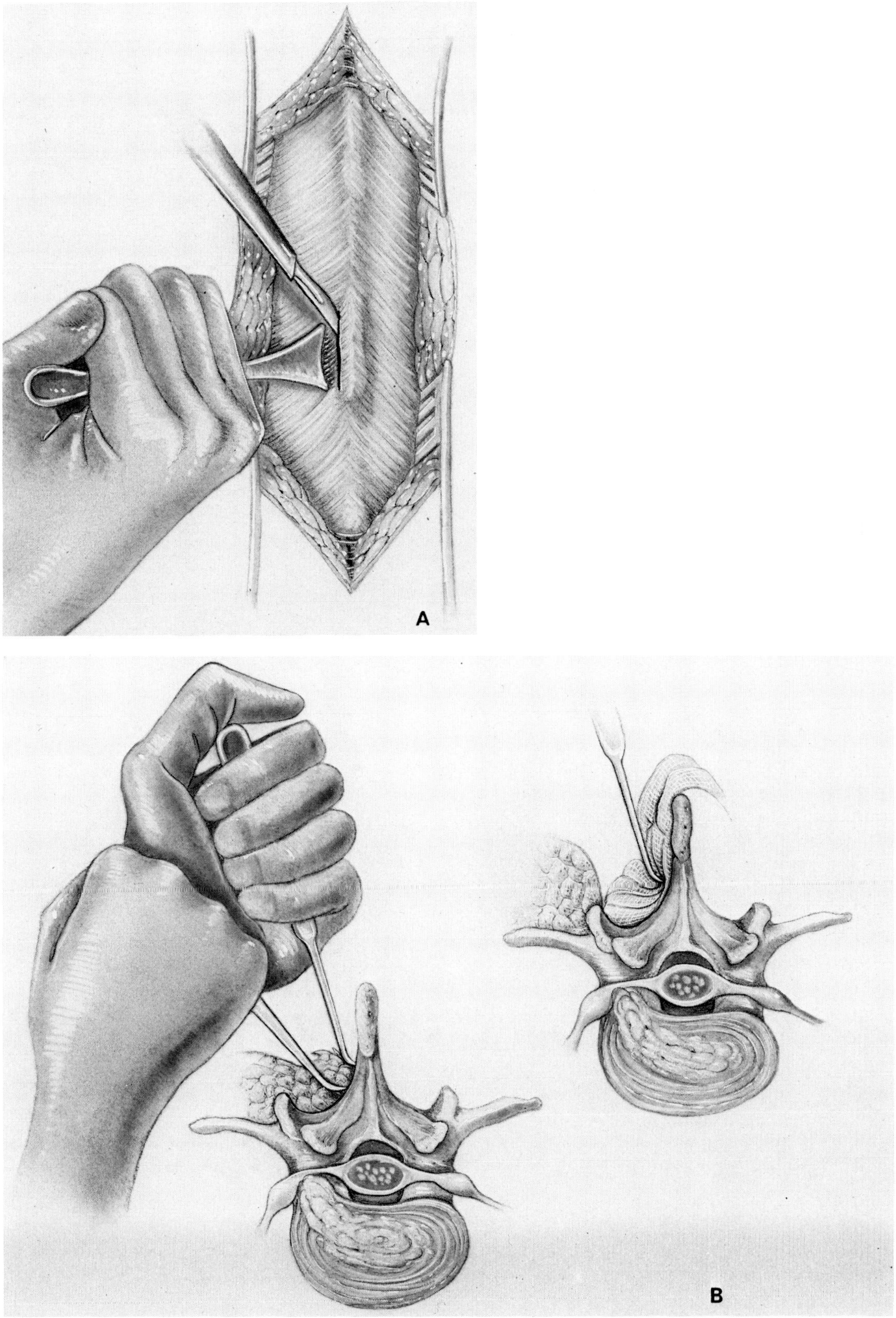

Fig. 25-10 A and B. Subperiosteal dissection technique (Reprinted from Finneson BE: *Low Back Pain.* Philadelphia, Lippincott, 1973, with permission).

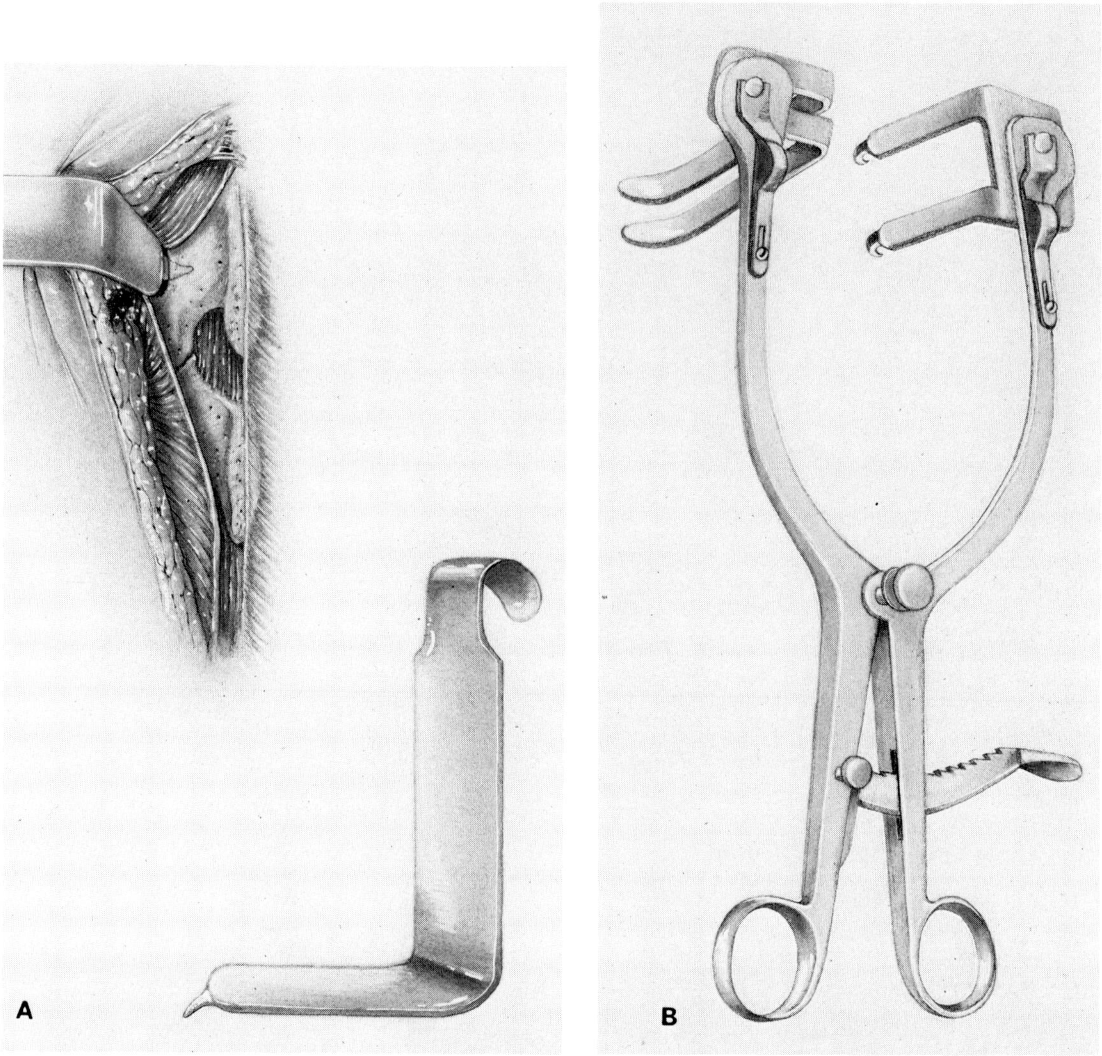

Fig. 25-11. A. Taylor hemilaminectomy retractor. **B.** Hoen hemilaminectomy retractor. **C.** If the hemilaminectomy retractor blades are longer than necessary, the depth through which the surgeon must work is increased (Reprinted from Finneson BE: *Low Back Pain.* Philadelphia, Lippincott, 1973, with permission).

spinous processes and lamina, using the bimanual 2 periosteal method. One periosteal elevator is used to retract the muscle mass laterally, while the other is performing a careful subperiosteal dissection (Fig. 25-10 A and B).

The hemilaminectomy retractor of my choice is the Hoen (Fig. 25-11 A, B and C), but I am fairly comfortable with the Scoville. Once the retractor is in place, all bleeding from skin, muscle, and fascia must be controlled. It must be emphasized that the rest of the surgery takes place in a small keyhole of space, and bleeding from any of these structures will funnel directly into the work area. If the assistant has to provide suction to remove the blood, either his head is in the way, obstructing the surgeon's vision, or the assistant is poking the suction tip into the wound blindly, which also has its disadvantages. The other alternative is the surgeon holds the suction with one hand while operating with the other which is not really satisfactory. Therefore control of bleeding at this stage is a must for smooth, safe surgery.

Strenuous manual work tends to create a perceptible hand tremor immediately afterward, so I prefer using airpowered rongeurs for much of the bone work. The Leksell or

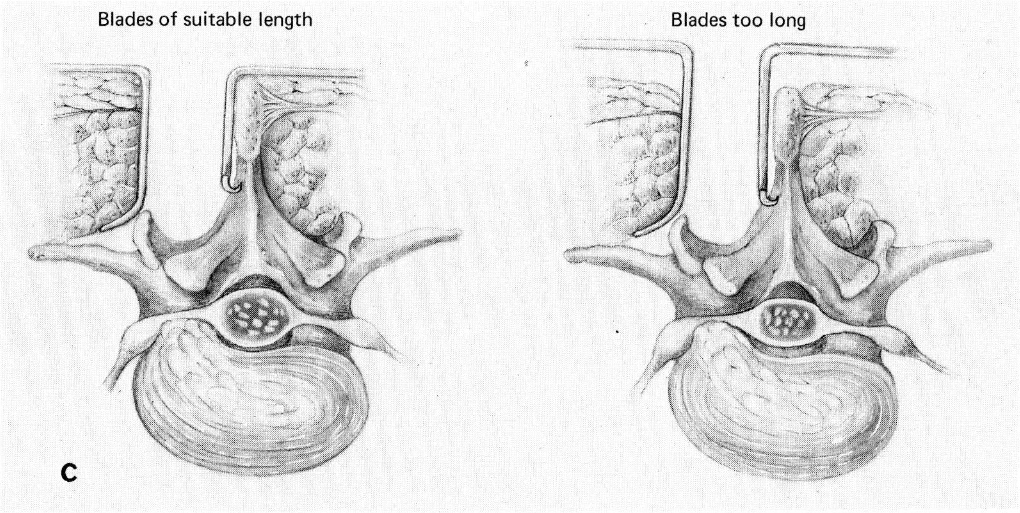

Fig. 25-11. (continued)

Duck-bill rongeur is used to remove the overhanging edge of the superior lamina, removing one-third of the lamina (Fig. 25-12). This bone will invariably bleed, and bone wax is used to provide complete hemostasis before the yellow ligament is excised. Some surgeons prefer rongeuring away half of the superior lamina, which exposes the superior border of the yellow ligament. This can then be grasped with an Allis tissue forceps and, using a scalpel, the remainder of the ligament can be excised by sharp dissection. I prefer to remove only one-third of the superior lamina so that the edge of the yellow ligament is not exposed. I use the Allis tissue forceps to grasp the yellow ligament and tug it laterally. Then I use a No. 11

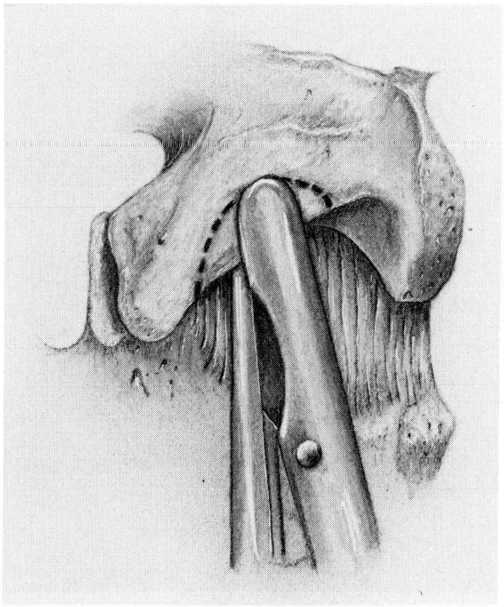

Fig. 25-12. The overhanging edge of the superior lamine is rongeured (Reprinted from Finneson BE: *Low Back Pain.* Philadelphia, Lippincott, 1973, with permission).

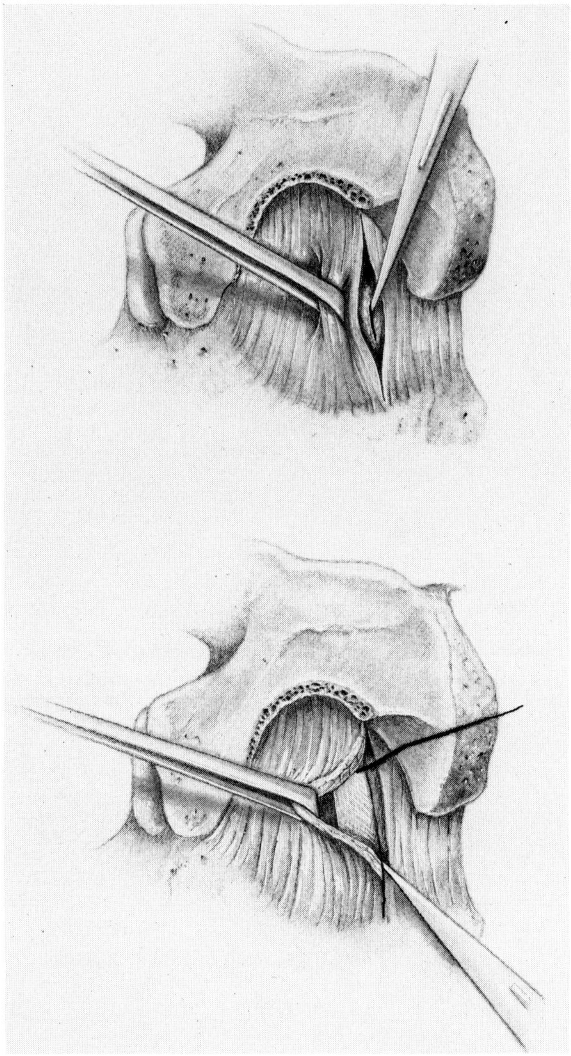

Fig. 25-13. The yellow ligament is cut (Reprinted from Finneson BE: *Low Back Pain.* Philadelphia, Lippincott, 1973, with permission).

blade to carefully cut the ligament along the direction of its fibers, until the dura and epidural fat can be visualized (Fig. 25-13). The point of the blade is used to dissect away the superior edge of the yellow ligament, so that it can be reflected laterally. A small curette can now be used to peel the yellow ligament away from the top of the inferior lamina, after which the epidural tissues can be clearly visualized and not traumatized (Fig. 25-14). Once the yellow ligament has been excised, the dura must be clearly visualized.

If epidural fat obscures the dura and nerve root, it is gently teased away with a fine forceps, since good visualization of the dura and root is a must for the next step. A 15° angled Schlesinger cervical punch is used to completely expose the lateral border of the nerve root. For this lateral exposure, the medial half of the facet joint must be removed. This can only be done safely when the dura and root can be clearly visualized and are not obscured by either blood or epidural fat.

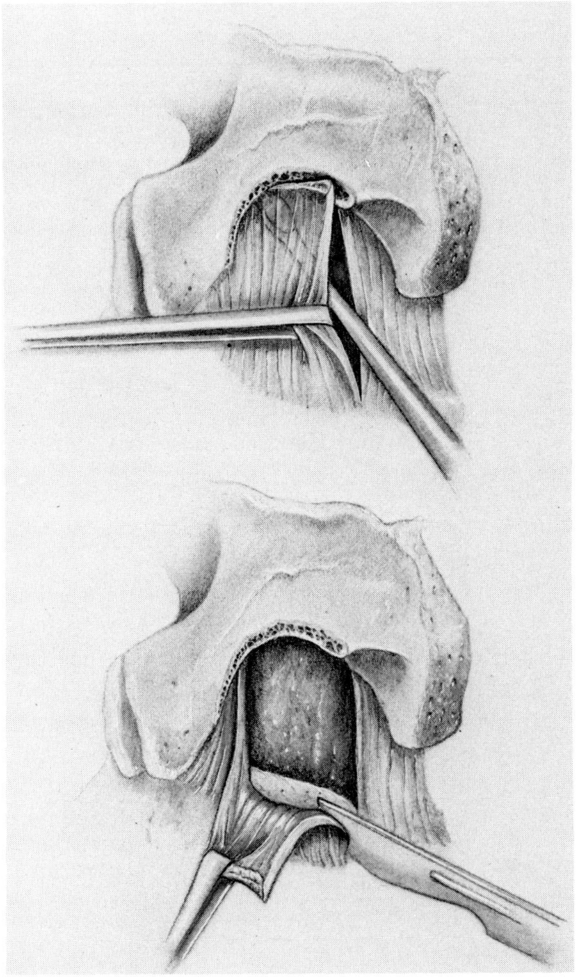

Fig. 25-11. The yellow ligament is curetted (Reprinted from Finneson BE: *Low Back Pain.* Philadelphia, Lippincott, 1973, with permission).

This is as good a time as any to remind ourselves that the goal of surgery is adequate decompression of the root, while assuring gentle safe handling of the root. At this point in surgery root damage is likely to occur in two ways. One common error is to mistake the lateral reflection of the yellow ligament immediately over the root for the root. Sometimes these form a band-like cylindrical appearance, which is quite deceptive (Fig. 25-15). If this band is retracted medially, the underlying root may be mistakenly identified as a bulging disc, which is then attacked with vigor. Another error is to insert the tip of the Schlesinger too deep so that it grasps a bit of the root along with the edge of the yellow ligament and bone. As the surgeon tugs on the instrument, a fairly long glistening piece of tissue, resembling spaghetti, comes out, followed by bloody spinal fluid. These errors are classifiable as surgical tragedies and can usually be avoided by proper hemostasis, good visualization, and by avoiding speed at this point in the operation.

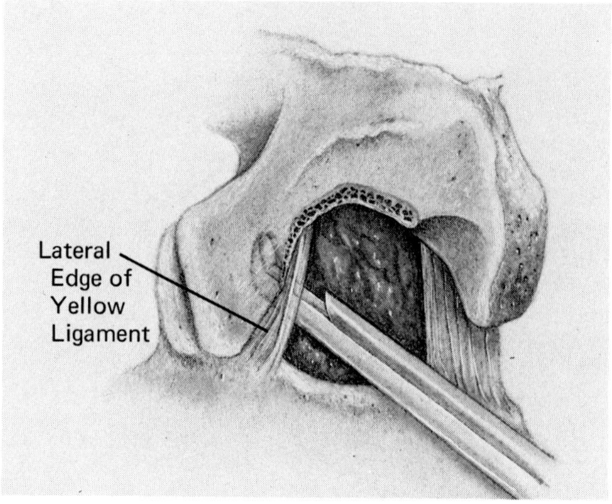

Fig. 25.15. In widening the interspace, do not mistake the rolled up lateral edge of yellow ligament for the root (Reprinted from Finneson BE: *Low Back Pain.* Philadelphia, Lippincott, 1973, with permission).

Once the dissection has been successfully carried out and the lateral border of the root is exposed, the surgeon uses a narrow blunt elevator to gently mobilize the root medially. Sometimes the root is under too much pressure to perform this with ease. In that case do not retract the root but work lateral to it to decompress it. If extruded disc fragments are free within the canal, they can usually be manipulated laterally, grasped with the pituitary forceps, and gently removed. If the disc is not extruded but is bulging so much that the nerve cannot be easily mobilized medially, work lateral to the disc, introducing the pituitary forceps into the intervertebral disc space, and remove disc fragments piecemeal until the root can be more easily retracted over a partially decompressed shell. The major error at this point comes under the heading of *grandstanding*. There is a temptation to demonstrate the pathology to any and all present in the operating room. The overstretched root is retracted over a large disc and maintained in that position while residents, interns, nurses, and visitors are invited to inspect the protruding disc. This is not the time to entertain ''the troops,'' and a herniated disc is not very spectacular looking in any event (Fig. 25-16).

Once the disc has been adequately excised, there is little difficulty retracting the root medially. A nerve root retractor can then be used to expose the disc space more completely. A No. 11 blade is used to make a rectangular slab-shaped window through the annulus, and this opening is used to remove the disc contents as completely as possible (Fig. 25-17). I use pituitary forceps of various sizes and shapes as well as a curette to free up loose fragments of disc material. Excision of a rectangular slab of annulus may prevent the remaining shell of annulus from buckling as the disc space collapses. This buckling may, in time, fibrose and provide a source of root compression a year or two postoperatively.

I do not think that any disc should be violated unless it can be seen to be causing nerve root pressure. However, once the disc is violated, thorough disc excision is required.

A bulging annulus does not have to be removed, particularly if the nerve root can be adequately decompresed. The root can easily go over a slight hump, as long as there is no bony counterpressure above it. Sometimes a generous foraminotomy alone is adequate. In equivocal cases saline injection into the disc, using a 10-ml syringe, may be helpful. If the bulging disc does not take more than 1 or 2 ml of saline without a great deal of pressure, it might be tempting to limit the approach to a decompressive foraminotomy; whereas, if the entire 10 ml can be injected into the intervertebral disc space without a great deal of diffi-

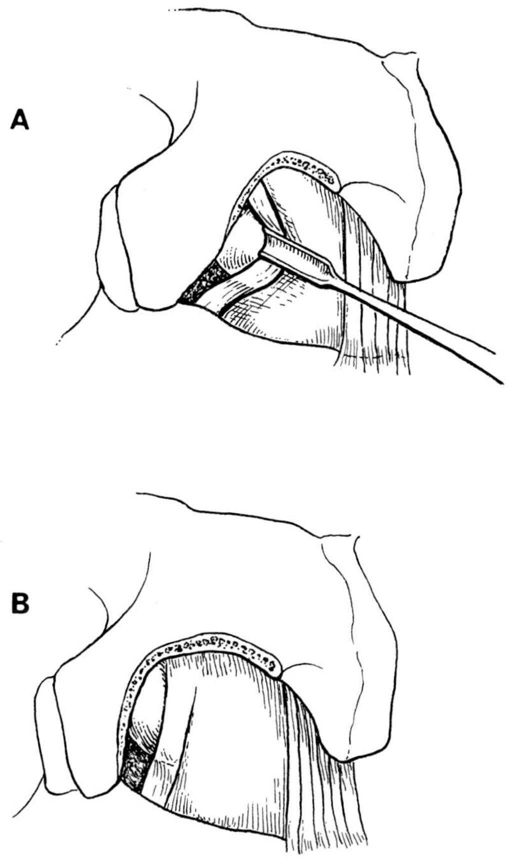

Fig. 25-16. A. Overstretched root and dural sac with an inadequate lateral bony exposure. **B.** Very little root retraction is necessary with adequate lateral bony exposure (Reprinted from Finneson BE: *Low Back Pain.* Philadelphia, Lippincott, 1973, with permission).

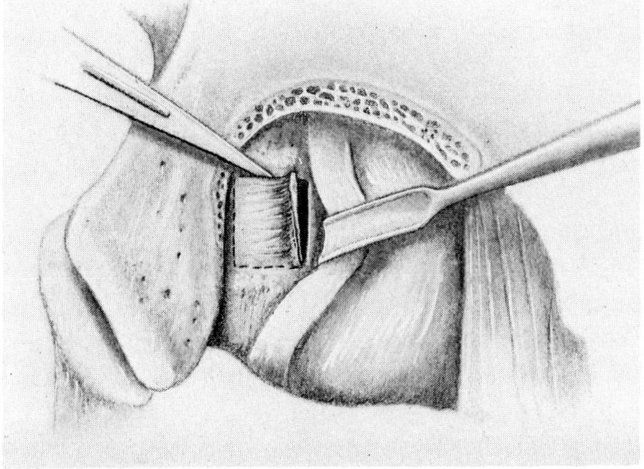

Fig. 25-17. Incision of rectangular window through the annulus fibrosus (Reprinted from Finneson BE: *Low Back Pain.* Philadelphia, Lippincott, 1973, with permission).

culty, such a disc could be considered more pathologic. Occasionally, two roots come out of the same foramen or separate foramina are encountered. The root above, instead of following the usual course, will come down very close to the root below so that when the dura and its root are exposed, there will be a second root just lateral to the first root. If it is recognized as a root there is no problem, but occasionally the laterally positioned root is mistaken for a bulging disc and attempts are made to excise it. In doing so the root may be destroyed beyond repair. There is no substitute for good lighting and magnification. In addition the operation should always be done questioningly, since the surgeon is working through a "keyhole" and identification of tissues is extremely important.

When venous bleeding becomes a problem, cottonoids placed above and below adequately control the bleeding at times, and when the table is flattened, should be satisfactory. Once the dissection is completed, merely releasing the root and dura stops the bleeding. If this is inadequate, a very small piece of Gelfoam, no larger than a match head, soaked in thrombin may be satisfactory if it can be placed right over the bleeding site. I prefer this to cauterizing the veins or using silver clips, since these measures do destroy the vein and stop venous flow, and I am never sure exactly what harm this may cause.

Transdural Exploration

Transdural exploration, described in the neurosurgical literature, is a technique for opening the dura, separating the roots to either side, and excising a lumbar disc through an anterior dural incision. I think this technique is to be condemned, and although I described it in my book, I will rectify this point in the next edition. The entire idea of excising an extradural structure by transdural exploration is not sound. Once the dura is opened, the fluid-filled sac collapses, resulting in increased venous bleeding once this support has been reduced. Some blood is invariably introduced into the subarachnoid space, which, because of this foreign material, must lead to some degree of adhesive arachnoiditis. Very little benefit is derived from looking into the cauda equina, suspected of having adhesive arachnoiditis, other to satisfy one's curiosity. If the dura must be opened for some reason, such as assuring that there are no varicosities or to rule out neoplasm, I would suggest that the arachnoid be left intact. This does not provide a very good view of the roots, because the arachnoid, which is filled with fluid, is like a curved lens that distorts the image. However, if a sterile glass microscope slide* is pressed against the rounded arachnoid, it will flatten out. The roots will be seen clearly, unless, of course, the arachnoid is milky, which would then confirm the diagnosis of adhesive arachnoiditis. In this case, there is not much point in opening the arachnoid because little would be achieved by trying to comb out the roots to dissect away the adhesive arachnoid film binding them together. Even the most experienced operator may accidentally open the dura, particularly if it is thin, which it often is in elderly individuals with a stenotic lumbar spinal canal in addition to a bulging lumbar disc. Sometimes it appears as though the dura will tear just as soon as it is visualized. This is apt to occur when a bone-biting instrument is used at the upper border of the inferior lamina. A slight fold of dura may bulge and be caught in the jaws of the instrument. A tiny pinch of dura caught by the bone-biting instrument will tear it (Fig. 25-18). Most of the fibers in the dura are longitudinal, running up and down; if the instrument catches a fiber and the operator pulls, the dura will rip like a seam. Just a small bite of bone can unknowingly cause an inch-long tear of dura. If the dura is opened, a small hole is much easier to close than a large one. Therefore dissection should proceed cautiously on the inferior lamina. Do not take a bite of bone and rip it out. Close the instrument carefully and ease the bone out very slowly so that if the dura is tugged even slightly, release the instrument and inspect the area carefully before removing the bone further. This type of complication always occurs before adequate exposure has been obtained.

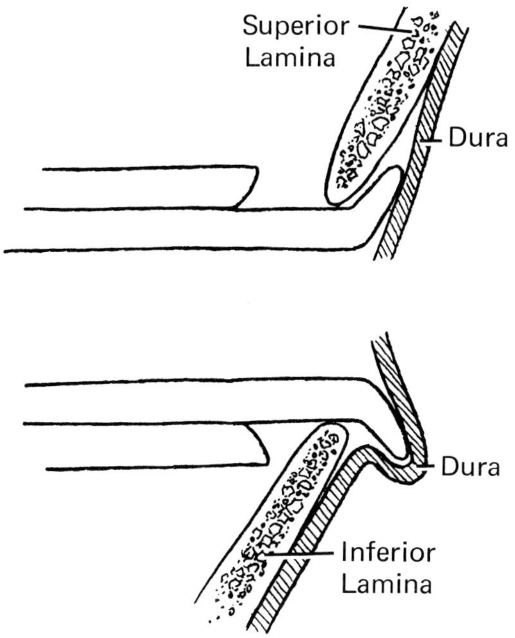

Fig. 25-18. The laminectomy punch with a 40 angled jaw is helpful when working on the superior lamina, but is not suited for the slope of the inferior lamina and may produce a dural tear (Reprinted from Finneson BE: *Low Back Pain.* Philadelphia, Lippincott, 1973, with permission).

Cerebrospinal fluid may fill the wound suddenly, becoming tinged with blood, so that it is impossible to see the area. There is a tendency to try to close this opening immediately, which is a mistake. It is also a mistake to try to see the damage and to put a sucker into the area, because the roots will come out through this hole, invariably catch on the sucker, and be damaged, sometimes severely. Instead, insert a cottonoid into the opening and suck only on the cottonoid until the structures can be seen. Then place a square of Gelfoam over the dural opening, place a cottonoid on top of the Gelfoam square, and tilt the table head down so that spinal fluid pressure decreases in the lumbar region. If the table is flexed, it should be flattened. At this point proceed as though the dura had not been opened.

Before closing the dural tear, it is necessary to expose both sides and both ends of the tear. Dural closure must be watertight, using 4-0 or 5-0 suture material.

Degenerative disc disease does not necessarily confine itself to the posterolateral portion of the disc. It may involve the entire disc, including the anterior portion of the annulus, which may lead to accidental perforation through the degenerated and nonresistant structure. If the iliac artery is grasped and torn by the pituitary forceps, a surgical crisis is created (Fig. 25-19). Various methods have been advocated to avoid this problem, including marking the instruments 1½ inches from the tip, which may keep the surgeon's depth perception. Hopefully, with good lighting and magnification, the interior of the disc space can clearly be seen during the dissection, also helping immeasurably with depth perception. After the disc has been adequately excised, it is usually easier to retract the dura and root medially, without stretching these structures unduly. Exploration should be continued cranially, caudally, and laterally, searching for any free fragments that were not visible because the bulging disc precluded adequate retraction and visualization. If the nerve root is swollen, a foraminotomy

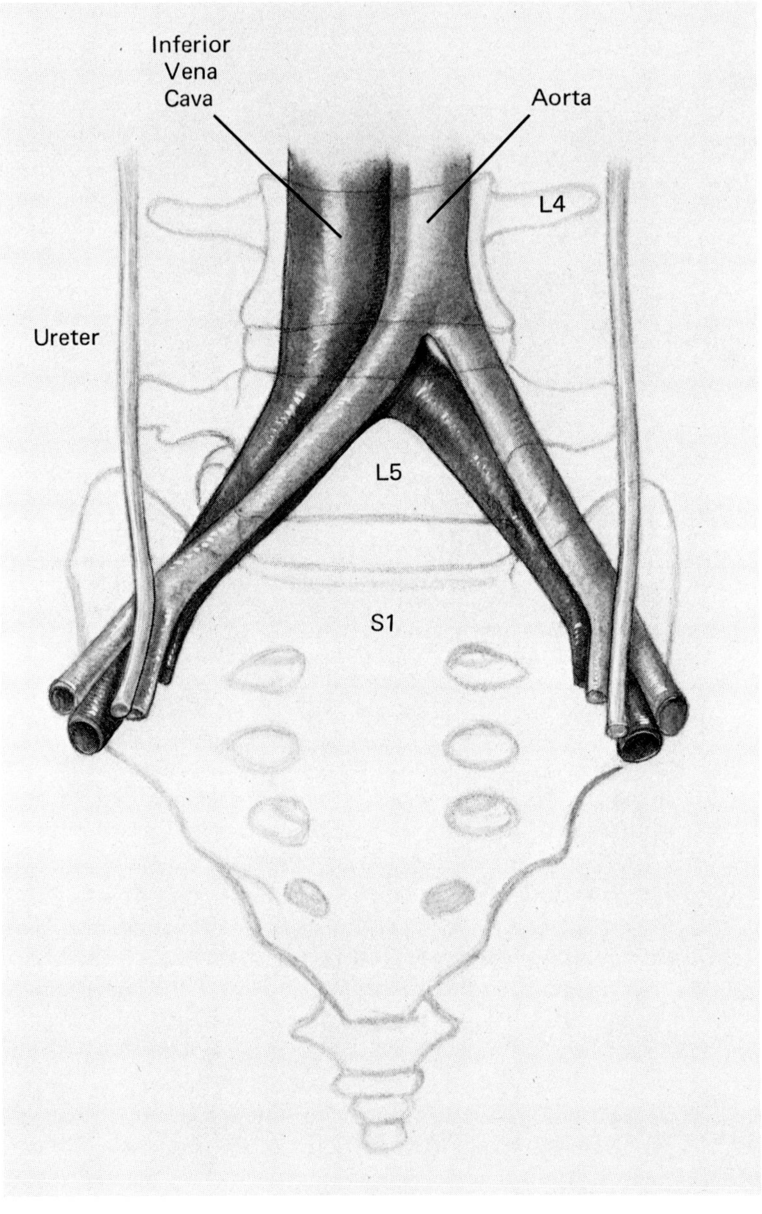

Fig. 25-19. The major vessels and ureters and their relationship to the anterior lumbar spine (Reprinted from Finneson BE: *Low Back Pain.* Philadelphia, Lippincott, 1973, with permission).

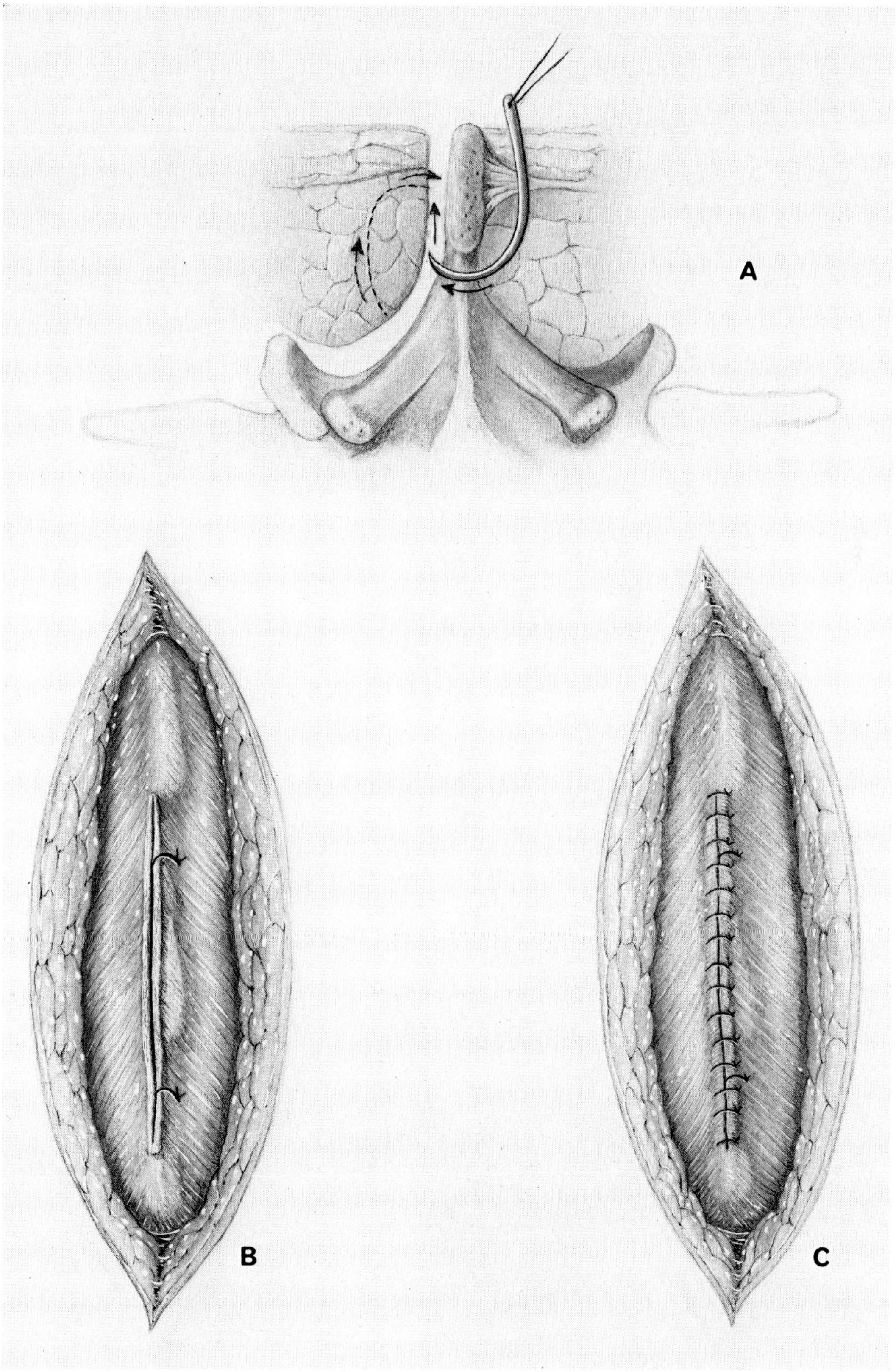

Fig. 25-20. A and **B.** Muscle closure to eliminate "dead space." **C.** fascial closure (Reprinted from Finneson BE: *Low Back Pain.* Philadelphia, Lippincott, 1973, with permission).

may help to free the swollen nerve root. If the operation was done with the patient in flexion, it is well to flatten the table out and reinspect the anatomy, since this change in position may allow detection of a free fragment that had previously gone unnoticed. I prefer not to leave any foreign substances within the area of the dura or root. Some surgeons electively place Gelfoam membrane over the dura; others excise a bit of subcutaneous fat and place it over the nerve root. I prefer not to place anything over the nerve root, but irrigate the wound with dilute Bacitracin solution and close with interrupted chromic catgut for muscle and fascia and the stainless steel technique for skin (Fig. 25-20).

CHAPTER 26

Posterior Lumbar Intervertebral Fusion

Paul M. Lin

THE CONCEPT OF INTERVERTEBRAL (intercorporal) fusion in the cervical area has gained wide acceptance in recent years.[1-3] In 1945 Cloward devised a workable technique of posterior lumbar intervertebral fusion (Fig. 26-1) and first reported "the treatment of ruptured lumbar disc by intervertebral fusion—report of 100 cases" at the Harvey Cushing Society meeting at Hot Springs, Virginia, in November 1947. His description of the technique of posterior lumbar intervertebral fusion predated his more popular cervical anterior interbody fusion by 12 years. With the exception of Christoferson[4] (Fig. 26-2), Wiltberger[5,6] (Fig. 26-3) and Cloward's own publication,[7-9] there has been astonishing little enthusiasm for posterior lumbar interbody fusion. Recent survey of all training programs in neurosurgery in the United States indicated only two institutions are doing Cloward's lumbar posterior intervertebral fusion and a third institution performs the Christoferson-type of implant intervertebral fusion. The practice of posterior lumbar intervertebral fusion is more popular outside of the United States, especially in Germany,[10] England,[11] and Australia.[12] The lack of enthusiasm could be due to fear of technical difficulty and inherent complications associated with posterior lumbar intervertebral fusion.

Anterior lumbar intervertebral spinal fusion has supporters among our orthopedic colleagues.[13-19] However, complications from transabdominal approach are high, especially vascular injuries and sexual incompetence.[20] With improve illumination and better technique in controlling epidural hemorrhage by proper position of the patient and the use of Surgicel* as a tampon, the author believes that this operation is technically feasible for any skillful neurosurgeon.

Junghanns[10] described lumbar intervertebral disc as part of a *motor segment* that consists of the intervertebral disc, intervertebral foramen, facet, interlaminal space, ligamentum flavum, spinous processes and its adjoining ligaments (Fig. 26-4). When a lumbar disc is degenerative, or if the disc is removed surgically, the intervertebral disc space narrows. There follows a sequential change of the motor segment (Fig. 26-5). It could be a recurrent disc herniation, posterior spur formation of the vertebral body, facet overriding, spur formation of the facet, or internal invagination of the ligamentum flavum. In various combination it

*Surgicel, oxydized regenerated cellulose, Johnson and Johnson Laboratories, New Brunswick, N.J.

Department of Neurological Surgery, Temple University Health Sciences Center, Philadelphia, Pennsylvania

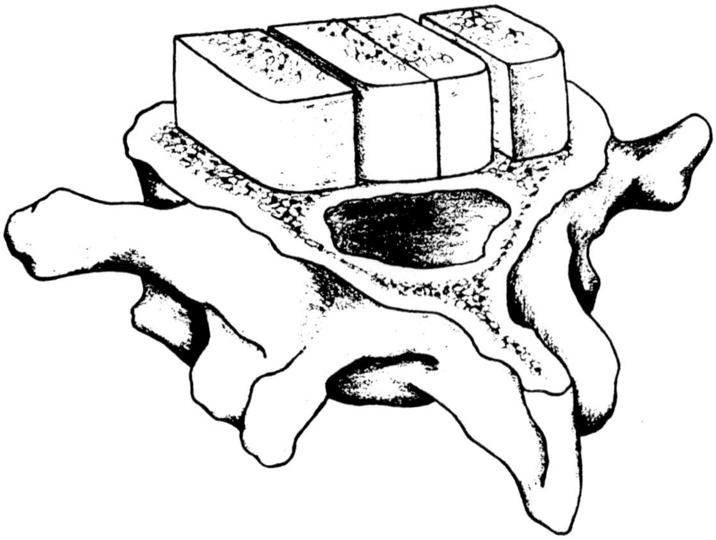

Fig. 26-1. Cloward's posterior lumbar intervertebral fusion using rectangular bone graft.

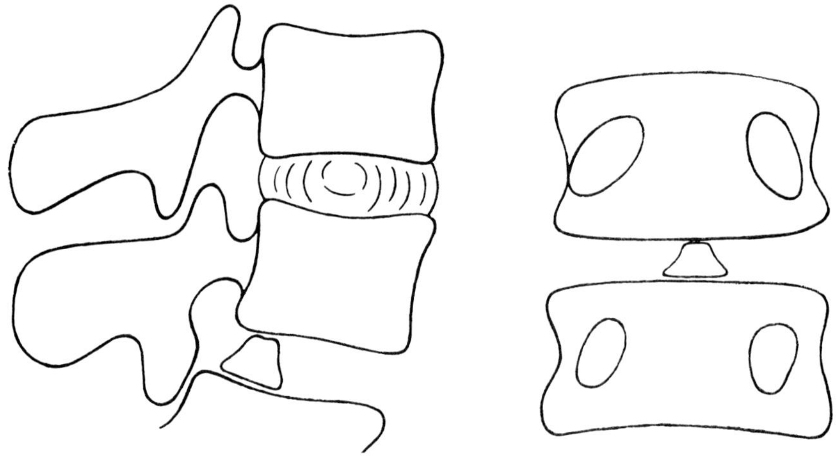

Fig. 26-2. Christoferson's posterior lumbar disc space bony implant after partial discectomy.

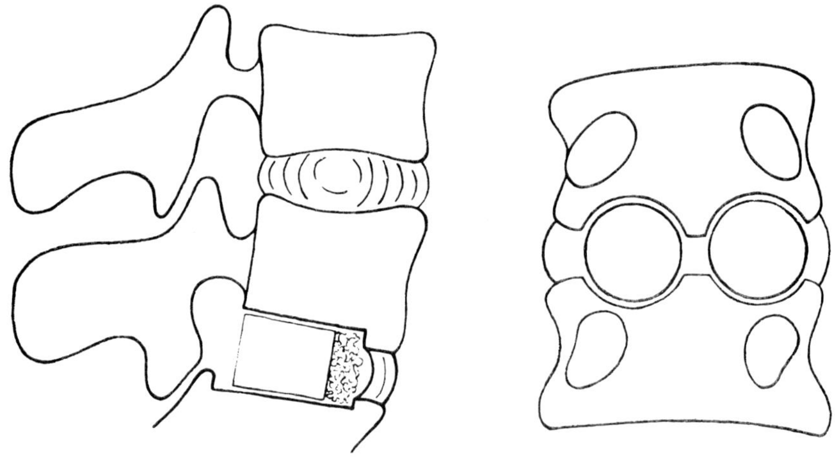

Fig. 26-3. Wiltberger's posterior lumbar intervertebral fusion using drill and dowel technique.

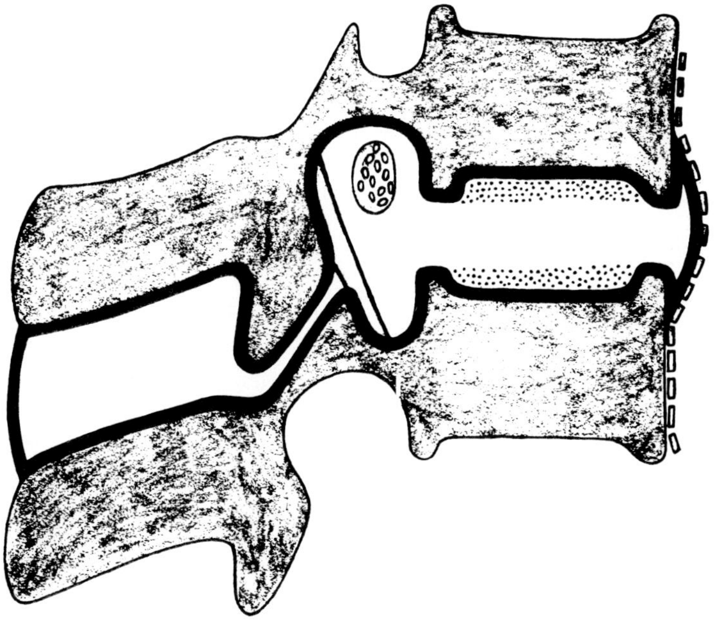

Fig. 26-4. Junghanns' concept of "motor segment" with disc and facet working as a signle motion unit. Note the ligamentum flavum covering the anterior portion of the facet.

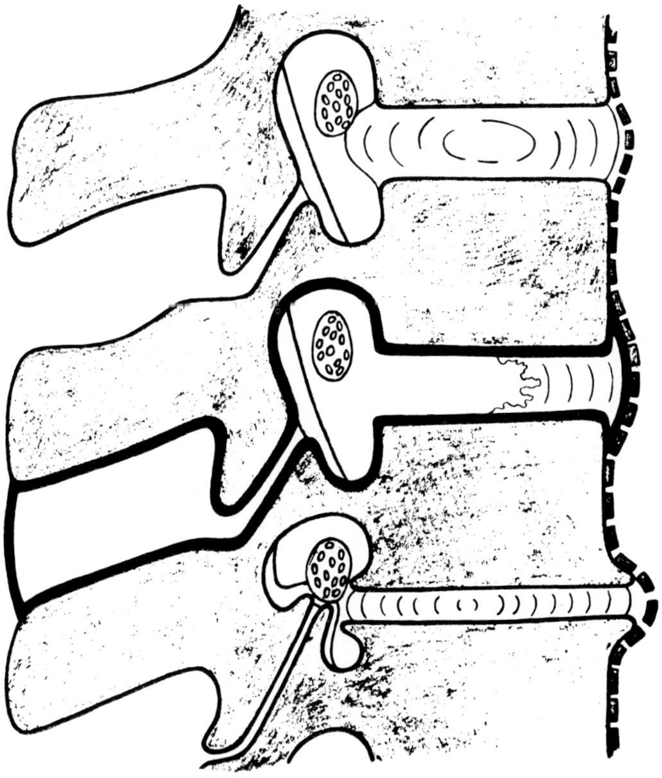

Fig. 26-5. Sequential changes expected in a "motor segment" when disc material is extruded or removed surgically. Laterally ligamentum flavum lies anterior to the facet and is generally not radiologically identifiable.

would result in spinal stenosis both at the intervertebral foramen and also at the spinal canal. The degenerative changes of the motor segment and the settlement of the disc space are the most common causes of failure or recurrent symptomatology of herniated nucleus pulposus treated by simple discectomy.

Indications

The advantages of posterior lumbar intervertebral fusion (PLIF) are:

1. PLIF reconstitutes the normal anatomic relationship between the motor segment and the neural structures. The narrow disc space and the motor segment are unfurled or restored back to its normal anatomic alignment.
2. Successful PLIF would arrest further degenerative process of the fused motor segment. However, there are indications that because of increased range of motion of the adjoining vertebral disc spaces, their degenerative processes could be enhanced by PLIF.
3. Total discectomy needed for PLIF prevents recurrent lumbar disc herniation at that level.
4. The PLIF would prevent painful nerve irritation from postoperative perineural adhesions; lack of motion after a successful PLIF prevents mechanical pulling of the nerve root from the surrounding scar tissue.
5. Wide laminotomy in PLIF relieves all neural compression from structures other than the disc.

Spangfort,[21] analyzing the results of 2,504 lumbar discectomies in Sweden, indicated that those with complete disc herniation had satisfactory results in about 90% of the cases. Those with incomplete herniation gave only 80% improvement, whereas bulging discs without herniation had 60% improvement. Of those with no disc herniation at the time of surgery, only 30% were improved. Assuming that all patients had similar preoperative indications, then in the categories where a bulging or no disc was found, there must be another cause for patient's back pain and sciatica.

Spinal stenosis, defined by Kirkaldy-Willis and McIvor[22] as narrowing of the intervertebral foramen, the nerve root canal or tunnel, and the spinal canal. The most important structure responsible for spinal stenosis is degenerative change or tropism of the apophyseal joint. The superior facet encroaches on the nerve root canal and the intervertebral foramen, whereas the inferior facet narrows the spinal canal. Each facet that produces spinal stenosis may compress the nerve at the same level at the intervertebral foramen or encroach on the intervertebral nerve root that leaves one space below (Fig. 26-6). Nerve root or cauda equina compression by deformed arthrosis of the facet has long been recognized, but from a group of early spinal stenosis, facet root syndrome appeared to be a clearcut clinical entity characterized by:

1. Low back pain and sciatica mimicking herniated disc syndrome.
2. Bilateral disc or root defect on AP myelogram even though symptoms may be unilateral (Fig. 26-7).
3. Lateral myelogram showed little or no anterior dural indentation (Fig. 26-8).
4. Oblique radiogram shows intervertebral foramen encroachment, the superior facet approaching or eburnating the inferior portion of the pedicle (Fig. 26-9).
5. Hypertrophic changes of facet, tropism, or inversion of facets are seen on AP radiogram (Fig. 26-10).
6. Spur formation or overriding of facet associated with the narrowing intervertebral foramen is seen on lateral radiogram (Fig. 26-11). Lateral extension of ligamentum flavum lies anterior to the facet, thus further narrowing the anterior foramen, as seen on the radiogram (Fig. 26-4).

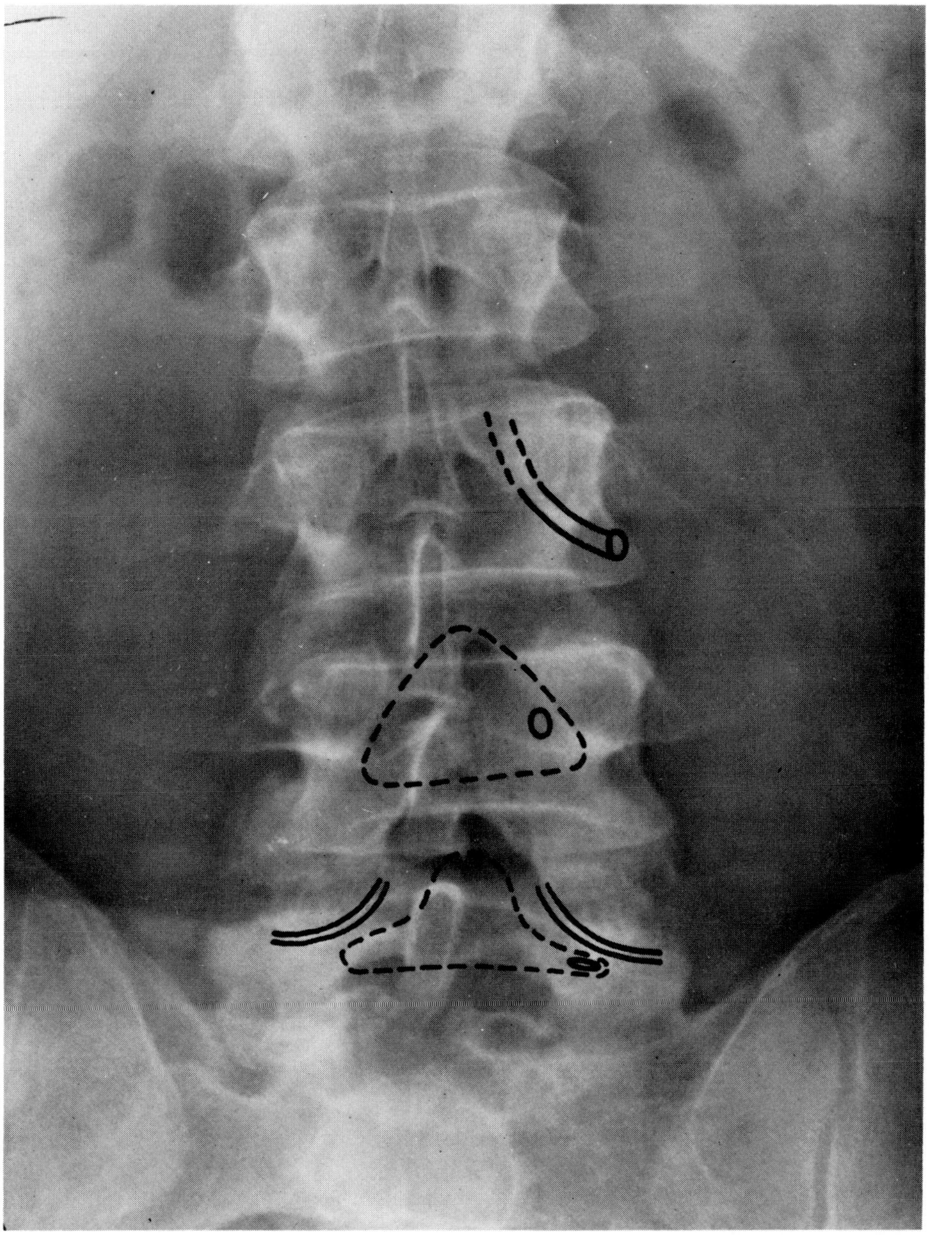

Fig. 26-6. A-P lumbar radiogram. Dotted lines indicate superimposed cross section of the spinal canal. Deformed arthrosis of facet compreses the spinal canal laterally (Napoleon's hat configuration) and note compression of L-5 nerve root before exiting from the intervertebral foramen.

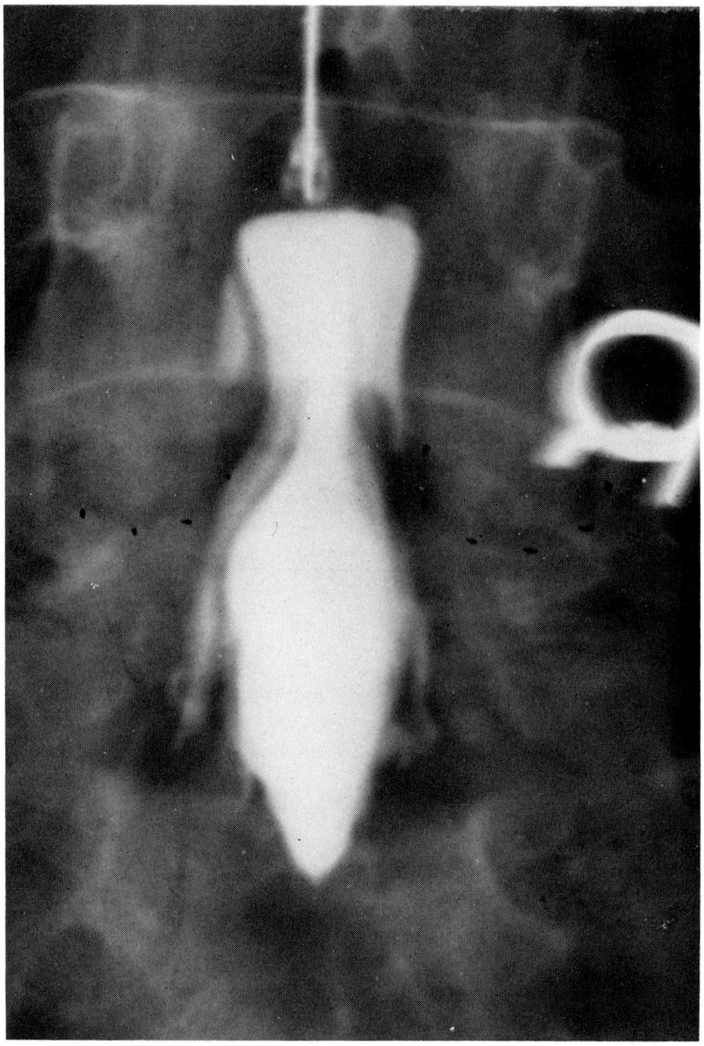

Fig. 26-7. A-P Myelogram in facet root syndrome. Waist-like defect and deformed arthrosis of the facet. The dural sac and nerve roots are compressed laterally and dorsally.

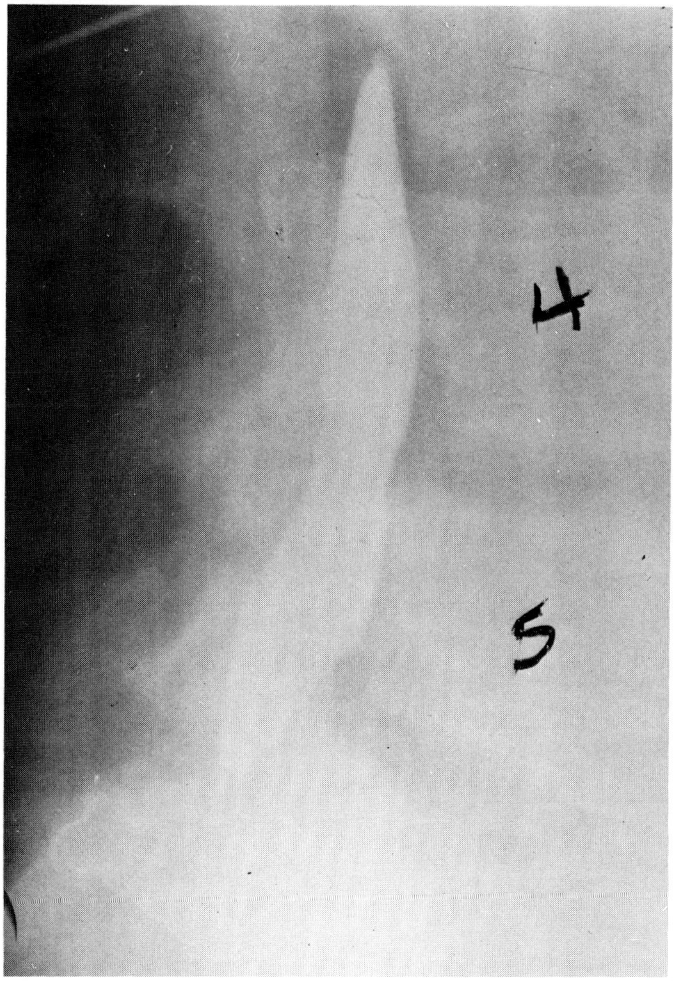

Fig. 26-8. Lateral myelogram. Note little indentation anteriorly from disc herniation. Dorsal indentation from facet, laminae, and ligamentum flavum noted.

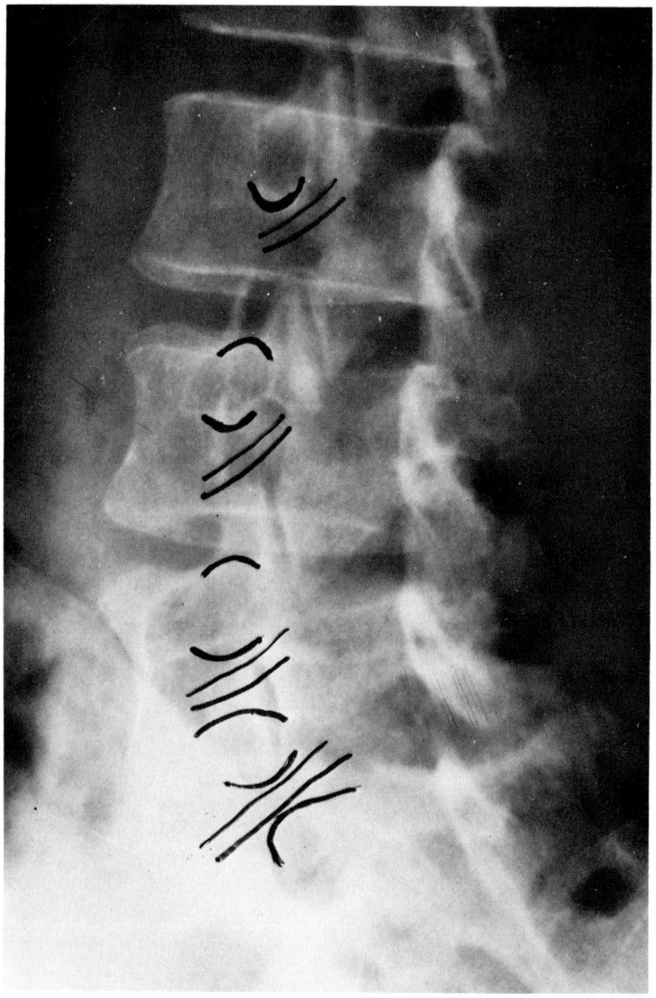

Fig. 26-9. Oblique view of lumbar radiogram showing the relationship of inferior border of pedicle, nerve root and facets. Bony encroachment on the nerve roots are noted in the lower two levels.

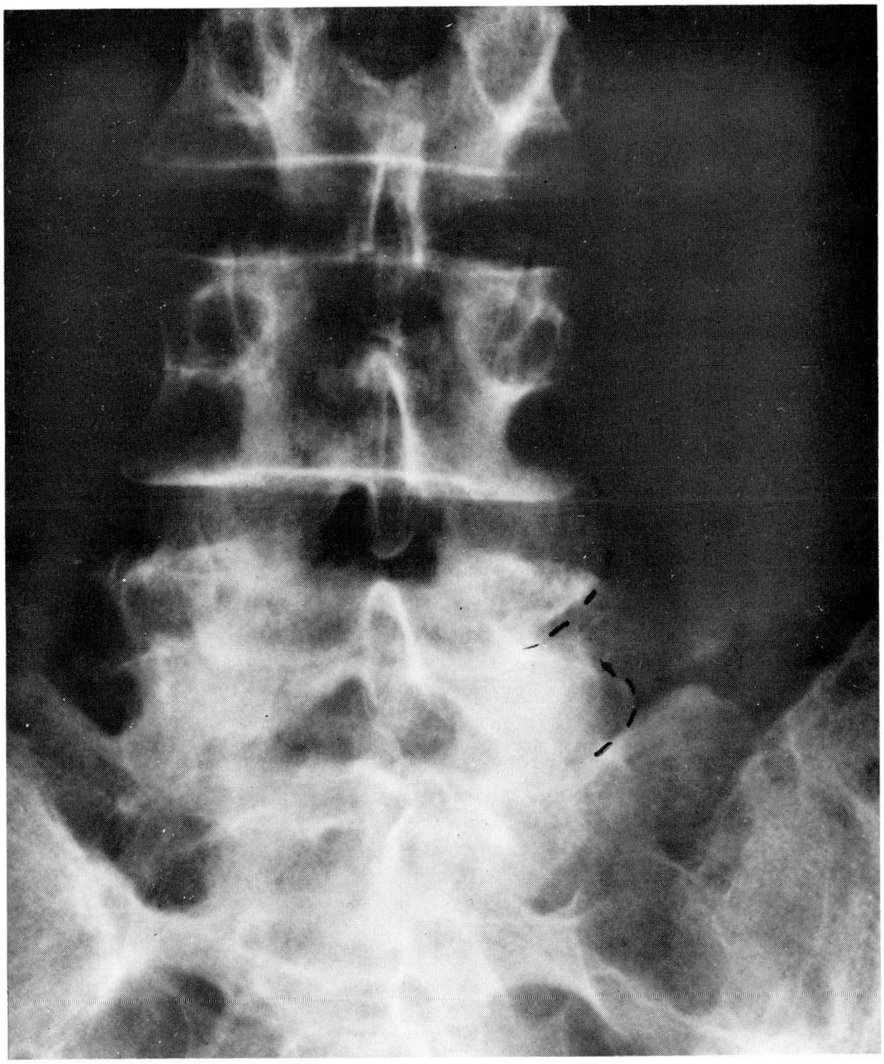

Fig. 26-10. A-P Lumbar Radiogram. Deformed arthrosis of L4-5 and L5-S1 facets.

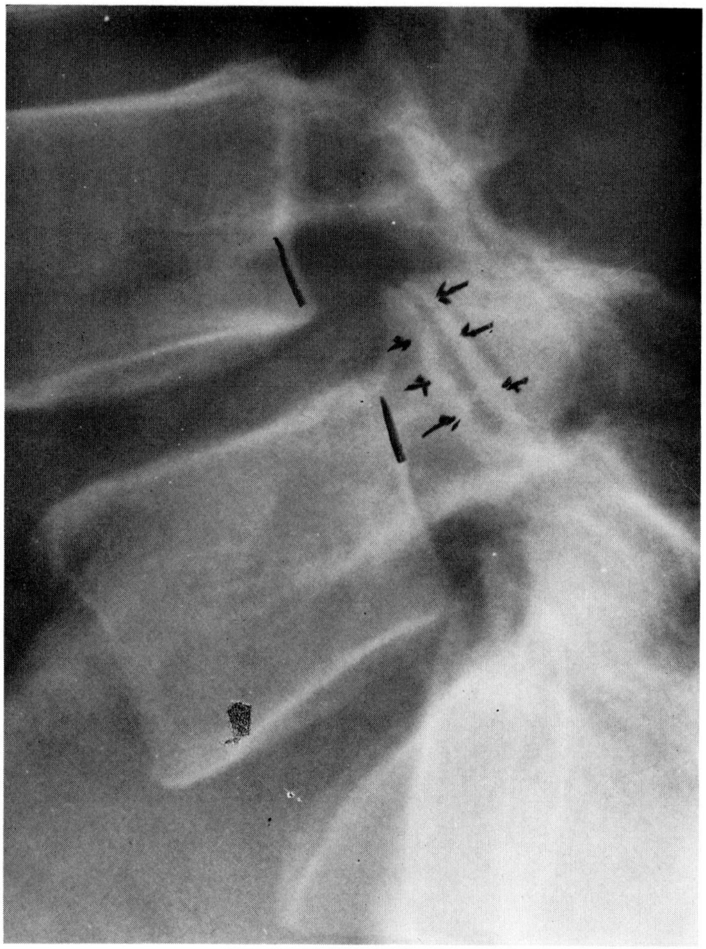

Fig. 26-11. Lateral lumbar radiogram. Overriding of L4-5 facet and slight degenerative spondylolisthesis noted.

7. At the time of surgery no significant disc herniation is found. As a result of foraminotomy and nerve root decompression, the surgical result is variable.
8. Recurrence or progression of symptomatology with slight physical provocation.

Failure of simple discectomy to fully relieve the patient's symptoms in this group is quite obvious.

Indications for PLIF are:

1. Facet root syndrome clincially diagnosable. PLIF is the surgery of choice.
2. An acute midline disc with bilateral symptomatology without the associated facet changes also could be treated by PLIF, especially if the person is likely to remain physically active both in the recreation field and employment.
3. In a person who has recurrence after initial satisfactory excision of an extruded or partially herniated disc, the PLIF is a better alternative than a repeat discectomy with or without perispinal fusion (lateral or posterior lateral).
4. In a selective group of patients with obvious lumbar disc herniation, such as young male patients who need to do heavy work for a living, the PLIF could be used as a primary operative procedure even though there is no evidence of spinal stenosis.
5. In chronic spondylosis with localized degenerative changes producing mainly back pain with little radicular pain, a successful PLIF does eliminate symptoms derived from the dysfunction of narrow degenerative disc.

Operative Technique

With few modifications, the technique described follows Cloward's approach of posterior lumbar intervertebral fusion.[7-9]

Anesthesia

General anesthesia and endotracheal intubation are preferred. Anectine is used routinely to facilitate muscle relaxation for adequate exposure. Antibiotic, 2.0 g Keflin, is given intravenously either just before the operation or intraoperatively. The same dose is repeated four times every 6 hours. The patient then receives Keflex, 500 mg, every 6 hours for 3 more days.

Positioning

Proper positioning of the patient, especially by placing firm rolls on each side of the body from the clavicle to the iliac crest is of the utmost importance (Fig. 26-12A). Care must be taken not to permit direct pressure on the abdomen or on the femoral veins. Compression of the inferior vena cava would increase venous pressure and bleeding from the epidural veins. Improper placement of the rolls may also tense up the abdominal wall and indirectly increase the venous pressure of the inferior vena cava (Fig. 26-12B). When the abdominal rolls are properly placed, the epidural veins should be collapsed. Compression of femoral veins would also increase epidural venous engorgement, since venous blood from the lower extremities must return through posterior pelvic or perispinal venous plexus. With the use of the laminae retractor, it is not necessary to flex the abdomen or the knees. Most surgeons flex the lumbar spine for lumbar discectomy. Finneson[23] indicated that if epidural bleeding became too profuse, flattening the table would decrease epidural bleeding. We routinely avoid any flexion of the table, and this decreases the problem of excessive epidural venous hemorrhage during

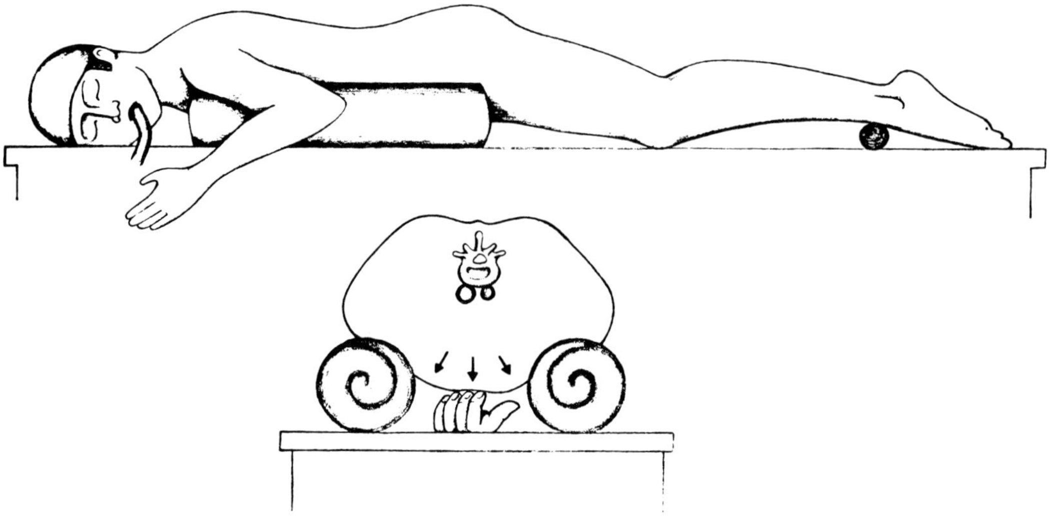

Fig. 26-12. A. Positioning of posterior lumbar intervertebral fusion. Rolls are firm. Flexion of table not needed. **B.** Testing the tension of anterior abdominal wall.

surgery. Positioning of the patient flat also avoids dependency and stagnation of venous blood in the lower extremities during the long procedure. This rigid observance of proper placement of firm rolls should decrease the incidence of postoperative thrombophlebitis and substantially decreases epidural venous bleeding during surgery.

Incision and Exposure

A horizontal incision is used routinely (Fig. 26-13). It gives ample exposure to the lamina and to the posterior iliac crest where bone grafts are removed. Cloward utilized a bone bank, and in his experience the degree of assimilation is the same as an autogenous bone graft. However, there is increased back pain during the postoperative period, apparently the result of a host-immune response.[8] To avoid inherent complications associated with the bone bank, autogenous bone grafts are removed after discectomy. Lamina retractor, placed at the base of the spinous processes, does help in gaining adequate exposure without excessive removal of the lamina or facet. The amount of lamina removed is no more than usual for interlaminal laminotomy for herniated lumbar disc. The only difference is that the lamina should be removed laterally up to the limitation of the pedicle. We believe the integrity of the facets must be preserved, although it may be necessary to remove the medial portion of the facet to gain adequate exposure.

Control of Epidural Veins

The control of epidural venous bleeding perhaps is the most notorious problem of this procedure. Success in mastering the proper technique to control eipdural venous bleeding is the key to the operation. With the advent of bipolar coagulation and better illumination, one or two vertical intervertebral veins could easily be coagulated and sectioned. It is not necessary to coagulate all veins within the exposure. Once the vertical veins are sectioned, they could be pushed above and below the interspace by Surgicel (1 × 2 inches) followed by cottonoid. After a minute or so, cottonoid can be removed and the hardened Surgicel not only controls the epidural bleeding by tamponade effect, it also keeps all vessels out of the way. Two Surgicel tampons, one above and one below the disc space, also push the nerve

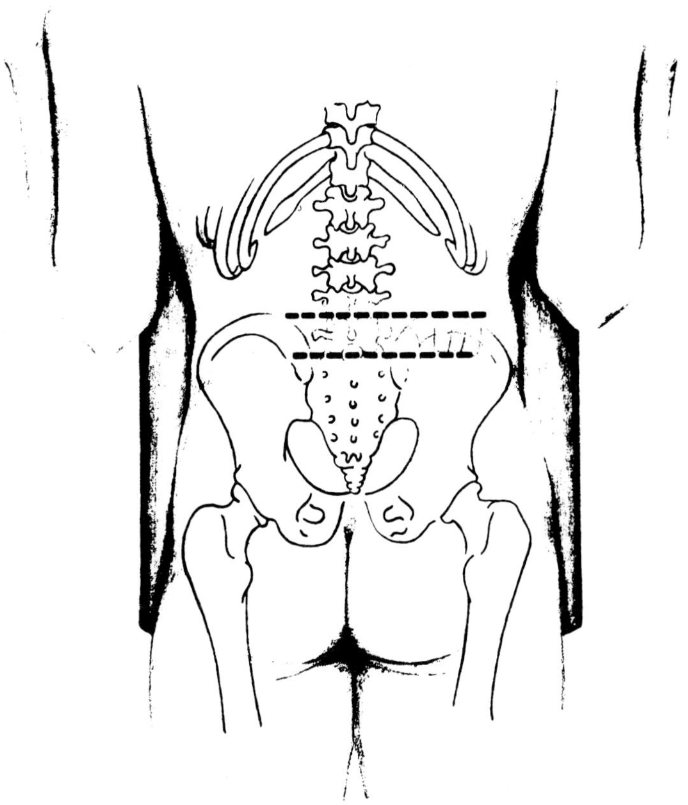

Fig. 26-13. Incision for posterior lumbar intervertebral fusion. Upper dotted line is for L4-5 disc and lower dotted line is for L5-S1 disc.

root and dura medially so that the use of nerve root retractors could often be avoided. In persons who have had previous surgery, identification of the longitudinal veins could be difficult. All epidural venous bleeding could be controlled with Surgicel alone without coagulation (Fig. 26-14). One should avoid the use of cottonoid in the epidural space during the graft insertion for fear of introducing the cottonoid with the graft into the intervertebral disc space. After the grafts are inserted, the impacted Surgicel should be removed with the help of a nerve hook and the epidural bleeding then controlled with Gelfoam.

Total Discectomy

Total discectomy includes removal of all disc material, the nucleus pulposus, the annulus fibrosus, and also the thin cartilaginous plate. The Scoville's horizontal downbite disc curette is most helpful to free subchondral cortical bone of all its attachments. The annulus fibrosus of the lateral wall of the disc space should best be removed by using an upbite curette and a small upbite pituitary rongeur. A larger straight or curve curette could be used to strip the cartilaginous attachment from the subchondral cortical bone simply by rotating the instrument within the disc space. With the good illumination presently available, total discectomy can be faithfully carried out up to the level of the anterior limiting membrane (Fig. 26-15). The midline bar is difficult to remove. In order to attain satisfactory intervertebral fusion, that portion of the disc material must be thoroughly denuded from its attachment to the posterior limiting membrane. A sharp pointed dissector or Cloward's osteophyte periosteal elevator is first used to strip the disc material from its attachment to the posterior

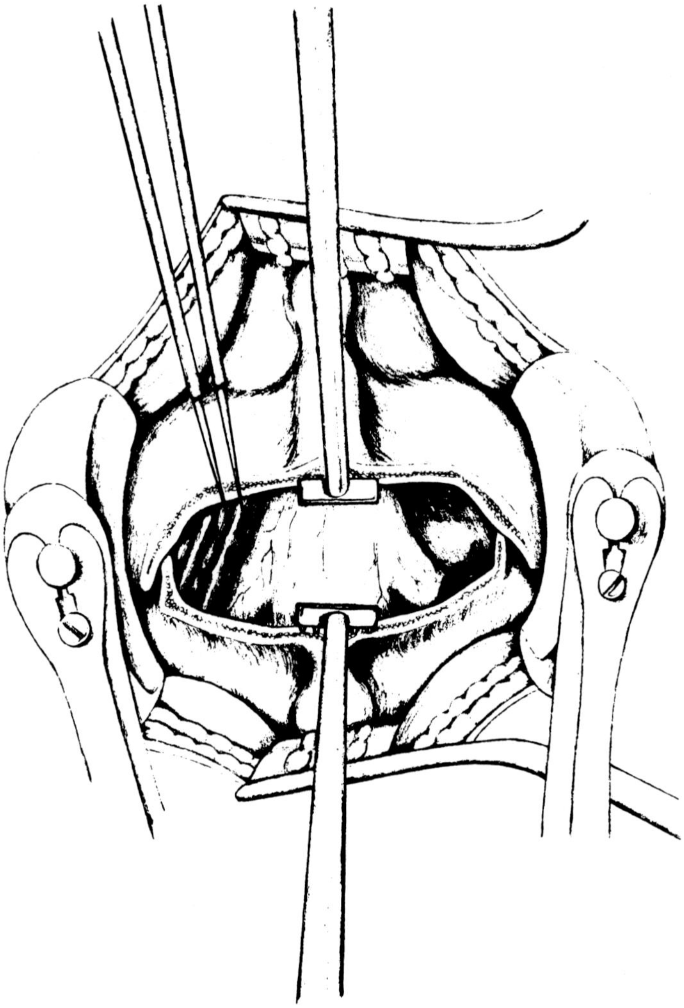

Fig. 26-14. Control of epidural hemorrhage. Bipolar or insulated coagulation forceps are used on the left side. On the right side epidural hemorrhage is controlled by impacted Surgicel tampons. Impacted Surgicel tampons also push the nerve root medially and expose the disc space without the need of nerve root retractor.

limiting membrane. A sharp downward dissector or downbite curette is then used to push the disc material downward, which is removed with a short upbite pituitary disc rongeur (Fig. 26-16). The integrity of the middle section of the posterior limiting membrane should be preserved so as to avoid posterior slipping of the central two bone pegs. The central portions of the adjoining vertebral bodies are concave. It is essential that an 8 to 10 mm width of the hard bony rims or epiphyseal rings of the adjoining vertebral bodies be chiseled away with an osteome (Fig. 26-15). A 1 to 2 mm thick slice of bone is removed from the superior lips, but a thicker wedge of bone, about 3 to 5 mm in thickness, is removed from the lower lip. With these osteotomies, the enlarged opening to the disc space affords direct visualization of the cleavage between cortical bone and the cartilaginous plate. The cartilaginous plate must be removed thoroughly and completely. When the cartilage is thoroughly removed, scraping the bone produces a hard metallic noise, in contrast to a squeaking feeling when the cartilage is scraped. Experience with Robinson's technique[2] of intervertebral fusion in the cervical area

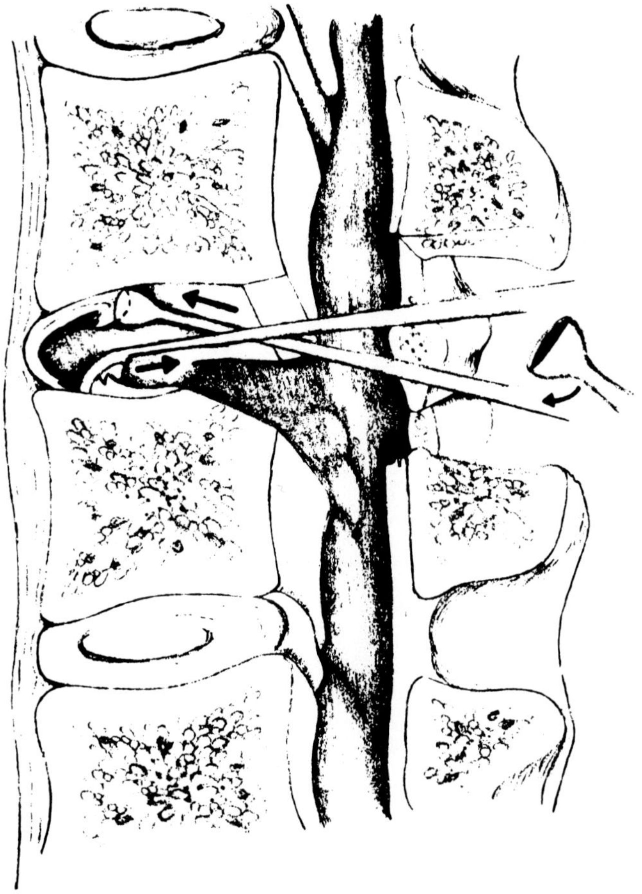

Fig. 26-15. Total discectomy down to subchondral cortical plate. The vertebral rims are chiseled away to gain maximal entrance to the disc space and also to delineate cleavage of cartilage from cortical bone.

indicated that it is not necessary to remove all the subchondral cortical bone to achieve a solid bony fusion. However the cortical plate is penetrated at several points by a chisel (Fig. 26-17) to enhance revascularization of the grafts. Cloward's osteophyte periosteal elevator, which is a right-angle pointed instrument, can be used conveniently to penetrate the cortical bone by gentle hammering. In fact, preservation of the cortical bone helps to maintain the height of the disc space that was unfurled by the laminal retractor and insertion of the bone grafts. Generous fenestration of the cortical plate definitely improves the quality of grafts.

Grafts Removal

The bone grafts are removed from the posterior iliac crest (Fig. 26-13). One can remove the iliac bone in full thickness, then split it equally in two. This would be preferable when two levels are fused or if the distance lateral to the nerve root in an exposed disc space is small. However, when there is a wide exposure lateral to the nerve root, a wider graft is desirable. A thick split-thickness graft from the iliac crest should be removed by chiseling technique, and the initial piece should be wide enough to cover the distance equivalent to at least four times that of the height of the retracted disc space. The height of the graft should be 1.0 inch

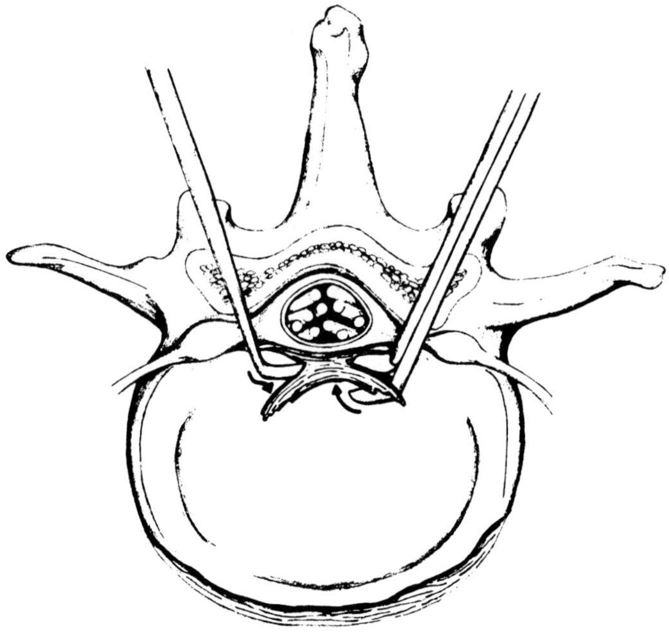

Fig. 26-16. Removal of midline bar of annulus fibrosus. Sharp pointed osteophyte periosteal elevator is used to separate the disc material from posterior limiting membrane and then removed by either a sharp angled upbite disc rongeur or "peapod" pituitary rongeur.

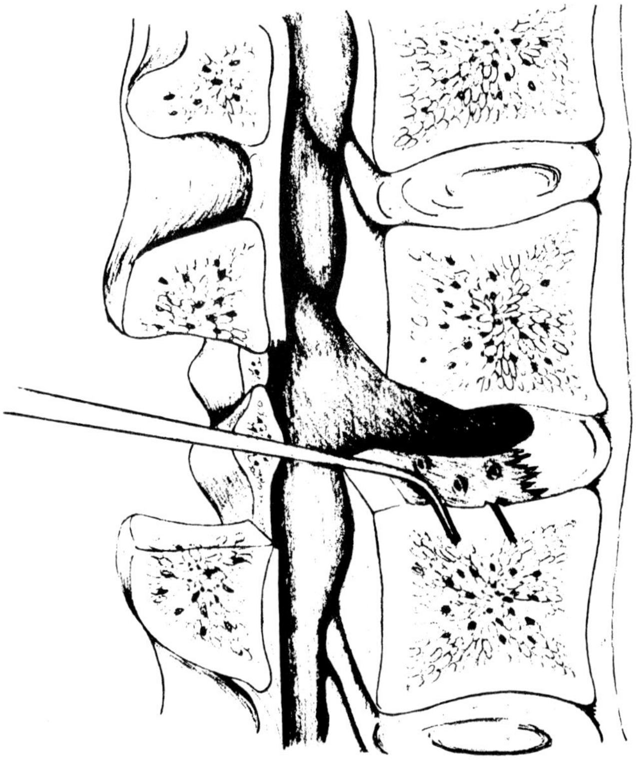

Fig. 26-17. Preparation of graft site—osteotomy of the epiphyseal ring, preservation of central cortical plate, and penetration of cortical plate to enhance revascularization of grafts from the cancellus bone.

long. The graft is then freed of its periosteum attachment, attached to the visor and, utilizing vibrator or pneumatic saw, cut into four equal size pegs. The width of each peg should be equal to the height of the disc space, when maximally distracted by the laminal retractor. In most cases the disc space after distraction should easily accept a graft of 10 mm in height. The width of the graft depends on the available space between the nerve root and the lateral bone pedicle.

Introduction of Grafts

After grafts are removed from the posterior iliac crest, the discectomy portion of the operative area is reentered. The disc space is maximally distracted by the laminal retractor. It is suggested that the cortical surface of the first graft be placed medially and the graft be pushed toward the midline by a swiveling action of a proper size chisel or curved curette (Figs. 26-18 and 26-19). However if the first graft is firmly impacted within the disc space, the medial displacement of the graft requires the employment of Cloward's ''PUKA'' technique by using two blunt-ended chisels. The swiveling action of the smaller chisel against a larger laterally impacted chisel propels the bone graft toward the midline (Fig. 26-20). The second graft should be placed with the cancellus bones toward the middle so that the cancellus bones of the adjoining bone grafts are in firm contact to assure solid fusion. With maximal distraction by laminal retractor, grafts should slip easily into the disc space with gentle tapping. Once impacted, the graft could still be moved by using a wood screw, penetrating the cortical surface of the graft, and the graft removed by pulling on the wood screw. In the absence of a laminal retractor the disc space could be enlarged by plying action of a blunt-end osteotome. The grafts used should be 2 mm wider than the available disc space. The central grafts are

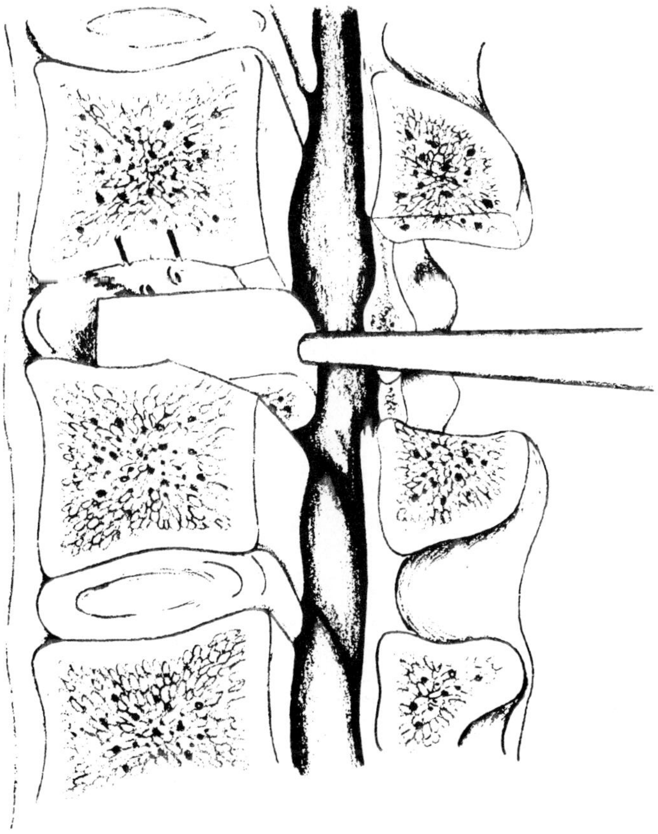

Fig. 26-18. Introduction of graft.

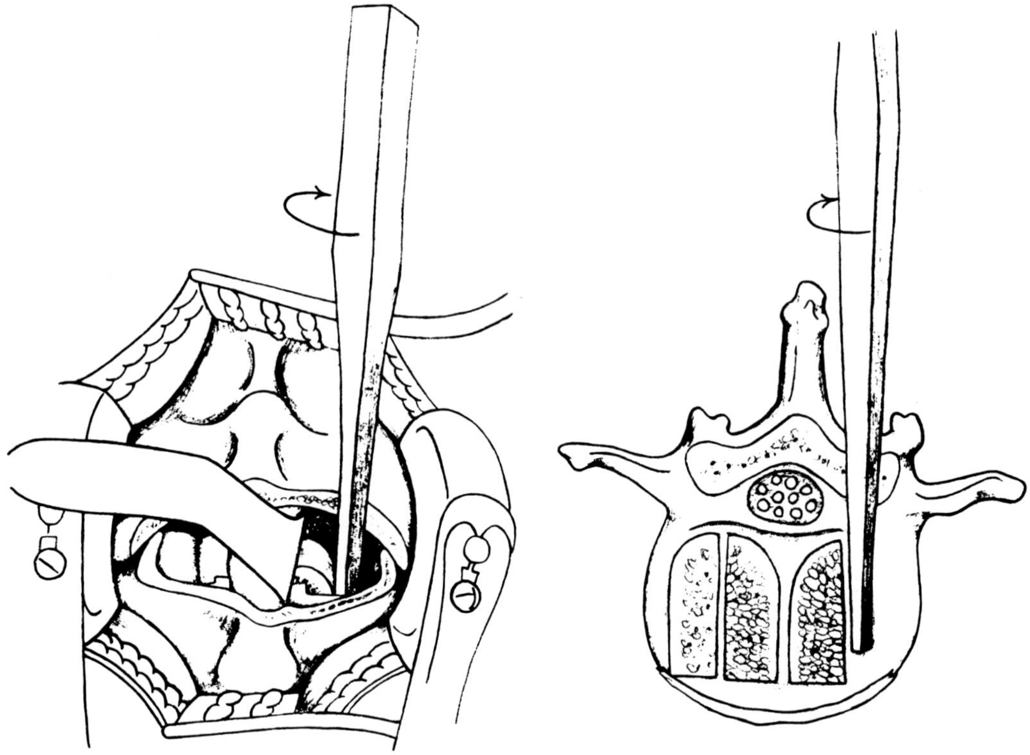

Fig. 26-19. Medial graft advancement with single chisel.

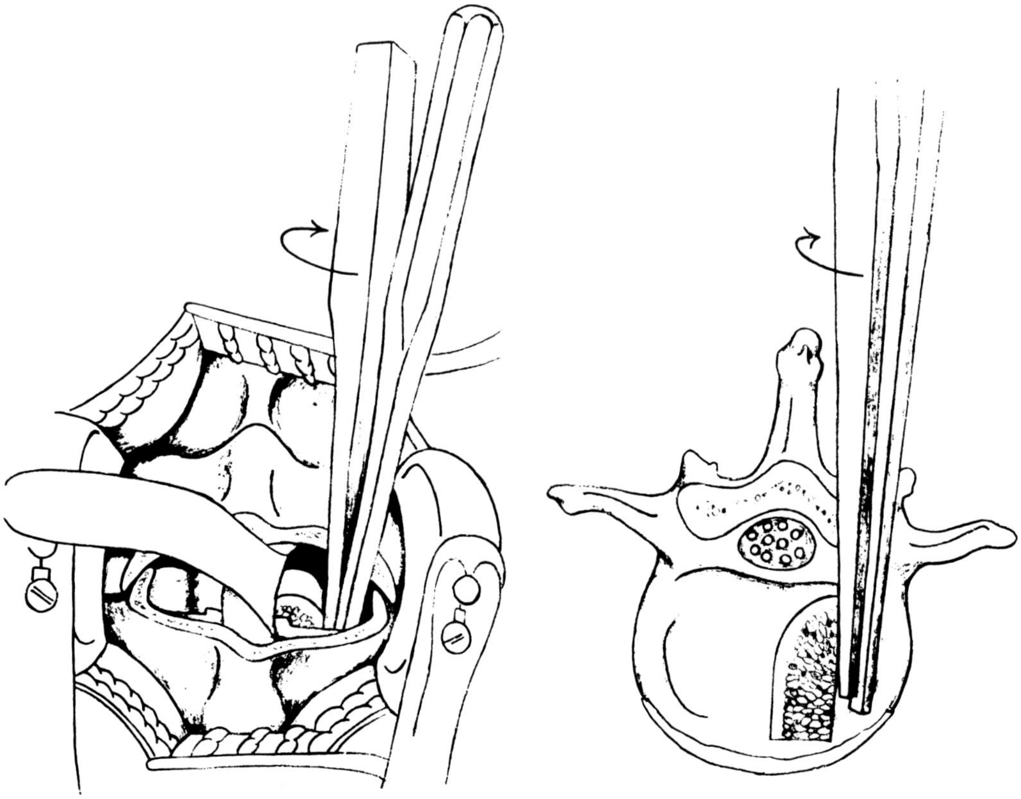

Fig. 26-20. Medial graft advancement with Cloward's "Puka" technique.

inserted first by plying the disc space with a blunt instrument on the opposite side while the larger size graft is introduced and "PUKA" to the center. The retained two large central grafts would then keep the disc space distracted and the two lateral grafts could be inserted with minimal impaction. Generally four pegs of graft are used but one may use up to five or six grafts to fill up the entire disc space compactly with bony material.

Cloward's lumbar intervertebral fusion technique, unlike other intervertebral body fusion techniques, does cover more than half of the available disc spaces with the bony grafts. Cloward[24] indicates that "pack them full with bone pegs" is the most important single factor in assuring a solid bony fusion. When the laminal retractor is removed, locking mechanism of the adjoining vertebral bodies from the natural curvature of the lumbar spine should assure solid contacts of the grafts with the adjoining intervertebral bodies (Fig. 26-21). When grafts are firmly impacted, the natural curvature of the lumbar spine also prevents the grafts from displacing posteriorly into the spinal canal. In cases of spondylolisthesis, attempts should be made to lift the lower vertebral body upward when the laminae are being held by laminal retractors. In spondylolisthesis with extremely narrow disc space or with slippage beyond 25% (stage I), this procedure may not be feasible. Intraoperatived irrigation with Neomycin, 0.5%, is used freely.

With improved illumination and better control of epidural bleeding, a skillful neurosurgeon should be able to perform single-level intervertebral fusion between 2½ and 3 hours. It

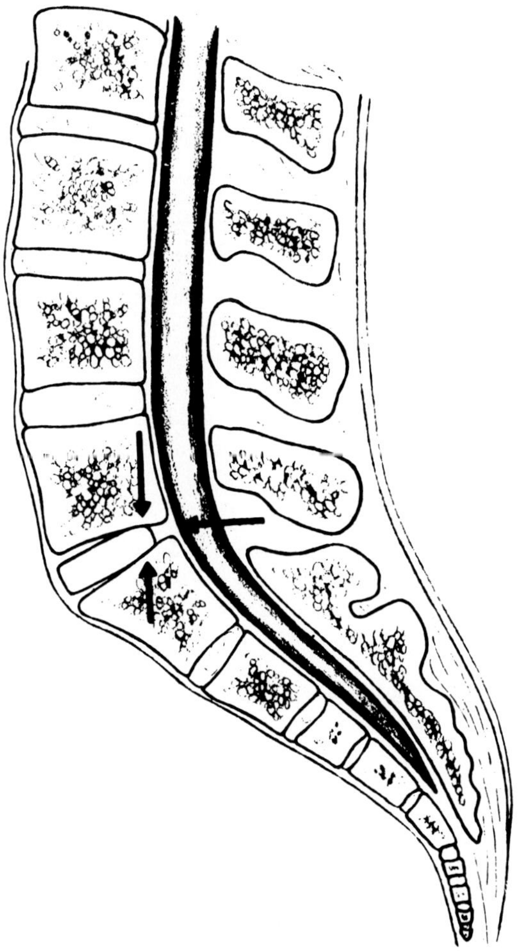

Fig. 26-21. Normal lumbar curvature enhances locking of graft pegs in Cloward's posterior lumbar intervertebral fusion.

is estimated that the operating time for a posterior lumbar intervertebral fusion would be three times that of a simple discectomy done through fenestration or interlaminal technique. This procedure does present a time limitation for slow meticulous surgeons. If the usual time for a single discectomy is 2 hours, then the estimated time needed to complete the posterior lumbar intervertebral fusion would approximate 6 hours. A long disc procedure does increase the chances of disc space infection.

Since the inception of using Surgicel as a tamponade to control eipdural bleeding, the average blood loss has dropped from 1,000 to 300 to 500 ml. In most instances it is now no longer necessary to consider transfusion for a single-level PLIF.

Drains are not used. Less than 10% of the patients have varying degrees of subcutaneous serous collections, which generally disappear without aspiration. Avoidance of wide subcutaneous dissection and careful attempt to obliterate all dead spaces should prevent subcutaneous serous collections.

Postoperative Care

The patient is usually out of bed 2 or 3 days after surgery. The average length of stay after surgery is 12 days. All participating or referring orthopedic surgeons have indicated that the postoperative disability related to this operation is less than any other form of lumbar spinal fusion. Thirty-five percent of the patients who had previous simple discectomy volunteered that PLIF gave less discomfort during the immediate postoperative period than the previous simple discectomy. A Knight's spinal brace is used for 3 to 4 months. If patient has nocturnal discomfort, a brace is used at night.

Results

Of the 50 patients that were operated, with more than 6 months followup over a 4-year period, the distribution was 31 males and 19 females, ranging in age from 20 to 59 years. All had varying degrees of narrowing disc space, and all had low back pain that in most cases was chronic. Ninety percent had midline disc with bilateral or unilateral leg pain, 18 had previous surgery with recurrent symptomatology, 3 of the procedures were done for spondylolisthesis.

Satisfactory clinical results were obtained in 44 (88%). Thirty-three (66%) were excellent, ie., total recovery with relief of chronic back pain and able to enjoy full physical activity. Eleven (22%) are classified as good results with mild residual symptomatology. Four (8%) had fair results and 2 (4%) had no improvement. It is within normal expectations that all 6 patients in the groups with fair and poor results are Compensation cases (Table 26-1). Ninety-two percent had solid bony assimilation with the adjoining vertebral bodies (Figs. 26-22, 26-23, and 26-24). In 1 case there was evidence of pseudoarthrosis with forward slipping because of facet removal but eventually fused in a forward slipped position. There

Table 26-1. Results of 50 Posterior Lumbar Intervertebral Fusions 6 Months Followup

	Patients		
Result	No.	%	
Excellent	33	66	
Good	11	22	
Fair	4*	8	
Poor	2*	4	(1 adhesive arachnoiditis)

*Compensation cases.

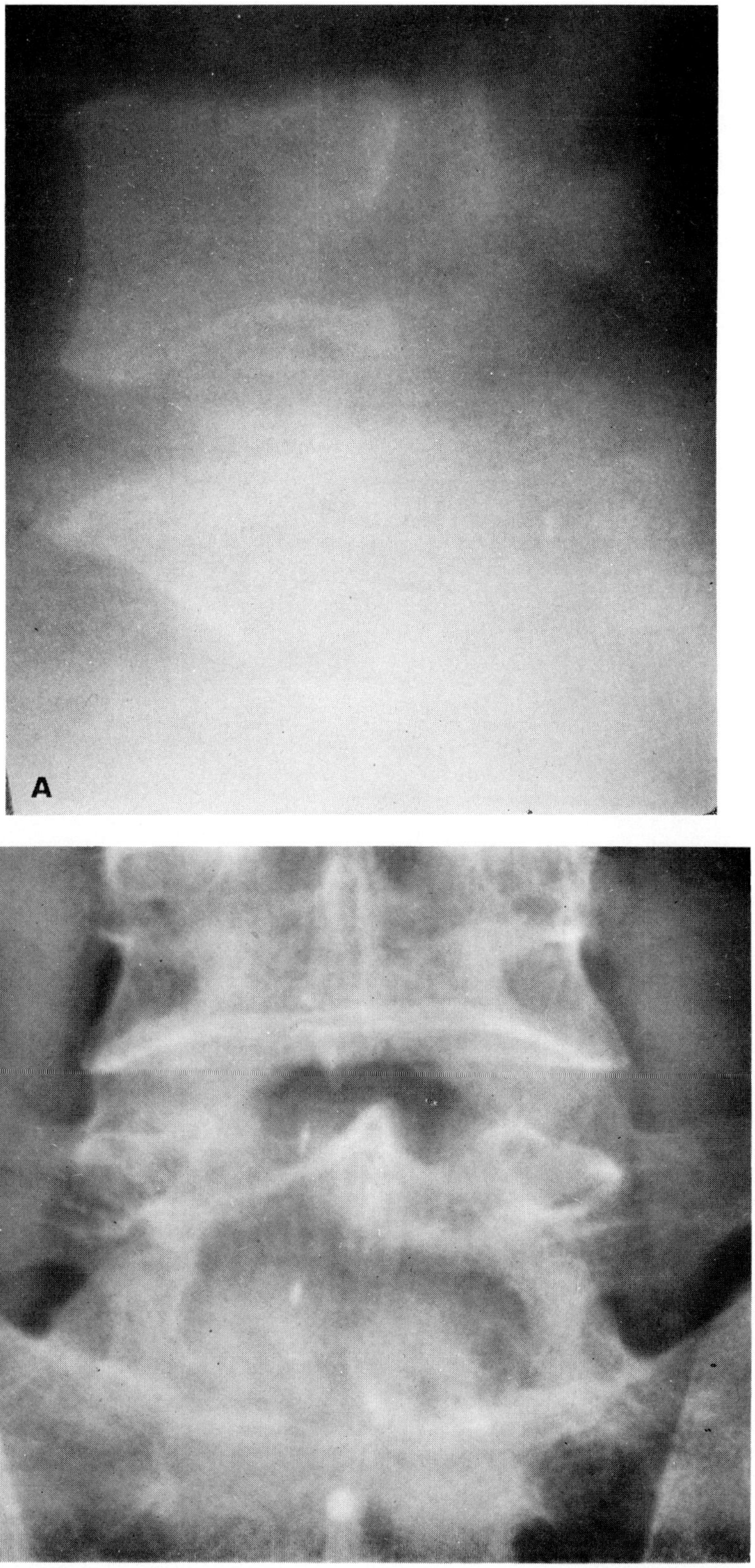

Fig. 26-22. L5-S1 single level fusion. **A.** Lateral view, larger disc space. **B.** AP view showing homogenous solid fusion at lumbosacral interspace.

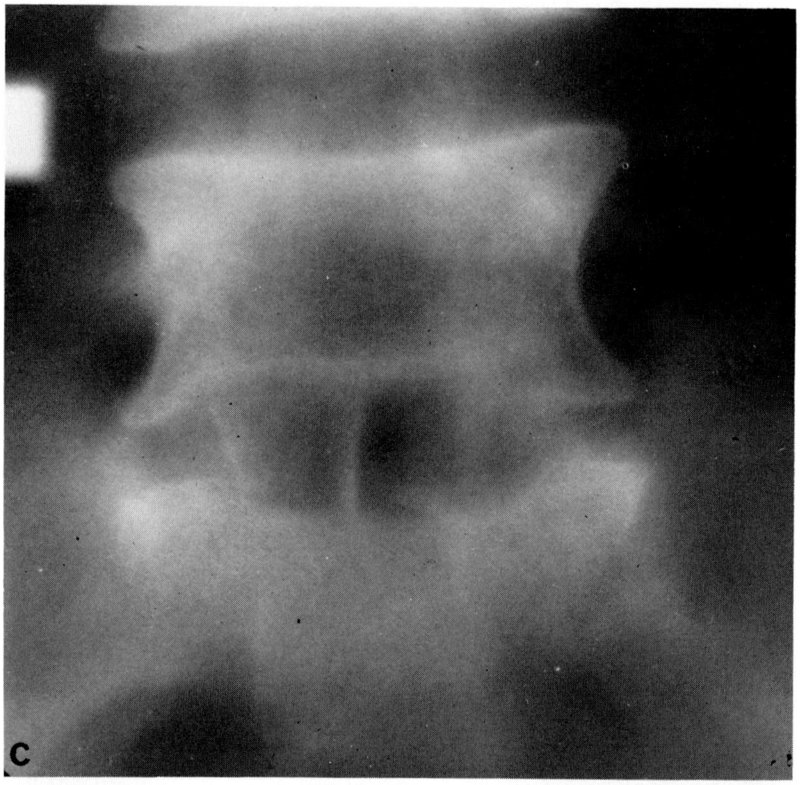

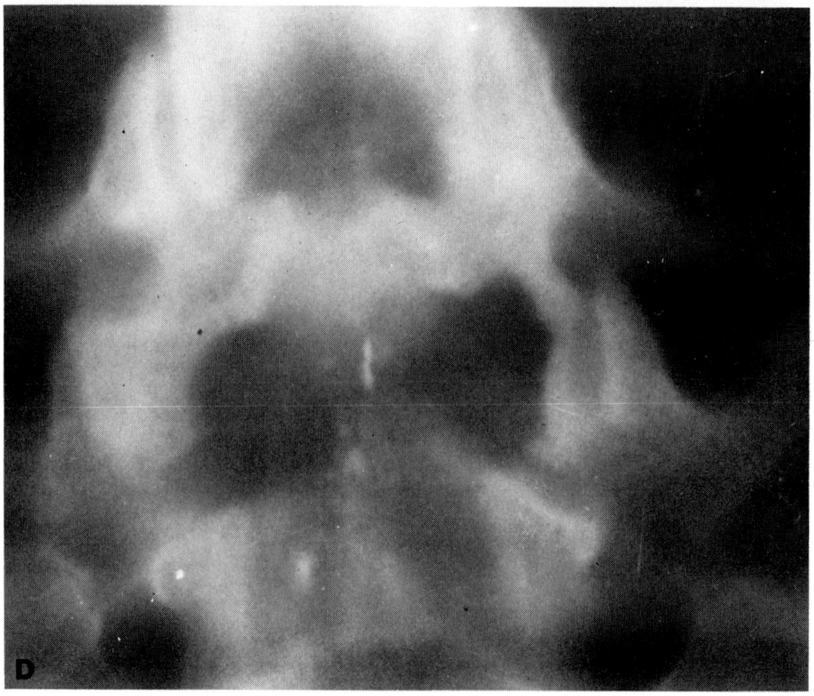

Fig. 26-22. **C.** AP planogram shows larger size peg-graft. **D.** AP planogram shows the extent of laminotomy. Note preservation of posterior neural arch and facets.

Table 26-2. Radiologic Result of Posterior Lumbar Intervertebral Fusion—50 Cases

	Cases	
	No.	%
Bony fusion	46	92
Pseudoarthrodesis	1	
Settlement	2	
Slight motion	3	

were 2 cases in which the grafts settled with further narrowing of the disc space, although the patient had a satisfactory result. Three had measurable movement of less than 3° in flexion-extension lateral radiograms (Table 26-2).

There were no postoperative wound infections, no postoperative thrombophlebitis, and no increased neurologic deficit. One Compensation patient who continued to have postoperative pain had myelographic evidence of adhesive arachnoiditis.

Conclusion

Froning[25] demonstrated limitation of flexion and extension in a majority of patients who had a successful discectomy. Persistence of mobility, comparable with that expected in a normal individual, was usually found in patients judged to have poor results. This collaborates with the contention of posterior intervertebral fusion advocates in that to achieve best results in disc prolapse surgery, there should be minimal motion of the *motor segment* after surgery.[7,8,16]

Modern improvements in operative illumination, better control of epidural hemorrhage by proper positioning of patient, and the use of Surgicel as a tamponade in retracting epidural veins and dura definitely improve the technical feasibility of PLIF. Compared with the complications encountered in anterior transperitoneal lumbar intervertebral fusion, the posterior lumbar intervertebral fusion is infinitely safer.[13-19] Goldner,[20] in his series of 50 cases of anterior intervertebral fusion, reports 13 different types of complications.

All too often, neurosurgeons are happy and anxious to do a simple discectomy in order to bring about quick short-term relief. When the pain recurs, neurosurgeons usually transfer the patient to orthopedic colleagues, hoping they will do a spinal fusion and assume the responsibility for future care. If our orthopedic colleague fails to restore the patient's usefulness, we get the patient back and then proceed to consider various forms of electrical stimulation or nerve severance procedures.

Neurosurgeons who perform surgery through the routine interlaminal discectomy approach must bear the responsibility for continuing care when a patient requires a spinal fusion procedure at a later date. Considering the difficulty and failure associated with other types of spinal fusion done by our orthopedic colleagues,[25,26] neurosurgeons must apply themselves to accept Cloward's posterior lumbar intervertebral fusion as a standard neurosurgical procedure.

Long-term followup is needed to assess the deleterious effect of a solid fusion on the adjoining disc spaces. Experience with the cervical interbody fusion has shown that the incidence of degenerative disc of the adjoining disc spaces appeared to be hastened by a solid interbody fusion. Nevertheless if one is to aim for a good reconstructive procedure for a diseased lumbar disc, posterior lumbar intervertebral or intercorporal fusion deserves wider acceptance.

Posterior lumbar intervertebral fusion not only has the advantage of avoiding collapse of

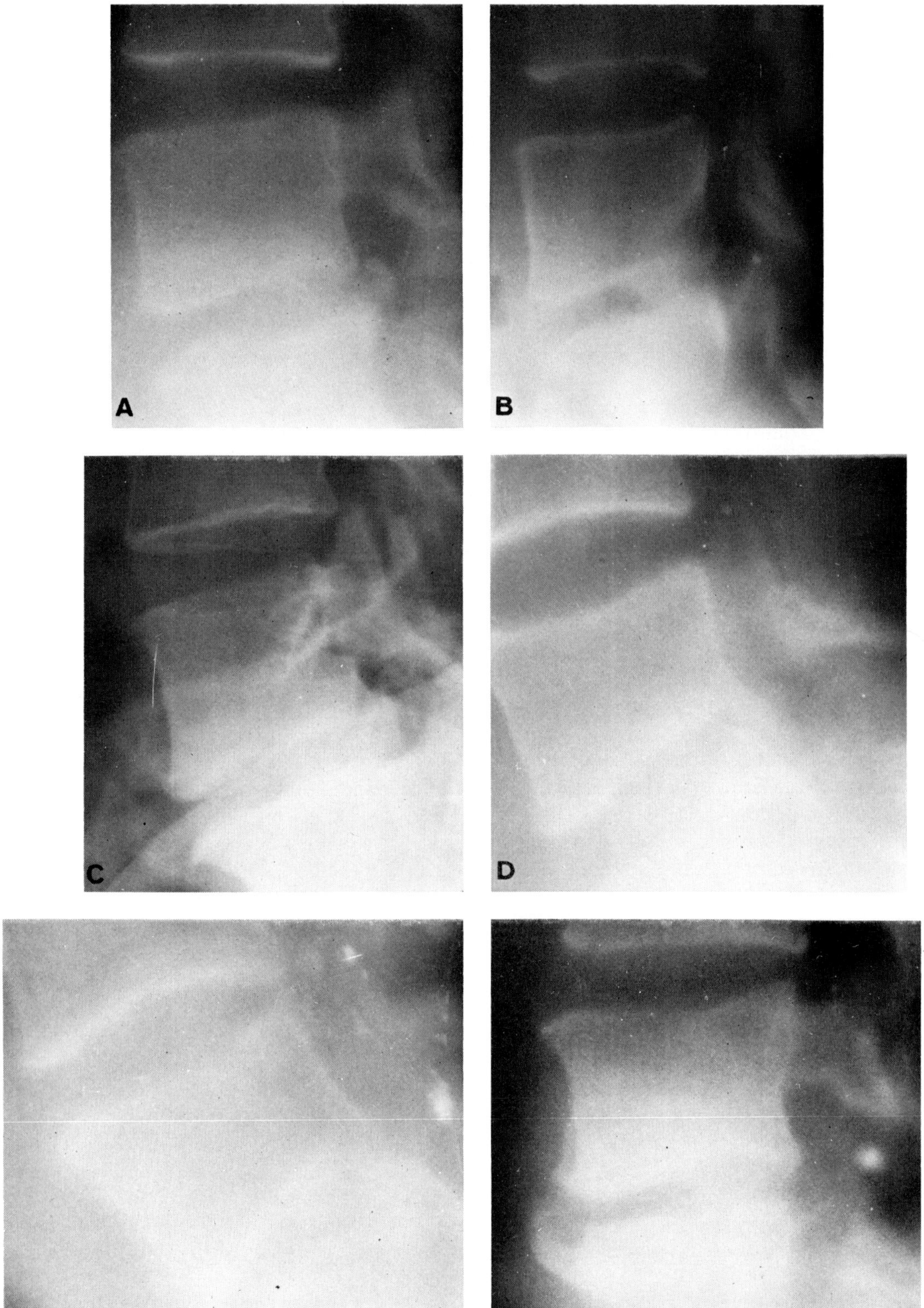
A
B
C
D
E
F

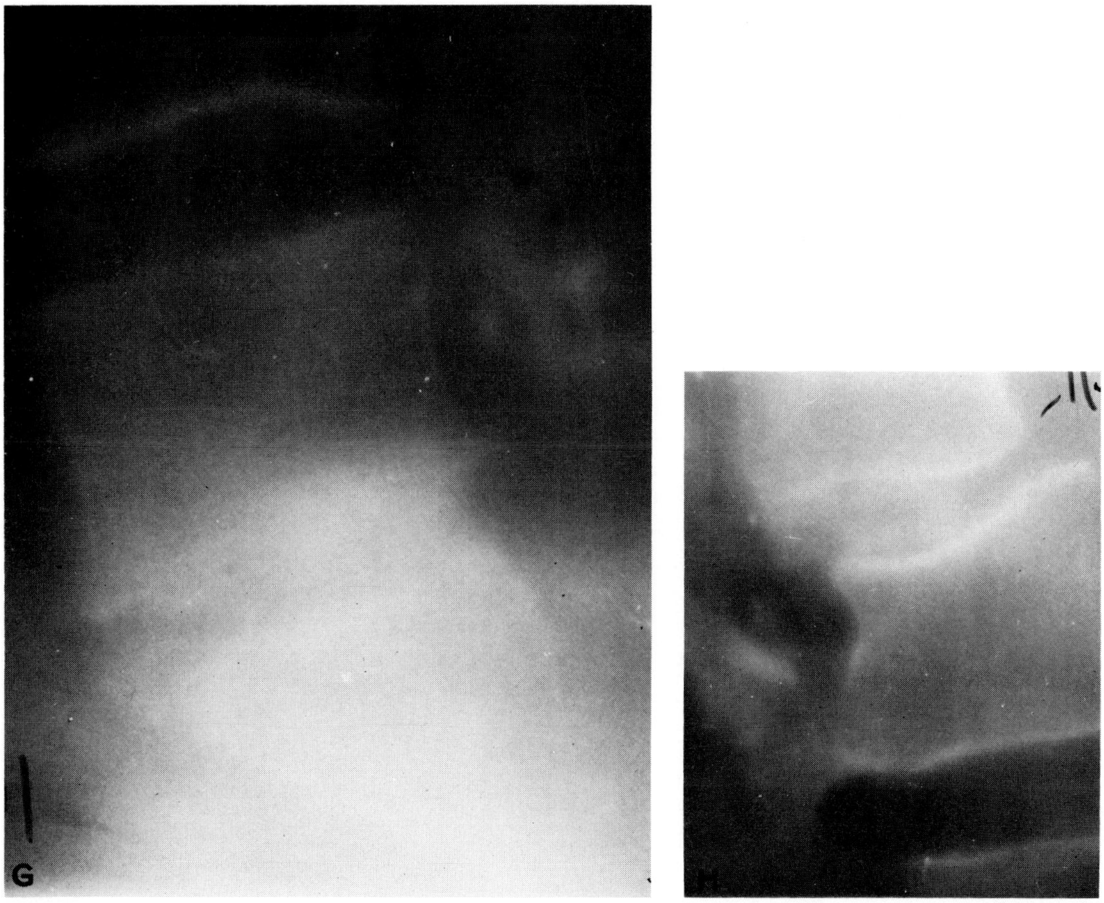

Fig. 26-23. Eight cases of single level PLIF. All show good solid fusion after 6 months. 8-H represents a case of spondylolisthesis (Grade I).

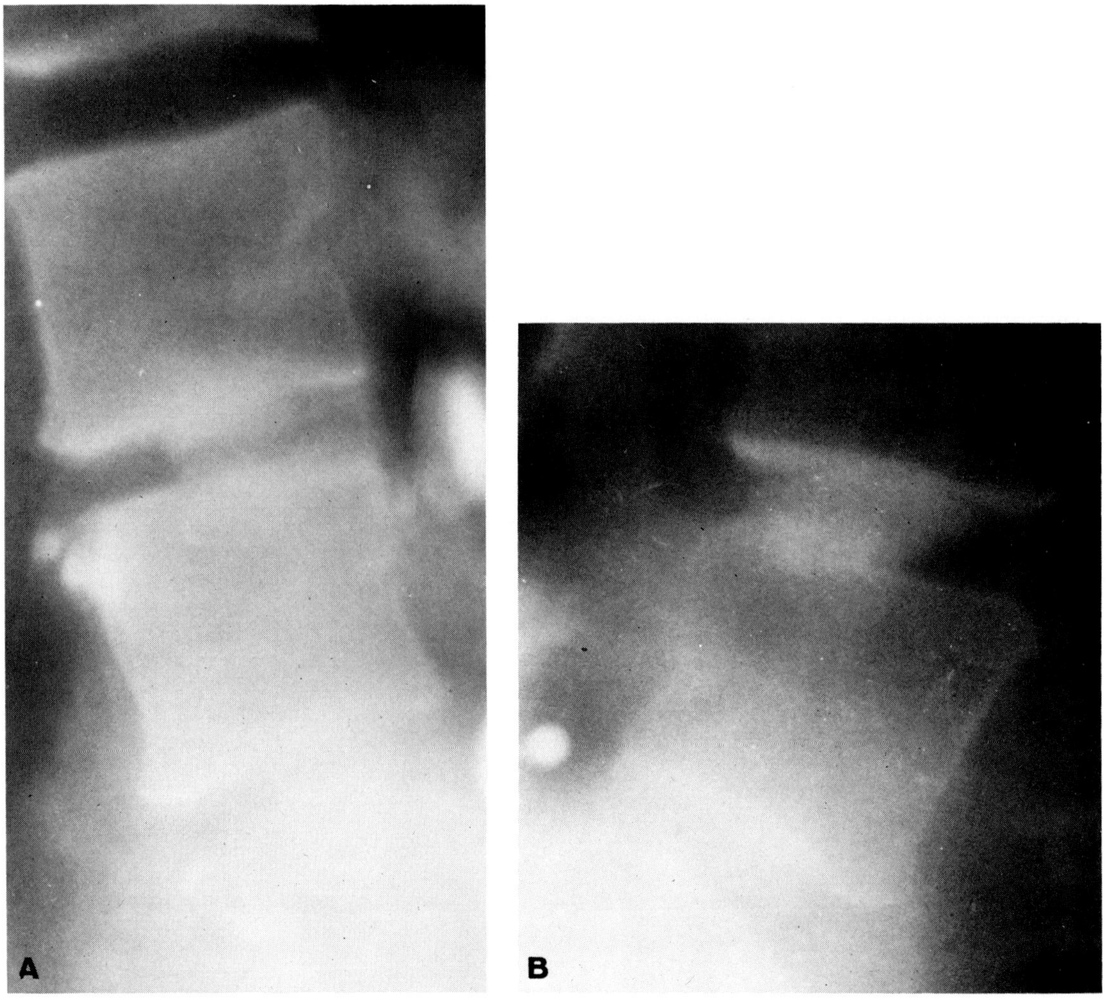

Fig. 26-24. Three cases of two-level fusion. Six months postoperative lumbar lateral radiograms show solid bony fusion.

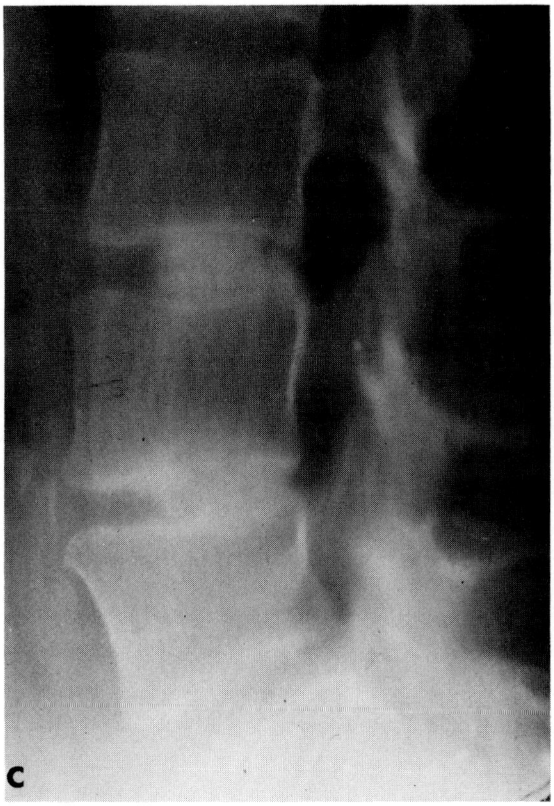
c

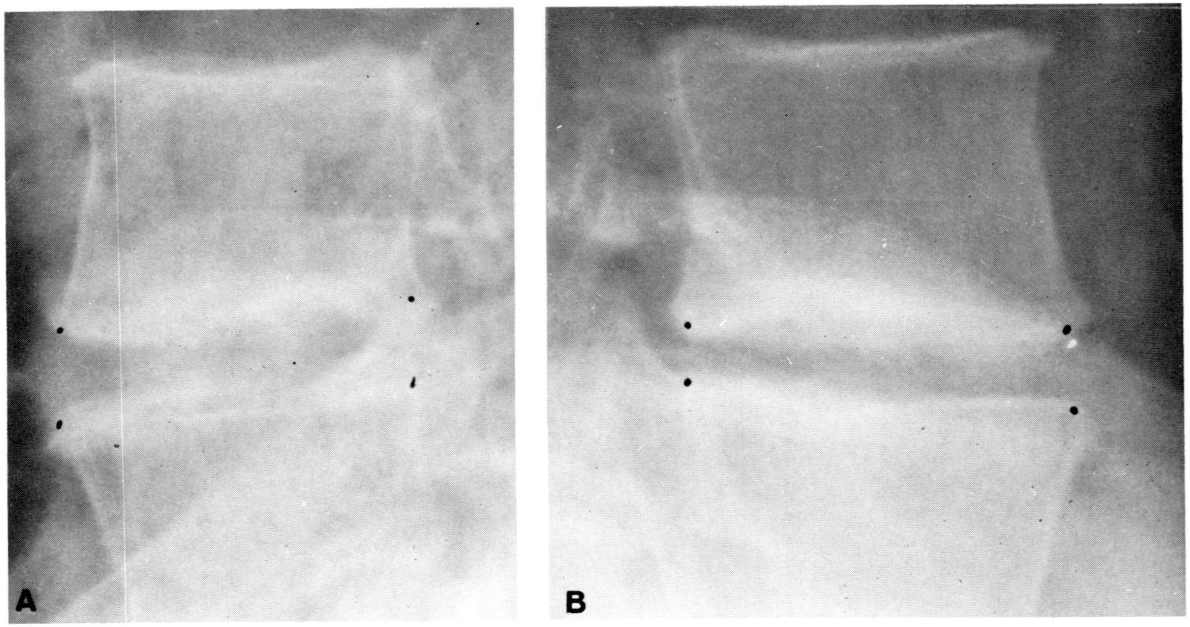

Fig. 26-25. **A.** Lateral lumbar radiogram, preoperative film. **B.** Lateral lumbar radiogram, postoperative film. Note the distraction of the disc space by PLIF.

the disc space, it assures stability of the motor segment. It also accomplishes wide decompression of all neural components. Distraction of the intervertebral disc space (Fig. 26-25) and the natural posterior concavity of the lumbar spine produce a firm locking mechanism of the graft within the disc space and enhance solid bony fusion (Fig. 26-21). Thus the posterior lumbar intervertebral fusion fashioned by Cloward more than 30 years ago remains theoretically superior to all other forms of spinal fusion. No longer should we defer lumbar spinal fusion to our orthopedic colleagues. Posterior lumbar intervertebral fusion is definitely a standard neurosurgical procedure that all neurosurgeons should include in their repertoire.

REFERENCES

1. Riley LH, Jr, Robinson RA, Johnson KA, et al: The results of anterior interbody fusion of the cervical spine. Review of ninety-three consecutive cases. *J Neurosurg 30*:127-33, 1969
2. Robinson RA, Riley LH, Jr: Techniques of exposure and fusion of the cervical spine. *Clin Orthop 190*:78-84, 1975
3. Simmons EH, Bhalla SK: Anterior cervical discectomy and fusion. A clinical biomechanical study with eight year follow-up. *J Bone Joint Surg 51*:225-37, 1969
4. Christoferson LE, Selland B: Intervertebral bone implants following excision of protruded lumbar disc. *J Neurosurg 42*:401-405, 1975
5. Wiltberger BR: The prefit dowel intervertebral body fusion as used in lumbar disc therapy. A preliminary report. *Am J Surg 6*:723-27, 1953
6. Wiltberger BR: Intervertebral body fusion by the use of posterior bone dowel. *Clin Orthop 35*:69-79, 1964
7. Cloward RB: The treatment of ruptured lumbar intervertebral discs by vertebral body fusion. Indications, operative technique, after care. *J Neurosurg 10*:154-68, 1953
8. Cloward RB: Lesions of intervertebral discs and their treatment by intervertebral fusion method. (The painful disc) *Clin Orthop 27*:51077, 1963
9. Cloward RB: The Cloward technique, chap 7, *Low Back Pain.* Edited by BE Finneson. Lippincott, Philadelphia, 1973, pp 217-235
10. Junghanns H, Schmorl G: *The Human Spine In Health And Disease.* Second edition. Grune and Stratton, New York, 1971, pp 35-37
11. LeVay D: A survey of surgical management of lumbar disc prolapse in the United Kingdom and Eire. *Lancet 1*:1211-3, 1967
12. Clock, HV: Isolated lumbar disc resorption as a cause of nerve root canal stenosis. *Clin Orthop 191*:109-115, 1976
13. Benton RB, Calandruccio RA: Surgical technique of anterior lumbar fusion. *Am Surg 32*:134-6, 1966
14. Calandruccio RA, Benton BF: Anterior lumbar fusion. *Clin Orthop 35*:63-8, 1964
15. Freebody D, Bendall R, Taylor RD: Anterior transperitoneal lumbar fusion. *J Bone Joint Surg 53*:617-27, 1971
16. Harmon PH: The removal of lower lumbar intervertebral discs by the transabdominal extraperitoneal route. Permanante Found Med Bull *6*:169-174, 1948
17. Lane JD, Jr, Moone ES, Jr: Transperitoneal approach to the intervertebral disc in the lumbar area. *Ann Surg 127*:537-51, 1948
18. Sacks S: Anterior interbody fusion of the lumbar spine. Indications and results in 200 cases. *Clin Orthop 44*:163-70, 1966
19. Stauffer RN, Coventry MB: Anterior interbody lumbar spine fusion. Analysis of Mayo Clinic Series. *J Bone Joint Surg 54*:756-68, 1972
20. Goldner LP, McCollum DE, Urbaniak JR: Anterior intervertebral discectomy and arthrodesis for treatment of low back pain with or without radiculopathy, Chap 16. *Clinical Neurosurgery* Vol 15. Williams and Wilkins, Baltimore, 1968, pp 352-383
21. Spangfort EV: The lumbar disc herniation. A computer aid analysis of 2504 operations. *Acta Orthop Scand* (Suppl 142):1972
22. Kirkaldy-Willis WH, Mclvor GWD: Spinal stenosis. *Clin Orthop 115*:2-3, 1976
23. Finneson BE: *Low Back Pain.* Lippincott, Philadelphia, 1975 Chapter VI, pp 139-215
24. Cloward RB: Personal communication
25. Froning EC, Frohman B: Motion of the lumbosacral spine after laminectomy and spine fusion. Correlation of motion with the result. *J Bone Joint Surg 50*:897-918, 1968
26. Rothman RH, Booth R: Failures of spinal fusion. *Orthop Clin North Am 6*:299-304, 1975

CHAPTER 27

Anterior Lumbar Discectomy and Interbody Fusion: Indications and Technique

J. Leonard Goldner
Kenneth E. Wood
James R. Urbaniak

IF SPINAL FUSION IS required for the management of patients with intervertebral disc disease, then anterior lumbar discectomy and fusion have a place in the management of patients with chronic low-back pain. We believe that regardless of the technique used certain patients are relieved of pain if the spine is stabilized. After one operation has failed to relieve intervertebral disc symptoms, spine fusion should be seriously considered as a part of the second operative procedure. This is a generality and exceptions do exist, but that philosophy has been helpful in managing patients with recurrent low-back pain who are candidates for operative treatment.

Those who believe in anterior cervical discectomy and fusion should also recognize the value of the same procedure in the lower lumbar and lumbosacral segments. Removal of an intervertebral disc from the anterior approach, in either the cervical or lumbar regions will decompress nerve roots without actually manipulating them. Immobilization is almost complete immediately postoperatively, and relief of nerve-root irritation is, temporarily, prompt.

This anterior procedure is not currently popular. It is reserved for *salvage* patients and considered a last resort. Our experience is that it will resolve the problem of failed discectomy at one or two interspaces, and that it might be the procedure of choice in certain patients prior to posterolateral fusion, and certainly before wide extensive laminectomy is done posteriorly to relieve patients who have nerve-root irritation and who do not have free fragments compressing the roots.

Historical Review

Anterior lumbosacral fusion was first used in the mid-1930s for spondylolisthesis.[1-5] In 1948[6] the procedure was used for lumbosacral intervertebral disc disease.

Sacks,[7] in 1961, reported 150 patients treated by anterior arthrodesis. He stated that 26% of these patients were asymptomatic, 62% were improved, and 12% were unchanged. In 1970

Department of Orthopaedic Surgery, School of Medicine, Duke University, Durham, North Carolina 27710 this same author[4] indicated that the functional results of the anterior lumbar fusion series were "about the same," as those for his posterolateral fusion series. Our experience has been similar. The arthrodesis rate of posterolateral fusions at Duke University Medical Center is only slightly better than the rate of healing of anterior interbody fusion.[8-10]

In 1972 Stauffer and Coventry[11] reported on 77 patients treated by anterior lumbar fusion. They observed a single interspace fusion rate of 68% and reported 36% "good clinical results." They stated that they reserved the procedure for salvage. They do not indicate why 64% were considered failures.

Kotcamp[12,13] has used anterior lumbar fusion in the management of over 500 patients. He states that he frequently uses this operation as a primary method of managing discectomy, and indicates that he has observed a fusion rate of 90% for a single interspace.

Several years ago the results of this procedure and the fusion rate obtained by authors using calf bone[14-16] and by a technique using circular plug grafts were thought to be very high. Harmon[17] has altered his reported technique and more recently obtained a higher fusion rate by using fibular graft and screw fixation.

Indications for Anterior Discectomy and Lumbar Fusion

The nonoperative treatment of intervertebral disc disease has a high priority in our management of patients with chronic low-back pain. We apply all currently available nonoperative techniques in an effort to "avoid the first operative procedure." If this treatment fails, then posterior nerve-root decompression and hemilaminectomy after myelography is the program selected for treating the patient with persistent radiculopathy. If this treatment fails, then reoperation and possibly posterolateral fusion are considered. The latter approach depends on whether or not the nerve roots require reexploration and further decompression or whether the interspace, proximally or distally, requires exploration. Patients in this first category have also been managed by anterior discectomy and fusion. They have had one or more prior operations, but pain has not been relieved.[8-10]

A second group of patients may have persistent pseudoarthrosis, if fusion has been attempted, or instability, incongruity, or nerve-root irritation secondary to specific pathologic conditions.

A third group is the fourth-decade female with a narrow lumbosacral joint, sclerosis of the interspaces, chronic severe low-back pain, and intermittent radiculopathy. The myelogram has usually been negative, but the patient does have evidence of buttock, thigh, and calf pain. Anterior discectomy and fusion usually relieve the back pain and radiculopathy without interfering with the nerve roots.

A fourth indication is seen in patients who have had posterior operations and developed infection. Persistent back pain and radiculopathy in these patients should be managed by anterior removal of the residual intervertebral disc material and localized arthrodesis. The interspace may or may not have been affected by the prior infection, but tissue is usually sterile after antibiotic therapy has been given.

The fifth group includes patients who have had posterolateral fusion and laminectomy for management of spondylolisthesis and who still have pain and pseudoarthrosis. They can usually be managed successfully by anterior discectomy and fusion. As a primary procedure for management of spondylolisthesis, however, this is not recommended.[16,18]

In the sixth group patients with proven spinal stenosis and arachnoiditis have been improved by anterior discectomy and fusion, particularly if the myelogram showed anterior indentations rather than posterior compression (Figs. 27-1A, B, and C). A second-stage posterior laminectomy was done, with less instability resulting if vertebral bodies were fused.

Diagnostic Studies

Usually information obtained from history, physical examination, and roentgenograms is essential to the decision concerning which approach to utilize for spine stabilization. Other studies selected, as indicated, are listed and the particular reasons for each are mentioned briefly.

1. *Laboratory studies* should include a battery of chemical analyses, including enzymes, uric acid, and blood sugar to detect any subtle systemic disease and, particularly, to determine any elevation of liver enzymes. This may be the best way to avoid general anesthesia. Studies related to rheumatoid arthritis or ankylosing spondylitis are important, as, occasionally, the patient with chronic back pain has a primary condition other than intervertebral disc disease.
2. *Roentgenograms* should be taken in multiple planes and, if the patient has been operated upon previously, a lateral flexion and extension as well as an anterior, posterior right, and left lateral bending-stress exposure should be done. This will give information about motion at the interspaces and aid in determining whether or not pseudoarthrosis exists. Tomography also helps to determine the latter.
3. *A differential spinal* test will aid in determining whether the patient has total relief of extremity or back pain at certain concentrations of injected anesthetic. If the patient's pain is relieved by saline, then the severity of this complaint is questioned. If pain is not relieved by a total motor and sensory block, then other considerations concerning its origin are considered.[18]
4. *Psychiatric consultation* is important in managing the patient who has had multiple operations and is being considered for another operation. Reactive depression, frank neuroses, or subtle psychoses may exist, and the psychiatrist can recommend appropriate medication and proper timing of an operation, if indicated, in this particular patient. The psychiatrist may be able to give advice to the family through the social worker and information to the employer, which are helpful in rehabilitating the patient.
5. *Clinical psychologic* studies have proved valuable in assessing the patient's behavior profile, response to injury and operation, and characteristics as they appear on the scale of conversion hysteria, hypochondriasis, or depression. This information is very important in postoperative management and in deciding whether or not the operative procedure, if not clearly indicated, should be done at all.
6. *Discography* has proven to be valuable for us in reproducing pain at a space that has not been operated upon, in providing information about the amount of fluid that can be injected into an interspace, and for providing information about a normal intervertebral disc that takes a minimal amount of contrast and does not result in pain at the time of the injection. An intervertebral disc that appears abnormal but does not cause pain at the time of injection usually can be ignored. Abnormalities seen by discography are not an indication for operation.[19]
7. *Electromyography* by a trained observer, if used to sample enough muscles, will provide invaluable information about the condition of the lower extremities. There is a high correlation between positive electromyography and positive myelography and discography. If the electromyogram is positive and the myelogram is negative, that information is particularly helpful. If the electromyogram is negative and the myelogram is positive then the electrical studies should be repeated by a more experienced electromyographer.
8. *A pantopaque myelogram* is helpful in localizing root-compression lesions and in ruling out a significant posterior block or posterior compression. A large defect, noted at the time of the initial myelogram, was usually a contraindication to anterior discectomy.

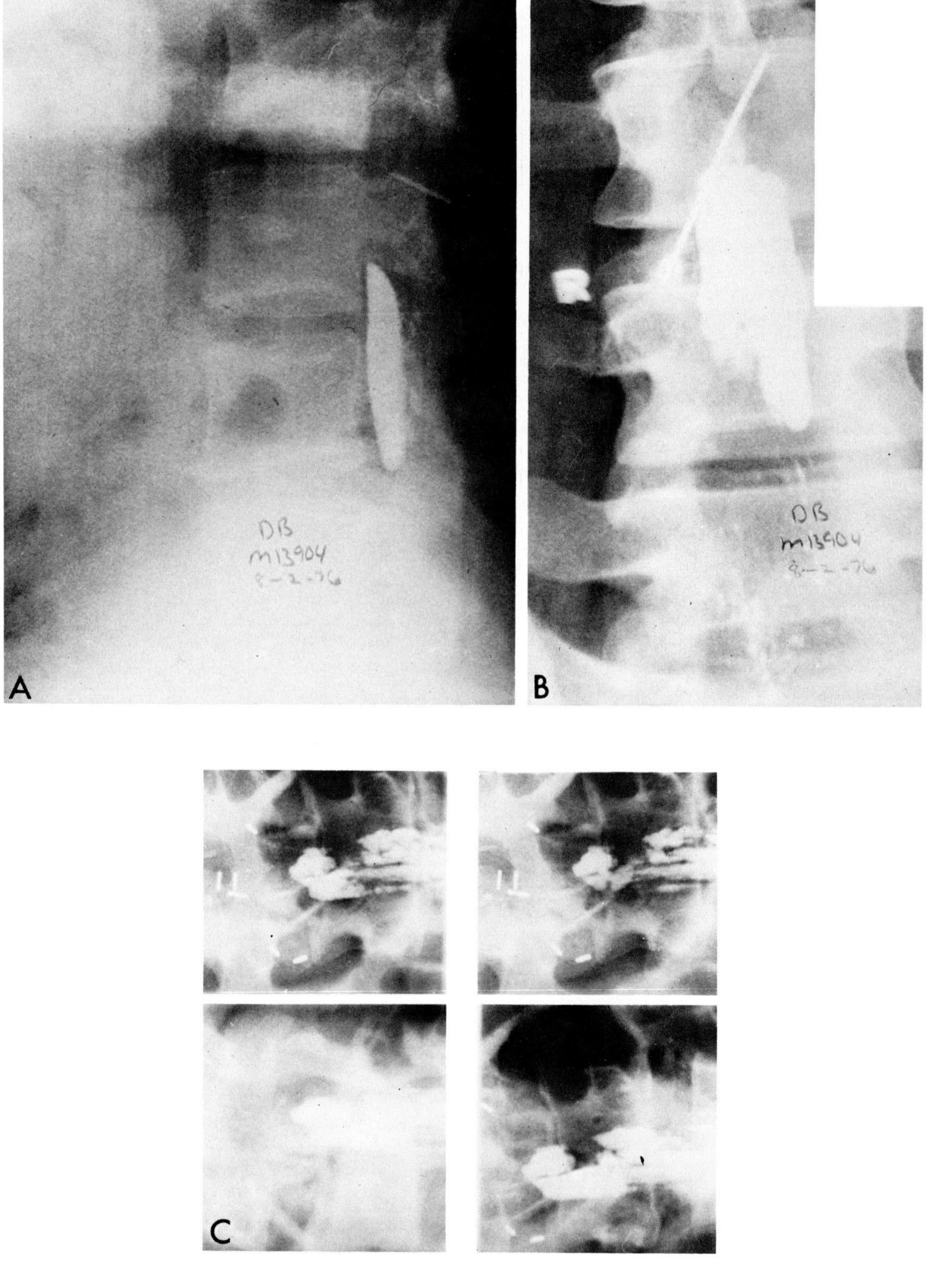
DB
M13904
8-2-76
A
DB
M13904
8-2-76
B
C

However, patients who have had multiple operative procedures and who had perineural fibrosis or arachnoiditis demonstrated that the block was not a contraindication to anterior discectomy and fusion.

9. *Nerve-root block* has been helpful in localizing the pain and the particular nerve root that required decompression. This test is an adjunct to the differential spinal in that it provides information about complete or partial relief of pain.
10. *Thermography* has provided some information about the inflammatory aspect of the patients' complaints. A positive thermogram suggests the process may be inflammatory rather than a primary mechanical deficiency. Occasionally this test has suggested ankylosing spondylitis and has resulted in other studies that aided proper diagnosis.
11. *Epidural venography* aids in localizing a compression lesion and may provide evidence of nerve-root involvement when the myelogram is negative. False-negative venograms may be a problem and the data must be interpreted in conjunction with other findings.

Contraindications to Anterior Lumbar Discectomy and Fusion

1. If nerve-root exploration is essential, then the posterior approach is desirable. We have not depended on nerve-root decompression from the anterior approach, as we have in the cervical spine.
2. Other contraindications are multiple interspace, advanced intervertebral disc disease (more than three interspaces), particularly in a patient over 50 years of age and in those with severe osteoporosis.

Operative Technique

Patients have usually been operated upon under general anesthesia supplemented with muscle relaxants. The Trendelenburg position, with the head down about 10°, is desirable as it allows displacement of the abdominal contents proximally and reduces venostasis in the lower extremities. This position is arranged after induction. A thin, folded sheet is placed under the left buttock to elevate the iliac crest. The upper extremities are placed so as to avoid stretch on axillary structures and compression on ulnar nerves at the elbows.

The anethetist is then asked to locate handles on the table that provide hyperextension of the lumbar spine. This position is not used when the incision is made, but is used while a discectomy is being done.

The abdomen and iliac crest are prepared with soap, water, and Betadine, and the skin is covered with a transparent adhesive dressing. The patient is also tilted to the left side 10°, if the surgeon is standing on the left while exposure is being made, or to the right side 10°, if the surgeon prefers to stand on the right while the *left* retroperitoneal exposure is performed.

The left paramedian incision is made through the skin and superficial fascia, the anterior rectus sheath is opened, and the muscle belly is retracted laterally to the lateral gutter (Fig.

Fig. 27-1A. Lateral x-ray film of a 20-year-old male who has had three operative procedures of discectomy and hemilaminectomy for management of back and lower extremity pain. This myelogram shows the column of contrast blocked at the L4-L5 interspace. Two years have elapsed since the original operation was done. The patient was almost completely incapacitated because of back and lower extremity pain. **B.** The anterior-posterior view showing the column of contrast blocked at the L4-L5 level. The presumptive diagnosis was arachnoiditis and perineural fibrosis. The appearance of the myelogram was the same after the second and the third operative procedures. Note that the spinous processes have been removed and that a segment of the laminal arches have been removed from the fifth lumbar vertebra and the inferior segment of the fourth lumbar vertebra. The facets are intact. **C.** Shows a postoperative AP view of the L4-L5 interspace with the bone grafts visible between the verebral bodies and the contrast at the same level as preoperatively.

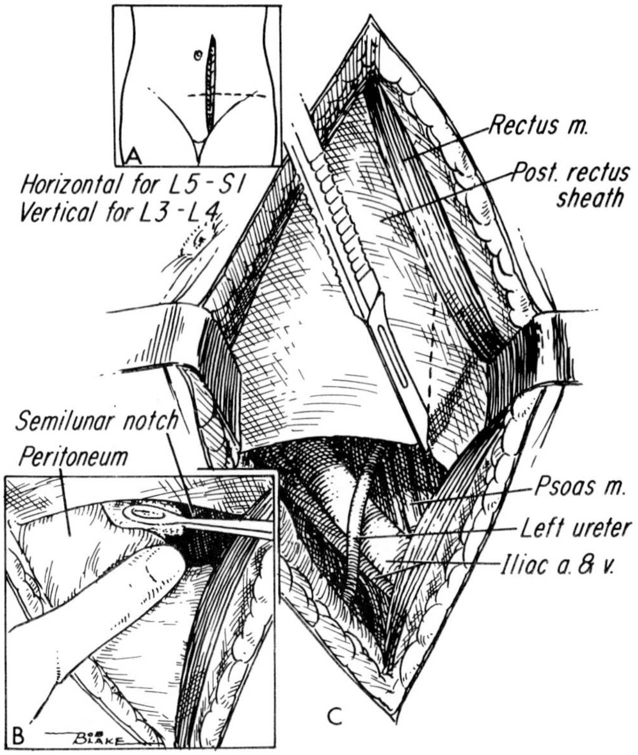

Fig. 27-2. A periumbilical incision has been made, the anterior sheath of the rectus has been incised and the rectus muscle retracted laterally. The posterior rectus sheath is identified anteriorly and far laterally. The semilunar notch is used as a guide for reflecting the peritoneum from the undersurface of the rectus sheath. The peritoneum and abdominal contents are swept medially. The posterior rectus sheath is incised laterally and proximally and these same flaps are sutured with nonabsorbable suture at the time of closure.

27-2). If the rectus sheath is incised in the midline, the peritoneum will be entered. The retroperitoneal space is entered, initially, inferiorly at the linea semilunaris, and the peritoneum is carefully and slowly separated by blunt dissection from the undersurface of the rectus sheath. The proximal incision into the posterior sheath should not be made until the peritoneum is separated from the fascia. Small peritoneal tears may occur during this step in the procedure, and they should be repaired with chromic catgut. The rectus sheath is incised from the semilunar notch inferiorly to its superior border proximally. The psoas muscle is identified and the iliac artery and vein are then palpated or visualized on the left side. The left ureter is located, after which the lumbosacral interspace is palpated. This space is identified between the right and left iliac arteries and veins (Fig. 27-3). The sacral promontory is identified by palpation without disturbing the sympathetic nerves crossing over the sacral promontory or the major sympathetic nerves on either side of the lumbar vertebrae. The soft tissue over the interspace of the vertebral and lower half of the fifth lumbar vertebral body is dissected off with a small dissector, and the venous tributaries from the iliac vein and vena cava are clamped with silver clips. The lumbosacral interspace is exposed by retracting the left iliac artery and vein to the left side and the right iliac artery and vein to the right side with blunt vein retractors (Fig. 27-4). Spike retractors, driven into the body of the fifth lumbar

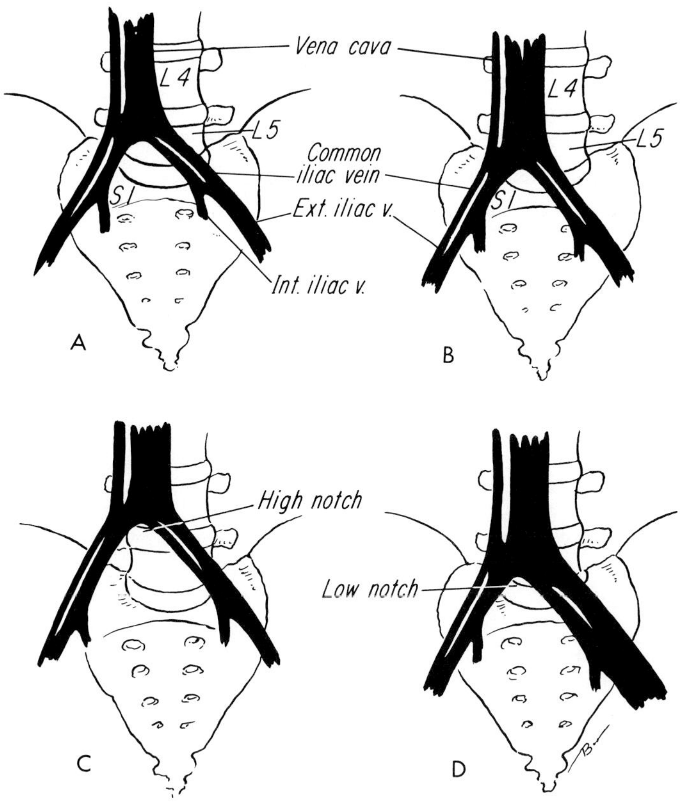

Fig. 27-3. Several patterns of bifurcation of the vena cava into the iliac veins exist. The bifurcation may be opposite the middle of the fifth lumbar vertebra, at the level of the last intervertebral disc space or even as high as the middle of the fourth lumbar vertebral body. The decision to reflect the artery, vein and ureter to the right, in order to expose L4-5, depends on the height of the notch. Over 90% of the time this reflection is necessary and makes the exposure easier. In each instance, isolation of the L5-S1 interspace has been possible just below the bifurcation.

vertebra, are helpful in maintaining the exposure (Fig. 27-5A). The vessels are protected from the spike by a small abdominal pack, and the peripheral pulse is palpated distal to the spike, indicating that excessive tension is not placed on the artery or vein. No dissection is done on the first sacral segment. Bleeding and the decussating fibers of the sympathetic chain, which control ejaculation, are avoided.

In exposing the fourth lumbar interspace, the left iliac artery and vein and the ureter are displaced to the right side of the spine and held in place by spike retractors. During exposure of this interspace, there is even more likelihood of obliterating the left iliac artery with retraction, if excessive tension is placed on the retractor.

The anterior longitudinal ligament at the L4-S1 interspace is elevated from the annulus as a flap, with the base attached at the left (Figs. 27-4 and 27-6). This flap, when tagged with sutures, affords additional retraction and protection for the vessels. Hyperextension of the operating table brings the spine closer to the surface of the wound and affords better exposure of the interspace (Fig. 27-7). The intervertebral disc and the annulus are separated from the cartilagenous plates of the vertebra with a knife or a thin osteotome. Once detached from

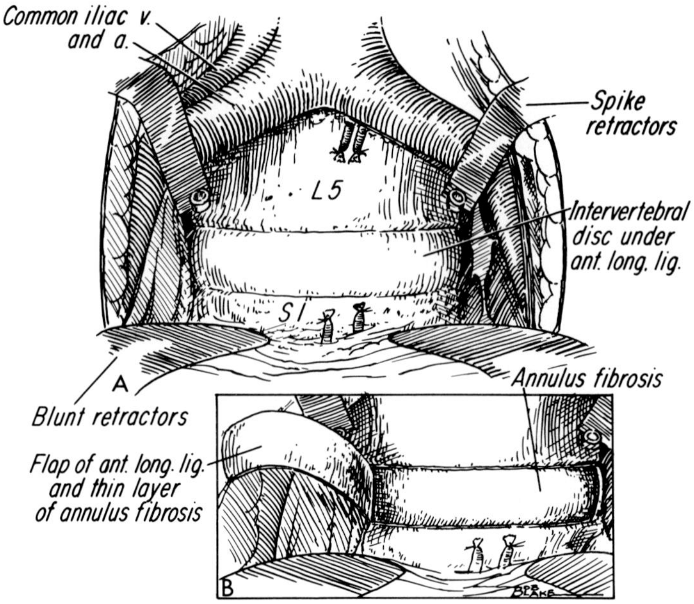

Fig. 27-4. The notch of the vena cava, where it divides into the iliac veins, may be high or low. In this instance the midportion of the fifth lumbar vertebra is clearly visible, the intervertebral disc is exposed widely to the right and left, and no dissection is carried out over the sacral prominence other than to interrupt the veins and arteries with silver clips. Spikes are not inserted into the sacrum, since this may result in additional dissection and cause trauma to the decussating nerve fibers over the first sacral segment. These fibers should be avoided. A long flap of anterior longitudinal ligament, to which is attached a thin layer of the annulus fibrosis, is isolated and reflected either right or left, depending on which interspace is involved. This flap will protect the artery and vein at the fourth interspace.

the vertebral body above and below, the disc complex can be removed easily with a large pituitary rongeur and large curettes (Fig. 27-5B). The space is cleaned out thoroughly, back to the posterior longitudinal ligament, before any bone is removed. In this way, bleeding is minimal and dissection can be done under direct vision. The lateral recesses are cleaned thoroughly. Cartilage surfaces are removed from the vertebral bodies with an osteotome until bleeding bone is encountered. Vigorous bleeding may occur from the posterior aspect of the vertebral bodies and can be controlled with small amounts of bone wax or cautery. The undersurface of the L5 vertebra is concave and requires special attention in removing soft tissue.

After the soft tissue and cartilage have been removed from the interspace, dimensions of the interspace are measured with a caliper and ruler. The grafts are then cut individually from the left ilium, which is prepared by subperiosteal dissection so that full-thickness grafts, with inner and outer cortex of the ilium, can be obtained.[11] The graft is cut slightly larger than the height of the interspace so that firm impaction can be obtained (Fig. 27-8A and B). The lateral recesses of the intervertebral space are packed first with short vertical struts, with the cortices at right angles to the vertebral bodies. The central graft is usually 3.5 cm deep and the width varies from 0.8 to 1.0 cm. After the lateral grafts are placed, the center graft is then

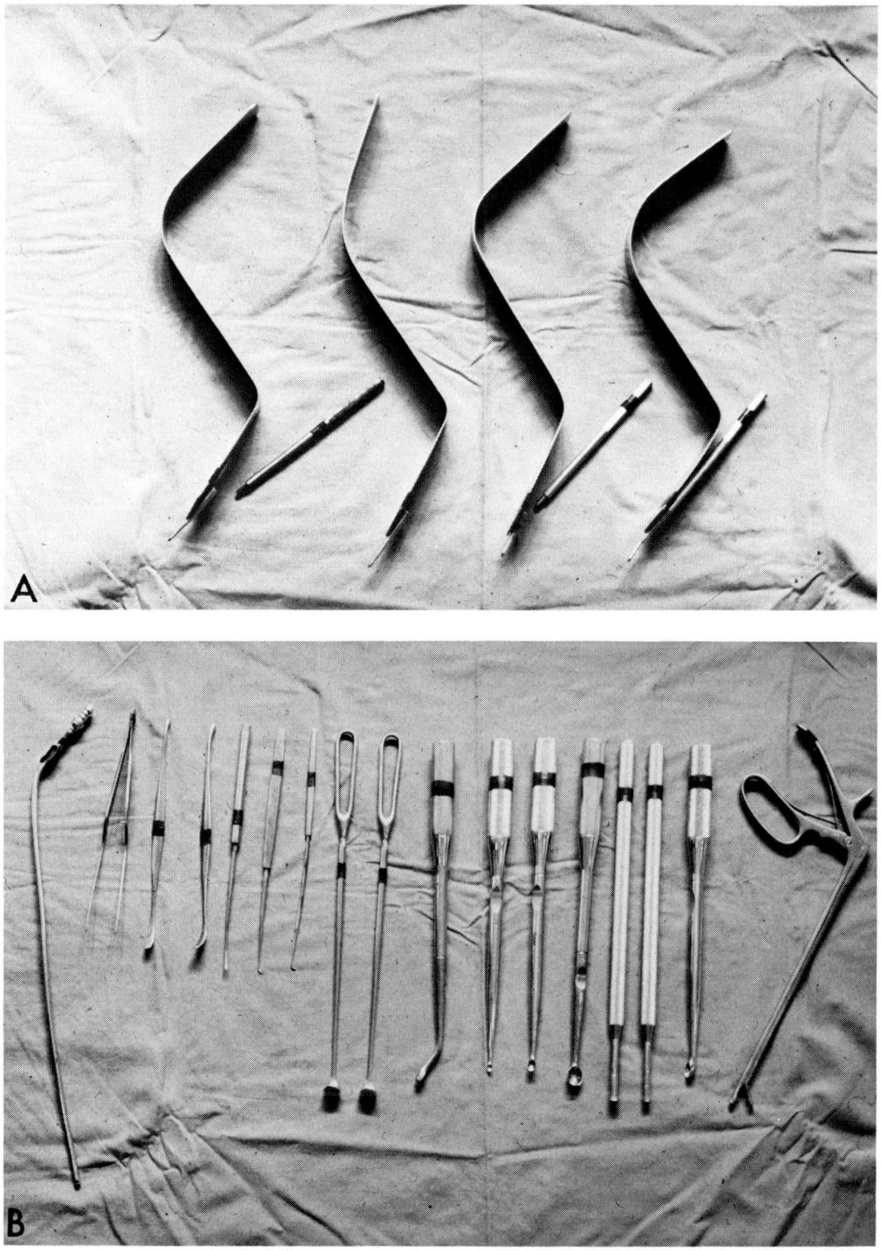

Fig. 27-5A. The spiked retractors are very helpful in doing the procedure. The extension screws on and off and is used to impact the spike into the vertebral body. Two retractors are usually used with one being placed on the right and one on the left in order to retract the artery and vein. The spike should be covered with a sponge pack on one side so that pressure from the metal does not irritate the vessels. When the spikes are removed, a small amount of bone wax is used to fill the bone hole in order to diminish bleeding. **B.** Special instruments used in doing anterior lumbar discectomy and fusion. The large pituitary ronguer was made by an instrument company at our request. The large curettes and long-handled impactors are helpful in cleaning out the interspace and in placing the bone grafts. The long-handled vein retractors are helpful in displacing the iliac vein and the vena cava while silver clips are used to clamp the small tributaries.

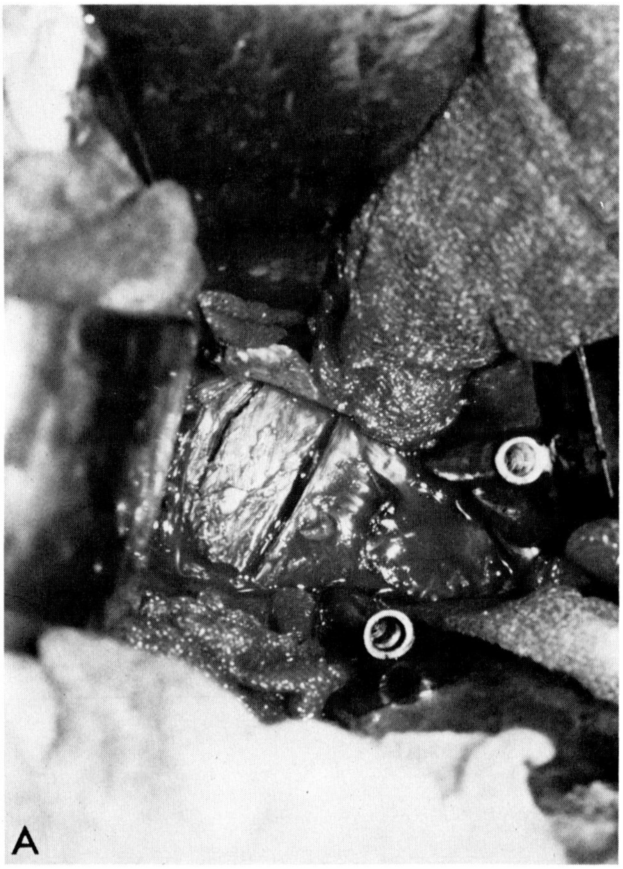
A

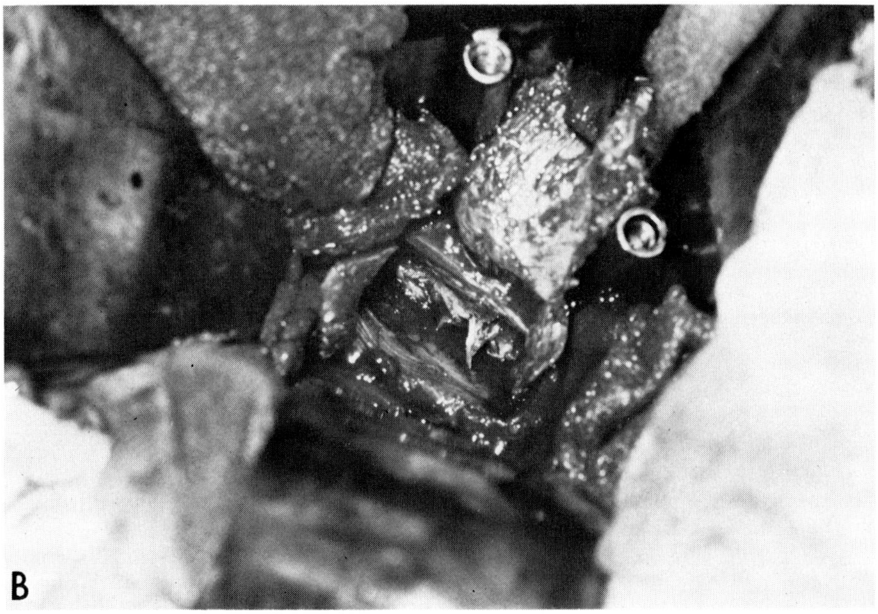
B

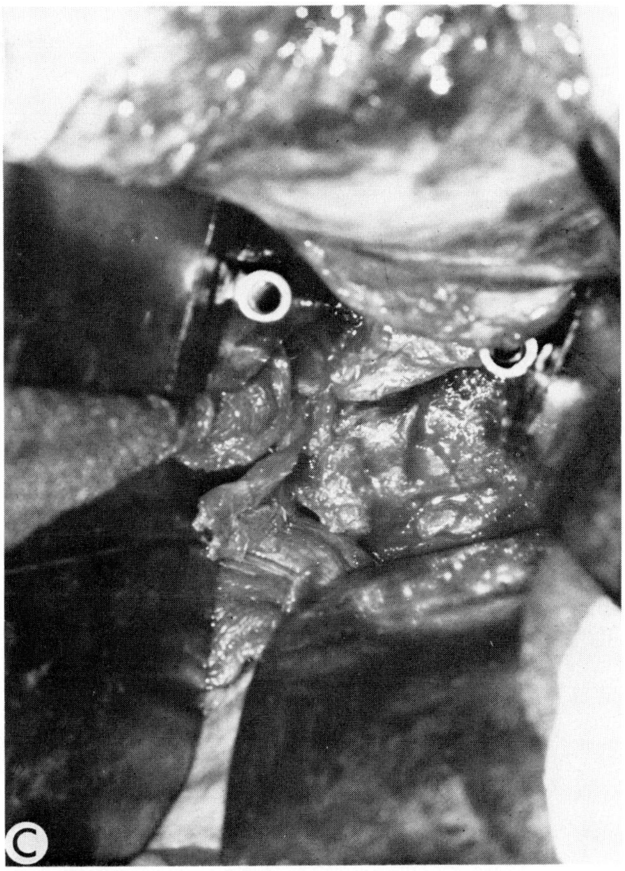

Fig. 27-6A. The anterior ligament has been removed and the annulus incised. The soft tissue remaining in the interspace made up of residual fragments of annulus, fibrous tissue, cartilaginous fragments, and minimal nucleus. All of this material is removed completely until the cartilage plates are clearly visible. **B.** The metallic retractor's 2.0-cm spikes projecting are driven into the L5 vertebral body. Cuts have been made into the anterior longitudinal ligament superiorly and inferiorly. A flap of anterior longitudinal ligament has been elevated and retracted to the patient's right. Packs are used to protect the vessels, the ureter, the sympathetic chain and the presacral decussation. **C.** Anterior longitudinal ligament flap has been elevated, the anterior and medial and lateral segments of the annulus have been removed and the remaining soft tissues superiorly, inferiorly and posteriorly must be removed so that good bone contact can be obtained between the autogenous bone graft and the vertebral bodies.

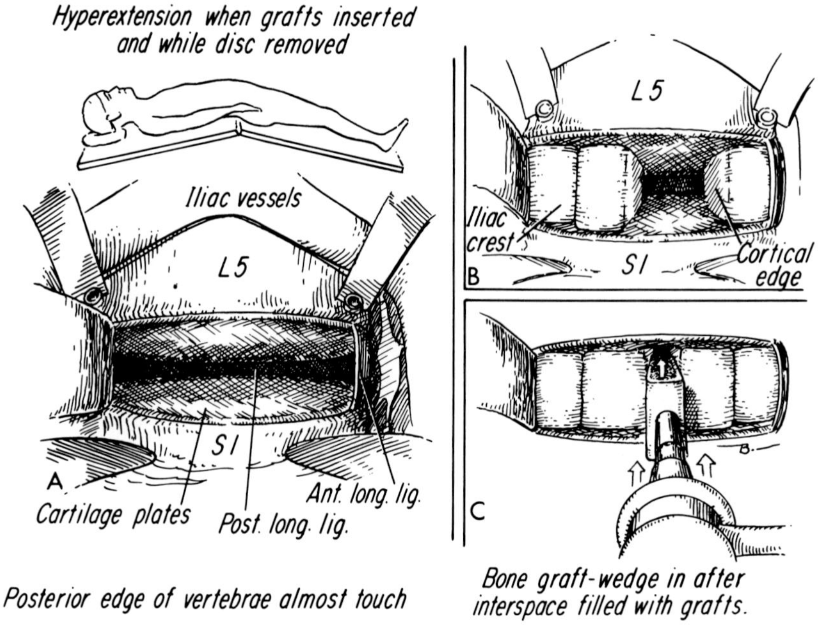

Fig. 27-7. The intervertebral disc, which is relatively avascular, has been removed without breaking through the cartilage plates. After the annulus and nucleus have been excised, then the cartilage plates are partially removed, perforated and roughened, so that bleeding bone surfaces exist. Lateral bone grafts are impacted so that the right and left edges of the interspace are filled with a graft. Additional bone grafts are then placed in the center of the interspace and the last bone graft is wedged in between the seemingly tight impacted grafts.

impacted so that the anterior edge is countersunk about 2 mm. The second center graft is then inserted and compressed, both to the right and to the left sides. A wedging technique is used by inserting two osteotomes between the center grafts and spreading the osteotomes to the right and to the left, thereby compressing the grafts and allowing space for an additional piece of bone (Fig. 27-7C). Small segments of cortical and cancellous bone can be impacted between the grafts. The grafts should not be countersunk excessively as they may extend posteriorly through holes in the posterior longitudinal ligament and irritate the nerve roots.

The spine is then straightened by correcting the hyperextended position of one table. This holds the grafts in place by wedging the vertebral bodies.

The L4-5 interspace is exposed by retracting the left iliac artery, vein, and ureter toward the right side and replacing the spike retractors in the L5 vertebral body. The spine is then hyperextended and the L4-5 interspace is cleaned out and prepared for insertion of the iliac bone graft (Fig. 27-9). If the L3-4 interspace is to be done, the dissection is completed proximally and the lumbar artery and vein ligated.

After the bone grafts are in place, a small piece of Surgicel is placed over the graft, and the anterior longitudinal flaps are replaced with a single nonabsorbable suture. All deep fascia layers are closed with nonabsorbable suture and subcutaneous tissues with absorbable suture. Four tension sutures of nylon are placed through the skin, subcutaneous tissue, and fascia and the dressing is sutured in place in order to absorb hematoma. This is removed at 5 days.

The average blood loss for one interspace has been 500 ml and for two interspaces 1200 ml. Replacement is done during the operative procedure, and packed cells may be given postoperatively as indicated.

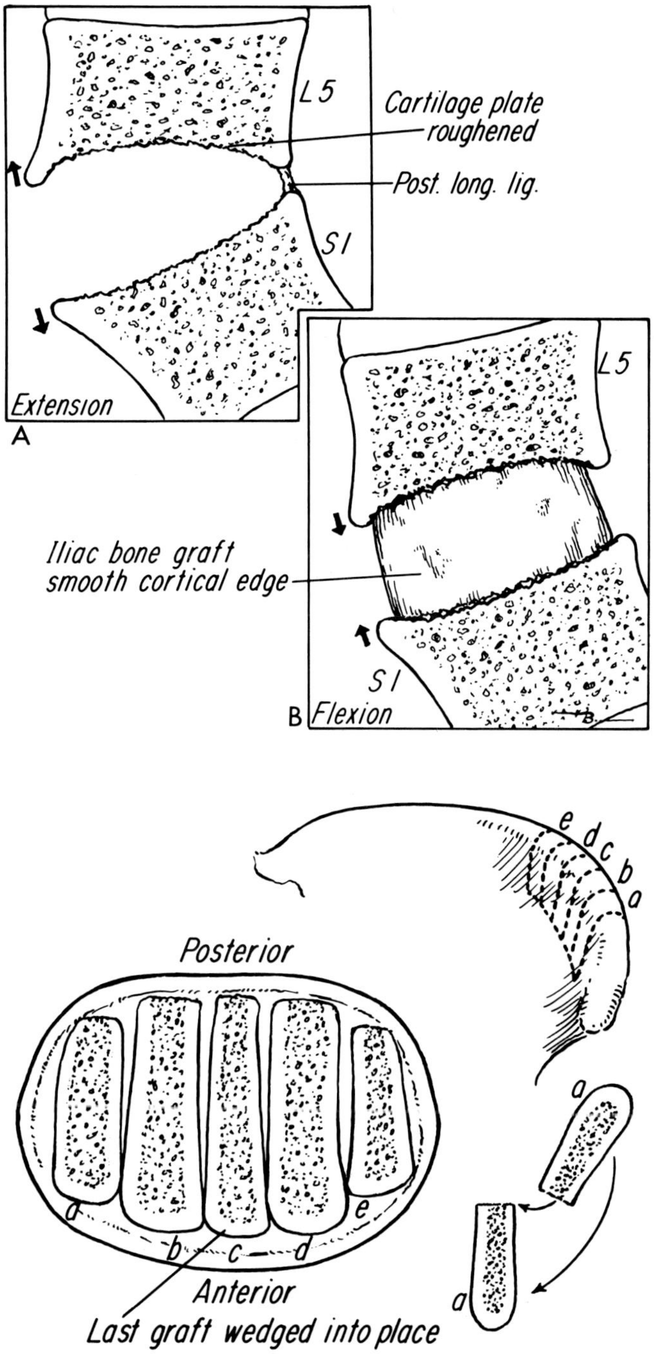

Fig. 27-8. A and **B.** Lateral view showing the vertebral bodies in the hyperextended position with the posterior longitudinal ligament intact, the roughened edges of the cartilage plates and perforations into the subchondral bone. After the bone graft is inserted, and the convex edge is placed into the inferior surface of the upper vertebra, the trunk is flexed for impaction and compression. The graft is countersunk with the anterior edge resting just deep to the edge of the verebral bodies. The muscle origins attached to the anterior iliac spine are left in place and the anterior-superior iliac spine is not removed. The full-thickness grafts are then rotated prior to insertion, so that the cortical edges provide vertical support for the vertebral bodies. The bone grafts are contoured so that there is a convex edge superiorly and a straight edge inferiorly. The iliac crest eventually rests in the outer two-thirds of the interspace and the narrower portion of the graft is deep. Wide exposure of the interspace is needed in order to place bone at the periphery of the interspace.

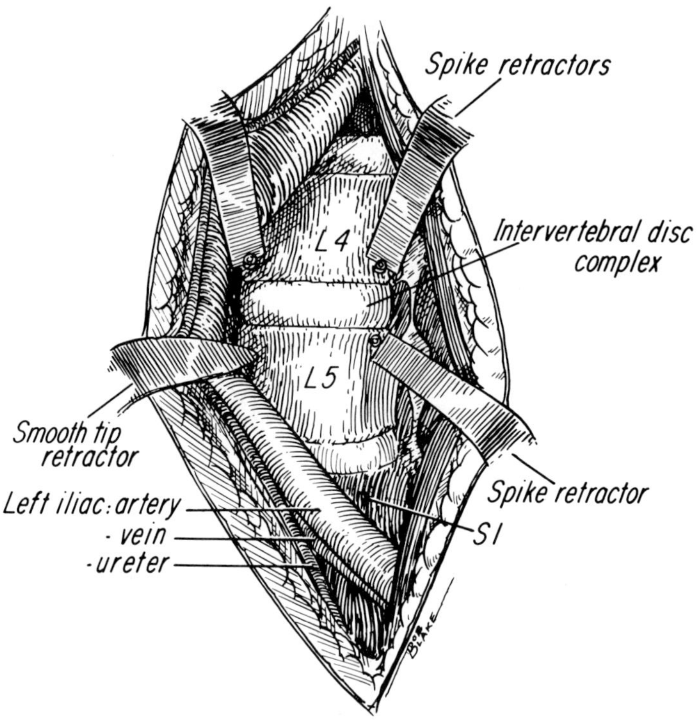

Fig. 27-9. Retroperitoneal exposure of L4, L5, and S1, through a retroperitoneal incision. The iliac artery, vein, and ureter have been displaced medially, the left sympathetic chain is recognized and avoided, and the spike retractors are used to provide exposure of the intervertebral disc complex. Compression of the artery and vein by the retractors must be avoided and the pulsation of the vessels should be felt from time to time. If L3 is to be exposed, the lumbar artery and vein must be ligated and the vessels dissected to the level of the upper edge of the third lumbar vertebra.

Postoperative Management

Nasogastric intubation is not always necessary but is used in some patients for maximum abdominal comfort, even though the tube itself may be uncomfortable. A low negative pressure is connected to the nasogastric tube until active peristalsis occurs, which is usually within 36 to 48 hours. The patient's head and chest are elevated slightly; the lower extremities should also be higher than heart level. Elastic stockings are used immediately postoperatively, but no elastic wrappings are used during the operation. The patient is encouraged to initiate active motion of the feet immediately upon awakening. The patient should be encouraged to turn frequently, to place a pillow on the abdominal wall in order to decrease pain of coughing, and to breathe deeply several times each hour. A trapeze is placed on the bed and the patient encouraged to use it.

Anticoagulation has been used in all patients who have anterior lumbar fusion. Our current anticoagulation routine is therapeutic low-dose heparin, giving 5,000 units subcutaneously on call, and 3,000 subcutaneously postoperatively, with the first dose beginning about 6 hours after the operation has been completed. The heparin is monitored daily by partial thromboplastin or clotting time. High therapeutics levels are not necessary. The level should be prolonged only slightly more than normal. Heparin is continued about 7 days, the platelet count is observed every third day, and the patient is then changed to Coumadin. Coumadin is monitored for a total of 3 weeks. Prothrombin time is maintained at 1½ times normal level. The patient may leave the hospital 10 to 14 days after the procedure, and the family physician is asked to monitor the anticoagulant. Certain medications alter the prothrombin time and the physician should be familiar with these.

Straight-leg raising is started on the third postoperative day and continued for several months. By the fifth postoperative day, the patient is allowed to sit and to walk. A low-back corset has been used to support abdominal muscles and to encourage deep breathing and coughing. The iliac donor site is usually more painful than the abdomen or back.

The pain relief associated with radiculopathy has been consistently noted on the day after operation. Because of early relief of pain, many patients tend to overexert physically and they must be warned that total pain relief will not persist and may not be present for several months. Recurrent episodes of discomfort are to be expected.

Patients are asked to avoid automobile driving for 6 to 8 weeks. Walking should be increased in a graduated way and the patient should attempt to go 2 to 3 miles daily after 4 to 6 weeks have passed. Isometric, abdominal and gluteal exercises are encouraged.

AP and lateral x-ray films of the lumbosacral spine are taken just before the patient leaves the hospital. These provide a baseline for judging the appearance of the graft, psoas shadows, bone density, and the height of the interspace. Three months after operation lateral flexion and extension x-ray films are taken with the patient in the standing position. X-ray studies are again repeated at 6 to 12 months. A solid fusion cannot be confirmed until at least a year after the operation, and even at that time trabeculations across both sides of the interspace are not always present.

Complications-Sequelae

Immediate complications have occurred infrequently. These diminished as experience with the procedure increased. Complications that have occurred are listed and a brief note concerning avoidance or prevention is made.

Thromboembolism

This has been avoided by anticoagulation of all patients done during the past 4 years. Low-molecular weight or regular dextran were used for 3 or 4 years, with a diminished incidence of venous thrombosis. About 1970, therapeutic low-dose heparin was introduced. After 7 to 10 days of receiving heparin, the patient was given coumadin and maintained on a limited anticoagulation regimen for a total of 4 weeks. Coumadin alone, or dextran and aspirin, or aspirin alone are also used by certain members of the staff. A recent review of all patients who had major orthopedic operations and received anticoagulation showed that therapeutic low-dose heparin had a predictable protective effect against thromboembolism.

Pseudoarthrosis

If the number of spaces operated upon increases in a particular patient, the pseudoarthrosis rate also increases. Studies of successful fusion in the first 100 cases operated upon in our series are listed in Table 27-1. Patients with successful fusion cannot be determined for at least 1 year after the operative procedure has been completed, and, preferably followup should be at least 2 years; non-union not evident at 1 year may be evident at 2 years.

Table 27-1. Anterior Discectomy and Fusion: Incidence of Successful Fusion

	Patients	Successful fusion	% Fusion
Single-space	46	42	91
Two-space	46	33	72
Three-space	8	5	62
Total	100	80	

Likewise, what appeared to be an early pseudoarthrosis may progress to a stable spine at about 1 year.

The arthrodesis rate has been reviewed for the second 100 cases and patients who have had one interspace arthrodesed showed a rate of fusion of about 80%; those who had two spaces arthrodesed had a fusion rate of about 70%. Individual surgeons, however, demonstrated smaller series in the group with a higher fusion rate, indicating that there is a direct relationship between the technique utilized, placements of bone grafts, stability of the interspace after the operative procedure has been completed, and the patient's activities during the next several months.

Our analysis of the last 200 patients reviewed shows a definite correlation between successful spine arthrodesis, subsequent relief of symptoms, and diminution of pathologic physical findings. A few patients who were relieved of radiculopathy did not have a solid fusion. Their back pain usually persisted. Other patients obtained a solid fusion and were not relieved of all their complaints. Factors known to be related to the persistence of pain, such as perineural fibrosis, intraneural fibrosis, and involvement of areas outside the spine as well as the interspaces proximally, must be considered in the total management of these patients.

When arthrodesis failed in patients who had undergone a two-space fusion, the pseudoarthrosis was usually in the upper interspace. Stress, torque, and abnormal motions persist at that space, whereas the L5-S1 interspace is compressed more readily. Almost all patients who developed pseudoarthrosis were managed by posterior lateral fusion. A combination of prior anterior and additional posterior fusion provided a high degree of success in obtaining fusion in these patients (95%). A prior ununited anterior fusion always showed evidence of union, with trabeculations crossing the vertebral bodies within a year after the posterior lateral fusion was done. Anterior fusion enhanced a failed posterior fusion as well. Reoperation anteriorly was done only if there was a contraindication to posterior exposure, such as prior infection or small transverse processes.

We prepare those patients who are to have an anterior discectomy and fusion to expect about a 20% chance of having to have an additional operative procedure in order to obtain a solid fusion. Considering the fact that many of these individuals have anywhere from two to five prior operations, we feel that this is an acceptable method of management.

Discussion of Other Complications and Sequelae

Donor Site Disturbance

This can be avoided if the anterior superior spine is not removed when the bone graft is taken. The lateral femoral cutaneous nerve should not be subjected to traction or laceration, as this is the most common cause of postoperative discomfort. Pain at the bone graft site after operation is usually more noticeable than abdominal pain. Gluteal and abdominal muscles should be removed with a small flake of bone attached to them. An osteotome is used to do this. This allows firm closure of periosteum with a bone attachment. There is usually quicker recovery of muscle tone and less pain if this is done. Suction draining is always used. Bone wax is used to cover the bleeding surfaces.

Thromboembolism

This has been avoided by administering anticoagulants as mentioned, elevating the foot of the operating table during the procedure, maintaining the lower extremities higher than heart level postoperatively, active motion of the patient in bed postoperatively using foot exercises, overhead trapeze, frequent coughing, blow bottles, and adequate hydration. Antithromboembolic stockings are used and these must contour above the knee, or below knee stockings are selected. Acetylsalicylic acid is used for several weeks after the primary anticoagulant is stopped.

Urinary Tract Disturbance

Indwelling catheters are avoided. Preoperative assessment for bacterial infection is done and the patient is not operated upon if there is evidence of a symptomatic bacterial infection. These infections are treated initially. Postoperatively urecholine, manual compression and other methods are used to maintain adequate bladder tone. One patient in 200 received a small puncture wound of the left ureter. This was demonstrable postoperatively by retroperitoneal urinoma. This was treated by an indwelling catheter and healed.

Impotence

In none of the 200 patients, both males and females, and in no instance in the management of a male was impotence related to neurogenic involvement recognized. Those patients who had difficulty with erection several weeks or months postoperatively had the same problem preoperatively. Three of the 200 patients demonstrated retrograde ejaculation. They were included in the first 30 patients done and more extensive dissection over the first sacral segment anteriorly had been performed. The decussating fibers of the upper sacral plexus may have been involved in this dissection. No dissection is carried below the anterior edge of the L5-1 interspace. Hand-held blunt-nosed retractors are used over the superior body of S1. No cauterization is done over the superior sacral segment and none over the body of L5. Soft tissues are swept aside with blunt dissectors and silver clips are used to manage the venous collaterals. We are confident that if this technique is followed, this procedure can be done in male patients of any age, without affecting sexual function.

Fear of sexual dysfunction associated with anterior lumbar fusion has been emphasized in the literature. This possibility, of course, does exist because of the anatomic location of the operative procedure. However, our experience has shown that this is not an expected or necessary complication of this operative procedure.

Infection

Bacterial infection occurred in 2 patients, both of which were accounted for by Gram-negative involvement from the urinary tract. Infection was controlled by draining the hematoma and by antibiotics. The fusion rate was not affected.

Postoperative Hematoma

Bleeding from a persistent epigastric vessel resulted in a large progressive retroperitoneal hematoma, which was managed by evacuation and by ligating the vessel on the sixth postoperative day. The patient's progress was satisfactory subsequent to that. If the hematocrit drops and if the patient shows evidence of enlarged abdominal girth, then reexploration is essential for the bleeding point, either from the branch of the iliac artery, a branch of the vena cava, or an abdominal vessel. Reexploration was required in 2 of 200 patients.

Prolonged Abdominal Ileus

This is prevented by inserting a nasogastric tube if the patient does not show rapid recovery of bowel sounds after the operative procedure. We do not use the nasogastric tube routinely, although there is much less likelihood of ileus if this is done. The patient is encouraged to assume a sidelying position and to avoid intake by mouth until bowel sounds occur and flatus is passed. A rectal tube is helpful.

Problem-Oriented Patients

Case 1. A 22-year-old nurse gave a history of having had acute back and lower extremity pain, initially treated by bedrest and antiinflammatory agents. Recurrent radiculopathy was followed by a myelogram by her attending neurosurgeon, who subsequently performed a hemilaminectomy and removed a soft, bulging intervertebral disc. The patient's symptoms improved during the subsequent 4 months, but back pain and buttock aching persisted. Serial x-ray studies showed rapid narrowing of the interspace. Her pain worsened, straight-leg raising tests became strongly positive, and a second myelogram was done. A decompressive laminectomy was performed as the second operation, and spine fusion was not done at that time. Improvement was slight. Several months elapsed, and she was unable to work at her nursing occupation. She continued to have evidence of nerve-root irritation and facet joint and interbody pain. One and one-half years after her initial onset of pain and radiculopathy she was still disabled.

Diagnostic studies included electromyography, which showed abnormal polyphasic action potentials in the S1 root distribution. The differential spinal gave a physiologic response and the clinical psychologic studies showed the patient was not an hysterical type, nor was she somatizing. A discogram was done at the L4-5 level while the patient was awake. There was no pain associated with injection of the contrast and only 0.8 ml could be injected. The retroperitoneal approach was selected for the anterior discectomy and fusion. Only the L5-S1 interspace was included because of the normal discogram. Postoperatively the straight-leg raising tests were possible to 70° as compared with 30° preoperatively. Her relief of extremity pain was almost immediate. The nerve root that is fibrotic or compressed in a small canal can be decompressed by immobilizing the interspace and distracting it minimally with the bone graft. By 3 months, her back pain had been eliminated and by 6 months she was doing limited nursing. Within 1 year there were trabeculations across the interspace, and she was fully active in her occupational and social life.

There are many advantages to directly decompressing a nerve root. Spinal fusion will not cure a nerve root with intraneural fibrosis, but perineural fibrosis may be helped by immobilization. At least the constant trauma of incongruity and instability are removed and the root is protected somewhat.

If we compare the anterior discectomy and fusion to posterior discectomy and fusion, we will note the greater ease in cleaning out the intervertebral space, placing the bone grafts under compression, and placing the grafts in such a way that they follow the contour of the vertebral bodies. If the nerve roots do not have to be retracted, then there is much less chance of involving the dura or roots during the operative procedure.

If there continues to be evidence of anterior-posterior spinal canal narrowing or nerve-root compression, then appropriate decompression can be done posteriorly at a time when the vertebral bodies are relatively stable.

Case 2. A 19-year-old male developed acute back pain with radiculopathy and had the physical findings and myelographic defect compatible with ruptured disc at the L4-5 interspace. A hemilaminectomy was done by the attending neurosurgeon and a soft bulging disc was removed. Temporary improvement occurred, but with increased physical activity, pain recurred in approximately 6 months. A second myelogram was done followed by a second decompression, and neurolysis was performed. Temporary improvement occurred while the patient was at bedrest, but within 4 months severe back pain and lower extremity radiculopathy were present. The x-ray films showed gradual narrowing of the L4-5 interspace and the myelogram showed a partial block and a defect at L4-5 (Figs. 27-1A, B, and C). The patient had a physiologic response to the differential spinal, the electromyogram was positive, involving the L5 root on the left, and a discogram at L3-4 was normal, but resulted in pain at both L4-5 and L5-S1.

An anterior discectomy and fusion through a retroperitoneal approach were done at L4-5 and L5-S1. Full-thickness iliac bone grafts were used and both spaces were adequately immobilized by the procedure. Immediately postoperatively, straight-leg raising was possible to 70° on the left and was painful on the right at about 60°, which had not been the case preoperatively. After 6 months, straight-leg raising was possible on both sides to 70° and back pain was eliminated about 80%. The x-ray study shows fusion is progressing satisfactorily.

The diagnosis was arachnoiditis and perineural fibrosis, and incongruity and instability secondary to removal of the intervertebral disc in the young male.

Spinal fusion is recommended in young people, particularly if the first operation for bulging or soft intervertebral disc fails. Discography is helpful, if performed properly and interpreted correctly. Abnormal discogram means that a pathologic lesion exists, but this does not mean that an operative procedure is necessarily indicated. If the clinical findings are abnormal, however, and if the electromyogram coincides, then treatment may be indicated. Furthermore, a normal discogram is much more helpful in many instances than an abnormal one.

Case 3. A 28-year-old female pharmacist with an intervertebral disc syndrome at L4-5 had a 4-year history of back pain with radiculopathy. A bulging disc had been removed initially with temporary relief. Six months later the persistent pain resulted in reexploration of the lower two interspaces posteriorly. Minimal improvement occurred temporarily and worsened as time passed. Serial x-ray studies showed moderately rapid narrowing of both lower interspaces. Because of her slow response, the question of emotional problems and the influence of possible litigation had been introduced by the attending neurosurgeon.

Our studies included an electromyogram, which was positive for S1 nerve-root irritation. The differential spinal was physiologic, a selective nerve block gave temporary relief of pain in one extremity, and the discogram was normal at the L3-4 space. We do not usually include spaces operated upon previously in the discogram procedure, although this is done occasionally to determine if pain can be reproduced. A selective nerve block will provide the same information by encouraging the patient to undergo physical activity in order to aggravate the pain and then attempt to relieve it with the nerve block.

A two-space anterior lumbar discectomy and fusion was done. Radiculopathy was diminished, back pain improved gradually, and by 1 year after the procedure, the L5-S1 interspace was solid but a fibrous union was present at L4-5 space. The patient had buttock and thigh pain on the left side after standing and walking for moderately long distances. This root was decompressed by hemilaminectomy and neurolysis with unroofing of the foramen. A posterior lateral fusion was then done from L4 to L5 using iliac bone. The patient's radiculopathy was improved within 2 months and the back pain improved during the next 6 months. Both interspaces were solid at 1 year, and the patient was back at work.

Case 4. A 21-year-old doctor's daughter with back pain and radiculopathy was treated by excision of a bulging intervertebral disc at L5-S1. Pain and limitation of motion persisted and several months later the myelogram showed a bulging intervertebral disc at L4-5. This was excised with temporary relief but back and buttock pain persisted. A third exploratory operation was done at the lower two spaces, four nerve roots were decompressed, and hemilaminectomies were done bilateral. Subsequent to this procedure, the patient was unable to sit more than 30 minutes without developing severe pain, she walked with the trunk flexed about 30° and she was comfortable only when lying flat on her back with the hips and knees flexed.

We performed a discogram at the L3-4 level, which was normal. An electromyogram was positive with abnormal action potentials at the L4-5 and L5-S1 roots. X-rays showed the interspaces to be narrowed about 70% of normal, and flexion-extension stress x-ray studies showed distinct motion at the interspaces. A two-space anterior discectomy and fusion through a retroperitoneal approach, using iliac bone graft, was done. Recovery was moderately slow, and pain, although improved, persisted for 4 additional months. However, the patient could sit for longer periods of time, could stand erect, and by 4 months after operation was able to drive her car. X-ray studies showed evidence of a solid fusion by 1 year; the radiculopathy had been eliminated and she returned to school.

Case 5. A 35-year-old female physician had been partially incapacitated because of chronic low back and lower extremity pain for over 5 years. She had been managed by laminectomy, attempted stabilization by posterior lateral fusion with a total of four previous operations. She was using two canes, was required to spend half the day in bed, and was carrying out limited general practice. The physical findings showed positive stretch tests, pain on manipulation of the spine and weakness of dorsiflexion of the foot.

She was taking Urecholine, 25 mg three times a day, for management of her atonic bladder. Cystometrogram showed minimal neurogenic involvement.

A differential spinal was physiologic, the discogram was negative at L3-4 and electromyogram was strongly positive involving the L4-5 and L5-S1 nerve roots bilateral. There was no evidence of spine infection.

A psychiatric assessment and clinical psychologic testing showed that the patient did need treatment for reactive depression and anxiety.

Stress x-ray studies in the right and left lateral position and forward flexion and extension showed definite motion at both spaces with evidence of pseudoarthrosis and incongruity.

Anterior discectomy and fusion were done through a retroperitoneal approach including the L4-5 and L5-S1 interspaces. A minimal amount of material was found at L5-S1 but considerable amount of annulus and fibrous tissue was removed from the L4-5 interspace. Full-thickness iliac bone grafts were used to stabilize the two lower intervertebral spaces.

Postoperatively, the straight-leg raising improved, over a period of 2 weeks, to about 60°. Bladder function improved to where Urecholine was reduced to 10 mg/day. During the next 3 months, the patient's progress was one of slow but steady improvement, with diminution of pain, increased strength, and increased activity. By 6 months after the operation, she was ready to return to work for half a day. Foot dorsiflexion had improved and bladder control was almost normal.

Results

In 100 patients anterior discectomy and fusion were included as part of their total management. The results were based on the patients' subjective descriptions, the physician's objective findings, and the patients' activity pattern at least 2 years after treatment was completed. The results of this study were based on an assessment of the degree of relief of back or lower extremity pain and rated as excellent, good, fair, slight, or none, or worse.

Table 27-2 can be interpreted as showing that 78% of the patients had moderate or complete relief of low-back pain, and 85% had complete or moderate relief of lower extremity pain. No patients were worse after treatment. Eighty-five percent of the patients who had one or two interspaces fused as shown to have had complete or moderate relief. Eighteen of the 100 patients continued to have pain and accepted additional back operations after the anterior discectomy and fusion. Fifteen of these had posterior lateral fusions and some had nerve root decompressions.

Table 27-2. Overall Results of Anterior Lumbar Fusion 100 Patients

	Complete relief	Moderate relief	Slight relief	No change	Worse
Low back pain	47	31	15	7	0
Lower extremity pain	58	27	12	3	0

Accessory characteristics, such as personality and occupation, of 200 patients were reviewed in 1975. Patients who were considered to have good results were analyzed from an occupational as well as an emotional standpoint. About one-half of those with good results were sponsored by Workmen's Compensation. About one-half had abnormal clinical psychologic findings, even though the result was satisfactory, and about two-thirds of the total patients had a "normal" emotional profile.

Conclusions

1. No single method of treatment is sufficient to successfully treat all patients with low-back pain and radiculopathy.
2. There is a direct relationship between patients who obtain a solid fusion and those who show improvement or relief of pain. Patients with persistent pseudoarthrosis have a greater chance of having persistent pain.
3. Detailed preliminary assessment utilizing several diagnostic studies aid in determining the proper method of management and prognosis.

4. Anterior discectomy and arthrodesis with autogenous bone is a safe procedure that allows the diminution of radiculopathy and back pain by removing fragments from the interspace and stabilizing the vertebral bodies.
5. The pseudoarthrosis rate associated with anterior lumbar fusion has been diminished by meticulous removal of the intervertebral soft tissue, by shaping the bone graft, and by the addition of a maximum amount of autogenous bone wedged into the interspace under compression.
6. Bone union as determined by roentgenography may not be accurate with plain films or stress x-rays until at least 1 year after the interbody fusion.
7. Spondylolisthesis, in our experience, should be managed by nerve root decompression and posterior lateral fusion at a single interspace. If pseudoarthrosis develops then anterior interbody spinal fusion can be done provided that the degree of displacement is not excessive.
8. Anterior discectomy and fusion have been helpful in diminishing pain and radiculopathy associated with perineural fibrosis and arachnoiditis.
9. Anterior interbody fusion is helpful in treating spinal stenosis and nerve root stenosis. A stable spine anteriorly allows wide decompression posteriorly without causing incongruity and instability. We have observed several patients who have had direct midline posterior fusions, who subsequently developed napkin ring constriction at the upper end of the fusion, encroachment of the fusion on the superior facets, and stenosis of the meninges associated with overgrowth of bone from the laminal arches.
10. Sexual dysfunction associated with anterior discectomy and fusion has not been a problem for the patients.
11. A meticulous operative technique is essential in order to obtain a high rate of fusion of the vertebral bodies.

REFERENCES

1. Burns BH: An operation for spondylolisthesis. *Lancet 224*:1233, 1933
2. Capener N: Spondylolisthesis. *Br J Surg 24*:80-85, 1936
3. Hartman JT, Kendrick JI, Lorman P: Discography as an aid in evaluation for lumbar and lumbosacral fusion, *Clin Ortho Related Res 81*:77-81, 1971
4. Sacks S: Anterior spinal surgery and ballarat. *J Bone Joint Surg 52-B*:392-393, 1970
5. Speed K: Spondylolisthesis. Treatment by anterior bone graft. *Arch Surg 37*:175, 1938
6. McCollum DE, Stephen CR: The use of graduated spinal anesthesia in the differential diagnosis of back and lower extremities, *So. Med J 57*:410-416, 1964
7. Sacks S: Intervertebral disc excision and lumbar spine fusion by transperitoneal approach. *J Bone Joint Surg 43-B*:401, 1961
8. Goldner JL, McCollum DE, Urbaniak JR: Anterior disc excision and interbody spine fusion for chronic low back pain. American Academy of Orthopaedic Surgeons, Symposium on the Spine. CV Mosby Company, St Louis, 1969
9. Goldner JL, McCollum DE, Urbaniak JR: Anterior intervertebral discectomy and arthrodesis for treatment of low back pain with or without radiculopathy, Chap 16. *Clinical Neurosurgery,* vol 15. Edited by RJ Ojemann. The Congress of Neurological Surgeons, 1968, pp 352-383
10. Goldner JL, Urbaniak JR, McCollum DE: Anterior disc excision and interbody spinal fusion for chronic low back pain. *Orthop Clin North Am 2*:543-567, 1971
11. Stauffer RN, Coventry MB: Anterior interbody spine fusion. *J Bone Joint Surg 54-A*:756-768, 1972
12. Kotcamp WW: Indications for anterior spine fusion. *Clin Ortho Related Res 70*:235, 1970
13. Hodgson AR, Stock FA: Anterior spine fusion for treatment of tuberculosis of the spine. *J Bone Joint Surg 42-A*:295, 1960
14. Harmon P: Anterior extraperitoneal disc excision and vertebral body fusion. *Clin Orthop 18*:169, 1961
15. Harmon P: Anterior disc excision and fusion of the lumbar vertebral bodies. *J Int Col Surg 40*:572, 1963
16. Shanewise RP: Anterior intervertebral lumbar spine fusion. *West J Surg 71*:212, 1963
17. Harmon P: Personal communication, 1975
18. Freebody D: Motion Picture shown at the Vancouver Meeting of the American Orthopaedic Association, 1965
19. Collis JS, Jr: *Lumbar Discography.* Charles C Thomas, Springfield, Illinois, 1963

CHAPTER 28

Percutaneous Rhizotomy in the Treatment of Intractable Facial Pain (Trigeminal, Glossopharyngeal, and Vagal Nerves)

John McLellan Tew, Jr.

Trigeminal Neuralgia

SURGICAL TREATMENT OF TRIGEMINAL neuralgia continues to stimulate controversy despite the fact that this condition has been recognized and treated surgically for centuries. A totally satisfactory method of treatment has never been devised. Section of a peripheral branch of the trigeminal nerve was probably the earliest form of surgical therapy. Later, intracranial section of peripheral branches,[1,2] ganglion resection,[3] and retrogasserian rhizotomy were developed.[4-6] Some questioned the need for destructive procedures[7-10] and developed techniques for decompressing or compressing the posterior rootlets.

Peripheral procedures are still effective for the temporary control of chronic trigeminal pain, particularly as an early measure that provides the patient an opportunity to test the effect of sensory deprivation.[11,12]

Recently, the need for destructive procedures has again been questioned by Jannetta,[13] who supports Dandy's[14] observation that trigeminal neuralgia is caused, in most instances, by vascular compression at the brain stem. While this hypothesis remains an attractive suggestion for treatment, the results of its application are still being tested.

The tactic of electrocoagulation of the trigeminal nerve was originally proposed by Kirschner in 1932.[15] Despite a report of favorable results,[16] this procedure gained no practitioners in this country until Sweet refined the technique,[17,18] with the following modifications: (a) a short-acting anesthetic agent, which permits the patient to awaken rapidly for sensory testing during the operation; (b) a reliable radiofrequency current for lesion production; (c) electrical stimulation for precise localization; and (d) temperature monitoring for precise control of lesion configuration. This procedure has been extremely safe and has gained considerable acceptance as a method for partially destroying the sensory root.

Mayfield Neurological Institute, Cincinnati, Ohio

Patient Selection

Much of the enthusiasm for percutaneous trigeminal rhizotomy has been engendered by patients who were relieved from pain after many years of suffering. While the patient's acceptance of a new surgical procedure is important, its ultimate value must depend on assessments of the duration of relief and the incidence of morbidity and mortality, compared with other surgical and medical treatments.

Presently, it is our practice to consider all patients with intractable trigeminal neuralgia, who failed to achieve long-standing control with medical therapy, candidates for percutaneous rhizotomy. A person less than 50 years of age, who has any indication of atypical pain is offered the alternative of posterior fossa exploration of the trigeminal root. These patients are also studied with tomography of the petrous bone, computerized axial tomography, and selective angiographic studies.

If surgical treatment is elected, the patient and family are required to read and listen to a full explanation of current procedures available for the control of trigeminal neuralgia. Frequently the patient is advised to discuss results with others who have undergone major trigeminal surgery. This tactic reinforces the patient's understanding and appreciation of possible undesirable sensory loss. Differential sensory block enables the patient to experience the effect of sensory deprivation and may aid in the decision concerning operation for atypical facial pain.

A carefully educated patient is better able to accept side effects, thus greatly reducing the incidence of postoperative disappointment. It has been our policy to let the informed patient make his own decision regarding the mode of treatment. If the patient elects a destructive procedure, such an electrocoagulation, he is encouraged to indicate the degree of sensory deficit he would like to acquire. While partial sensory loss is associated with a higher incidence of recurrence, patients are usually not reluctant to undergo repeat percutaneous rhizotomy.

Technique—Percutaneous Trigeminal Rhizotomy

The rationale for electrocoagulation of the trigeminal rootlets is based on the premise that differential thermal destruction of the small, finely myelinated fibers that conduct pain can be achieved.[19,20]

A preliminary submentovertex radiograph of the skull is obtained to demonstrate the foramen ovale and adjacent bony landmarks (Fig. 28-1). The procedure is conducted in the radiography suite after the patient is given an intravenous injection of 30 to 50 mg of methohexital (Brevital, Lilly, Indianapolis, Indiana). A hollow 19-gauge needle is used to penetrate the foramen ovale and serves as the lesion-making electrode. A needle tip, with the terminus bare for 5, 7.5, or 10 mm, depending on the number of trigeminal divisions involved in the painful condition, is selected. Generally, a 7.5-mm electrode is chosen for a patient with neuralgia involving two divisions of the nerve; patients suffering from pain in three divisions or those who have had a previous alcohol injection or intracranial rhizotomy require a larger tipped electrode. If a lesion patient is to made the first division of the nerve, a 2.5 or 5 mm electrode may be selected.

Electrode Placement. The patient is positioned on the x-ray table with the neck parallel with the body. Three landmarks are marked on the face (Fig. 28-2):

1. A point 3 cm anterior to the external auditory meatus.
2. A point beneath the medial aspect of the pupil.
3. A point 2.5 to 3 cm lateral to the oral commissure.

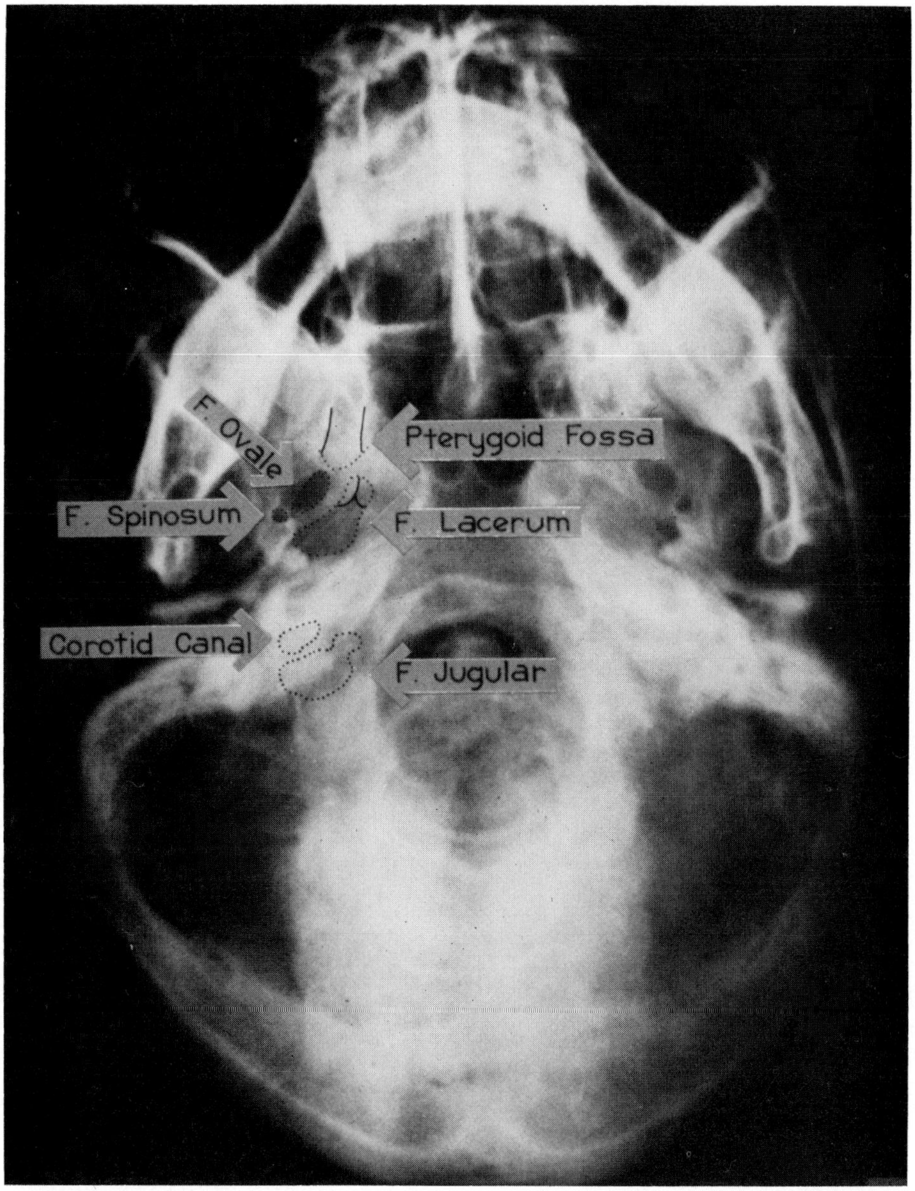

Fig. 28-1. Submentovertex view of the skull illustrating the basal foramina.

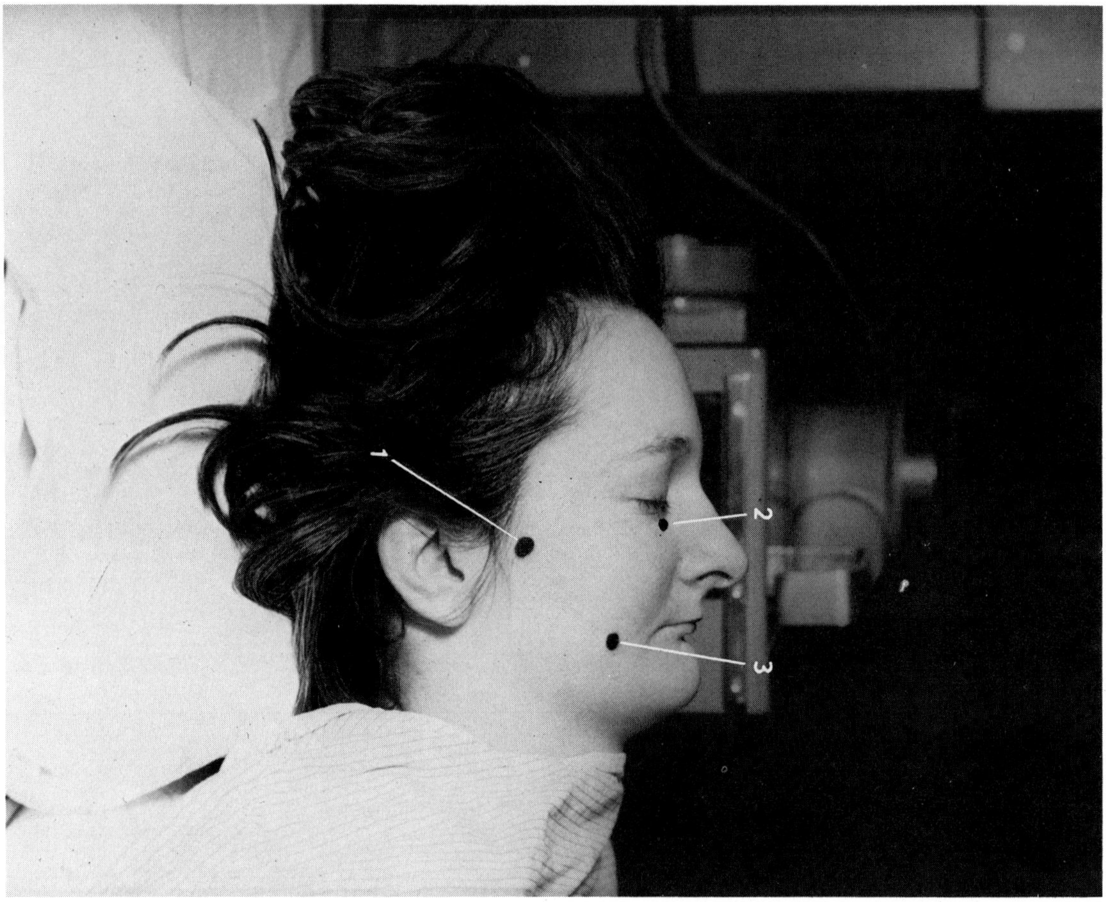

Fig. 28-2. Anatomic landmarks for electrode placement.

The first two points indicate the site of the foramen ovale and the third is the point at which the needle penetrates the skin of the jaw. The anterior approach to the foramen ovale, as advicated by Härtel[21] is used (Fig. 28-3). A free-hand technique is used to explore the area of the foramen ovale. We have not found simultaneous radiographic control[22] of value and prefer to rely on the medial and lateral anatomic landmarks of the external auditory meatus and pupil. Utilizing these landmarks, we have been able to penetrate the foramen ovale on the first attempt in most cases and after a simple adjustment in all instances.

The index finger of the gloved hand is placed just inferior to the lateral ptergoid wing, and the electrode is directed into the medial portion of the foramen ovale (Fig. 28-4). If a needle enters the posterolateral aspect of the foramen, it may not lie within the dural investment of the trigeminal ganglion and, if advanced, probably will not reach the maxillary or ophthalmic divisons of the rootlet of the nerve. As the electrode is advanced, an oral airway is placed between the jaws to prevent involuntary biting of the guiding finger. Intravenous methohexital is injected as the foramen is neared. Entrance of the needle into the foramen is signaled by a wince and a brief contraction of the masseter muscle, indicating contact with the mandibular sensory and motor fibers. Before the electrode is advanced any further, a second series of radiographs is obtained to confirm proper placement of the electrode (Fig. 28-5A and B). The stylet is withdrawn to determine whether the carotid artery has been penetrated. In our experience, this circumstance has occurred on one occasion only.

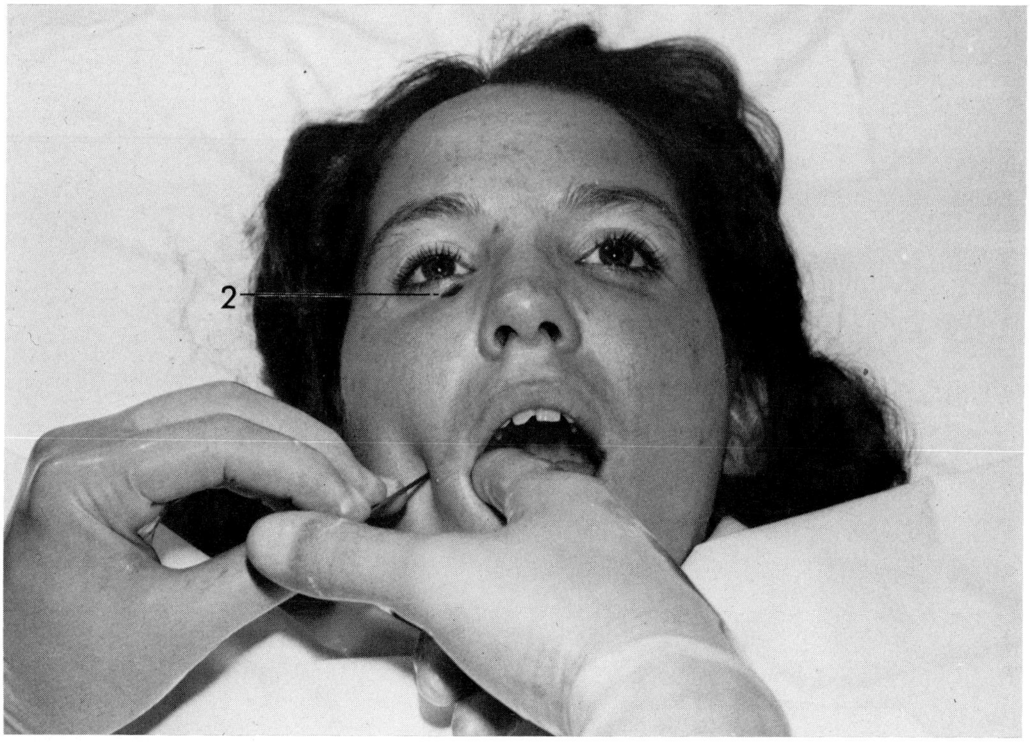

Fig. 28-3. Illustration demonstrating needle placement according to the technique of Härtel.

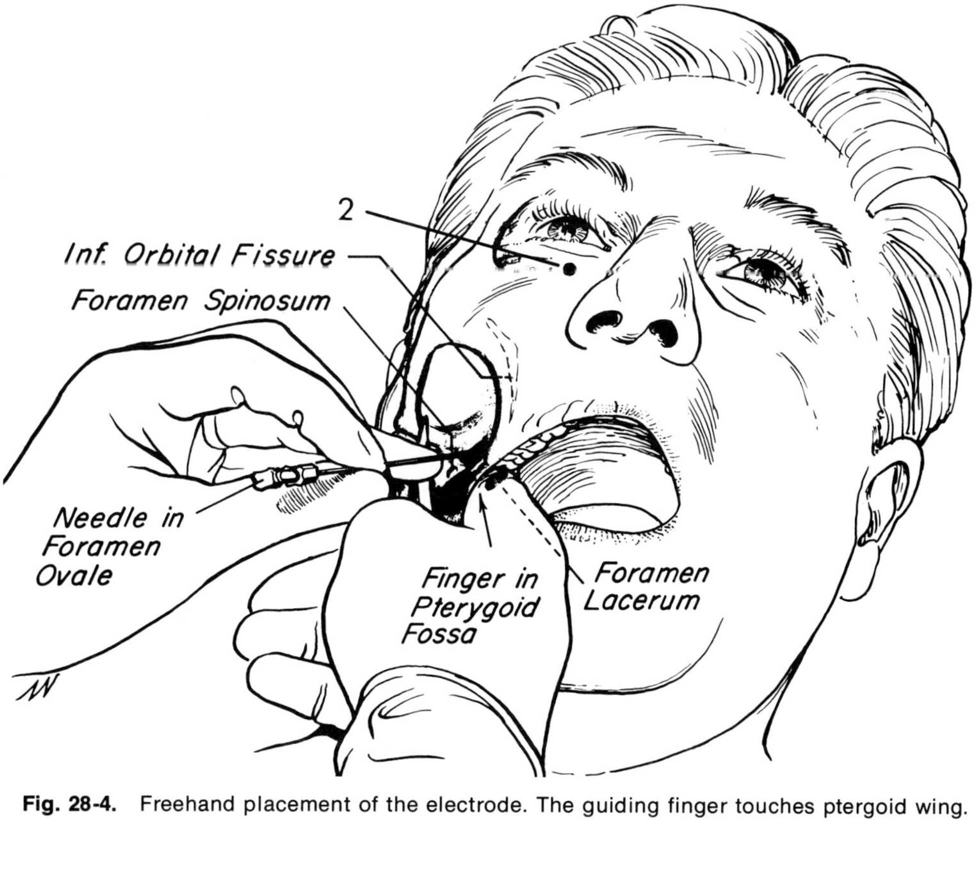

Fig. 28-4. Freehand placement of the electrode. The guiding finger touches ptergoid wing.

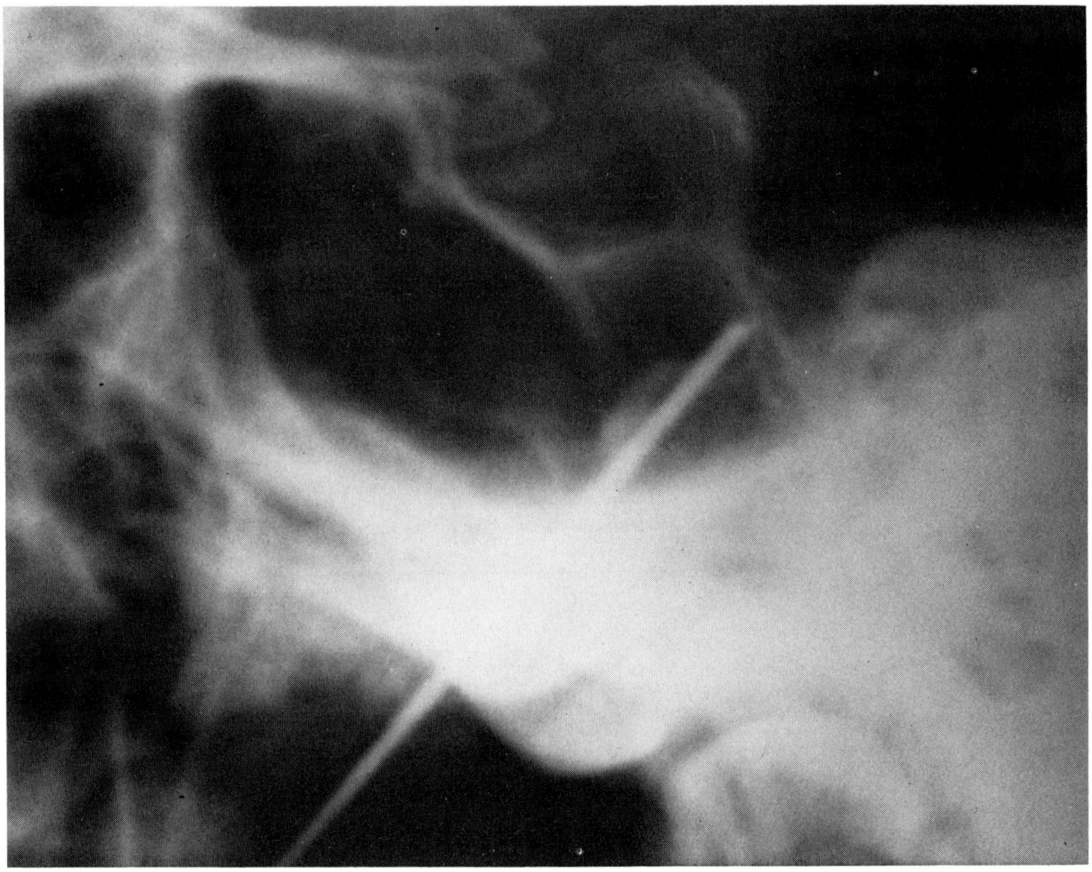

Fig. 28-5A. Submentovertex radiograph confirming electrode placement in the foramen ovale.

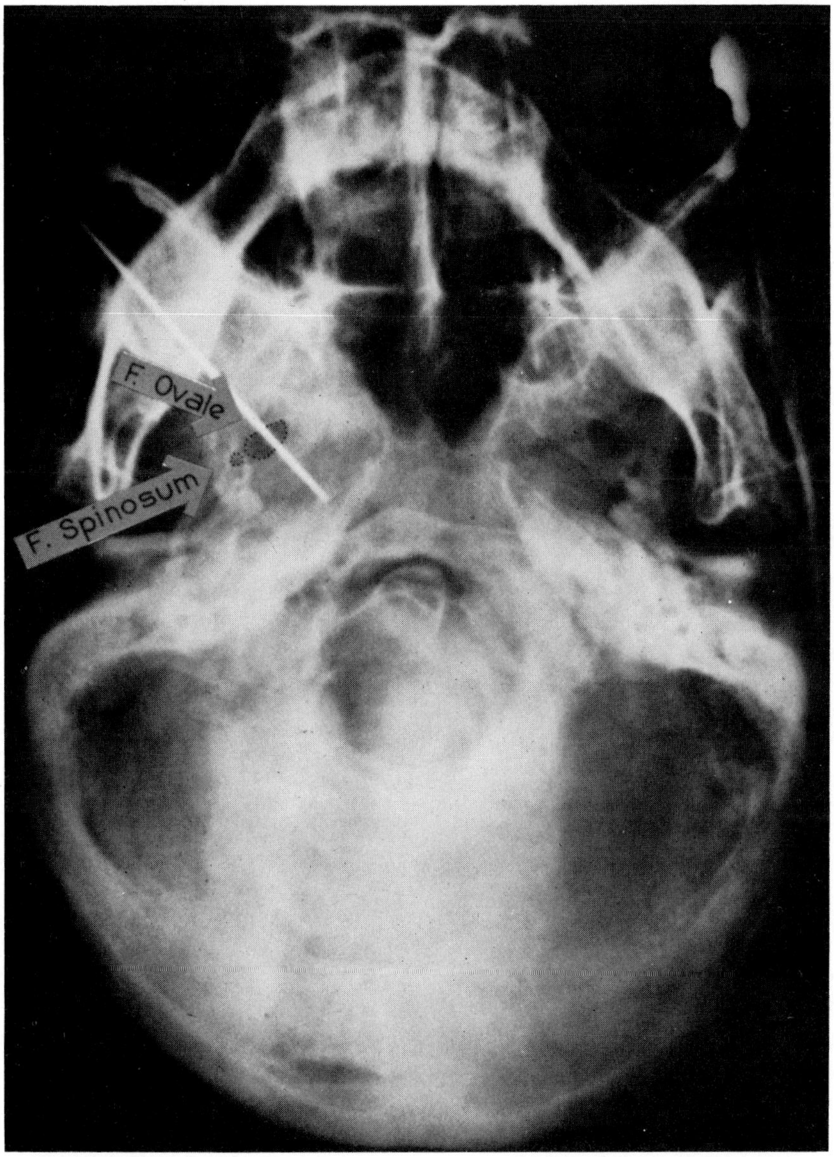

Fig. 28-5B. Lateral radiograph demonstrating trajectory of electrode.

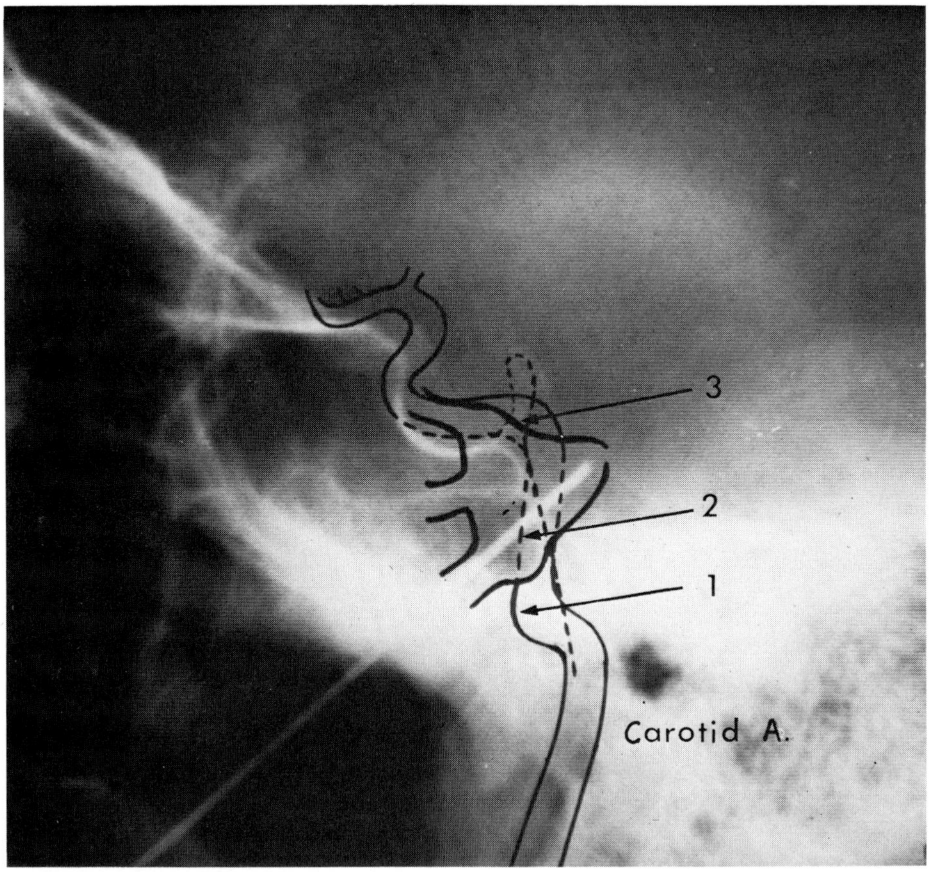

Fig. 28-6. A composite illustration demonstrates the relationship of the carotid artery to the trigeminal ganglion and posterior rootlets. Note the location of three points of possible carotid penetration.

If the carotid artery is penetrated, the needle should be promptly withdrawn and manual pressure applied over the posterior pharyngeal space. The procedure should be discontinued for 24 to 48 hours. Ischemic complications, such as hemiparesis, have resulted from internal carotid puncture.[23] The electrode may penetrate the cartilaginous covering of the foramen lacerum, if deviated medially, and puncture the carotid artery. If the electrode is directed posterolaterally, it may pierce the carotid artery at its entrance into the petrous bone. Finally Rish[23] suggests that after the electrode passes through the foramen ovale, it may penetrate the carotid artery. This may occur if the electrode was directed anteriorly and medially into the area of the cavernous sinus (Fig. 28-6). Our anatomic studies illustrate that the carotid artery is frequently devoid of bony covering deep to Meckel's cave.

Electrode Localization. Final placement of the electrode tip is determined by the response to electrical stimulation. A current of precisely 0.2 to 0.3 V at 50 to 75 cycles/sec will reproduce the paroxysmal bouts of pain reminiscent of trigeminal neuralgia. Higher voltage stimulation, 1.0 to 2.0 V, may be required in patients who have had previous intracranial rhizotomy or repeated alcohol injections. The response evoked serves as a reliable indicator of probe temperature required to produce a lesion.

After the hollow tip of a needle reaches the trigeminal cistern, stimulation should elicit a paroxysm of pain in the mandibular distribution. Lateral radiography at this time will indicate

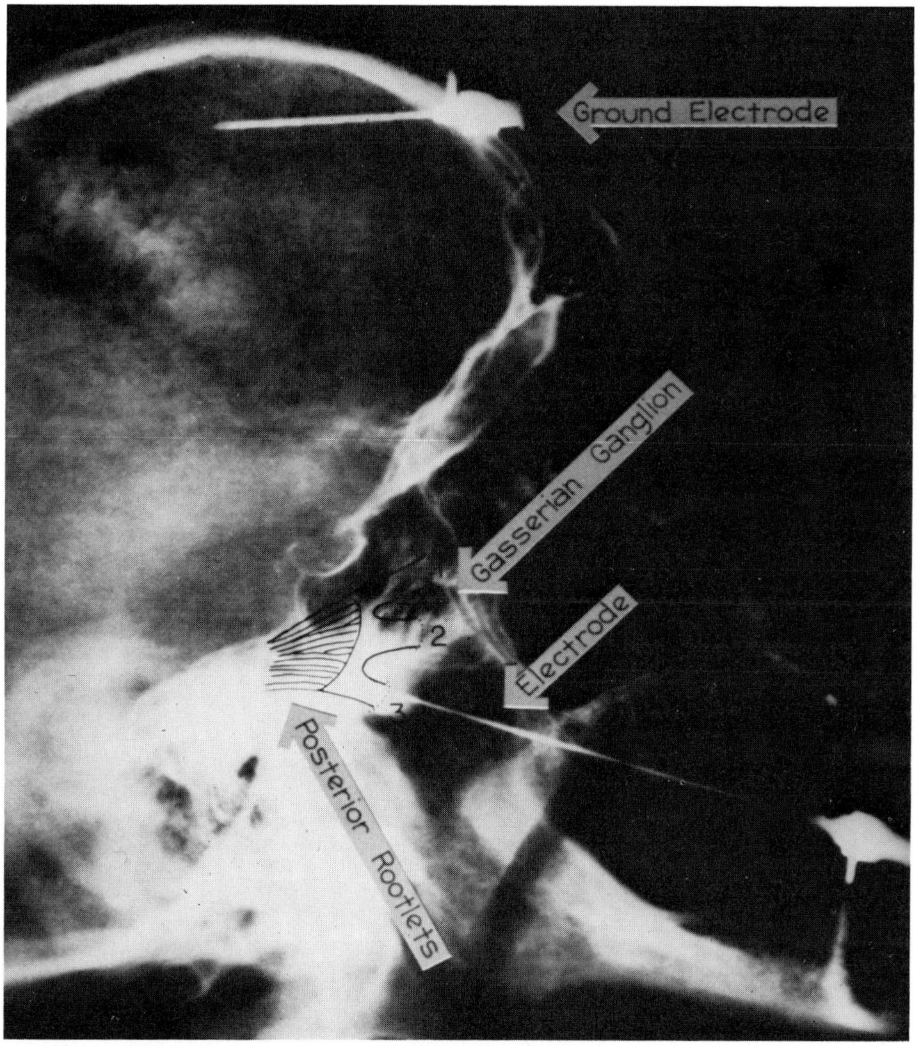

Fig. 28-7. A lateral composite illustrates the relationship of the electrode tip and its trajectory to the mandibular nerve, ganglion, clivus, and posterior rootlets.

whether the tip of the electrode lies at a point 4 to 5 mm external to the profile of the clivus (Fig. 28-7). If the needle is advanced 5 mm, its tip should lie at the level of the clivus, where stimulation will elicit paresthesias in the second-division rootlets (Fig. 28-8A and B). The needle tip should not advance more than 8 mm deep to the profile of the clivus, since it may injure the abducens nerve in this region. If the proper response is not achieved in the ophthalmic division, the needle should be withdrawn and directed more medially to bring the tip closer to the posterior clinoid process.

Lesion Production. Additional intravenous anesthetic is administered and a preliminary lesion produced at 60°C for 60 seconds. A facial blush usually appears at this point and helps to localize the region of the nerve root undergoing thermal destruction.[24] When the patient has fully awakened, careful sensory testing of the face is conducted. Repeat lesions are produced until the desired effect is achieved. Generally sequential lesions of 60-seconds duration are made by increasing the temperature 5°C with each lesion. When analgesia is

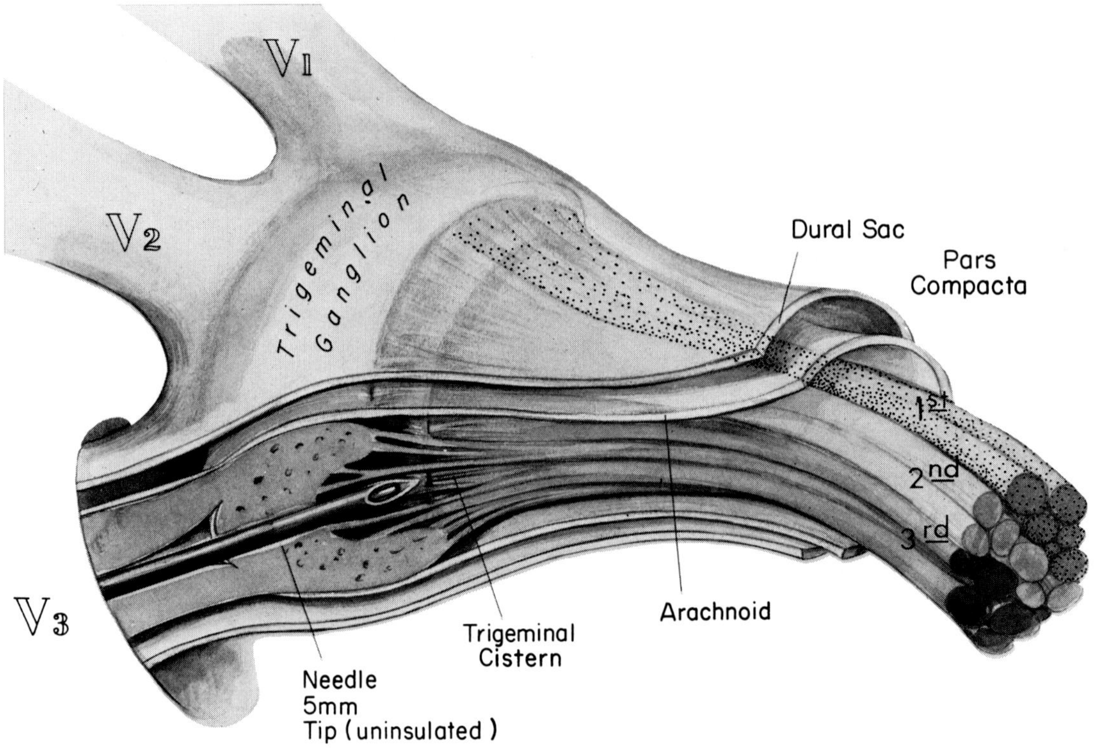

Fig. 28-8A. Illustration of lamination of the trigeminal rootlets and location of the trigeminal cistern.

approached, great care is exercised to avoid overshooting the desired result, which includes preserving the sense of touch. After a partial lesion has been produced, it is frequently possible to complete it without an anesthetic agent. This tactic is particularly valuable when partial sensation of a cornea or other radicular zones is to be preserved.

Once the desired sensory deficit has been achieved, the patient is observed for an additional 15 minutes to determine if a fixed lesion has been produced. If the examination indicates a stable level of analgesia, the distribution and degree of deficit are determined by careful sensory testing. Touch perception is recorded in grams of pressure, using calibrated Von-Frey hairs. Masseter, ptergoid, facial, and ocular muscle function is recorded. The patient is then returned to his room and observed for 24 hours. During this period he is informed of the necessity for eye care, for avoiding jaw strain, and of the consequences of facial analgesia.

Results

At the time of this report, 450 patients with typical trigeminal neuralgia were treated surgically by the percutaneous rhizotomy approach. A thorough follow-up evaluation, extending over a period of 1 to 7 years, has been completed for 400 of these patients (Table 28-1).

The average age for the group was 63 years and 60% were female. In 60% the pain was located on the right, and the second and third divisions of the trigeminal nerve were commonly involved. Isolated pain in the first or third division was less frequent than in the second division. It is notable that 21% of patients had a significant degree of pain in the first division, although pain was isolated to this division in only 2% of patients.

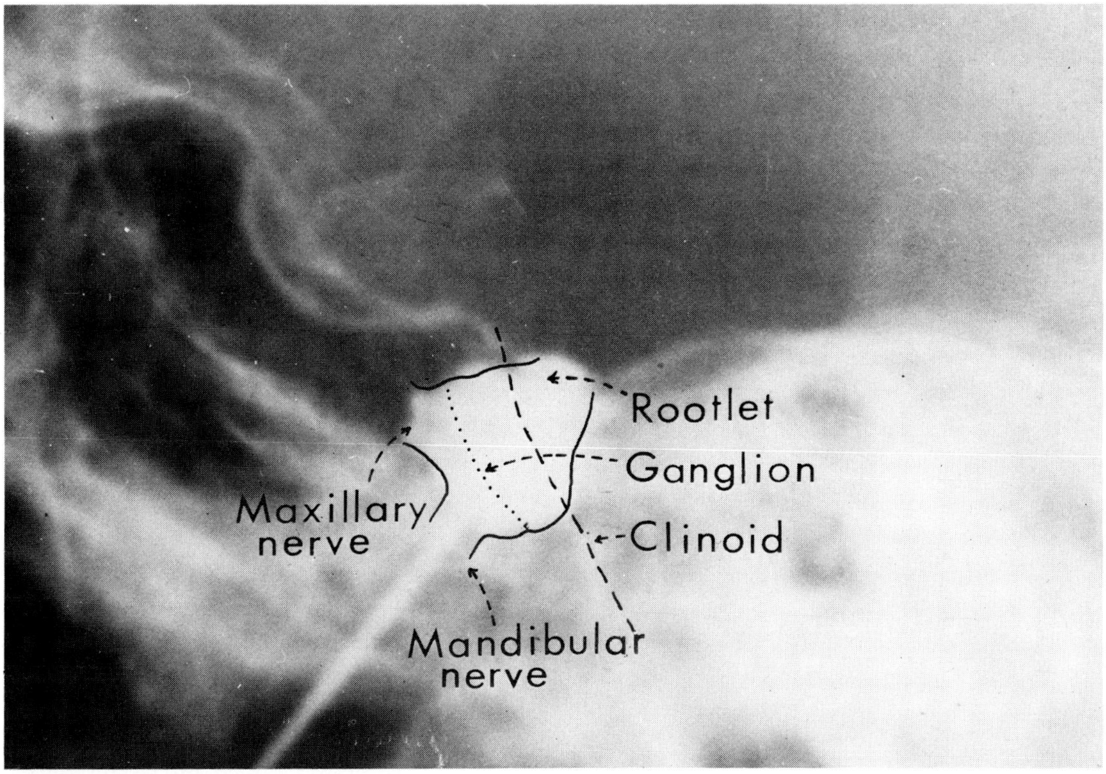

Fig, 28.8B. Composite illustration of a trigeminal cisternogram (Pantopaque®). Note the outline of the peripheral nerves and nerve rootlets.

The disease had been present for an average of 8 years and was characterized by increasingly severe episodes of paroxysmal pain and progressively shorter periods of remission. Many patients had been treated surgically, usually by nerve avulsion or alcohol injection (32%), while 11% had a prior intracranial procedure, usually subtotal rhizotomy. Nearly all patients had been treated with either diphenylhydantoin (Dilantin) or carbamazepine

Table 28-1. Characteristics of 400 Patients Selected for Electrocoagulation

		Percent of patients
Average age	63 years	
Sex	60% female	
Side of coagulation:		
Right		60
Left		39
Bilateral		1
Division of trigeminal Nerve involved:		
V-1		2
V-2		20
V-3		17
V-1, V-2		14
V-2, V-3		42
V-1, V-2, V-3		5

In preparation for writing a book on trigeminal neuralgia or tic douloureux, we are asking your cooperation in answering the following questions concerning the treatment of this condition by percutaneous electrocoagulation. We are particularly interested in knowing if the original pain for which you were treated has been controlled and if any side effects have developed as a result of this treatment. Your assistance by answering the following questions would be helpful.

1. What is the present status of your facial pain?
2. Has there been any recurrence of pain since the operative procedure?
3. To what extent is your face numb?
4. Is the numbness or loss of feeling troublesome?
5. Do you have difficulty chewing or eating food? If so, please explain.
6. Do you have double vision?
7. Do you have blurring of vision or difficulty with your eye?
8. Have you suffered any complications as a result of the procedure?
9. How do you rate the result of the operation?
   Excellent—no pain, no side effects ____________
   Good—minimal pain, minimal side effects____________
   Fair—recurrence of pain no major side effects ____________
   Failure—original pain never relieved ____________

Fig. 28-9. Evaluation protocol form

(Tegretol), as well as other forms of medical and physical remedies. While diphenylhydantoin was effective in over 50% of patients, the effect was seldom lasting or satisfactory. Carbamazepine was considered more effective: 92% of patients reported significant relief of a lasting nature but efficacy was limited by the tendency of most patients to develop increasing side effects to the drug as higher doses were required.

A response to followup was obtained for all 400 patients. However, many of the patients were not recalled for personal examination because of advanced age, disability, distance from the examining clinic, death, or other reason. However, all were contacted by questionnaire (Fig. 28-9) or phone, and a family member was contacted if the patient had died. At the time of evaluation, 92% of patients reported excellent to good results. The remaining patients obtained only fair results (5%) because of undesirable side effects or recurrent pain. Four patients (1%) reported that their pain had never been relieved satisfactorily at any time after the coagulation procedure.

Side Effects

Sensory. Troublesome numbness and paresthesias from the sensory deficit proved to be the most consistent adverse side effect. Commonly, an intermittent crawling, burning, or itching sensation was described. Most patients readily adjusted to the sensory deficit, and the paresthesias usually diminished with time. The more active and mentally alert the patient, the fewer the disturbances of sensation reported. Older patients were more prone to this complication. Constant, severe dysesthesias in an anesthetic or analgesic zone (anesthesia dolorosa) rarely occured. One patient reported a severe burning pain that improved considerably after several months. Forty-five patients reported a significant problem with paresthesias and 11 additional patients complained of other symptoms related to sensory deprivation. Five patients reported a troublesome aching pain in the jaw region.

Five aged patients developed persistent excoriation of the skin about the face, nostril, or scalp. Many traumatized the skin by frequent scratching or manipulation, which could be controlled, in most cases, by applying mittens at bedtime.

Eye. Eye complications occurred in 8% of patients; 8 (2%) developed neurolytic keratitis. Thirty percent of this group had corneal analgesia, indicating that touch perception in the absence of pain perception does not necessarily protect against corneal ulceration. The corneal lesion was reversed in all patients by early ophthalmologic treatment. Application of a soft contact lens, meticulous eye care, and occasional tarsorrhaphy prevented permanent visual loss. Intermittent blurred vision was reported by 12 patients (4%). In 7 of the 12 touch perception of the cornea was preserved, but the corneal reflex was markedly diminished. Again, this finding suggests that preserving touch perception of the cornea does not necessarily protect against keratitis and visual clouding. Our experience indicates that persons with some sensory preservation of the cornea adjust more rapidly to the deficit and rarely develop ulceration. Similarly patients with corneal anesthesia seldom develop keratitis during the later postoperative period. Patients or their relatives must be given meticulous instructions about all aspects of eye care. By carefully adhering to this practice, I suspect that serious eye complications, sometimes seen following this procedure, have been prevented. Seventy patients in this group had neuralgia involving or limited to the ophthalmic division; 72% achieved pain relief without losing corneal sensation and only 6% developed neurolytic keratitis.

Transient diplopia occurred in 7 patients (2%). In 5, the double vision could be explained by abducens nerve palsy and in 2 the cause was trochlear palsy. The deficit was transient in all patients. The most persistent diplopia lasted for 4 months, while in all but 1 patient it disappeared in a few weeks. This complication was seen only in patients undergoing treatment for neuralgia involving the ophthalmic division. Abducens nerve palsy may be produced if a thermal lesion is created with the tip of the electrode extending more than 6 to 8 mm past the profile of the clivus, as measured on a lateral film of the skull (Fig. 28-10).

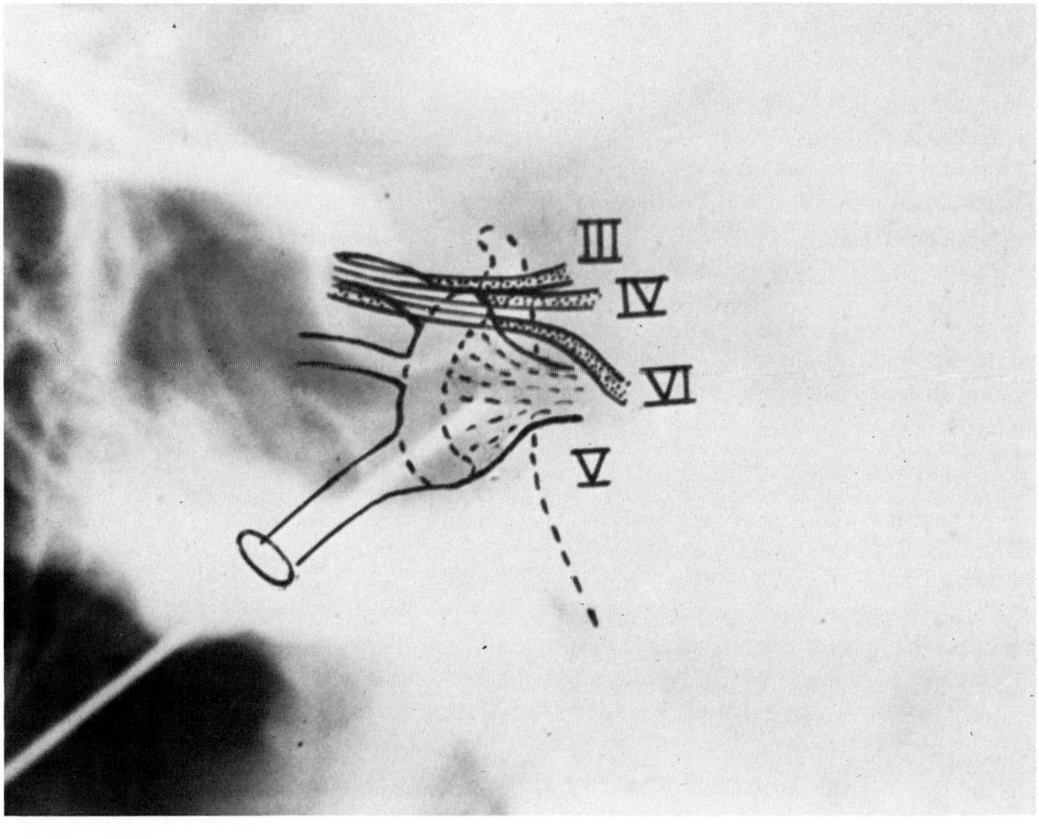

Fig. 28-10. Lateral radiograph demonstrates course of the oculomotor, abducens and trochlear nerves and their relation to electrode trajectory. The electrode tip should not extend more than 8 mm deep to the profile of the clivus.

Trochlear palsy is apparently minimized if the electrode trajectory is not aimed toward the posterior clinoid process, where the tip may encounter the cavernous sinus.

The incidence of unwanted loss of corneal sensation and paresis of ocular nerves has been greatly reduced in recent years by performing electrocoagulation with the patient alert and cooperating in the evaluation during the final stage of lesion production.

Motor Paresis. Paresis of muscles innervated by the motor root of the trigeminal occurred in 22% of patients. In most instances the deficit was partial and transient. Weakness of masseter, temporalis, and ptergoid muscles causes a mild degree of disability due to jaw deviation and loss of chewing power. Trismus was a more troublesome problem but it could be avoided or eliminated by placing the patient on a soft diet and instructing him to exercise his jaws frequently in the presence of pain or muscle weakness.

Hearing difficulties related to inconstant roaring, popping sounds, or fullness in the ear, were reported by some patients. These symptoms are attributable to paresis of the small muscles about the eustachian tube (tensor veli palatini) and tympanic membrane (tensor tympani).

Many patients, who did not have motor paresis had difficulty chewing. They related this difficulty to sensory loss in the mouth. However, most did not find it significant, since they had become accustomed to chewing on the nonpainful side.

Herpes Simplex. Lesions of herpes simplex were noted in 3% of patients. Since most were not examined more than 48 hours postoperatively, this figure is undoubtedly low.

Recurrence of Trigeminal Neuralgia

The follow-up period varied from 1 to 7 years. Recurrent pain sufficiently severe to require repeating the procedure developed in 37 (9%); 13 (3%) had some recurrent pain that was adequately controlled with medication; and 6 (2%) had minor recurrent pain that did not require additional medical or surgical treatment.

Recurrent pain after percutaneous rhizotomy of the trigeminal nerve developed more frequently during the early years of our experience. At that time we tried to make minimal lesions, hoping to limit the degree of sensory deficit. However the recurrence rate was too high in patients with minimal sensory deficit. Subsequently we advised patients to have lesions that would induce analgesia in the zones of pain and hypalgesia in adjacent painful zones. As a result the frequency with which pain recurred was significantly reduced, but as expected the patients complained more of numbness.

Comparisons of Percutaneous Rhizotomy with other Major Surgical Procedures

Percutaneous rhizotomy can be compared with other major surgical procedures on the basis of complications and incidence of recurrent pain. No attempt was made to compare our results with all series reported but selected only those that appeared to be representative. Followup for percutaneous rhizotomy has not been as long as for intracranial rhizotomy; therefore, recurrence data may not be comparable. However, data for mortality and morbidity should be significant (Table 28-2).

Analysis indicates that the percutaneous approach is associated with the lowest mortality and morbidity. Recurrence rates compare favorably with those following intracranial rhizotomy, if analogous portions of the root are destroyed in both operations. Facial palsy has been eliminated, but ocular palsy occurs more frequently than in any other major procedure. The incidence of troublesome numbness ranks favorably with that reported for other forms of rhizotomy. However, this major side effect has been eliminated in decompression procedures. Temporal decompression is associated with a prohibitive recurrence rate but

Table 28-2. Analysis of Comparative Techniques and Results in 1930 Cases

	Recurrence rate (%)		Patients (%)	Complications (percent of patients)							
Technique	Recurrence (%)	Surgical followup (yr)	Relief of pain (%)	Mortality	Ataxia	Corneal ulcer	Facial palsy	Ocular palsy	Motor palsy	Paresthesia	Anesthesia dolorosa
Percutaneous rhizotomy											
Tew 400 cases	14	4	98	0	0	2	0	2	22	19	0.3
Sweet[17] 274 cases	22	4	91	0	0	NR (1 pt blind)	0	0	43	2	1
Mengel[25] 315 cases	80	12	97	0	0	0	0	NR	50	93	2
Decompression											
Svien[9] 100 cases	84	4	24	1.0	0	0	NR	0	0	0	0
Transtemporal rhizotomy											
Peet[26] 553 cases	14	8	95	1.6	NR	15	6	NR	NR	55	4
Posterior fossa rhizotomy											
Dandy[27] 88 cases	NR	2	100	2.0	NR	0	1	2	0	0	0
Vascular decompression											
Jannetta[13] 200 cases	4.5	4	98	0.5	2	0	0	1	0	0	0

NR—Not reported

vascular decompression, as described by Jannetta[13] appears to provide an attractive alternative to percutaneous rhizotomy, particularly in the young patient. As more experience is gained with this method, the incidence of successful pain relief and the freedom from recurrence can be better defined.

Percutaneous Coagulation in Other Painful Conditions

The percutaneous approach to the trigeminal nerve has been used to treat several other conditions. In facial pain due to multiple sclerosis (8 cases) and invasive carcinoma (8 cases), results are promising. The technique has considerable advantages in patients with either condition. In multiple sclerosis, touch sensation and masseter function should be preserved, since pain on the opposite side may require a contralateral procedure. In the debilitated patient with invasive carcinoma, percutaneous coagulation for complete sensory denervation of the face and lasting pain relief, is a simple procedure.

Atypical facial pain was treated by percutaneous rhizotomy in 11 patients. In most instances the pain resembled trigeminal neuralgia in some respects but features of an atypical nature were noted. Several patients with dental neuralgia were included in the group. In all of these, a preliminary differential xylocaine block was performed to familiarize the patient with sensory deprivation and to determine if pain relief could be achieved. Despite careful appraisal, the results were considerably less satisfactory than those reported by patients treated for typical trigeminal pain.

Long-standing cluster headache (periodic migrainous neuralgia) was treated in 6 patients by denervation of the ophthalmic and maxillary zones. Four of the 6 reported satisfactory relief, and 2 failed to respond. The failures could not be predicted from the history of their disease or the preoperative differential block.

Postherpetic neuralgia was treated by electrocoagulation of affected rootlets in 3 patients. The response was poor in each instance and this procedure is no longer offered in this affliction.

Pain in the Throat and Ear

Pain due to involvement of the vagus and glossopharyngeal nerves was treated in 6 patients by percutaneous electrocoagulation of the nerve rootlets at the jugular foramen. Four of the 6 patients had intractable pain due to invasive tumors and the remaining 2 had idiopathic neuralgia but were too debilitated to undergo intracranial section of the glossopharyngeal and vagus nerves.

The technique used to place an electrode in the neural portion of the jugular foramen was learned serendipitiously, when it accidentally entered the posterior fossa through the jugular foramen, in 2 early cases treated for trigeminal neuralgia. During subsequent studies a minor change in electrode placement was made so that the neural portion of the jugular canal (Fig.

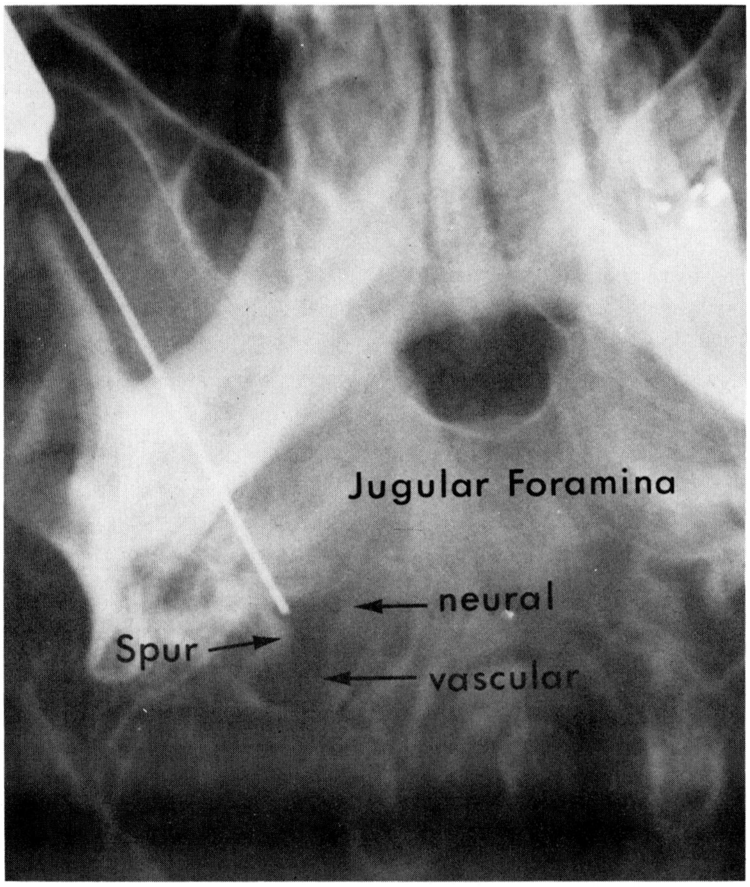

Fig. 28-11. Needle penetrating the neural portion of the jugular foramen. Note the bony spur which divides the neural from vascular portion.

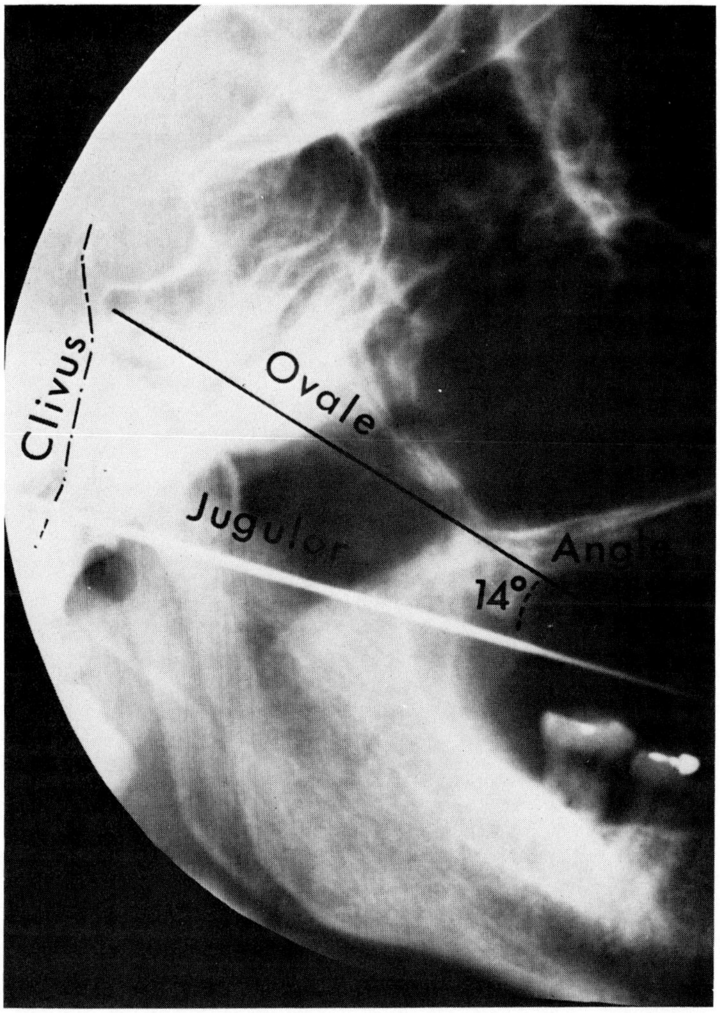

Fig. 28-12. This composite illustration demonstrates the trajectory of approaches to the foramen ovale and jugular foramen. The sagittal plane is identical for both procedures.

28-11) is consistently penetrated. The needle is directed posteriorly, 14° from the angle used to penetrate the foramen ovale; the sagittal direction is unchanged (Fig. 28-12). Stimulation provokes pain in the ear and throat. Coughing and contraction of the sternocleidomastoid muscle may be induced.

Pain in 4 patients with invasive carcinoma was relieved until their death 4 to 11 months later. Two patients with idiopathic vagoglossopharyngeal neuralgia were relieved of pain but vocal cord paralysis was produced in each. The procedure is not advisable in patients with intact vocal cord function, who can tolerate intracranial section of the glossopharyngeal and the upper fibers of the vagus nerves.

Conclusion

Percutaneous rhizotomy of the trigeminal nerve is a safe procedure that can produce long-standing relief from intractable trigeminal neuralgia. The incidence of recurrent pain is greater than that observed after intracranial section of posterior rootlets, but the lower morbidity makes the procedure more acceptable to most patients. Postoperative sensory complaints are similar to those associated with intracranial rhizotomy but can be nearly eliminated by preserving touch perception. Extratrigeminal complications are rare and reversible in most instances.

Percutaneous rhizotomy is applicable in selected types of facial pain, other than typical trigeminal neuralgia. A technique for eliminating pain caused by neoplastic invasion of the trigeminal, vagus, and glossopharyngeal nerves is described.

Percutaneous rhizotomy is a destructive procedure. It is not the ideal treatment for facial pain. Therefore a more acceptable nondestructive form of therapy continues to be our goal.

REFERENCES

1. Hartley F: Intercranial neurectomy of the second and third divisions of the fifth nerve. *NY J Med 55*:317-319, 1892
2. Krause F: Resection des Trigeminus innerhalb der Schadelhohle. *Arch Klin Chir 41*:821-832, 1892
3. Krause F: Entfernung des ganglion gasseri und des central daron gelegnen trigemenusstammes. *Dtsch Med Wochenschr 19*:341, 1893
4. Horsley V: Remarks on the various surgical procedures devised for the relief or cure of trigeminal neuralgia. *Br Med J 2*:1139, 1891
5. Spiller WG, Frazier CH: The division of the sensory root of the trigeminus for the relief of tic douloureux. *Univ Pa Med Bull 14*:341, 1901
6. Spiller WG, Frazier CH: An experimental study of the regeneration of the posterior spinal root. *Univ Pa Med Bull 16*:126-128, 1903
7. Shelden CH, Pudenz RH, Freshwater D, et al: Compression rather than decompression for trigeminal neuralgia. *J Neurosurg 12*:123-126, 1955
8. Taarnhoj P: Decompression of the trigeminal root. *J Neurosurg 11*:299-305, 1954
9. Svien HS, Love JG: Results of decompression operation for trigeminal neuralgia four years plus after operation. *J Neurosurg 16*:653-663, 1959
10. Gardner WS: Concerning the mechanisms of trigeminal neuralgia and hemi-facial spasm. *J Neurosurg 19*:947-958, 1962
11. Harris W: Alcohol injection of the gasserian ganglion for trigeminal neuralgia. *Lancet 1*:218-221, 1912
12. Harris W: An analysis of 1433 cases of paroxysmal trigeminal neuralgia (trigeminal-tic) and the end results of gasserian alcohol injection. *Brain 63*:209-224, 1940
13. Janetta P: Microsurgical approach to the trigeminal nerve for tic douloureux, *Progress in Neurological Surgery* vol 7. Karger, Basel, 1976, in Press
14. Dandy WE: Concerning the cause of trigeminal neuralgia. *Am J Surg 24*:447-455, 1934
15. Kirschner M: Elektrocoagulation des ganglion gasseri. *Zentralbl Chir 47*:2841-2843, 1932
16. Kirschner M: Zur behandlung der trigeminusneuralgie. *Med Wochenschr 89*:235-239, 1942
17. Sweet WH, Wepsic SG: Controlled thermocoagulation of trigeminal ganglion and results for differential destruction of pain fibers. *J Neurosurg 39*:143-156, 1974
18. White JC, Sweet WH: *Pain and the Neurosurgeon.* Charles C Thomas, Springfield, Illinois, 1969
19. Letcher FS, Goldring S: The effect of radiofrequency current and heat on peripheral nerve action potential in the cat. *J Neurosurg 29*:42-47, 1968
20. Brodkey JS, et al: Reversible heat lesions with radiofrequency current. *J Neurosurg 27*:49-53, 1964
21. Härtel F: Ueber die intracranielle Injektionsbchandinng der Trigeminusneuralgie. *Med Klinik 10*:582-584, 1914
22. Tator CH, Rowed DW: Fluoroscopy of foramen ovale as an aid to thermocoagulation of the gasserian ganglion. *J Neurosurg 44*:254-259, 1976
23. Rish BL: Cerebrovascular accident after percutaneous thermocoagulation of the trigeminal ganglion. *J Neurosurg 44*:376-377, 1976
24. Gonzalez G, Onofrio BM, Ken FW: Vasodilator system of the face. *J Neurosurg 42*:696-703, 1975
25. Mengel J, Piotrowsin W, Penzholz H: Long-term results of gasserian ganglion electrocoagulation. *J Neurosurg 42*:140-143, 1975
26. Peet MM, Schneider RD: Trigeminal neuralgia. *J Neurosurg 9*:367-377, 1952
27. Dandy WE: Operation for cure of tic douloureux; partial section of the sensory root at the pons. *Arch Surg 18*:687-734, 1929

CHAPTER 29
Commissural Myelotomy

John E. Adams
Robert Lippert
Yoshio Hosobuchi

COMMISSURAL OR MEDIOLONGITUDINAL MYELOTOMY was first performed for the relief of pain by Armour in 1927.[1] The rationale for this operation is obviously based upon the traditional concept that finely myelinated and unmyelinated fibers of the lateral division of the dorsal root, which subserve nociception, cross in the anterior commissure of the spinal cord at the level of or up to three segments cephalad to their point of entry into the spinal cord. Thus, by sectioning the anterior commissure over several segments, the neurosurgeon should theoretically be able to bilaterally denervate relevant segments of the body from nociceptive input. This potential ability to relieve bilateral segmental pain during a single operation without compromising the function of the descending or ascending long tracts, presents obvious advantages over bilateral anterolateral spinal tractotomy at either the high thoracic or high cervical level. The naturally occurring model for spinal commissurotomy, of course, is the cystic lesion of syringomyelia, where the pathologic process interrupts the same decussating fibers as the surgeon does with his knife, producing an identical clinical result insofar as the segmental loss of nociception.

The operation has enjoyed moderate popularity in European centers,[2-5] but until recently has rarely been performed in the United States.[6] It is perhaps noteworthy, however, that the introduction of the operating room microscope has encouraged a revival of this operative procedure for the relief of intractable pain. This is no mere coincidence, since in spite of earlier successes achieved without benefit of the operating room microscope, it is clear that both the success of the procedure and prevention of postoperative complications are greatly enhanced by the microscopic technique.

We have employed commissural myelotomy primarily to relieve intractable bilateral pain in the lower abdomen, pelvis, perineum, and lower extremities. Most patients have suffered from malignant disease, but we have employed the procedure in patients whose pain is of nonmalignant origin, such as chronic adhesive arachnoiditis, trauma to the spinal column, etc. The majority of patients have had pain involving the lower segments of their body, but in a minority the pain has been mid or upper thoracic in origin.

Department of Neurological Surgery, University of California Medical Center, San Francisco, California 94143

Technique

The position of the incision in a caudad cephalad plane is dictated by the highest segment involved in the painful process. The myelotomy must extend at least three cord segments above this level. Thus, if the pain extends as high as the L1 dermatome, it will be necessary to carry the myelotomy as high as the tenth thoracic segment in the cord.

General anesthesia is usually employed, although the operation can be done under local anesthesia. The patient is operated upon in the prone position, since there is nothing to be gained by employing either the lateral or sitting position. A skin marker is placed over a designated spinous process, which is then identified by an intraoperative x-ray film (Fig. 29-1). After the laminectomy has been completed, if there is any doubt regarding the level, a further intraoperative film can be taken.

After the appropriate laminectomy has been performed and the dura opened, the operating room microscope is positioned and, at a magnification of four- to sixfold, the midline sulcus of the dorsal surface of the spinal cord is identified. This is accomplished by identify-

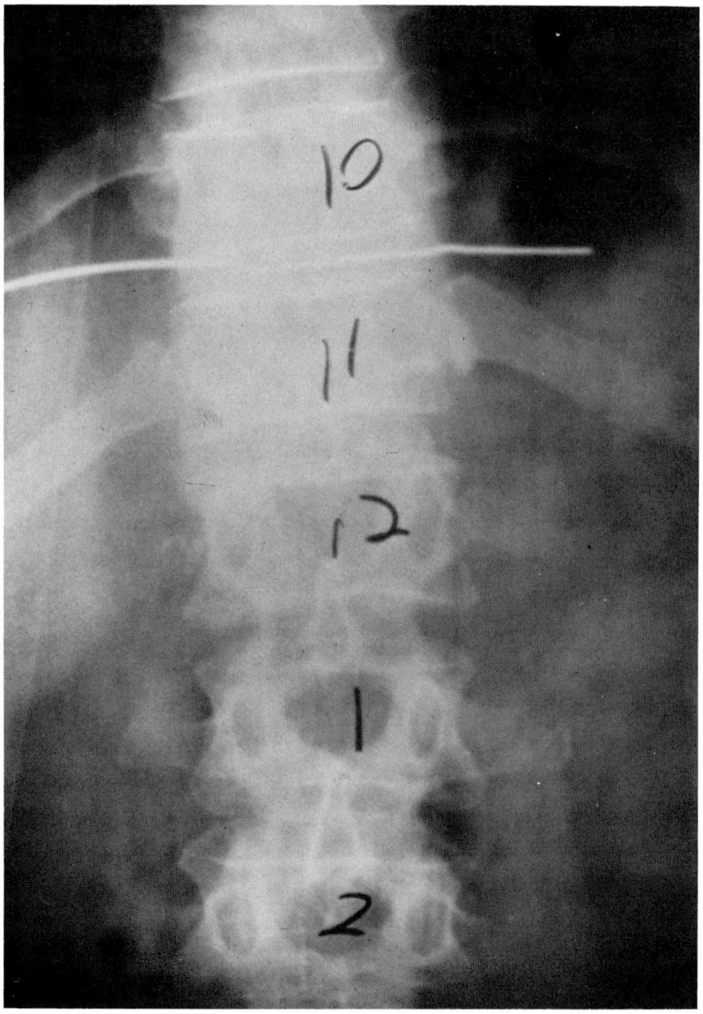

Fig. 29-1. Spinous process of T10 identified in roentgenogram by marker placed on skin.

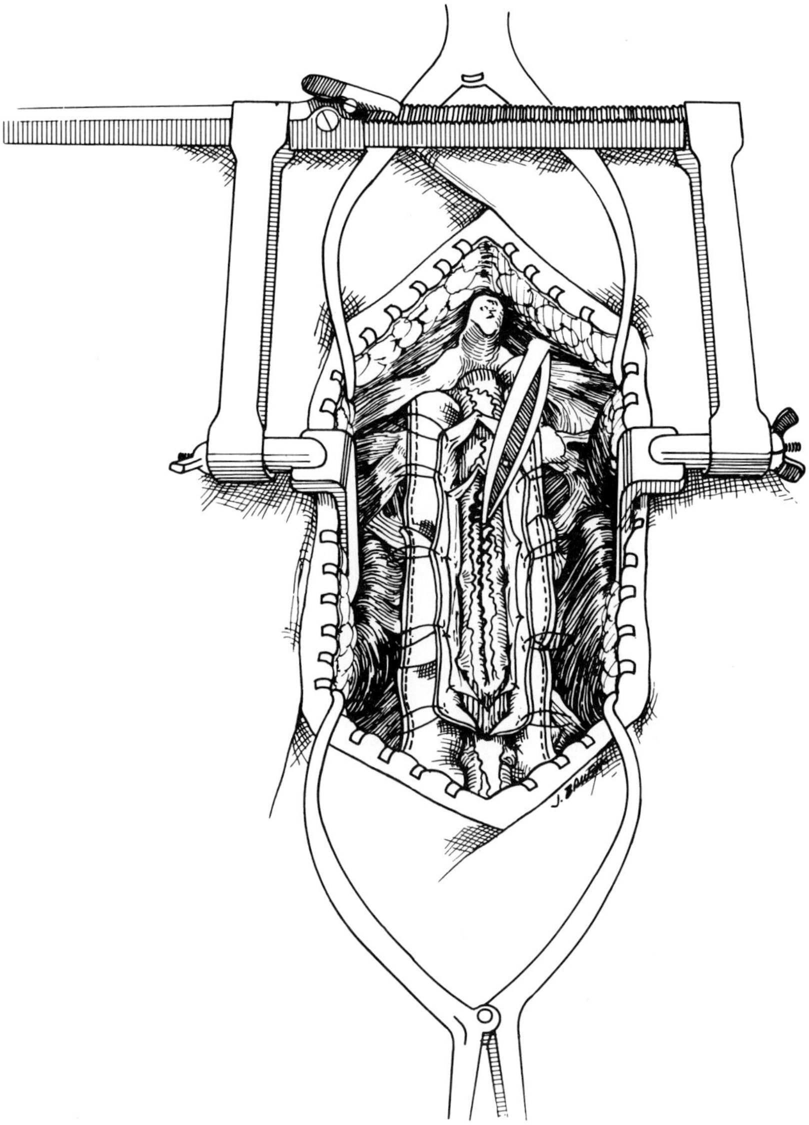

Fig. 29-2. Artist's drawing of bipolar coagulation of midline dorsal vein.

ing the midline dorsal vein and the fine arachnoidal septum. With microdissection, the midline dorsal vein is coagulated with bipolar forceps throughout the length of the proposed incision (Fig. 29-2). It may be necessary to coagulate one or two very small arterial radicals, which may cross the midline. King[7] has stressed the advisability of preserving not only the midline dorsal vein but even the smallest arterial branch. We have not, however, encountered any deleterious effects due to coagulation of these small vessels. The length of the proposed incision is thus prepared, varying from as long as 2.5 to 4 cm, depending upon the extent of the body involved in the painful syndrome.

Two methods have been used to carry out the section of the anterior commissure. Either an iridectomy knife or a No. 12 Bard-Parker blade held in a hemostat (Fig. 29-3) is used to penetrate the upper end of the median sulcus to a depth of from 6 to 7 mm. The knife is then

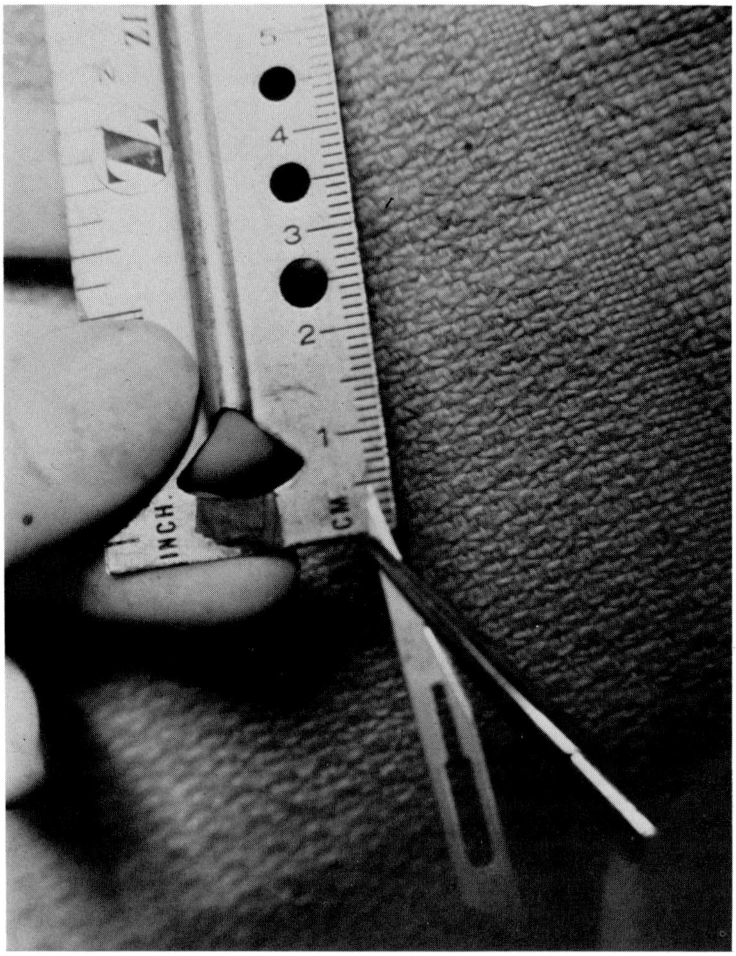

Fig. 29-3. Desired length of cutting edge of Bard-Parker blade is measured.

passed in a caudad direction, maintaining its position strictly in the midline, as viewed in the microscopic field, until the full length of the planned incision has been achieved (Fig. 29-4).

An alternative method, sometimes employed, is to develop the median incision through the pia-arachnoid with sharp section and then with a blunt microdissector, penetrate the midline cord through the anterior commissure, with gentle bilateral retraction of the incision to give visualization throughout.

At the present time we employ the former technique in most cases because we feel that the open technique involves more manipulation of the cord and consequently more risk of damage to the posterior columns and the lateral funiculus.

King[7] prefers the open technique to insure complete section of the anterior commissure, as well as to avoid coagulation of any blood vessels.

Postoperative Care

Postoperative mobilization and ambulation are dictated, to some extent, by the primary disease but can occur as early as the first or second postoperative day. Catheterization may be necessary, but often is not.

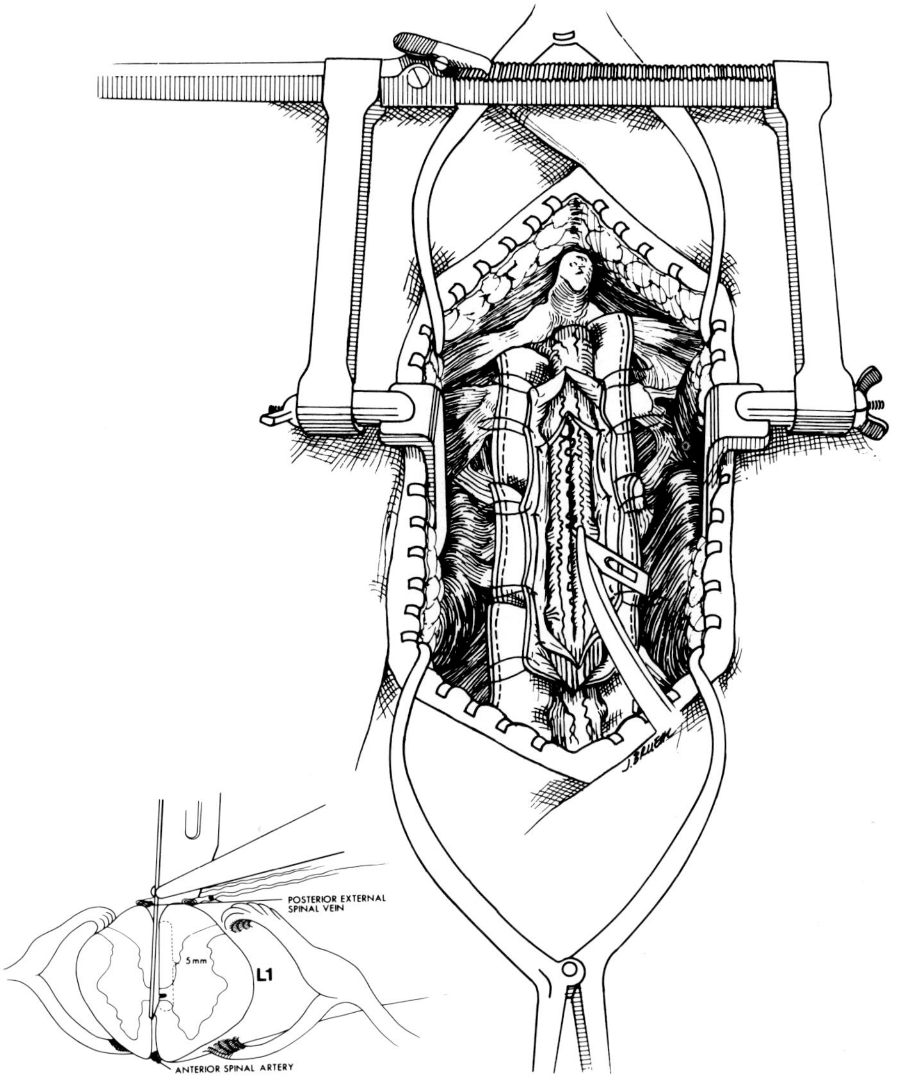

Fig. 29-4. Artist's illustration of technique of blind section through midline of spinal cord. Diagramatic representation of the section in the coronal plane (inset).

Results

Our results with 24 patients who have undergone this procedure are summarized in Tables 29-1 and 29-2. Table 29-1 gives the results in terms of the etiology of the painful syndrome. For simplicity, the clinical result has been designated as either complete, partial, or no relief of pain. In Table 29-2 the same data are tabulated in terms of the anatomic site of pain. Since many patients had pain involving more than one area of the body, the number of pain locations represented is greater than the actual number of patients operated upon.

There were no deaths in this series and complications were not serious. Bladder function, normal preoperatively, was altered in 3 patients, 2 of whom became unable to void and were discharged with a catheter in place. One patient developed partial incontinence. Weakness of the legs, present in 2 patients, appeared to be a lower motor neuron disturbance and

Table 29-1. Results of Commissural Myelotomy According to Etiology in 24 Patients

		Relief			Complications			
Diagnosis	No. of patients	Complete	Partial	None	Bladder	Leg weakness	Persistent dysesthesia	Comments
Carcinoma of:								
Rectum and colon	7	5	1	1	1	1	3	Pain due to pelvic extension
Cervix and uterus	4	3	1	—	—	1	—	Pain due to pelvic extension
Bladder	1	1	—	—	—	—	1	Pain due to pelvic extension
Breast	1	—	1	—	—	—	—	Metastatic to lumbar spine and pelvic mass
Prostate	3	2	1	—	—	—	—	Metastatic disease to the lumbar spine
Lung	2	—	1	1	1	—	—	Metastatic to the thoracic spine and sternum
Osteogenic sarcoma	1	1	—	—	—	—	—	Metastatic to the lumbar sacral spine
Transverse myelitis	1	—	1	—	—	—	—	Girdle chest pains
Medulloblastoma	1	1	—	—	—	—	—	Metastatic to cauda equina
Paraplegia traumatic	1	1	—	—	—	—	—	Burning leg pain
Multiple sclerosis	1	1	—	—	—	—	—	Constant sacral pain plus painful flexor spasms
Sacral Chordoma	1	—	1	—	1	—	—	—
Total	24	15	7	2	3	2	4	

Table 29-2. Results of Commissural Myelotomy According to Anatomic Site of Pain

Location of pain	No. of patients	Relief: Complete	Relief: Partial	Relief: None	Complications: Bladder	Complications: Motor loss	Complications: Persistent dysesthesia
Chest	2	1	—	1	1	—	—
Lumbosacral spine	3	2	1	—	—	—	—
Rectum and perineum	11	7	3	1	1	1	3
Buttock	2	1	1	—	1	—	—
Legs and hips	10	7	3	—	—	1	4
Suprapubic	1	1	—	—	—	—	1
Testicular	1	—	1	—	—	—	—
Total	30	19	9	2	3	2	8

was interpreted as due to damage to anterior horn cells in appropriate segments. Paresthesias or dysesthesias were temporarily encountered in most patients, but disappeared within a few days in all but 4. This complication was interpreted as the result of trauma to posterior columns of the cord. In the 4 patients in whom these symptoms persisted, there was also a concomitant loss of position sense in the lower extremities; this did not, however, interfere significantly with ambulation.

From these results, it can be seen that commissural myelotomy should be considered in the treatment of intractable pain, when it is primarily bilateral or involves midline structures of the body. With the advent of the operating room microscope and newer microsurgical techniques, it appears to be a relatively safe procedure. In this regard the operation was abandoned after its introduction into this country primarily because of fear of injury to the anterior spinal artery.[8] In none of our cases has this occurred.

In the reported series in the United States commissural myelotomy has been performed primarily in lower segments of the cord for midline pain involving the pelvis or for bilateral lower extremity pain. However, in Europe and in England, the operation has been employed more frequently for midline or bilateral truncal pain as well as for pain involving the lower cervical areas and the upper extremities.[4]

The sensory loss following commissural myelotomy is extremely variable. In our cases no reproducible pattern was evident. The loss of awareness to pain and temperature might erratically involve the appropriate segments, but in some instances there was only minimal loss of acute pain and temperature sensation, even though there was complete relief from chronic pain. This has been the experience of all surgeons who have performed this operation.

Discussion

As yet, there is no adequate explanation for the relief of pain obtained by this procedure. To consider that section of the decussating fibers in the anterior commissure is the sole explanation appears to be too simplistic, in view of the vagaries of the resultant sensory loss. Sourek[4] has hypothesized that the relief of pain is due to the involvement of two sensory systems subserving nociception. These are the slow conducting anterolateral system and the more rapidly conducting mediodorsal system. Hitchcock[9] has produced profound and extensive analgesia following a stereotactically placed small midline lesion in the anterior commissure at either the medullary cervical junction or at the C1-2 level. He suggests that not only pain relief, but also the extensive analgesia produced by lesions at this site may be due to interruption of decussations of both direct and crossed pain pathways ascending close to the gray matter of the spinal cord, or is possibly due to interruption of fibers in the spinal cervical tract (Morin), which decussate in the high cervical area.

Conclusions

On the basis of our experience and a review of the literature, it would appear that spinal commissurotomy has now become a relatively safe and effective procedure. It should be seriously considered as a method to manage intractable pain related to midline structures of the body, or bilateral pain. It may well become the procedure of choice for rectal and perineal pain. At the present time however, we would still recommend the use of other procedures for the relief of unilateral pain.

References

1. Armour D: Surgery of the spinal cord. *Lancet* 2:691-697, 1927
2. Guillain J, Mazars G, Movillae V: La myelatomie commissurale. *Presse Med* 49:666-667, 1945
3. Neansery B, Lecuire J, Acassat L: Technique de la myelatomie commissurale posterieure. *J Chir* 60:206-213, 1944
4. Sourek K: Commissural myelotomy. *J Neurosurg* 31:524-527, 1969
5. Wertheimer P: Posterior commissural myelotomy for relief of pain. *Acta Chir Belg* 54:28-29, 1946
6. Lippert RS, Hosobuchi Y, Nielsen SL: Spinal commissurotomy. *Surg Neurol* 2:373-377, 1974
7. King RB: Anterior Commissurotomy for intractable pain. *J Neurosurg* 47:7-11, 1977.
8. Putnam JJ: Myelotomy of the commissure. *Arch Neurol Psychiatr* 32:189-195, 1934
9. Hitchcock E: Stereotactic cervical myelotomy. *J Neurol Neurosurg Psychiatr* 33:224-230, 1970

CHAPTER 30

Longitudinal (Bischof's) Myelotomy

Leslie P. Ivan

THE MAIN FEATURES OF SPASTICITY arise from the exaggerated stretch reflex and the exaggerated flexor withdrawal. Any procedure that can disrupt the reflex arcs participating in these two basic spinal reflexes would relieve muscle spasm and flexor withdrawal reflexes. The methods listed in Table 30-1 all relieve spasticity, but each has some disadvantage. (a) Posterior rhizotomy has no lasting effect and produces complete sensory denervation in the segments involved, thus predisposing to the development of pressure sores in these areas. (b) Intrathecal alcohol injection gives temporary relief only and may aggravate the bladder problem. (c) Intrathecal phenol injection is somewhat unpredictable in its effects, but a satisfactory injection has the same disadvantage as alcohol. (d) Cordectomy is a major procedure and its finality makes both the patient and the surgeon uneasy. (e) Cauda equina transection, besides having the same finality, has the disadvantages of both anterior and posterior rhizotomy. (f) Anterior rhizotomy is followed by severe muscle wasting and exposure of bony prominences, increasing the risk of pressure sores either in the ischial region, from sitting, or in the lower extremities of patients who wear braces.

Bischof's myelotomy, on the other hand, produces permanent flaccidity without loss of muscle bulk and, except for segmental analgesia, should not affect other sensory modalities. With accurate technique, all long tracts, including the pyramidal, should remain intact following myelotomy. An important feature of longitudinal myelotomy is that after the operation

Table 30-1. Procedures for the Relief of Spasm

Procedure	Described by
1. Posterior rhizotomy	Foerster 1910
2. Intrathecal alcohol	Dogliotti 1930
3. Intrathecal phenol	Suvansa 1931
4. Cordectomy	MacCarty 1948
5. Transsection of cauda equina	Meriowsky 1950
6. Anterior rhizotomy	Munro 1945
7. Myelotomy	Bischof 1951

Department of Neurosurgery, Ottawa General Hospital; present address Children's Hospital of Eastern Ontario, Ottawa, Ontario, Canada

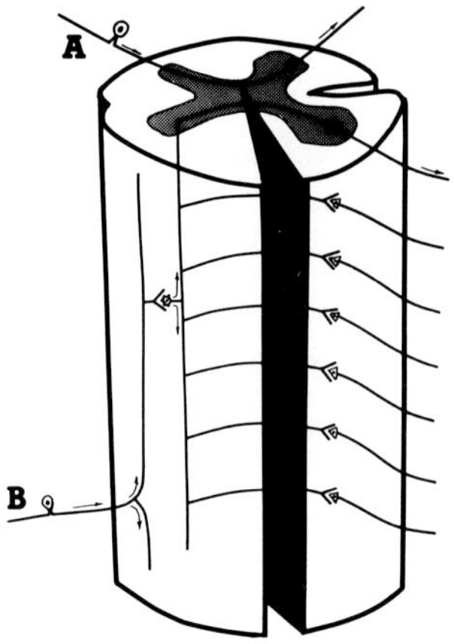

Fig. 30-1. Schematic representations of the original concept of Bischof's myelotomy. **A.** Monosynaptic reflex arc. **B.** Reflex collaterals with ascending and descending branches to motor neurons.

there is no late recurrence of spasticity because short propriospinal pathways and long collaterals were disrupted (Fig. 30-1). This disruption eliminates the influx of afferent impulses from higher and lower segments, which is the suggested cause of failure in some other methods.

Bischof[1] first described his procedure in 1951 and called it *longitudinal lateral myelotomy*. No response to his paper can be found in the medical literature until 1955 when Weber[2] reported the use of this technique in 2 patients, with good results. Nadvornik,[3] in 1961, reported one such case and commented favorably on the procedure. In 1962 Tonnis and Bischof[4] gave an account of 20 cases with a follow-up time of 2 to 8 years. Our papers with Paine and Hunt,[5,6] in 1966 and 1967, appear to be the first North American accounts of this operation. The procedure gained popularity in Canada, and the Canadian experience was summarized by Moyes in 1969.[7] Since then, several reports from various countries were published,[8-12] all authors commenting favorably on the method.

Technical Considerations and Modifications

The original Bischof's myelotomy involves separating the spinal cord longitudinally into an anterior and posterior half between L1 and L5 segments, to which unilateral separation between S1 and S3 can be added to decrease bladder spasticity. Bischof suggested severing the cord completely into an anterior and posterior half to preserve the pyramidal tract on one side (Fig. 30-2). Later Pourpe in 1960[13] and Bischof in 1967,[14] suggested an approach through the posterior median fissure (Fig. 30-3).

A further search for the ideal procedure resulted in the use of an L-shaped knife by the author, and this procedure was (Fig. 30-4) called *circular griseotomy*, which worked well in animal experiments (Fig. 30-5). During laboratory trials, it became obvious that both mechanical and radiofrequency destruction can be used (Fig. 30-6). It was recognized that for the relief of spasticity, the effective part of the surgery is *disruption of pathways inside the gray matter. This is why the term griseotomy (cutting the gray) was proposed.*[8,15]

In experiments on 43 dogs (Table 30-2), my colleagues and I made the following observations: lateral longitudinal myelotomy, circular griseotomy, T-griseotomy, and radiofrequency lesions would all relieve spasticity, however, myelotomy on intact animals caused more paraplegia than any of the other procedures. Radiofrequency heat could reduce or eliminate spasticity, provided lesions were made close (4 mm apart) to each other, at least

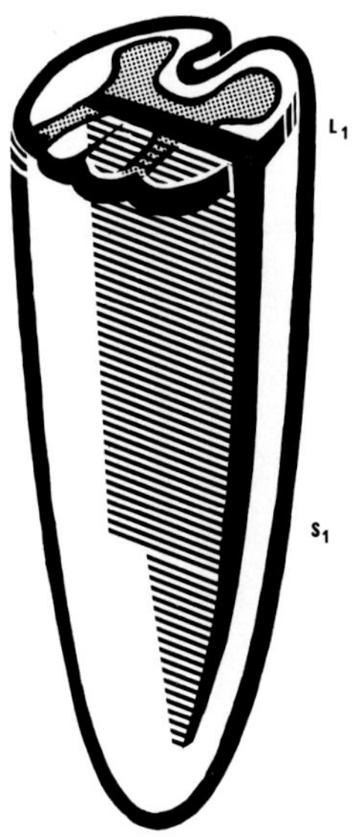

Fig. 30-2. Bischof's myelotomy. The original procedure.

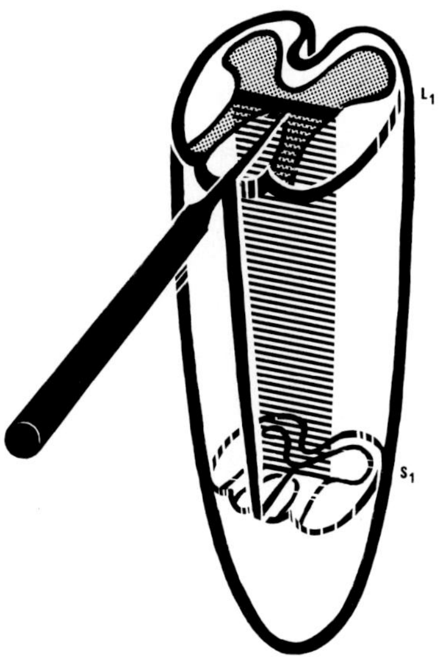

Fig. 30-3. T griseotomy.

Table 30-2. **Segmental Relief of Spasticity**

	No. of dogs	Postoperative paraplegia	Percentage
Group 1			
Lateral longitudinal myelotomy	4	4	100
Group 2			
Circular griseotomy	14	4	28
Group 3			
RF griseotomy	25	10	40
Total	43	18	

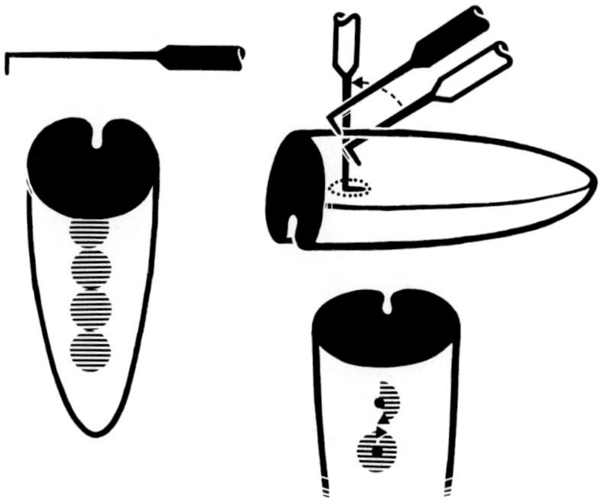

Fig. 30-4. Technique of circular griseotomy. An L-shaped instrument is inserted through the posterior midline sulcus and rotated 360° in the equatorial plane of the cord.

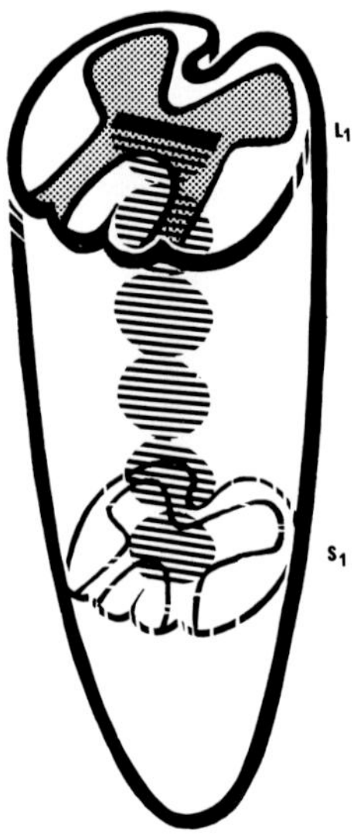

Fig. 30-5. The end result of circular griseotomy: a series of circular cuts within the gray matter.

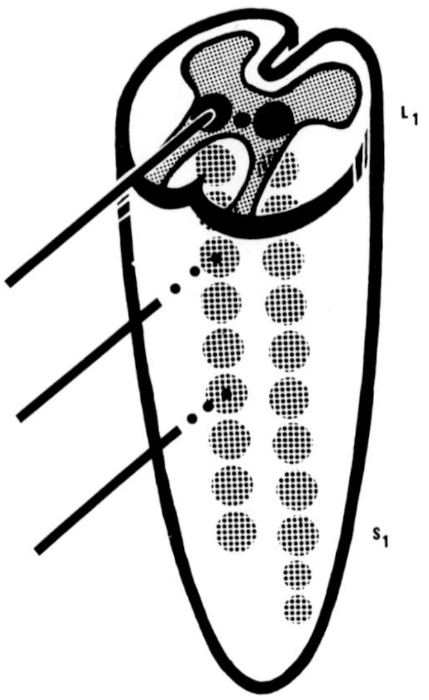

Fig. 30-6. Radiofrequency griseotomy. Radiofrequency heat microlesions within the gray matter through the posterior approach with a 0.5 mm bare tip electrode.

two lesions per segment. This would indicate that to achieve segmental relief of spasticity of the lower limbs in human beings, at least 14 to 18 radiofrequency lesions should be made on each side, in the equatorial line of the cord. The target area is within the gray matter, in lamina 6 and 7 of Rexed (Fig. 30-7).

Indications for Myelotomy

Myelotomy can best be used for patients suffering from spasticity of the lower limbs to such a degree that the spasms interfere with sitting in a wheelchair or lying comfortably in bed, and when there are some cord functions that are advantageous to preserve. *Without*

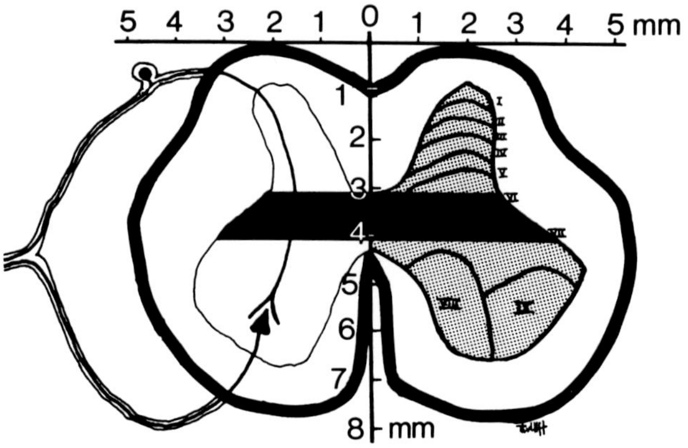

Fig. 30-7. The target area (blackened between 3 and 4 mm) within the gray matter for the relief of spasticity. The roman numbers indicate the laminar structure of the gray matter according to Rexed. The arabic numbers are reference points in millimeters.

further refinement of the present technique, myelotomy should not be performed on patients who are able to walk. In some patients the use of braces or the ability to walk may be restored following successful myelotomy, and it is possible to retain voluntary emptying of the bladder, if this was preserved in the original injury or disease.

If the patient has severe pain in the lower limbs, which is not infrequent in spastic conditions, relief of this pain might be an additional indication for this type of procedure.

Preoperative Management

Routine laboratory studies, x-ray films of the lumbosacral spine, cystometrogram, urologic assessment, exact charting of muscle-strength, muscle-tone, reflexes, sensory functions, and also measuring the degree of contractures, are required studies.

Most patients already have indwelling catheters. If not, a catheter should be inserted prior to surgery. During surgery, electrocystometrogram can be performed to ascertain whether bladder tone was reduced sufficiently.

Operative Exploration

The surgery is always performed under general endotracheal anesthesia. The patient is positioned prone on the operating table, with semiflexion in hip and knee joints, and draped in such a way that an observer can report movements when nerve root stimulation is done during surgery.

Spinous processes are counted from C7 and the count double checked by counting them from the L5 vertebra. The T10 vertebra is marked, and after the patient's back is cleansed with surgical soap and Betadine scrub, the operative field is draped between the T7 and L3 spinous processes. An incision is marked between the T9 and L2 spinous processes, and the subcutaneous tissue and paraspinal muscles are infiltrated with physiologic saline. The incision is made in the midline and through subperiosteal dissection the T9, T10, T11, T12, and L1 vertebrae (Fig. 30-8) are exposed. A laminectomy is done on T10, T11, T12, and L1

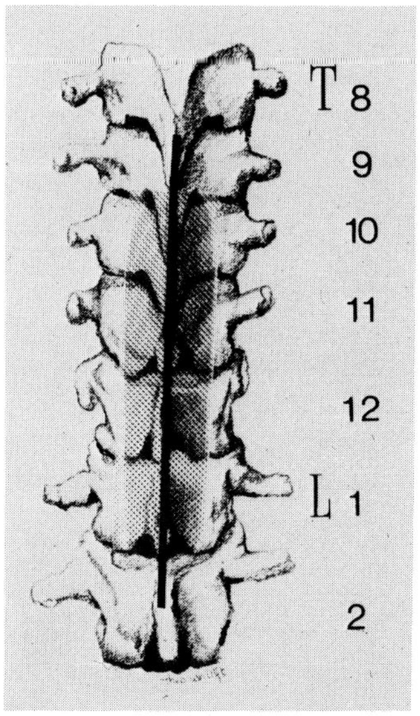

Fig. 30-8. Schematic drawing to show the extent of the incision and laminectomy.

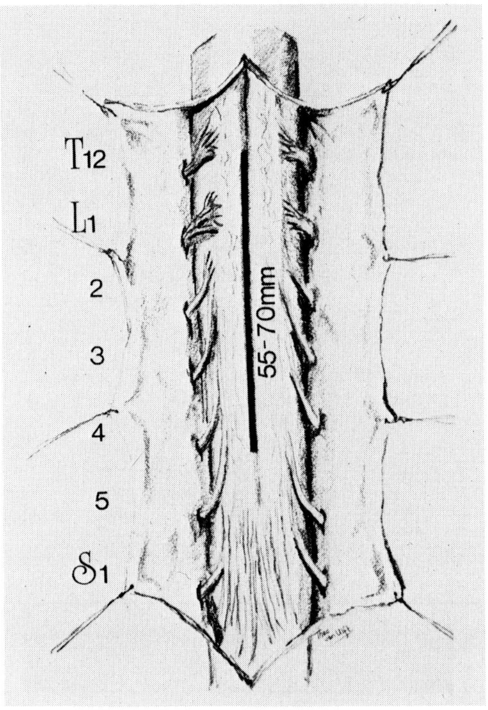

Fig. 30-9. Artist's concept of the exposed cord indicating the length of the cord between L1 and S1 segments.

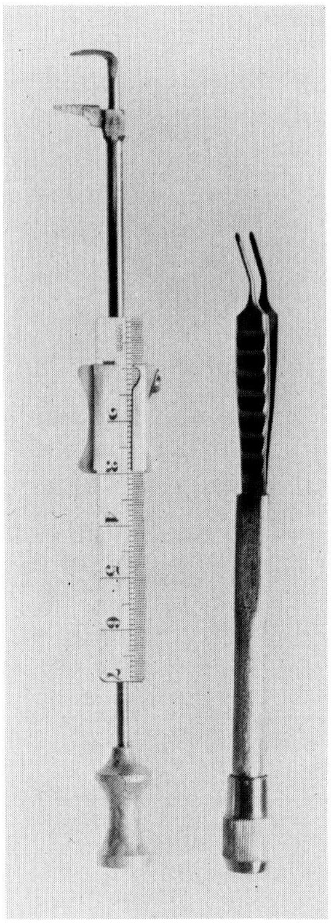

Fig. 30-10. Spinal cord gauges to measure the width and AP diameter of the cord.

vertebrae. After the dura is opened, the conus medullaris should be at the caudal part of the operative field and at least 80 mm of spinal cord should be visible. Holding stitches are placed in the dura, while the operative field is kept bloodless with the usual placement of cotton pledgets (Fig. 30-9).

Using a nerve stimulator with a 2 V 1 msec current, T12 and S1 nerve roots should be identified. THis is done by rotating the cord slightly and placing the stimulating electrode on the motor root of T12, while an observer identifies contraction of the lower abdominal muscles. Contraction can sometimes be felt by the operating surgeon through the draping. S1 nerve root is usually the thickest of the cauda equina fibers and when the motor root of S1 is stimulated, the foot should move into plantar flexion. After these two landmarks are identified, (the distance between them varies between 55 to 70 mm), the surgeon should prepare the cord and instruments for lesion-making. The width and AP diameter of the cord are measured with a spinal cord gauge (Fig. 30-10). The total length of the cord subject to lesion-making is also measured (Fig. 30-9).

Lesion-Making

Four methods of lesion-making will be described. The first three depend on mechanical instruments, used laterally on the cord or through a posterior approach. The fourth depends on radiofrequency heat and is done posteriorly.

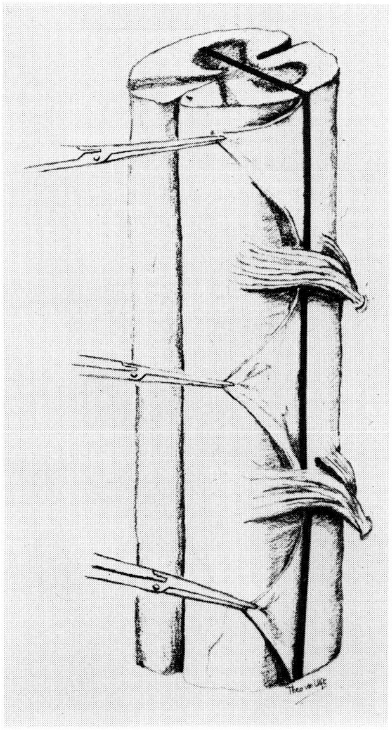

Fig. 30-11. Drawing to show the rotation of the cord and the plane of incision at the attachment of the dentate ligaments.

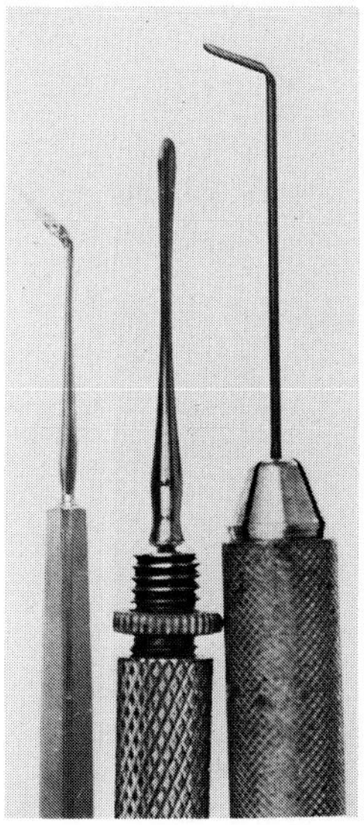

Fig. 30-12. Instruments used for the incision of the cord in lateral longitudinal myelotomy.

Lateral Longitudinal Myelotomy

This is the original Bischof's method (Fig. 30-11). In preparation for the myelotomy the cord is rotated sideways after the last three denticulate ligaments are cut. Some surgeons use a No. 11 blade or a keratome;[16] others, such as myself, use a slightly less sharp and smaller instrument (Fig. 30-12). If it is difficult to rotate the cord, transfix it with three, 20-gauge needles to make it easier to rotate and find the cutting plane. An incision is then made slowly just anterior to the attachment of the denticulate ligament in the equatorial line of the cord, in such a way that about 2½ mm of the cord is saved on the opposite side. This can be determined accurately by measuring the width of the cord (which may vary anywhere between 6 to 10 mm) and marking the knife with a hemoclip or a small piece of bone wax. The cutting (in a length of 55 to 70 mm) is done in small segments, because the space between the anterior and posterior roots prevents a continuous incision. Usually, some blood begins to ooze in the line of incision; the bleeding, however, stops when the wound is irrigated and small cotton pledgets placed. When the oozing stops, the dura is closed with interrupted 0000 black silk sutures and the muscle layer with 0 silk or 0 chromic catgut. The fascia, subcutaneous tissue, and the skin are closed with sutures, according to the surgeon's routine. There is no need for a drain.

Posterior Longitudinal Myelotomy

This procedure was first described by Pourpre, in 1960,[13] who called it *Myelotomy en Croix* and *T-griseotomy* by the author (Fig. 30-3). After the exposure described previously and after nerve stimulation and measurements, the posterior median sulcus of the cord is

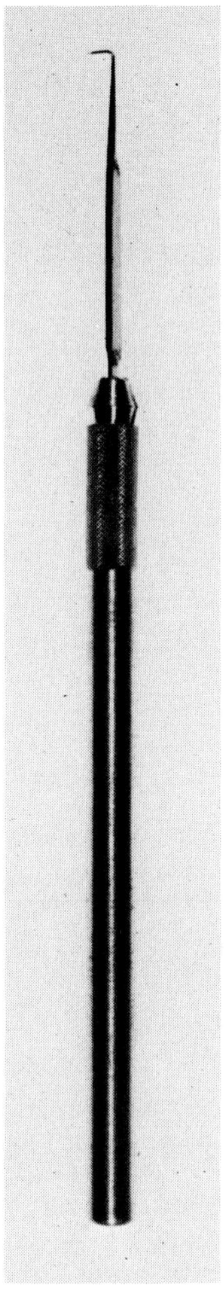

Fig. 30-13. L-shaped knife for T-griseotomy.

identified under magnification and, avoiding injury to the dorsal vein, the posterior median fissure is entered with a semisharp instrument to a depth half that of the AP diameter of the cord, using an L-shaped knife (Fig. 30-13). Separation is made in the usual myelotomy plane, 3 mm on each side, sideways from the midline. The final myelotomy is reached by proceeding with the separation in small sections to avoid injuring the usually tortuous dorsal vein. At the end of this procedure a T-shaped cleavage is left in the cord at a length of 55 to 70 mm. Slight oozing is easily controlled by irrigation with physiologic saline and placement of small cotton pledgets. The wound is closed as previously described.

Circular Griseotomy

This procedure (Figs. 30-4 and 30-5) was used only in animal experiments, with a special instrument and stereotaxic attachment. It was tried twice on human material by the author, but because of the toughness of the diseased cord, available instruments appeared unsatisfactory. It is suggested that by designing the right instrument for this purpose, a very simple and accurate method may evolve.

RF Griseotomy

After several years of experimentation and developing suitable electrodes, this procedure was performed on 5 adults. The technique depends on the same exploration as previous procedures. Special electrodes with an adjustable tip are used (Fig. 30-14). Fourteen to 18 pairs of lesions are necessary to obtain satisfactory results (Fig. 30-15). The tip of the needle should be inserted 2 mm from the midline on each side and a pair of lesions should be made at each 4 mm distance along the posterior aspect of the cord. Depending on the measurement of the cord, the half millimeter bare tip of the electrode should reach a depth of 3 to 4 mm (Fig. 30-16). Using the Radionics lesion-maker with a test lesion setting of 100 m amp, 50-m amp 10-second effective radiofrquency lesions are made at each insertion. Care should be taken to use a clean electrode for each lesion.

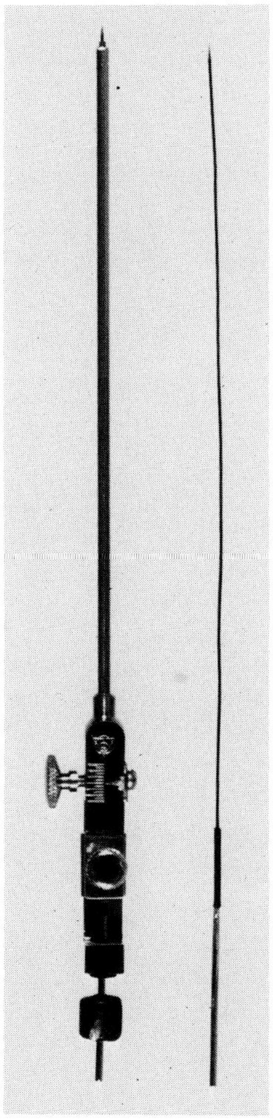

Fig. 30-14. Adjustable needle electrode with 0.5 mm bare tip. Depending on the AP diameter of the cord, the penetrating portion of the electrode can be adjusted with 0.5 mm accuracy.

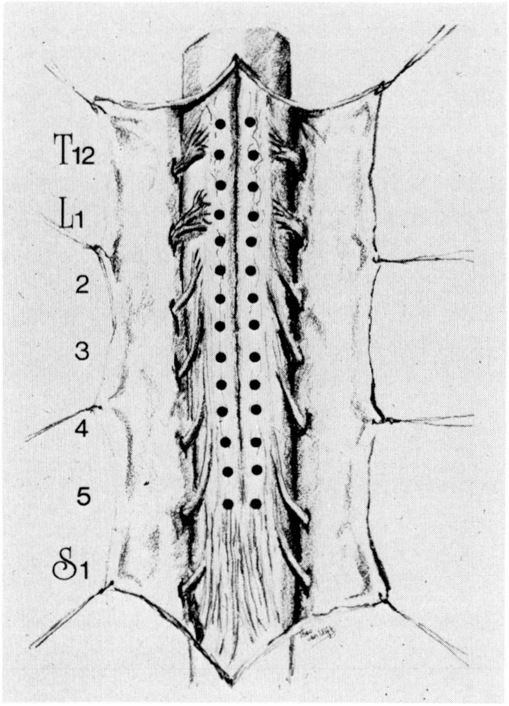

Fig. 30-15. Points of penetration on the dorsal aspect of the cord for RF griseotomy. The distance between the lesions is 4 mm, both in the craniocaudal and lateral direction.

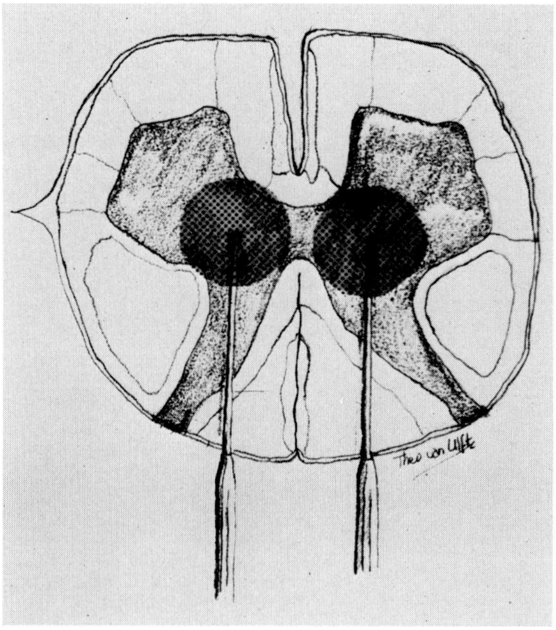

Fig. 30-16. Schematic drawing of the cord with two electrodes in position showing the approximate area of RF heat destruction in the intermediate gray matter.

Postoperative Care

The patient should be turned hourly and physiotherapy started the day after surgery. The patients are able to take solid food 24 hours after operation, although in some cases paralytic ileus may be a complicating factor. In case of preexisting pressure sores in the sacral areas, prophylactic antibiotic treatment is justifiable to prevent wound infection. A week after surgery, wheelchair routine may start and, if the patient's condition permits, learning self transfer from bed to wheelchair can be started. In case of remaining useful functions, 3 or 4 weeks after surgery, ambulation with long braces can be attempted.

Results

Most reports agree that myelotomy is one of the best available procedures for the permanent relief of spasticity. The question is which type of myelotomy should be performed so that spasticity recurs less frequently and a greater number of patients can ambulate after surgery? Unfortunately, on the basis of the available literature, including the author's material, this question cannot be answered with certainty.

The great majority of case reports comment on the *original Bischof's method*.[7,8,10,11,17] It appears that with unilateral longitudinal myelotomy, spasticity recurs on the opposite side through the cord incision in about 20% of the cases.[18]

Posterior commissural myelotomy (myelotomy en croix or T-griseotomy), on the other hand, seems to have definite advantages as compared to the original Bischof's method.[14,18] There have been only about 14 cases reported in all of the medical literature. The author's single experience showed that this was a time-consuming procedure, but the patient had good relief of spasticity; movements in the ankle joint were preserved on both sides. The paper by Laitinen and Singunas,[9] from Finland, reporting the results in 9 patients, gives a favorable impression of this method.

Circular griseotomy appeared a feasible procedure in animal experiments. Refinement of the instrumentation and adapting it for the characteristics of the human spinal cord may make this a very valuable technique in the hands of someone who sees a large number of patients.

Radiofrequency griseotomy worked very well in animal experiments and was performed five times on patients by the author. The last 3 patients treated by this method had excellent results. One of the patients who died, due to pulmonary embolism (the only fatality among 26 patients), provided us with a spinal cord specimen (Fig. 30-17). The histology showed that the lesions were surprisingly bigger than predicted from eggwhite experiments. The radiofrequency lesions of the cord are entirely bloodless, but the selectivity of the method cannot be judged from the small number of cases.

My colleagues and I have frequently found that a contracture that appeared fixed clinically, may entirely disappear under general anesthesia. A slight degree of contracture after myelotomy may resolve spontaneously. In a few cases we combine myelotomy with tenotomy of the hamstring muscles.

In my material, consisting of 26 cases, only 1 patient could walk with braces after surgery.

Spasticity recurs in about 20% of the cases. In half of these the recurrence is insignificant and not disturbing. In about 10% of the cases reoperation or intrathecal alcohol injection should abolish the remaining spasticity.

For those neurosurgeons who have an occasional case, probably the original unilateral longitudinal myelotomy is the most suitable method. For those who see many cases, a variety of modifications are available, as discussed earlier.

From the purely experimental circular griseotomy through the proved radiofrequency griseotomy to the quite well-accepted posterior commissural myelotomy, there are a variety

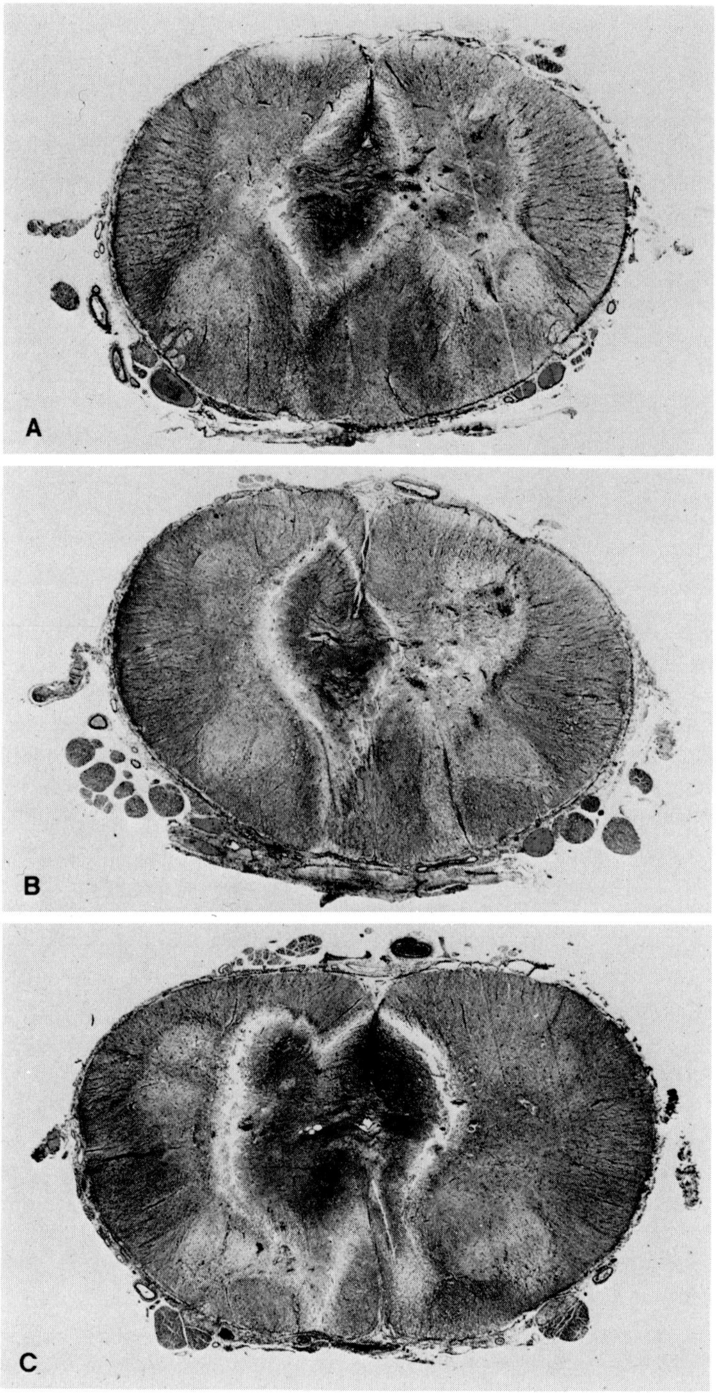

Fig. 30-17. Histologic appearance of human spinal cord 2 days after RF griseotomy. Death was due to pulmonary embolism. Note the lesions, which are considerably larger than expected from eggwhite experiments.

of lesion-making methods. With ultrasound and laser, a wide field of experimentation remains open. The target to be destroyed within the gray matter, corresponding roughly to lamina 6 and 7 of Rexed, is well established;[15,19] it is the intermediate gray matter around the equatorial plane of the cord.

Acknowledgment

The work appearing in this chapter was supported by grants from the Medical Research Council of Canada, from the Ontario Crippled Children's Society and from the Multiple Sclerosis Society of Canada.

Art work and photography was done by the Department of Medical Communication, Faculty of Medicine, University of Ottawa, Canada, and by the Department of Medical Illustration, Children's Hospital of Eastern Ontario.

The adjustable electrodes, the spinal cord gauges, and the special knives were developed by Mr. G. Zellerman, Accurate Surgical Instruments Company, Toronto, Ontario.

Special thanks are due to Maureen Melrose for assembling the references and editing the manuscript and to Lise Riffel for the numerous retypings.

REFERENCES

1. Bischof W: Die longitudinale myelotomie, *Zentralbl Neurochir 11*:79-88, 1951
2. Weber W: Die Behandlung der spinalen Paraspastik unter besonderer Berucksichtigung der longitudinalen Myelotomie (Bischof). *Med Monatsschr 9*:510-513, 1955
3. Madvornik P: Effect of longitudinal myelotomy on spasticity of lower limbs and urinary bladder. *Sb Ved Pr Lek Fak Karlovy Univ 2*:77, 1959, abstracted, *Excerpta Med VIII 14*:3876, 852, 1961
4. Tonnis W, Bischof W: Ergebnisse der lumbalen Myelotomie nach Bischof. *Zentralbl Neurochir 23*:120-132, 1962
5. Ivan LP, Paine KWE, Hunt TE: Experience with Bischof's myelotomy. *Can J Surg 10*:191-195, 1967
6. Paine KW, Ivan LP, Hunt TE: The Bischof myelotomy for treatment of spasticity in paraplegics. *Proc Annu Clin Spinal Cord Inj Conf 15*:72-86, 1966
7. Moyes PD: Longitudinal myelotomy for spasticity. *J Neurosurg 31*:615-619, 1969
8. Ivan LP, Wiley JJ: Myelotomy in the management of spasticity. *Clin Orthop 108*:52-56, 1975
9. Laitinen L, Singounas E: Longitudinal myelotomy in the treatment of spasticity of the legs. *J Neurosurg 35*:536-540, 1971
10. Schirmer M, Barz D, Wenker H: Longitudinal myelotomy—indication and results. *Acta Neurochir (Viënna) 31*:308-309, 1975
11. VanderArk MC, Kempe GL: Longitudinal myelotomy in spastic paraplegia. *Milit Med 134*:608-611, 1969
12. Virozue ID, Chipko SS: Experience with 60 frontal myelotomies in treatment of spastic manifestations in patients with injuries of the spine and spinal cord. Voprosy *Neurochir 2*:21-26, 1975
13. Pourpre MH: Traitement neuro-chirurgical des contractures chez les paraplégiques post traumatiques. *Neurochirurgie 6*:229-236, 1960
14. Bischof W: Zur dorsalen longitudinalen Myelotomie. *Zentralbl Neurochir 28*:123-126, 1967
15. Ivan LP: The segmental relief of spasticity. Read before the 7th Congress of the Canadian Neurological Society, Banff, 1972
16. Asenjo A: *Neurosurgical Techniques.* Charles C Thomas, Springfield, 1963
17. Galanda M, Nadvornik P, Frohlich F: Contribution to surgical treatment of spasticity in spinal cord injuries (critical remarks to longitudinal myelotomy). *Bratisl Lek List 61*:589-594, 1974
18. Gonsette R, André-Balisaux G: Contribution au traitement neurochirurgical de la spasticité des membres inférieurs dans la sclérose en plaque. *Acta Neurol Psychiatr Belg 63*:460-477, 1963
19. Fever H, Horner TG, De Myer WE, Campbell RL: Anatomical and histological lesions in Bischof's myelotomy in dogs. *Surg Forum 23*:438-440, 1972

CHAPTER 31
Percutaneous Cordotomy

William H. Sweet

WE OWE TO THAT remarkably innovative, thoughtful neurosurgeon, Dr. Sean Mullan of the University of Chicago, the entire concept and tactic for percutaneous cordotomy.[1] I have found this operation difficult to do and in this chapter emphasize the difficulties I am continuing to have with this procedure, although some progress is being made in resolving at least some of them.

Figure 31-1 points to a problem that was drawn to my attention in an unattractive way. After I made a T2 lesion at open operation in what I thought was the anterior half of the white matter of the cord of this patient with a cancer, she had an ipsilateral severe weakness of the right lower limb. This cleared enough in 10 days so that she could walk. But following her second operation, 79 days after her first one, for pain on the other side, this patient had almost complete paralysis of both legs, recovering active straight-leg raising against resistance to 90° on each side, with normal power of the feet and toes only by the end of 1 month. The postmortem specimen, 10 months later, showed similar lesions on both sides of the cord 1½ segments apart.

My colleagues, in analyzing this material, tactfully refrained from asking me how it happened that I had made the lesions so far posteriorly. I hated to look at these sections because they made it appear that I was too pathetically clumsy for words. However, Figure 31-2 shows what I saw when I examined sections of the cord far more caudal than the site of the original lesion, namely that the dentate ligament in this patient arose from the cord far dorsal to the midequatorial plane. The anteroposterior extent of the lesion was the same on both sides. Each lesion destroyed the anterolateral half of the lateral and all of the ventral corticospinal tracts. The most serious sequel in this patient, painful dysesthesias, came on gradually 5½ months after the first operation. These pains, the worst ever described to me after cordotomy, were perhaps related to destruction of the grey matter in the ventral parts of the posterior horns and the posterior white columns. They were not relieved by a succession of bilateral frontal inferior, medial lesions in the white matter of the cerebral hemispheres, so extensive that the patient was greatly reduced in her mentational level.

Figures 31-3A and B are from another patient in whom the unusually dorsal site of origin of the dentate ligament, bilaterally, led another member of our staff to make lesions that

It is a pleasure to acknowledge the kindness of the publishers Williams and Wilkins, the editors of *Clinical Neurosurgery,* and the Congress of Neurological Surgeons in permitting us to reproduce with only minor changes the entire Chapter 5 and 6 of volume 23 of *Clinical Neurosurgery,* 1976. The financial assistance of the Neuro-Research Foundation is also gratefully acknowledged.

Department of Surgery, Harvard Medical School and the Neurosurgical Service, Massachusetts General Hospital, Boston, Massachusetts 02114

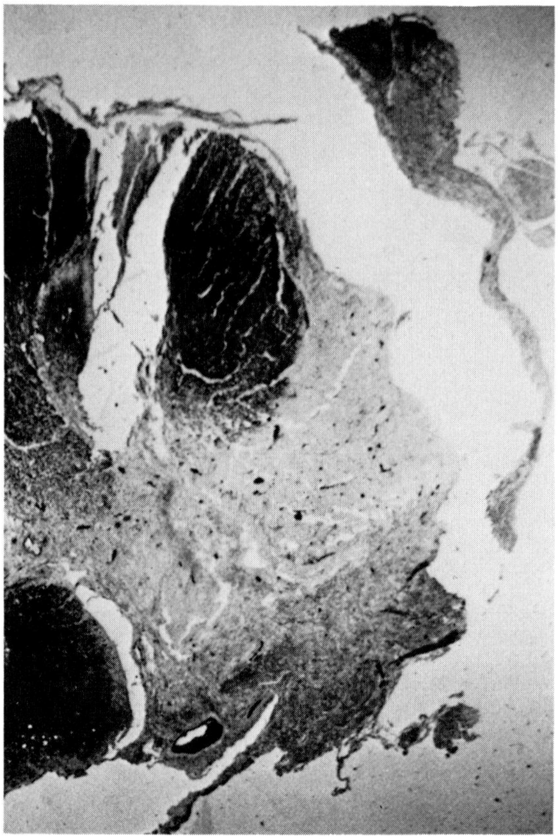

Fig. 31-1. Hazel P. Cross section at level of right incision showing major encroachment into posterolateral white matter. (The broad vertical cleft in the right posterior column is an artifact.) The site of origin of the dentate ligament from the cord cannot be seen. (Reproduced by permission from Sweet WH: Recent observations pertinent to improving anterolateral cordotomy, *Clinical Neurosurgery,* vol 23. Williams and Wilkins, Baltimore, 1976, p 81)

extended too far dorsally. The surgeon took as the landmark for discontinuing the lesion ventrally the sizable ventral rootlet pointed out in Figure 31-3B. Since this rootlet extended straight laterally instead of straight ventrally, the surgical lesion left intact much of the cord ordinarily considered the appropriate target area. Hence our so-called *landmarks* can be, at times, very misleading. Awareness of such problems makes their correction easy.

More serious is the growing evidence that the entire anterior quadrant of the cord may be neither as safe nor as appropriate a target as many of us had concluded. Through the decades, from the 1930s into the 1970s, most who ventured to write on the subject of anterolateral cordotomy felt that nearly all of the anterior quadrant had to be destroyed to get all pain and temperature fibers, not only the anterolateral but the anterior columns as well.[2-6] Figure 31-4 shows that even this extensive degree of destruction at the T3 level of incision into the cord, yielded analgesia only up to the T10 level at the umbilicus, probably because there was a delayed crossover of fibers from the secondary afferent neurons in the posterior horns. Indeed there may be only a partial crossover at the usual levels, so that bilateral cordotomy is

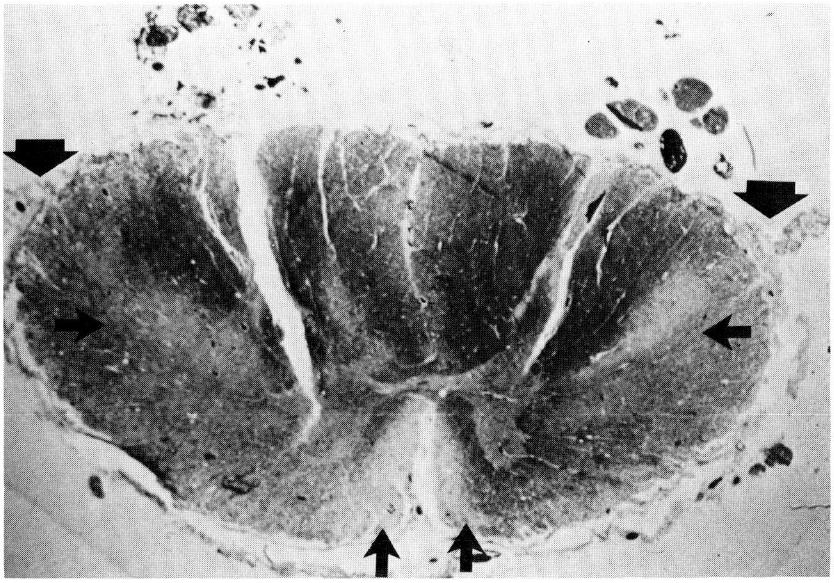

Fig. 31-2. Hazel P. Cross section of midthoracic cord (myelin sheath stain) below incisions at T2 and T3 levels. Downward directed arrows indicate origins of dentate ligaments in the plane through the apices of the posterior horns. Degeneration is most marked in the lateral and ventral corticospinal tracts, indicated, respectively, by horizontal and vertical arrows. (Reproduced by permission from Sweet WH: Recent observations pertinent to improving anterolateral cordotomy, *Clinical Neurosurgery,* vol 23. Williams and Wilkins, Baltimore, 1976, p 80)

required for unilateral pain.[7-9] In fact, French and Peyton[10] and Voris[11] have each reported one patient in whom no crossover at all occurred.

In the usual topographic distribution of the pain fibers the sacral segments lie most dorsolaterally. However, in some cases this is reversed, as Dr. White and I have shown at several open cordotomies with the patient awake. In these cases the last incision that produced a desired sacral analgesia lay far ventrally in the cord. Schwartz[12] has reported 3 such cases and Moossy and Rosomoff[13] add the postmortem findings in another (Fig. 31-5). Here there was relative sparing of the dorsal half of the left ventral quadrant, yet analgesia was maintained only below T11 on the right side.

Even the very extensive lesions of Figure 31-6[14] at the T5 level did not eliminate pressure pain, did not produce thermanesthesia, and did not help the gastric crises associated with this patient's tabes dorsalis. Cutaneous analgesia to pinprick was produced up to within one segment of the incisions in the cord. Foerster[14] made his incisions under local anesthesia, testing the patient as he steadily deepened his cut, until the desired contralateral cutaneous analgesia was secured. However, his thorough method at open operation may fail, because even his type of lesion may not cut all of the pain pathways. In this case, of course, both those fibers ascending ipsilaterally and those ascending contralaterally would be included. Clearly in that individual some of the pain fibers must have lain in the posterior half of the cord. That such may be the case has also been demonstrated as a consequence of the relative imprecision at times attendant on percutaneous cordotomy. We owe to Moossy and Rosomoff the startling findings related to the postmortem specimens of Figures 31-7 and 31-8. In their patients 2, 3, and 12 (Fig. 31-7) with lesions almost exclusively in the dorsolateral white matter and posterior horns, there was no hemiparesis, yet there was analgesia to pinprick and satisfactory pain relief of unstated duration. Kurze[15] has described to me a

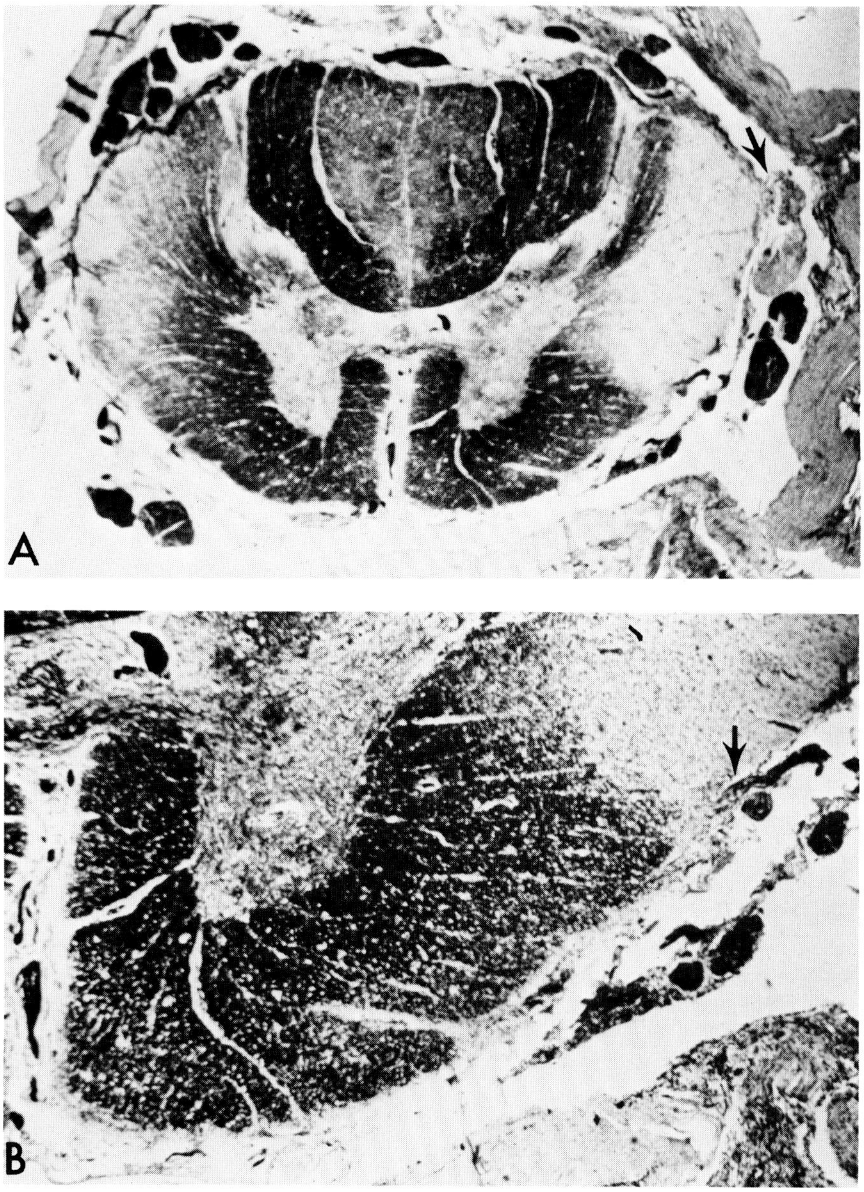

Fig. 31-3. Top. Cross section of midthoracic cord (myelin sheath stain). The upper thoracic incisions on each side were placed too far posteriorly, not only because of a posterior displacement of the origin of the dentate ligament (arrow on right), but also because a conspicuous anterior rootlet emerged from the cord straight lateral to the anterior horn. Bottom: Closeup of right anterior quadrant of the cord at the level of the above figure. Arrow indicates the large anterior rootlet whose emergence led to sparing of most of the anterolateral white matter. (Reproduced by permission from Sweet WH: Recent observations pertinent to improving anterolateral cordotomy, *Clinical Neurosurgery,* vol 3. Williams and Wilkins, Baltimore, 1976, p 82)

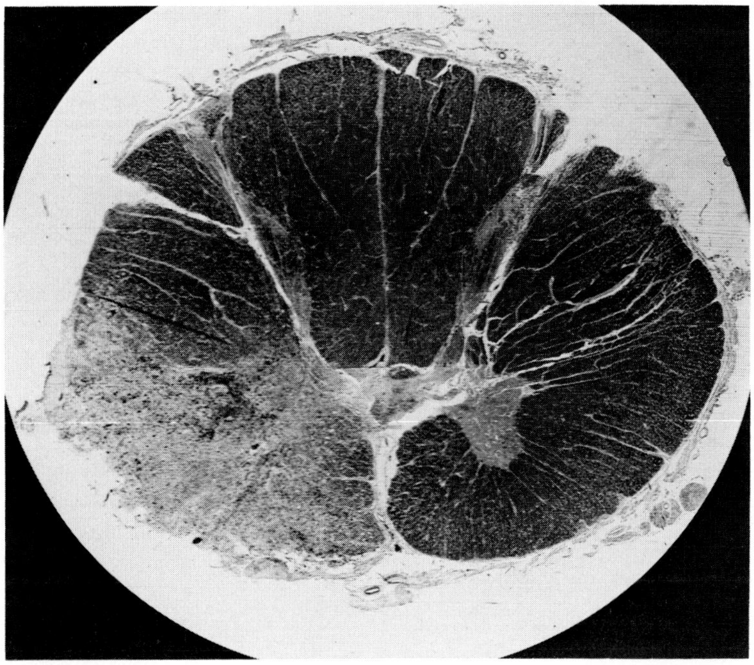

Fig. 31-4. Patient MB. Cross section of cord at T3 level of incisions. Despite destruction of one entire anterior quadrant, contralateral analgesia only to T10, indicating delayed crossing of fibers and need for making cord incision well above highest segmental level of pain. (Reproduced by permission from White JC, Sweet WH: *Pain: Its Mechanisms and Neurosurgical Control.* Charles C Thomas, Springfield, Illinois, 1955)

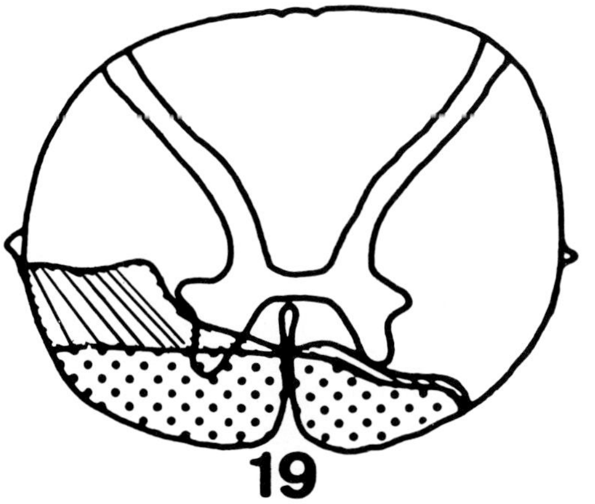

Fig. 31-5. This lesion, with relative sparing of the dorsal half of the left ventral quadrant, was accompanied by sensory loss maintained only below T11 on the right side. One would have expected the reverse, namely analgesia confined to the cervical and thoracic segments.

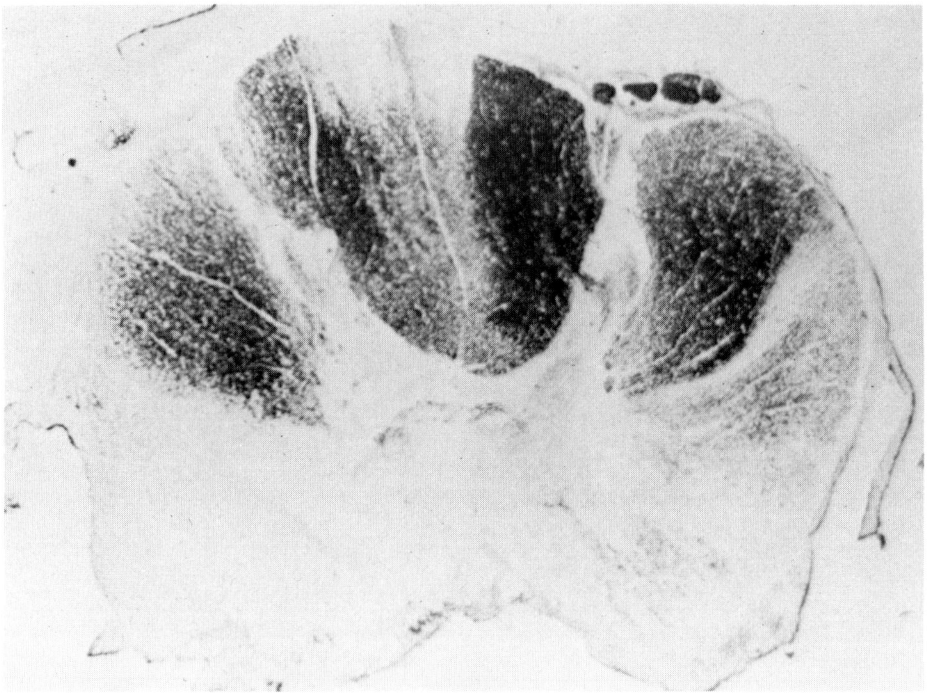

Fig. 31-6. Foerster and Gagel's Figure 29, showing cross section of cord at T5 level, indicating extent of bilateral incisions into anterior quadrants at same horizontal level. Today we would always stagger the two sides of such incisions at least 1 cord segment apart, making the lower incision no lower than T3. The surgical lesion produced analgesia of skin from T6 segment down, but senses of pressure pain, and temperature were not lost and the patient's spontaneous gastric crises continued. (Reproduced by permission from Sweet WH: Recent observations pertinent to improving anterolateral cordotomy, *Clinical Neurosurgery,* vol 23. Williams and Wilkins, Baltimore, 1976, p 83)

patient with such lesions, seen bilaterally at postmortem, who had had similar pain relief, analgesia, and normal strength in the limbs. Although Moossy and Rosomoff's cases 11 and 16 (Fig. 31-8) were not relieved of pain, no weakness of ipsilateral limbs was noted.

These unequivocal evidences of aberrant placement of motor pathways reminded me of the unexpected motor responses I was eliciting in single-shock stimulation inside the cord. In particular, I have evoked twitches in the *contralateral* forearm or hand near the lateral surface of the ventral quadrant of the cord, as judged by slight depth of penetration after an abrupt rise in impedance. The electrode was too superficial for the usual position of ventral corticospinal fibers. More striking, and of greater therapeutic importance, is evidence that the pain pathways may, at least in some patients, be confined to a smaller zone than we neurosurgeons have thought. The feasibility of protracted detailed sensory testing after each increment to the lesion at percutaneous cordotomy has permitted me to observe that either the initial few seconds of heating at 55°C, or some modest later increment of heating, may abruptly produce an extensive zone of analgesia.

My neuroscience colleague Dr. R. Sidman, hearing of my perplexity, advised me to consult Dr. P. Rakic. This investigator and Dr. P. Yakovlev had, by 1967, finished a comprehensive manuscript on variations in the anatomy of the pyramidal tracts in man. These tracts are the last to develop myelination and are still almost totally unmyelinated in the first month postpartum. Hence the absent myelination is striking in specimens stained for myelin.

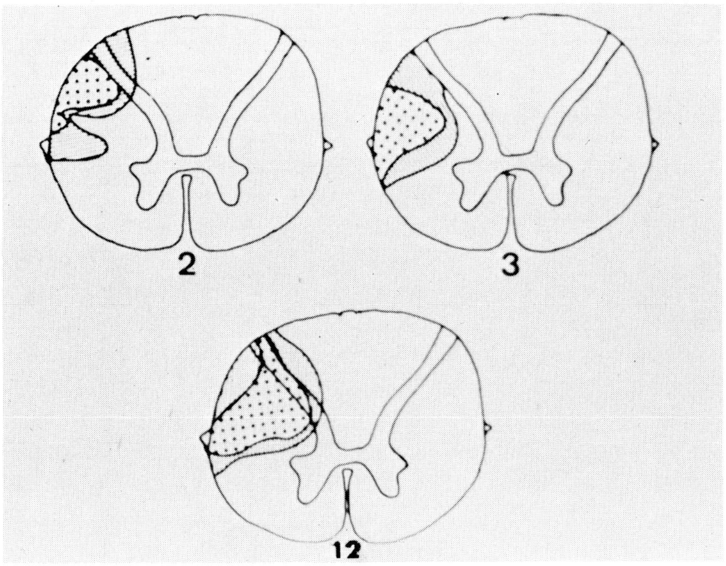

Fig. 31-7. Diagram of postmortem demonstration of cord lesions made at C1-2. All 3 of these patients had "an analgesic level to pin" and relief of pain of unstated duration, with no hemiparesis even though the lesion was confined to the posterolateral sector of the cord. (Reproduced by permission from Sweet WH: Craniospinal surgery for pain, AVENS. New York, NY)

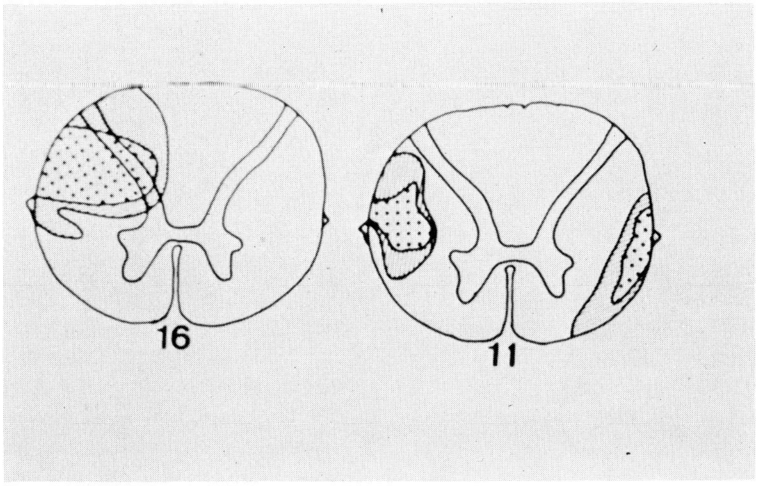

Fig. 31-8. Diagram of postmortem demonstration of cord lesions at C1-2. Similar lesions (noted in Fig. 31-7) in these 2 patients did not give pain relief but did not cause hemiparesis. (Reproduced by permission from Moossy J, et al: Percutaneous radiofrequency cervical cordotomy: pathological anatomy. J Neuropathol Exp Neurol 26:118, 1967)

These investigators studied serial sections of 144 specimens of human fetal or neonatal cords and/or brainstems. There were 94 specimens of medulla plus spinal cord, and 50 of spinal cord only. Rakic and Yakovlev managed an excellent summary of much of their study in the diagram presented as Figure 31-9. The textbook description of large crossed-lateral and smaller uncrossed ventral corticospinal tracts did indeed occur in 71.5% of the specimens. However, these tracts were usually far less symmetrical than illustrated in the diagram of pattern C; the authors state that the pyramidal tracts were patently unequal in 81 of the 103 pattern-C specimens. In 82% of these 81 the tracts were mainly on the right side. 66 of the specimens were of both medulla and cord; in 94% of these specimens the pyramid that began its decussation more rostrally continued this process to a more nearly complete crossing than did the other pyramid.

Even more important for the neurosurgeon are the major variations revealed in patterns A and B in which no uncrossed corticospinal tract occurred, respectively, bilaterally and unilaterally. This was seen in 36 (25%) of the specimens and, as shown in Figure 31-10, results in a grosser displacement of myelinated fiber tracts than the diagrams indicate. Both Figures 31-10 and 31-11 reveal the clarity with which the myelin stain depicts the anomalous distribution. Bok[16] in 1928 (Fig. 31-12), had described gross asymmetries in the pyramidal

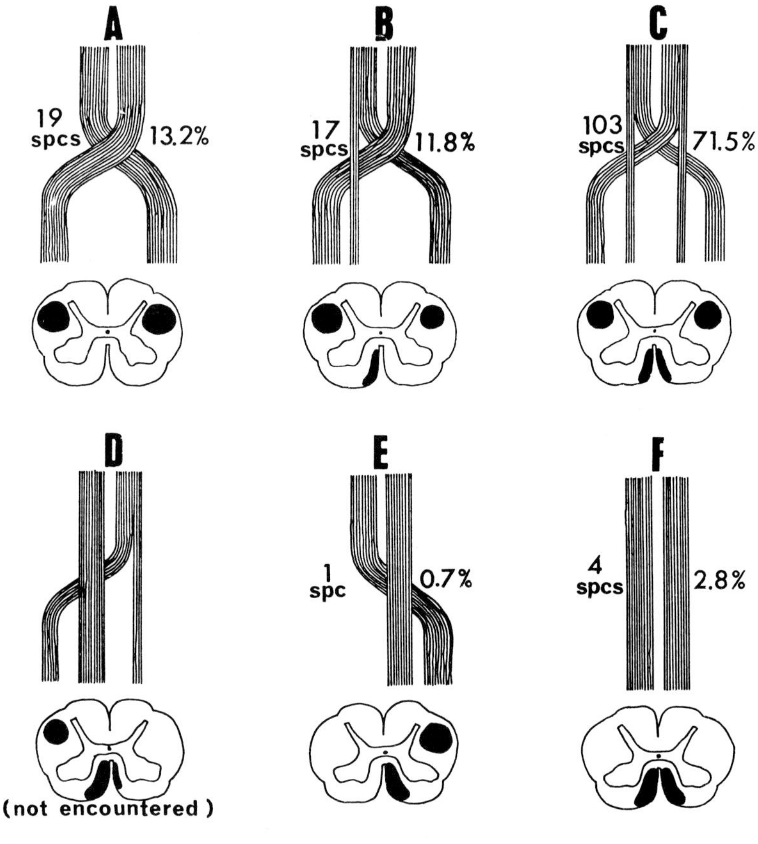

Fig. 31-9. Diagram of disposition of pyramidal tracts in cords of 144 specimens of human fetal or neonatal spinal cords and/or brainstem. Although pattern C is shown in the diagram as bilaterally symmetrical, the pyramidal tracts were "patently unequal" in 81 of 103 specimens. (Reproduced by permission from Sweet WH: Recent observations pertinent to improving anterolateral cordotomy, *Clinical Neurosurgery,* vol 23. Williams and Wilkins, Baltimore, 1976, p 86)

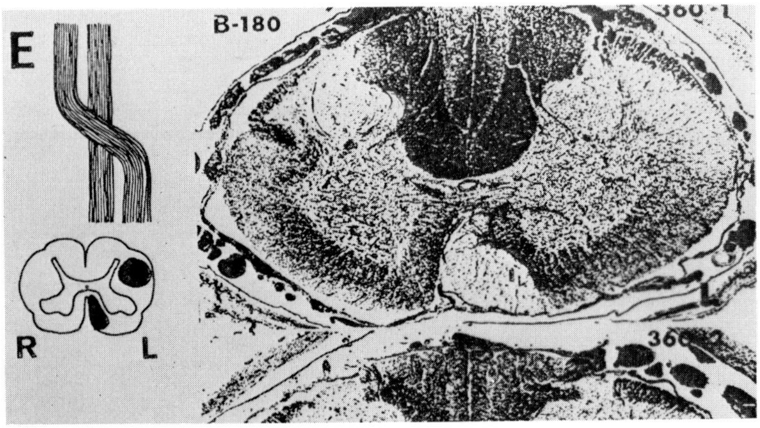

Fig. 31-10. Pattern E. All pyramidal tract fibers lie on one side of the cord. (Reproduced by permission from Sweet WH: Recent observations pertinent to improving anterolateral cordotomy, *Clinical Neurosurgery,* vol 23. Williams and Wilkins, Baltimore, 1976, p 87)

tract, but the great frequency with which these occur and, hence their significance for neurosurgeons, has been determined only by Rakic. It should be emphasized that Rakic's material did not contain a large number of anatomic congenital lesions. In fact in only 1 of his 36 specimens with pattern A or B were malformations described in the obstetric or autopsy record, and these were visceral and not neural. Although his work, at the present time, has been published only in abbreviated form without illustrations, Rakic has kindly allowed me to present his crucially important documentation to the neurosurgical fraternity.

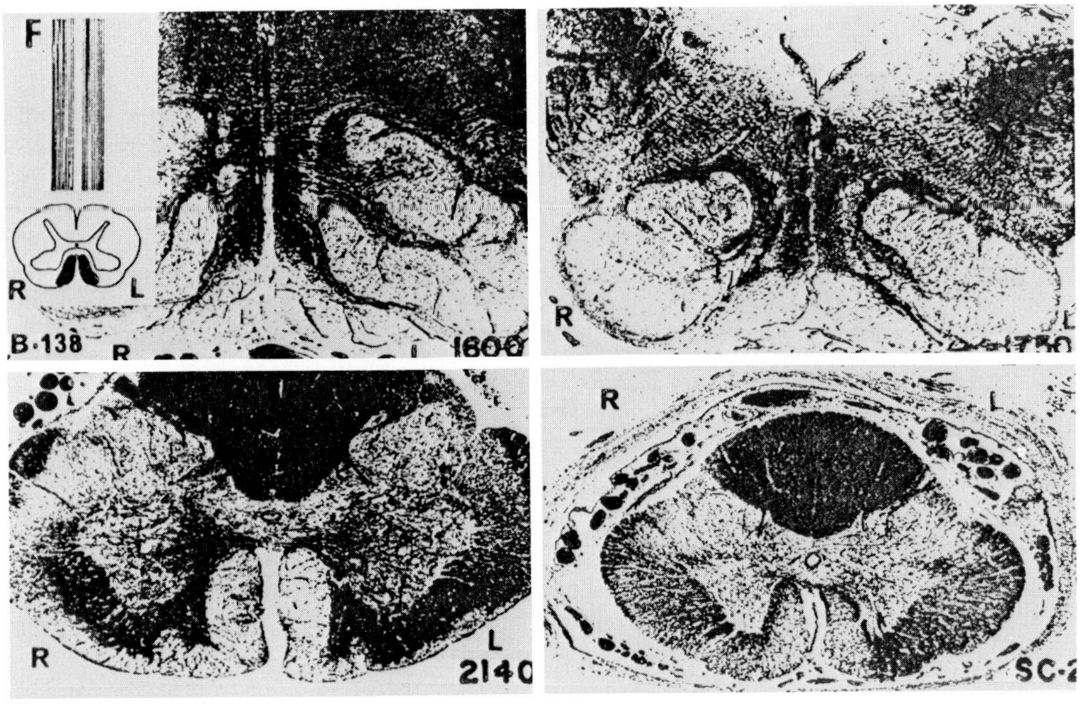

Fig. 31-11. Pattern F. All pyramidal fibers lie ventromedially. (Sections 2140 and Sc-2 Courtesy of Rakic and Yakovlev, unpublished data)

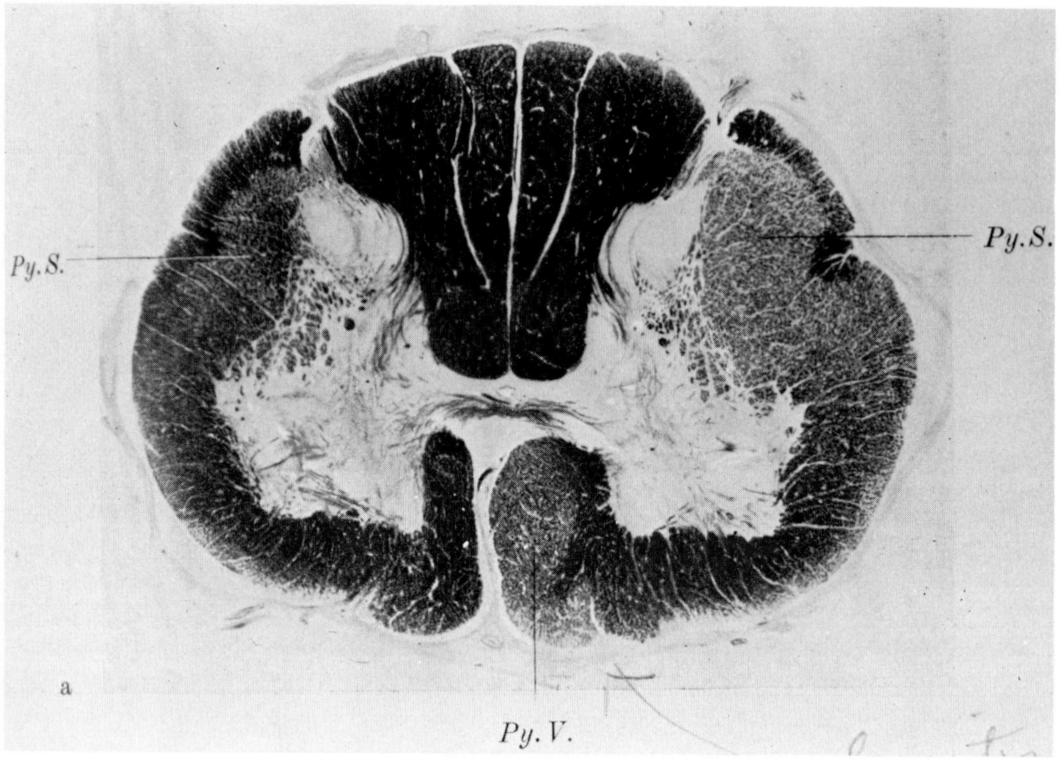

Fig. 31-12. Cervical cord of 6-month-old child. Py.S. and Py.V. on right side of illustration show gross enlargement of the unmyelinated tracts as compared with the tiny unmyelinated lateral pyramidal tracts and no ventral pyramidal tract on left. (Reproduced by permission from Sweet WH: Recent observations pertinent to improving anterolateral cordotomy, *Clinical Neurosurgery,* vol 23. Williams and Wilkins, Baltimore, 1976, p 89)

It seems unlikely that sensory pathways are distributed in a more stereotyped fashion than are motor pathways and, even if they are, the gross discrepancies in the motor tracts must push the sensory tracts into unusual positions. Hence, it is clear that in every patient we must seek to determine where pain pathways lie in the cord. A really satisfactory method for doing this remains to be developed.

Technical Details of Percutaneous Cordotomy

These are well described in the AVENS video-casette tape, monograph, and slides prepared by Mullan and Rosomoff; each gives an account of his technique. At first I used the relatively firm fixation of the patient's head and electrodes, developed by Rosomoff, but minor movements of the patient's head and neck worried me re a cutting movement of the fixed electrode shaft. This worry was crystallized into a change in technique when I learned of a patient who had casually but abruptly turned his head during the procedure and promptly died from a significant transsection of his cord. A shift to the absolutely firm fixation of the skull in the Todd-Wells stereotaxic apparatus was pursued for over a year. This inexorably firm fixation proved unattractive to enough patients so that I reverted to the Rosomoff head-holding equipment, but simply let the electrode rest on top of the post attached to a mechanical stage movable precisely in all three directions. If the patient does make a significant movement of his head, he carries the electrode with him, rather than use it as an internal guillotine. The head lies in sufficient extension so that subsequently injected air will remain in the spinal canal and not produce headache related to unwanted entry intracranially.

A few points about the electrode and its metal sheath are in order. We find that we must aim the 18-gauge, thin-walled, insulated sheath-needle in the proper direction to the very best of our ability before we ever penetrate the dura. It is not as easy to reguide it by markedly elevating or lowering the shaft as we had hoped. One aims 1 to 2 mm ventral to the midpoint of the anteroposterior diameter of the bony spinal canal. Injection of 1 to 2 ml of lidocaine 1% into the epidural space should precede penetration of the dura. Then I favor Mullan's method of injecting a mixture of air, Pantopaque, and cerebrospinal fluid (CSF). Once the subarachnoid space has been entered, the most reliable anatomic landmark is the ventral surface of the cord. I seek to delineate this both by air and Pantopaque. To do this the needle hub is temporarily depressed markedly so that the mixture of 1.0 ml of Pantopaque, emulsified with 0.5 ml of 1% lidocaine, in 2.0 ml of CSF, and 10 ml of air, will be directed ventral to the cord. Our initial reliance upon air at this stage has led us to presume that the front of the cord was more ventral than was the case. Mullan's use of Pantopaque lying on the dentate ligament, shows a less reliable landmark, as was pointed out at the beginning of this chapter.

As one seeks to determine the relation of the electrode to the cord, I find the measurement of impedance valuable as initiated by Becker and Nulsen.[17] On the Radionics impedance meter, with an electrode 0.5 mm in diameter, the impedance is around 200 to 250 Ohms in CSF, moving to between 500 and 750 Ohms within the cord. As Organ and Tasker[18] have pointed out, a pulsation of the reading with the heart beat indicates only partial engagement of the electrode with the cord. With their apparatus, the meter reads 350 to 550 Ohms with the electrode free in the cord and over 1,000 when it is completely within the cord. Since the cord may be pushed away by the advancing electrode and adhere to it as it is withdrawn, this delineation of the actual position of the electrode is most helpful.

Once the electrode is in the cord, opinions differ markedly as to the localizing value of sensations induced by electrical stimulation. Gentle electrical stimulation of primary afferent fibers yields a reference of sensation that on the whole is a reliable indicator of where the sensory loss will be after a radiofrequency (RF) heat lesion. This applies both to the posterior roots and to primary afferent fibers in the bulbar trigeminal tract. Thus, in one group of 158 consecutive procedures in which I stimulated posterior trigeminal rootlets with a 50-cycle square-wave pulse, in all but 8 patients subsequent analgesia after heating was in the same division of the trigeminal branches as the electrically evoked sensation. It was also in this same division in all but 9 of these same patients when gentle RF heat (42° to 50°C) was the stimulus.

For reasons that are entirely mysterious, either RF heating or surgical cutting of secondary afferent pain pathways in the cord or brainstem usually causes no sensation at all. While this fact permits one to enlarge lesions in the cord by minute increments, without intravenous anesthesia, its corollary of erratic responses to electrical stimulation in these pathways poses an as yet unresolved dilemma. Rosomoff decided that he got so little help from electrical stimulation that he does not do it as part of his operative procedure. Mazars[19] said he characteristically elicited no response to stimulation at sites wherein a lesion produces analgesia. Tasker[20] on the other hand has found that in 94% of his 240 percutaneous cordotomies at sites yielding satisfactory analgesia, prior stimulation had elicited a contralateral warm or cool tingle. However, the converse is also true, i.e., only patchy analgesia or loss of sensation confined to a leg is seen in a significant percentage of patients who had an appropriate contralateral sensation on stimulation. Mullan[21] also relies heavily on the results of square-wave stimulation. He states that when the electrode is on target, a stimulus of 0.25 V 20 pulses 75/sec produces a sensation of tingling, numbness, cold, or rarely heat at the appropriate area. When the threshold is above 0.75 V, he states that the electrode must be repositioned.

Mayer and others[22] found that 50 second, monophasic, rectangular wave cathodal pulses of 0.2 msec duration, delivered in 1-second trains, into the anterolateral quadrant of the cord caused pain referred to the contralateral side of the body. In 7 of their 13 patients in whom such pain occurred at a threshold of 300 μAmp or less, a complete analgesia from C3 to C5 was then produced by a radiofrequency signal at 50 mAmp for 5 seconds. In the 6 patients whose pain threshold was from 300 to 1,000 μAmp, the same radiofrequency parameters yielded a less complete sensory loss. I have found that the patient tolerates the added times required for such stimulation, if the analgesic fentanyl and the neuroleptic droperidol in the mixture called Innovar are given initially in a 1.0 or 2.0 ml dose intravenously. Since the analgesic effect of fentanyl lasts only 30 minutes to 1 hour, whereas the sedative and tranquilizing effects of droperidol last about four times as long, only the intravenous fentanyl will have to be repeated in doses of 0.05 mg intravenously at a time, unless the procedure continues for more than 2 hours.

There is, however, no question but that motor responses, best produced by single-shock stimuli, are of value. Typically of course, in the lateral corticospinal tract one elicits ipsilateral jerks and in the ventral corticospinal tract contralateral jerks in the limbs or torso, whereupon one moves the electrode. Of positive value are jerks of the ipsilateral neck muscles, usually the trapezius, indicating, when at ~0.5 V, that the electrode is near cells in the ventral horn or axons leading therefrom into the white matter. A lesion at this site or a little more superficial may be fruitful.

Unhappily, details of the anatomy, and especially the variation of motor pathways in man, are not known.[23] The ventral pyramidal tract may end anywhere from the highest thoracic to the upper lumbar segments. However, the fibers leaving the tract in the upper cord segments may not all innervate upper limbs or torso. Bok[16] has cited evidence that they may gradually pass to the lateral pyramidal bundle before they terminate. Moreover the anatomists are not certain how many ventral pyramidal fibers fail to undergo the typical crossover just before they terminate at a ventral horn cell. Hence an ipsilateral rather than a contralateral motor response in limb or torso may occur upon stimulation of the ipsilateral ventral pyramidal tract.

Even more confusing is the possibility of a "ventrolateral pyramidal tract" described by Barnes,[24] Swank[25] and others. This aberrant bundle moves laterally away from the pyramidal tract at the level of the twelfth cranial nerve. Both of the aforementioned observers have seen it extend in some cases as low as the lumbar region. The sort of motor function it has is unknown. Another complication is the evidence assembled by Nathan and Smith[26] for spinocortical fibers intermingling with motor lateral corticospinal fibers in the upper cervical cord. We do not know whether their stimulation causes any sensation in man. It is clear that there is an abundance of room for critical charting of our electrode positions and stimulation findings at percutaneous cordotomy if we are to improve the results of this procedure.

For the lesion itself, most workers have contented themselves with recording voltage, current, and time and have increased these stepwise. I have used thermistor monitoring of the temperature at the electrode just as in my method for trigeminal lesions. The Radionics Instrument Company has recently developed a cordotomy electrode of only 0.508 mm, which is equal to 0.0198 inch in diameter, containing a thermistor, so that such units are now generally available. As in the trigeminal lesions some individuals require much less of an increment in electrical parameters to produce a given rise in temperature than do others.

I have had one patient, who at 80°C for a few seconds, suddenly cried out that she felt a peculiar sensation all over her body. The heating was stopped but a bilateral analgesia gradually developed from the neck down, followed by a severe quadriparesis. At post mortem, 1 month later, a thrombosis of the anterior spinal artery was seen. I have avoided this and other major sequelae by heating no higher than 70°C, changing the position of the electrode if that temperature fails to give the required analgesia.

Radionics Instrument Company's latest radiofrequency lesion generator provides six different rates, from 5 to 100 per second, and five different durations of rectangular wave pulses, from 0.1 to 2.0 msec, so that there is ample opportunity to try for optimal parameters to elicit sensory responses as well as control temperature. An impedance monitor with audio control is included. During the making of each lesion, it is helpful to have the patient keep the ipsilateral limb elevated so that impending paresis can be detected at once.

Another troublesome problem seen is pain in the posterior cervical and/or occipital region as higher temperatures are used, even with the electrode in good position within the cord. Mullan[21] stated: "It may be that the patient will have to endure some of this severe pain in order to achieve a good sensory loss." We have dealt with this either by an intravenous injection of Brevital (methohexital) or preferably by an injection of 0.2 ml of 1% lidocaine into the lumen of the electrode sheath. The 0.5-mm electrode shaft does not completely fill the lumen of the 18-gauge, thin-walled electrode sheath needle and the Radionics unit includes a sidearm on that sheath needle which permits this injection into the spinal fluid without disturbing the correctly placed electrode. I assume, from the affect of lidocaine, that the pain is due to the spread of heat to the C2 posterior rootlets. We know that trigeminal posterior rootlets, when heated to ~50°C, give rise to intolerable pain. The fact that such spread of heat is occurring, however, is a warning that we may be injuring more of the cord than we wish, and the phenomenon is a further stimulus to achieve more precise localization of a hopefully concentrated pain fiber bundle.

The need for vigilant monitoring of all aspects of the procedure is crucial. In one patient the electrode extended more than the intended 4 mm beyond its sheath; the locking screw on the electrode collar was found to have loosened. After this radiograph had been taken, careful examination showed a little weakness of the opposite arm; presumably the electrode had penetrated the opposite lateral corticospinal tract. In the new Radionics unit the electrode cannot extend more than 4 mm beyond the 18-gauge sheath, and I now applied a spring clip to the shaft of the sheath, against the skin of the neck, to prevent the shaft from creeping in as well. That such precautions are not redundant is emphasized by the 2 postmortem specimens of Figure 31-13 from the work of Moossy and Rosomoff.[13] In both cases a unilateral lesion was intended, but the bilateral lesion made caused significant respiratory difficulties.

This leads to another important matter, ie., my impression that it is usually inadvisable to make a cord lesion on the other side at the C1-2 level, because of the danger of respiratory paralysis during sleep (Ondine's syndrome). Rosomoff had, by 1976, done 258 bilateral cordotomies and reassures us that "the syndrome is usually self-limiting, lasting up to 3

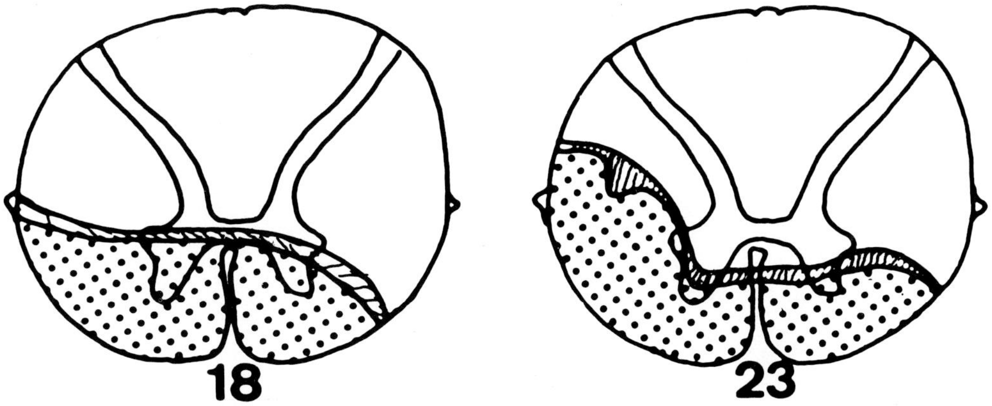

Fig. 31-13. Case of Moossy-Rosomoff. The white matter lateral to each ventral horn contains the respiratory regulating fibers relevant to preventing sleep-induced apnea. Its destruction on both sides was followed by this symptom in both patients in whom only a unilateral lesion was intended. (Reproduced by permission from Sweet WH: Craniospinal surgery for pain, Audiovisual Education in Neurosurgery [AVENS], 1973.)

weeks, and very occasionally, for longer." One patient who was brought through the initial first month of sleep-induced apnea in an intensive care unit was found dead in bed some months later after a dose of hypnotics the night before. Her relatives brought suit against the neurosurgeon for professional negligence in performing such operations and he settled the case out of court for several score thousands of dollars. Particularly troublesome is the fact that the areas containing the important fibers for reflex control of respiration appear to be just lateral to the ventral horns. In all but case 13 of Figure 31-14 both lesions included this area. The 4 patients whose cords are shown in this figure had had bilateral lesions and all developed sleep-induced apnea. Since the relevant fibers partially abut upon or may comingle with the fibers for pain, destroying the latter without destroying the former is hard to achieve. If the surgeon proposes C1-2 cordotomy on the second side, he would do well to explain in writing the special risks entailed by this procedure, not only to respiratory but to bowel and bladder function also.

Because dissatisfaction with the results of cordotomy has been such a prolific source of malpractice actions in this country, I discuss with the patients the document reproduced in the appendix to this chapter. It not only provides evidence that I have explained the risks of the operation but serves an even more important purpose of letting the patient know how helpful and important his cooperation will be during intraoperative testing.

Examples from my operative protocols explain my uncertainties. Patient Edward T. may have had an unusually large lateral pyramidal tract. In Figure 31-15A the electrode tip lies 4 mm on the film or 3 mm in vivo in front of the unusually clear line of Pantopaque on the

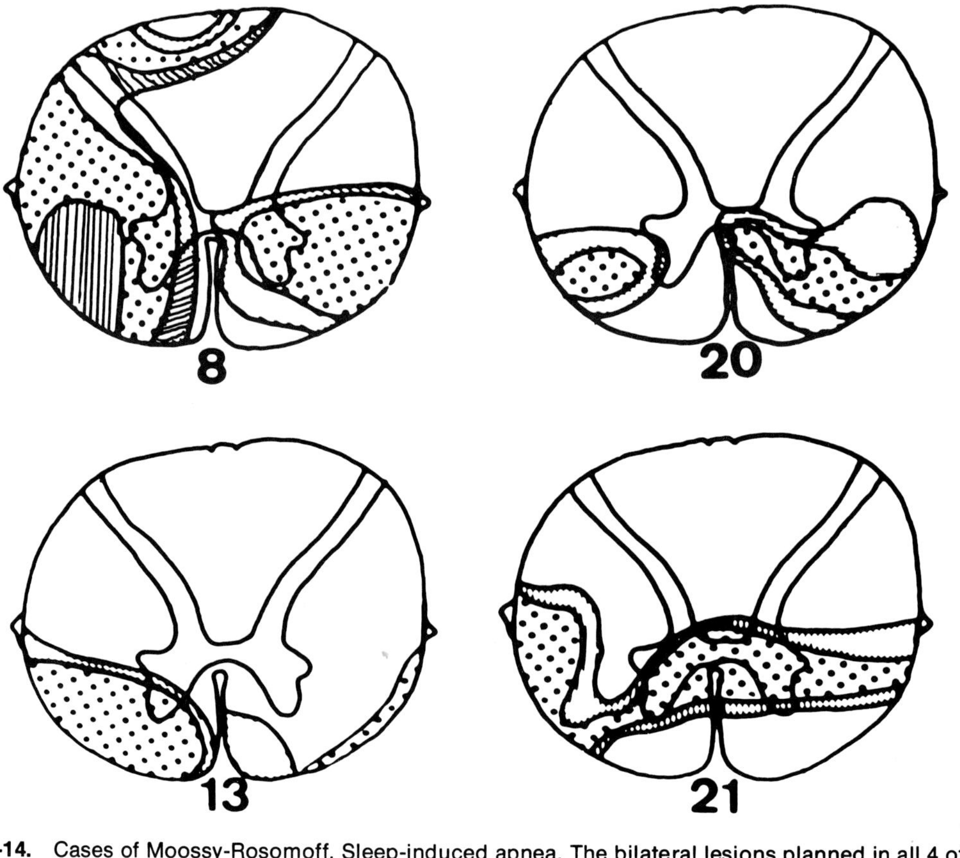

Fig. 31-14. Cases of Moossy-Rosomoff. Sleep-induced apnea. The bilateral lesions planned in all 4 of these patients were followed by respiratory difficulties. In all but case 13 there is a lesion lateral to each ventral horn.

dentate ligament. This ligament lies exactly at the midpoint of the anteroposterior dimension of the bony spinal canal and 11/25 of the distance from the anterior dura, shown by air, and the posterior dura, shown by the more dorsal of the two streaks of Pantopaque. At three different depths, 1.0 mm apart, along the same horizontal line, and all within the cord, as judged by the impedance, single shocks at 0.5 V caused only ipsilateral sternomastoid twitches. There was no other sensation on continuous stimulation at 50 cps. Assuming I had to be in or lateral to the anterior horns, I made six progressively larger lesions, the last at 60°C for 30 seconds. No sensation had been evoked at any interlesion stimulus. He now complained of numbness and was virtually paralyzed in his ipsilateral upper limb (the lower had already been paralyzed by his malignant tumor). There was no clearcut hypalgesia. I concluded that I was probably in ventrally placed lateral corticospinal fibers; the weakness would presumably have been in the contralateral arm had I destroyed ventral corticospinal fibers. So I placed the electrode 2.5 mm more ventrally in vivo—just within the cord—as judged by the pulsating air shadow at fluoroscopy (Fig. 31-15B). Here, at a threshold of 1.2 V at 50 cps, the *ipsilateral* leg at first felt pressure; later such a stimulus caused a "pulsing" sensation there. Soon the response changed to a cold tingle at 0.3 V in the *contralateral* forearm. Repeat radiographs revealed no clearcut change in the position of the electrode. The first lesion here, at only 55°C for only 5 seconds, produced unequivocal analgesia throughout the contralateral lower limb and nowhere else. One must conclude that the pain fibers from that limb were concentrated at that site, despite the different reference of sensation on stimulation. This lesion was gradually increased in size in eight small steps. Contralateral analgesia from C4-S5 had ensued after only 65°C for 15 seconds. Interlesion stimulations never evoked any sensation outside the contralateral shoulder and upper limb; yet the analgesia gradually increased from below upward.

Although the patient's pain was confined to the lower torso and lower limb, we sought to destroy all the pain pathways we could with a moderate degree of heating. *Even when the*

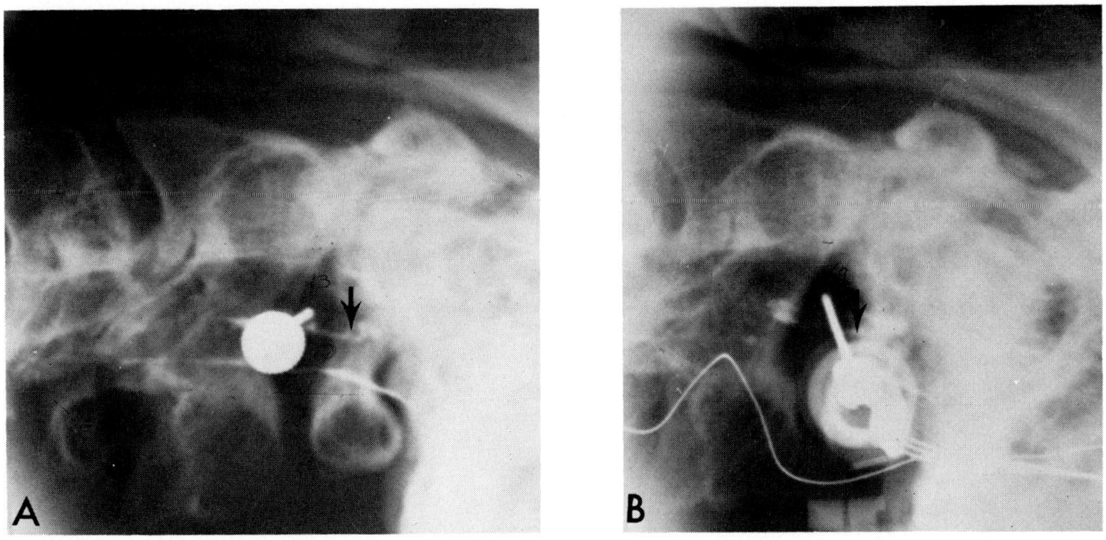

Fig. 31-15. Edward T. Lateral views upper cervical spine, patient supine, after injection through electrode sheath of 0.5 ml Pantopaque and 0.5 ml of 1% lidocaine emulsified with 3.0 ml CSF and 10 ml of air. **A.** Electrode tip 3 mm ventral to line of Pantopaque lying ventral to dentate ligament (arrow). In this position the electrode produced paralysis of the ipsilateral arm. **B.** Electrode tip 5.5 mm ventral to same line of Pantopaque (arrow). In this position the electrode heated to 55°C for 5 seconds produced complete analgesia of the contralateral lower limb. (Reproduced by permission from Sweet WH: Recent observations pertinent to improving anterolateral cordotomy, *Clinical Neurosurgery,* vol 23. Williams and Wilkins, Baltimore, 1976, p 91)

painful area has been differentially rendered analgesic, I think it better judgment to increase the analgesic zone, doing this gradually and stopping at any untoward sign and before intense heat is reached. A major problem with cordotomy in later follow-ups is the fading of analgesia and return of pain. This is more likely to occur with incomplete lesions of the whole pain bundle.

Even production of a contralateral warm or cool tingle is not an invariable harbinger of success. Thus in one patient with left midthoracic pain, we were delighted that he felt, at the start of the procedure, a warm precordial tingle at 0.5 V, or at 0.65 V an indescribable sensation in the left shoulder. Single shocks at 0.6 V caused jerks of the uppermost ipsilateral (right) trapezius. Yet increasing lesions, the ninth at 70°C for 10 seconds, achieved no maintained analgesia. Severe hypalgesia or analgesia in the same zone of upper or lower contralateral segments after a small lesion would be followed by fading of the sensory loss after the next larger lesion. Stimulation at 50 cps between lesions had caused sensations now on one side and now on the other in the upper torso or upper limb. Figure 31-16, showing the ventral aspect of the cord and the dentate ligament's origin, makes it clear that we had to be in the classical position of the pain pathways since no motor weakness developed. In this patient they must have lain more ventrally. The advantage of a clear picture with Pantopaque of the ventral surface of the cord is illustrated by the demonstration of a slight upward angulation of the cord impaled by the electrode in Figure 31-16A, whereas there is a slight concavity of the ventral surface later on in the procedure as the angle of the electrode shaft in the dorsolateral plane apparently changed (Fig. 31-16B). The distance between the ventral surface of the cord and the electrode tip remained the same.

I am now so convinced that we must maximize our efforts to make a small critically placed lesion that I have extended the tactic of controlled flexible search to open cordotomy. It is, of course, easier under direct vision to be certain of the exact electrode site. The principal problem has been to hold the electrode in precisely the desired spot once it has been

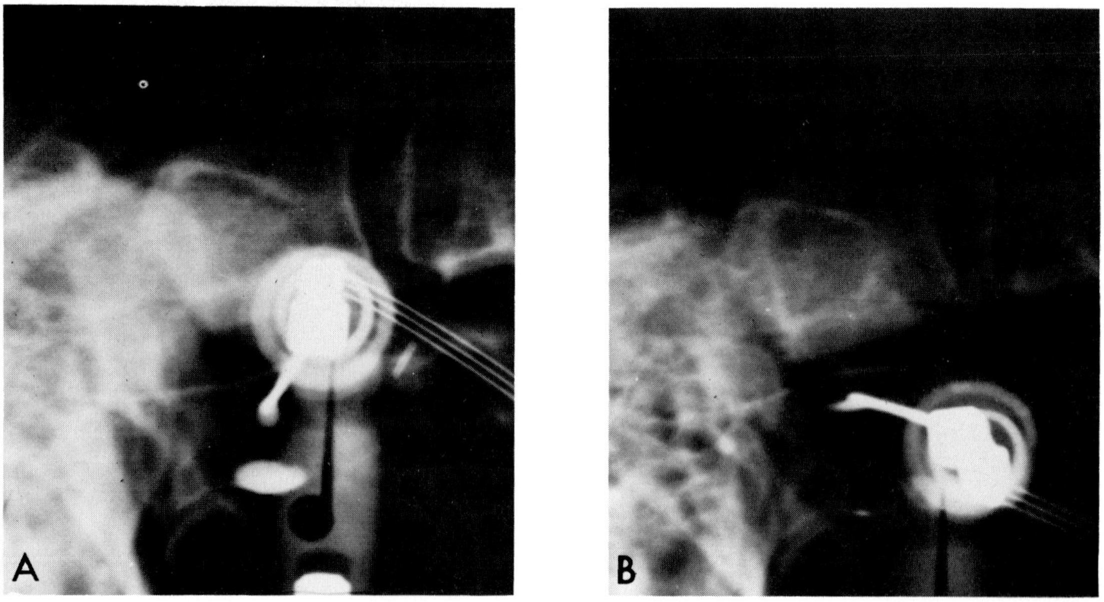

Fig. 31-16. Alexander T. C1-2 percutaneous cordotomy. Demonstration of ventral aspect of cord with emulsified Pantopaque (two arrows), showing how convincing this landmark is and how the cord can be deformed slightly by electrode insertion. **A.** At start and **B** at end of lesion-making sequence. A globule of Pantopaque lies ventral to dentate ligament and dorsal to electrode tip (arrow). (Reproduced by permission from Sweet WH: Recent observations pertinent to improving anterolateral cordotomy, *Clinical Neurosurgery*, vol. 23. Williams and Wilkins, Baltimore, 1976, p 93)

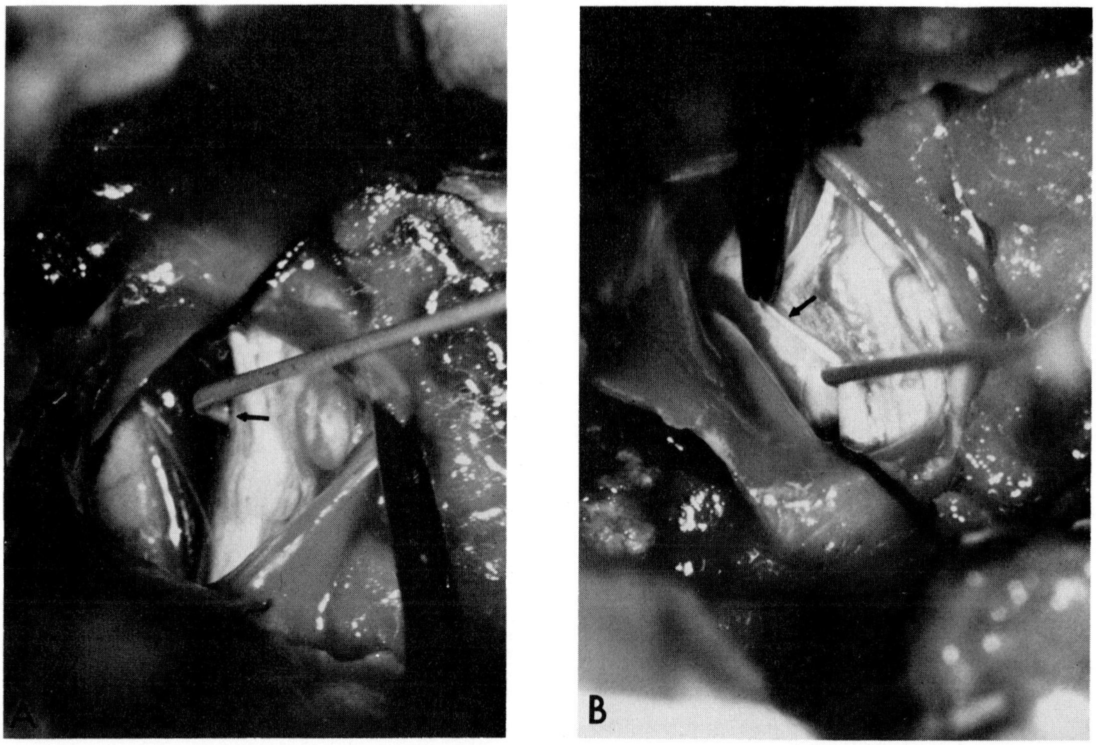

Fig. 31-17. Irvin F. Exposure left side of cord at T2 level. **A.** Bipolar electrode held firmly in Dott retractor clamps and tip inserted 2 mm ventral to origin of dentate ligament. **B.** Cord rotated back into normal position by drawing dentate ligament laterally during stimulation and lesion making. (Reproduced by permission from Sweet WH: Recent observations pertinent to improving anterolateral cordotomy, *Clinical Neurosurgery*, vol 23. Williams and Wilkins, Baltimore, 1976, p 94)

found. The Dott self-retaining retractor assembly accomplishes this. Figure 31-17A shows a right-angle electrode insulated, except at the tip, fixed a measurable distance into the cord through a pial opening 2 mm ventral to the origin of the dentate ligament. (The Dott retaining unit is not shown.) In Figure 31-17B the dentate ligament has been released, allowing the cord to fall back into its normal position. The fixation has maintained the electrode position within the cord as the awakened patient moves about during sensory testing. I use this procedure when a cordotomy is required on the second side and the pain does not involve segments above T4.

Summary

A fundamental change has occurred in my thinking about the tactics to be employed in cordotomy, ie., instead of making a maximal lesion in the anterior quadrant consistent with avoiding motor weakness, one should seek the precise location of the pain fibers and try to destroy them only. Evidence has been presented not only that these fibers are far more variable in their location than we had hitherto realized, but also that at least in some patients, they are probably compact. Methods have been suggested to improve the accuracy and safety of identifying these fibers, but it is clear that electrical stimulation, by any parameters as yet defined, is an inadequate solution. Innovative thinking is in order.

REFERENCES

1. Mullan S, Harper PV, Hekmatpanah J, et al: Percutaneous interruption of spinal pain tracts by means of a strontium[90] needle. *J Neurosurg 20*:931-939, 1963
2. Kahn EA, Barney BF: Anterolateral cordotomy for intractable pain of tabes dorsalis. *Arch Neurol Psychiatr 38*:467-472, 1937
3. Hyndman OR, van Epps C: Possibility of differential section of the spinothalamic tract. A clinical and histologic study. *Arch Surg 38*:1036-1053, 1939
4. Voris HC: Variations in the spinothalamic tract in man. *J Neurosurg 14*:55-60, 1957
5. White JC, Sweet WH: Pain: Its Mechanisms and Neurosurgical Control. Charles C Thomas, Springfield, Illinois, 1955
6. Mazars GJ: État actuel de la chirurgie de la douleur. *Neurochirurgie 22:Suppl 1*:1976
7. French LA, Chou SN, Story JL: Cervical tractotomy: technique and clinical usefulness, Pain. Edited by RS Knighton, PR Dumke. Little Brown and Co, Boston, 1966, pp 311-319
8. Sweet WH, White JC, Selverstone B, et al: Sensory responses from anterior roots and from surface and interior of spinal cord in man. *Trans Am Neurol Assoc 74*:165-169, 1950
9. White JC, Richardson EP, Jr, Sweet WH: Upper thoracic cordotomy for relief of pain. Postmortem correlation of spinal incision with analgesic levels in 18 cases. *Ann Surg 144*:407-420, 1956
10. French LA, Peyton WT: Ipsilateral sensory loss following cordotomy. *J Neurosurg 5*:403-404, 1948
11. Voris HC: Ipsilateral sensory loss following cordotomy: report of a case. *Arch Neurol Psychiatr J Neurosurg 14*:55-60,1957
12. Schwartz HG: High cervical cordotomy: technique and results. *Clin Neurosurg 8*:282-293, 1962
13. Moossy J, Sagone A, Rosomoff HL: Percutaneous radiofrequency cervical cordotomy: pathological anatomy. *J Neuropathol Exp Neurol 26*:118, 1967
14. Foerster O: Die Vorderseitenstrangleitung, Handbuch der Neurologie, vol 5. Edited by O Bumke, O Foerster. Springer, Berlin, 1936, pp 320-340
15. Kurze T: Personal communication, 1975
16. Bok ST: Das Ruckenmark, Handbuch der Mikroscopischen Anatomie des Menschen Nervensystem, vol 4. Edited by W von Möllendorf. Springer, Berlin, 1928, pp 562-567
17. Becker DP, Nielsen FE: Control of lesion making in percutaneous cordotomy. Presented at the 76th Meeting of the Society of British Neurological Surgeons jointly with the Neurosurgical Society of America, New York, October 10-14, 1967
18. Organ LW, Tasker R: Percutaneous cervical cordotomies: technique using the lateral high cervical approach. Communication from the Department of Neurosurgery, Toronto General Hospital, Canada, September 1972
19. Mazars GJ: Discussion of Tasker et al. September 1975
20. Tasker RR, Organ LW, Rowe IJ, et al: The human spinothalamic tract. Stimulation mapping in the spinal cord and brain stem. Presented at the First World Congress on Pain, Florence, Italy, Sept 5-8, 1975
21. Mullan S: Percutaneous cordotomy. *J Neurosurg 35*:360-366, 1971
22. Mayer DJ, Price DD, Becker DP, et al: Threshold for pain from anterolateral quadrant stimulation as a predictor of
23. Bucy PC, Keplinger JE, Siqueira EB: Destruction of the pyramidal tract in man. *J Neurosurg 21*:385-398, 1964
24. Barnes S: Degeneration in hemiplegia with special reference to a ventrolateral pyramidal tract, the accessory fillet and Pick's bundle. *Brain 24*:463-501, 1901
25. Swank RL: The relationship between the circumolivary pyramidal fascicles and the pontobody in man. *J Comp Neurol 60*:309-317, 1934
26. Nathan PW, Smith MC: Spinocortical fibers in man. *J Neurol Neurosurg Psychiatr 18*:181-190, 1955
27. Rosomoff HL: Percutaneous radiofrequency cervical cordotomy for intractable pain. Presented at the Neurosurgical Postgraduate Course of Dr. GR Nugent, Morgantown, West Virginia, December 1975

Appendix

Statement for Patient

Cordotomy

The operation called *cordotomy* has as its objective stopping pain by destroying those pathways in the spinal cord, which transmit impulses related to pain and temperature. (Extremes of hot and cold are also painful.) Fortunately nerve fibers that have this function tend to cluster together high in the spinal cord, so that it is usually possible to destroy them without taking away too many other important functions. After those fibers enter the cord, they cross to the opposite side, so that for example, to relieve left-sided pain, we destroy on the right side of the cord. Although we know roughly the location of these pathways in man, we also know that they vary in position from person to person and are, to a varying degree, mixed in with fibers that have other duties. Hence a major part of our task in any given individual is to determine exactly where these pathways lie in him or her. We seek to do this by the patient's responses to gentle electrical stimulation. Oddly enough, and for reasons we do not understand, this electrical stimulation within pain pathways of the spinal cord only infrequently causes pain! However, this fact makes the whole job of trying to locate these pathways much less of an ordeal for the patient. When the electrode lies in the area for pain, we find that the patient may feel any of a variety of sensations on the side of the body on which we are seeking to provide pain relief. Motor fibers that cause movement of muscle are also activated at low voltage. These fibers, on the way out of the cord toward the muscles they are going to supply, cross at right angles, passing through the sensory fibers for pain ascending to the brain. Consequently, if we see tiny muscle twitches at the level of and on the side of the body at which our electrode lies, this is evidence that the electrode is in the right place to turn on heating current and start to destroy that area. Conversely, if we provoke contractions in some other part of the body, we are warned that destroying here will produce an undesired paralysis.

As a result of these types of observations in the patient, we can usually destroy the pain and temperature pathways by a process of gradual and repeated heating of the electrode without causing a major undesired weakness. We cannot, unfortunately, guarantee that we shall be able to either destroy all pain pathways and give adequate pain relief or avoid destruction of motor pathways with resultant paralysis. When such paralysis occurs, it is usually on the side opposite the pain because the motor fibers normally do not cross in the spinal cord the way pain fibers do. The pathways concerned with bowel, bladder, and sexual sensation and function lie so close to those for pain, all of these faculties are usually impaired after cordotomy on one side, and more seriously and lastingly impaired if a cordotomy is carried out on the opposite side. We seek to produce a state in which a pinprick no longer feels sharp over much or most of the limbs and torso on the painful side. With this degree and extent of sensory loss, the person usually has a satisfactory degree of relief of his spontaneous pain.

In addition to the small risk of death, total paralysis, and other less severe complications, another major complication after cordotomy occurs to a varying degree in 5% to 10% of the patients. This consists of the development, weeks to even years later, of progressively more disagreeable and widespread sensations in the area that formerly could not feel a pin as sharp. These sensations may become severe pains and be worsened by even slight touch so that in their worst form the patient cannot even tolerate clothing touching any of that part of the limbs or torso.

After some years, about half of the patients recover some capacity to feel a pin as sharp. With this recovery, pain may, in some degree, reappear.

The more favorable side of the picture is that we can usually relieve the original pain to a helpful degree without taking away the ability to either make strong coordinated movements or to feel touch and to know automatically where the limbs are in space.

Understood and agreed to: ____________________
Patient signature

Witness: ____________________

CHAPTER 32

Percutaneous Electrothermocoagulation of Spinal Nerve Trunk, Ganglion, and Rootlets

Sumio Uematsu

Editorial Note: The editors think it important to draw the reader's attention to the fact that there are almost no reports of the results of radiofrequency heating to destroy *spinal* posterior roots. Hence it is impossible to assess definitively the place of such surgery (if it has any) in our therapeutic armamentarium.

SELECTIVE SURGICAL INTERRUPTION OF posterior roots was first carried out by both Abbe[1] and Bennett[2] in 1889. This technique was later extended to sections of anterior roots for the treatment of motor disorders. However, the open surgical technique limits its applicability to some debilitated patients. Therefore efforts have been made to develop a less traumatic rhizotomy technique. Scoville[3] described a simplified approach for extradural spinal sensory rhizotomy. Dogliotti[4] proposed injecting ethanol alcohol, via lumbar puncture, into the subarachnoid space, while Maher[5] advocated the use of phenol solution. However, these hypobaric solutions must be injected with extreme caution since their penetration is likely to be unpredictable and C-fibers as well as the larger myelinated fibers may be destroyed.[6]

Electrothermocoagulation of the Gasserian ganglion for trigeminal neuralgia was introduced by Kirschner.[7] Later, it was abandoned because of the high complication rate due to the uncontrolled effect of the diathermy current. In October 1965, Sweet[8] introduced an advanced technique for electrothermocoagulation of the trigeminal ganglion. Accumulated clinical experience has shown that it is possible to alleviate pain and still preserve proprioception and motor function in the trigeminal nerve.[8] Based on physiologic studies, it has been assumed that the less myelinated pain fibers were more easily destroyed by heat than are the larger fibers. However, a preliminary histologic study revealed indiscriminate destruction of both small and large fibers rather than selectively destroy smaller, less myelinated ones. In my opinion, it is therefore logical to believe that the proportional destruction of nerve fibers increases the pain threshold but also preserves enough fibers for satisfactory proprioception and motor function (Fig. 32-1).

Our first percutaneous radiofrequency spinal rhizotomy was carried out in 1971 on an 18-year-old girl with spastic paraplegia due to spinal cord injury. Bilateral L1, L2, and L3 roots were denervated to reduce spasticity of the hip joints. The first successful result with

Department of Neurosurgery, The Johns Hopkins University School of Medicine, Baltimore, Maryland 21205

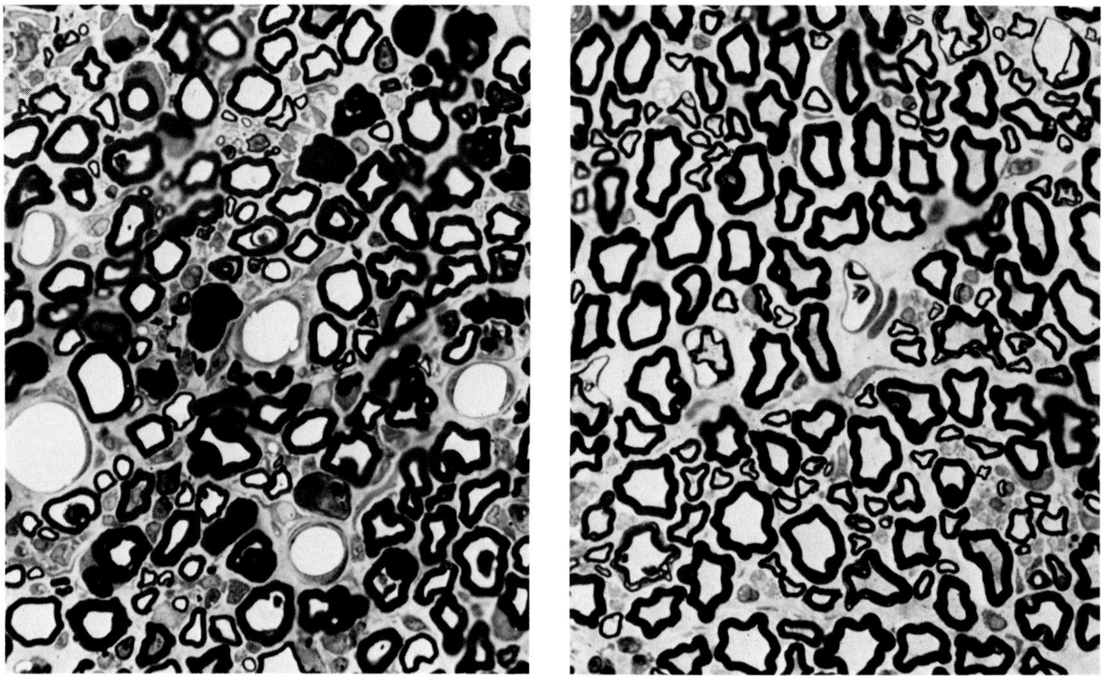

Fig. 32-1. Radiofrequency thermocoagulation of the sciatic nerve of a cat. **A.** Section taken at the site of the heat lesion. Note the indiscriminate effect of the heat on both the small and large myelinated fibers. The wall of the capillaries is well preserved. **B.** Control, proximal portion of same nerve, away from the heat lesion (Phosphotungstic acid hematoxylin, ×750).

this technique encouraged us to expand its use to other spinal levels for the treatment of pain and motor disorders.[9] Possibly, it could also be used to treat spasmodic torticollis,[10] cerebral palsy,[11] and spastic bladder dysfunction by differential denervation of sacral rootlets.[12]

The technique is relatively simple and definitely less invasive then surgical open rhizotomy. However, its success depends heavily upon the availability of a fluoroscopic x-ray monitor for precise stereotaxic introduction of the probe into the intervertebral foramen. The procedure should be carried out under local anesthesia. Careful observation of the response to electrical stimulation and the assessment of sensory and motor functions during the entire period of the procedure are essential to avoid undesirable complications.

Anatomy and Physiology

Rootlets, Ganglion, and Trunk

Each spinal nerve arises from the cord through two roots: a posterior sensory and an anterior motor root. These roots traverse the subarachnoid sac, penetrate the dura, and reach the intervertebral foramen, where the posterior roots swell into the spinal ganglion, which contains the cells of origin of sensory fibers. Distal to the ganglion, the posterior and anterior roots unite and emerge from the intervertebral foramen of a mixed spinal nerve or common nerve trunk, which contains both sensory and motor fibers (Fig. 32-2).

Each nerve root has the following five parts, based upon its meningeal covering and relationship to the intervertebral foramina.

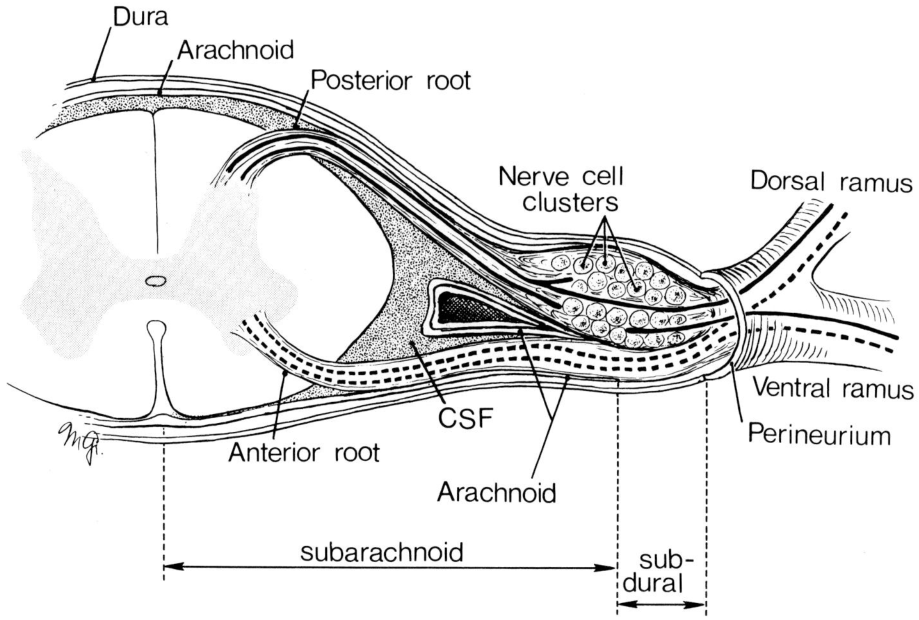

Fig. 32-2. Rootlets, ganglion and trunk. The subarachnoidal space stops at the proximal end of the ganglion.

1. Subarachnoid
2. Subdural
3. Extra dural
4. Intraforaminal
5. Extraforaminal

Dural and arachnoid sleeves surround both the anterior and posterior nerve roots. The nerves may sometimes be separated or fused, but the arachnoid membranes are definitely separated by the dura and each root is surrounded by its own extension of the subarachnoid space. The subarachnoid space stops at the proximal end of the ganglion on the posterior roots, and in the corresponding portion on the anterior roots. At this termination, there are three meningeal layers, which blend with the connective tissue of the peripheral nerves. The subarachnoid space is not believed to be continuous with either the perineural space or the lymphatic channels, but the subdural space is thought to be continuous with connective tissue of the peripheral nerves.

The posterior roots are, as a rule, thicker than the ventral ones and vary with the size of their respective ganglia. The only exception is the first cervical nerve, dorsal root of which is greatly reduced and often missing. The largest spinal nerves are the lower cervical and the first thoracic, which form the great nerve for the upper limbs and upper sacral nerve for the lower limbs. The smallest in size are the coccygeal nerve roots. Cervical nerve roots diminish in size from below and upwards.[13]

Radicular Artery

Most of the 62 embryologic radicular arteries regress during the course of development, and in the adult only six to eight functioning arteries supply the anterior while between 10 and 23 functioning arteries supply the posterior spinal artery. The radicular arteries, which actually supply the spinal cord, are called *radiculomedullary arteries*. They perfuse the cord via two terminal branches: the anterior and posterior radicular arteries (Fig. 32-3).

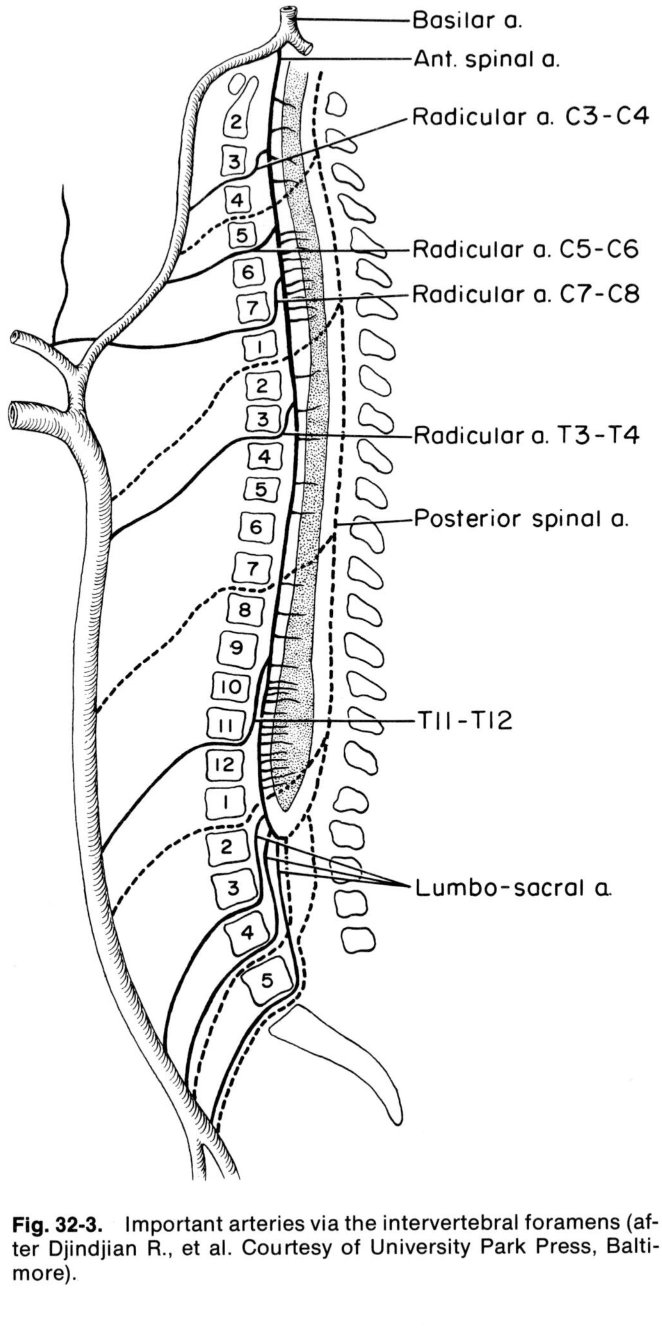

Fig. 32-3. Important arteries via the intervertebral foramens (after Djindjian R., et al. Courtesy of University Park Press, Baltimore).

The anterior radicular arteries run in the intervertebral foramina on the anterior surface of the dural investment of the spinal roots, and remain extradural until they reach the lateral border of the dural sheath proper. At this point they give off short to medium dural arteries. The anterior radicular arteries then pierce the dura anterior to, and slightly below, the nerve. The arteries then run upward at an angle that depends on the spinal level, always remaining anterior to the plane of the dentate ligament. The posterior radicular arteries, in general, run along the superior border of the nerve sheath, piercing the dura through the same opening as a nerve passing between the sensory nerve filaments, to reach the posterior spinal arteries, always remaining posterior to the plane of the dentate ligament.

The blood supply of the spinal cord may be jeopardized in certain transitional regions, where its arterial supply is derived from two different sources. Because the upper third of the spinal cord is supplied primarily by the anterior spinal artery, an occlusion of the C2 or C3 radicular artery, or an occlusion of the vertebral artery, can be revascularized effectively by the retrograde flow from the basilar artery. The inferior two-thirds, including the cervical enlargement, are supplied by a large artery, usually arising from the deep cervical artery, supplemented by a second artery, which is a branch of the first intercostal artery. In the presence of an obstruction of the subclavian artery, or an occlusion of the radicular artery at the interspace of C7 and C8, the only possible blood circulation comes from the contralateral subclavian system. The upper segment of the thoracic spinal cord, on the other hand, depends upon the radicular branches of the intercostal arteries. If one or more of the parent intercostal vessels is compressed, segments of the spinal cord, T1-4, could not be adequately maintained by the small branches of the anterior spinal artery. For this reason, thoracic segment T1-4, particularly T4, is considered a vulnerable area in the distribution of the anterior spinal artery. The posterior surface of the cord most susceptible to vascular insult is also in segment T1-4. Cord segment T11 and L1, in which the blood supply depends upon the Adamkiewicz artery, is an equally vulnerable region. Any vascular injury may result in necrosis of an entire segment of the cord.[14]

Indications and Selection of Patients

The largest series of patients treated by rhizotomy suffered from pain due to various causes. When pain is limited to a relatively localized area, use of the extremities as well as bladder and bowel function are not impaired when the nerve roots are cut. Rhizotomy has long been the standard operation for relieving pain from metastatic nodes in the neck, provided the trunk of the brachial plexus is not involved.[15]

Patients are selected for rhizotomy on the basis of a detailed history and a careful physical and neurologic examination. If indicated, a myelogram should be performed. Routine psychometric testing and psychiataric evaluation are necessary for patients with benign chronic pain before any procedure is undertaken.

Diagnostic Paravertebral Block

As a preliminary procedure, it is generally advisable to inject a local anesthetic into the spinal nerve that is being considered for sensory root section. This procedure should be carried out under fluoroscopic control. Anesthesia equipment should be on hand to treat serious respiratory or cardiac complications, if they occur. This temporary procedure serves a dual purpose: it shows to the patient what permanent sensory loss will be like, and it assures the surgeon that the given area of analgesia is likely to relieve his patient's discomfort. However, it does not guarantee the pain will not recur.

Extent of Posterior Rhizotomy

White and Sweet[6] stated that posterior rhizotomy would be effective when pain is limited to a localized area of the limb, so that an extensive rhizotomy can be avoided. With pain in the chest or abdomen, an extensive rhizotomy could be carried out (Table 32-1).

For occipital neuralgia, denervation of C2-3 is indicated. However, bilateral denervation of C3-4 should be avoided, since it could interfere with diaphragmatic respiration.

Pain in the anterior one-third of the tongue and mandibular portion of the neck could be successfully relieved by combined rhizotomy of the fifth cranial nerve and C2-3. Pain of the ear, secondary to infiltrated cancer, could be treated in the same way. However rhizotomy may not be technically feasible when pain is referred to the shoulder or lower neck. These areas are innervated by the lower half of the cervical and upper thoracic nerve (C4-T4). Denervation of C8 to T2 is required to relieve pain of ulnar nerve distribution.

To relieve intercostal neuralgia, two roots above and below the affected area must be interrupted. T11 to L2 denervation is recommended for a painful scar after herniorraphy.

Table 32-1. Extent of Posterior Rhizotomy Recommended

Origin or Site of pain	Involved nerves	Roots of origin	Extent of rhizotomy	Comment
Occipital scar	Greater or lesser occipital	C2-3	C2-3, C4 if present	Look for possible posterior root of first cervical
Carcinoma of cervical nodes	Superficial and deep cervical plexuses	C2-C4	C2-4, C5, and C4, if present	Eliminate cases of cranial nerve involvement. Include C5 when pain is referred to shoulder or lower neck
Epicondylar fractures and scars along medial side of forearm and hand	Ulnar	C8-T2	C8-T2	Occasional failures will result from C7 overlap
Scarring from chest wounds and thoracotomy operations	Inter-costals	Variable	Generally two roots above and below nerves caught in scar	After intercostal drainage for empyema cut 5 roots. After costectomy cut 6 roots
Sensitive scar after herniorrhaphy	Ilioinguinal and hypo-gastric	T12-L1	T11-L2	
Retroperitoneal scar and other injuries to nerve in lateral thigh	Lateral femoral Cutaneous	L2-L3	L2-L3	
Coccygodynia	S5 and coccygeal	Same	S4-Coc1	Pain following rectal resection requires additional rhizotomy of S3. This may impair detrusor activity of bladder
Angina pectoris	Thoracic cardiac rami	T1-T4	T1-T4	Bilateral rhizotomy necessary if pain radiates down both arms
Gastric, biliary, and pancreatic	Splanchnic rami	T5-T10	T5-T10	To be recommended only when splanch-nicectomy fails because of involve-ment of somatic nerves in posterior abdominal wall
Renal	Lower splanchnic rami	T10-L1	T10-L1	Preferable to sympathectomy after previous operations on diseased kidney

From White JC, Sweet WH: *Pain and the Neurological Surgeon, A 40-year Experience.* Charles C Thomas, Springfield, Illinois, p 653

However, care should be taken not to injure the Adamkiewicz artery. Pain in the lateral aspect of the thigh requires denervation of L2 to L3. Motor function should be monitored carefully during electrothermocoagulation. Denervation of S4 to the coccygeal nerve is necessary to relieve coccygodynia. Bladder or bowel function is not affected by this procedure; only the dermatome between the posterior portion of the perineum and the coccyx will be denervated. Interruption of S2 and S3, particularly if bilateral, will impair bowel, bladder, and sexual function.

To alleviate pain secondary to malignancy of visceral organs a combination of sympathectomy and rhizotomy may be required.[6]

Technique

Preparation and Anesthesia

The patient should have nothing by mouth. Heavy sedation should be avoided: the patient must be alert because his cooperation is needed to monitor motor and sensory functions during the procedure. A few milliliters of 0.5% or 1% lidocaine are injected subcutaneously at the needle-entering point. Particular caution should be taken to avoid injecting the anesthetic into the subarachnoid space, especially in the cervical region. During electrothermocoagulation, sodium methohexital (Blevital sodium, Lilly) can be given intravenously, by the anesthesiologist, for C2 rhizotomy. The patient may experience extreme pain in the area of C2 during treatment. Hence, it is important to explain the procedure in detail, particularly what the patient might experience and the need for his or her cooperation during the procedure. This significantly reduces the amount of premedication and anesthesia required.[16,17]

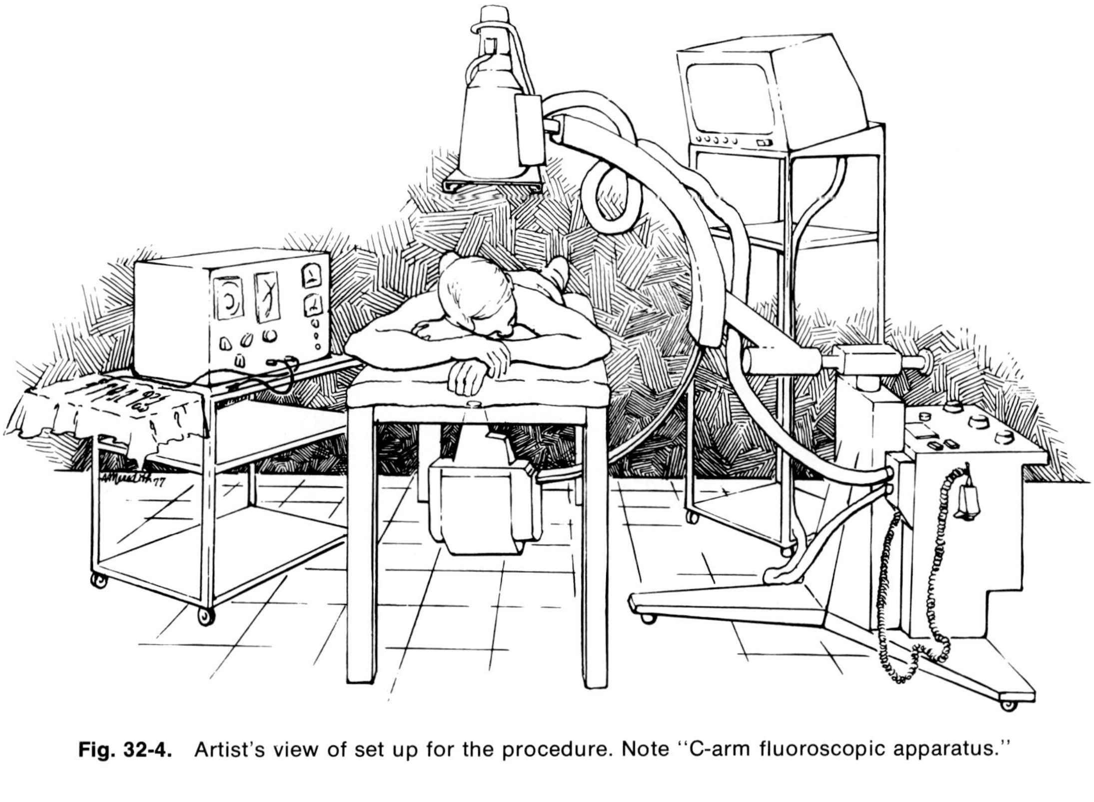

Fig. 32-4. Artist's view of set up for the procedure. Note "C-arm fluoroscopic apparatus."

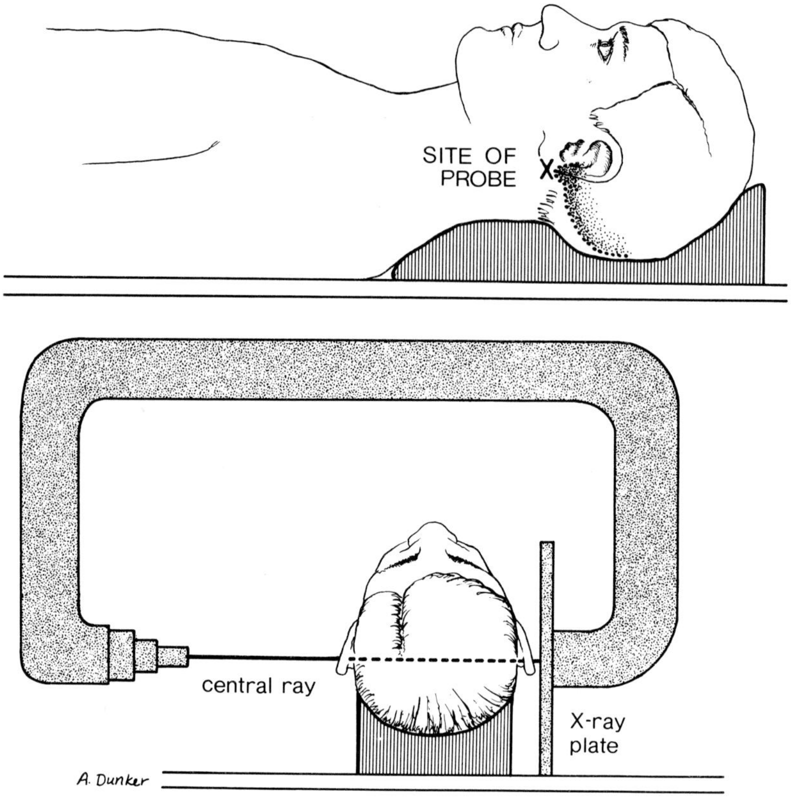

Fig. 32-5. The neck is slightly flexed for C2 rhizotomy. This moves the vertebral artery away from the intervertebral foramina.

Cervical Rhizotomy

The procedure is performed in a room equipped with radiologic image intensification. The patient is placed in the supine position, with the neck slightly flexed. The head and neck rest comfortably on a pillow of folded sheets. This position permits fluoroscopic examination of the lateral, oblique, and anteroposterior (AP) views of the cervical spine. The slight flexion, rather than extension, of the cervical spine moves the vertebral artery away from the intervertebral foramina. After the surgical area is prepared routinely, local anesthesia is injected at the entering point of the needle. The usual puncture site for the C2 foramen is located 1 cm below the mastoid process (Fig. 32-5).

A hollow 20-gauge needle with a short bevel and tip, completely insulated except for 5 mm of the tip,* is used. The position of the needle is adjusted and the needle advanced under fluoroscopic control in the lateral view. In this view the target posterior ganglion is the midpoint on the rostrocaudal axis and in the dorsal one-third of the foramen. On the AP view it is 0 to 2 mm medial to the medial edge of the facet (pedicle) and 2 mm caudal to the caudal margin of the inferior pedicle (Figs. 32-6 and 32-7). When the needle is placed in the target, it is gently aspirated. Occasionally, cerebral spinal fluid escapes through the needle, indicating that the tip of the needle is in the subarachnoid space. In this case the needle should be withdrawn about 1 mm and its position rechecked with the image intensifier. The stylet is then replaced with a thermocouple electrode and the nerve root electrically stimulated, twice per second, by a biphasic square-wave pulse, 1 msec in duration at less than 1.0 V. Appropri-

*Radionics, Inc., Burlington, Massachusetts 01803.

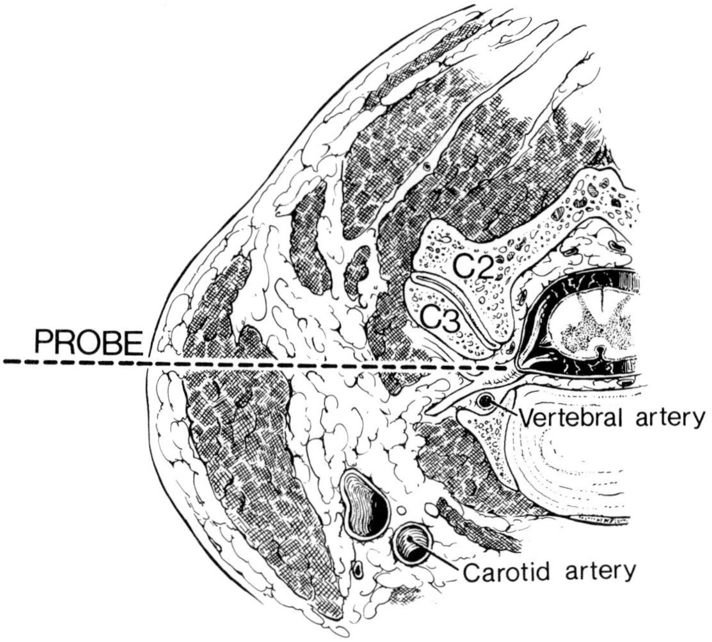

Fig. 32-6. Cross section at the C2 foramen and the direction of the needle.

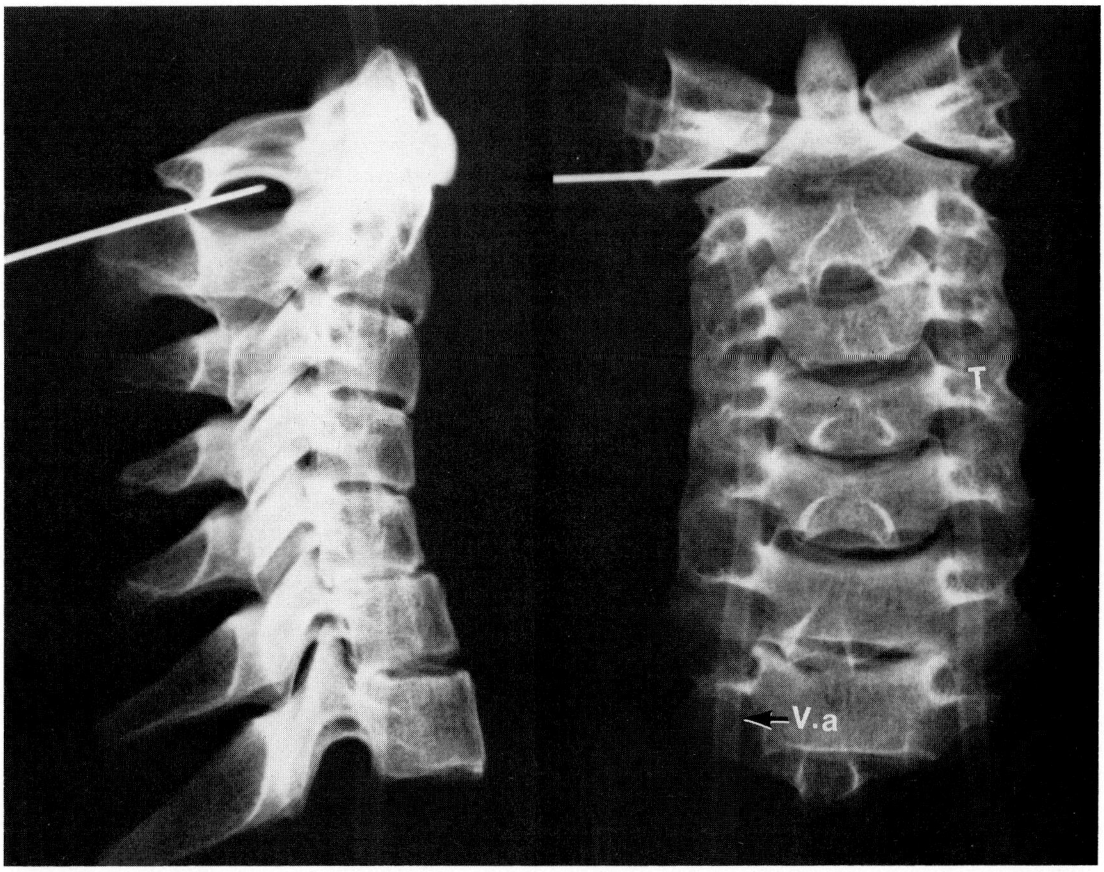

Fig. 32-7. Relationship of the needle to the C2 foramen (x-ray film of a specimen of the cervical spine). V.a=vertebral artery.

Table 32-2. **Sensory and Motor Responses at Less than 0.5 V with Probe in Direct Contact with Nerve Fibers**

C2	Trapezius
C3	Trapezius
C4	Supraspinatus
C5	Deltoid
C6	Biceps brachii
C7	Triceps
C8	Movement of thumb
T1	Movement of 5th finger
T2 to T5	Sensory response radiating pain to anterior chest wall at appropriate dermatome. Intercostal muscle contraction is often difficult to observe due to subcutaneous adipose tissue
T6 to T12	Abdominal muscle
L1 to L3	Iliopsoas and adductor muscle group of the thigh
L4	Hamstring, quadriceps femoris
L5	Peroneus
S1	Adductor hallucis
S2	Movement of 5th toe
S3 to S5	Sphincter ani

Modified from Raymond CT, Carpenter MB: Human Neuroanatomy. Sixth edition. Williams and Wilkins Company, Baltimore, 1969, pp 196-198

ate sensory or muscle responses should be obtained at less than 0.5 V, if the probe is in direct contact with nerve fibers (Table 32-2).

Ground electrodes are placed away from the affected dermatome or myotome. If muscle contraction is observed and the pain response is reproduced, the final position of the electrode is confirmed fluoroscopically. An initial trial at 50° to 70°C is used for a period of 15 seconds, with clinical monitoring. Then a total of 90 to 120 seconds is given. The electrode is then removed and a small pressure dressing applied to the puncture site.

When the electrode tip is in the subarachnoid space, it is difficult to generate a temperature sufficient for denervation. Care should be taken not to puncture the vertebral artery when the needle is advanced into the target, as described above, under careful fluoroscopic control. This technique cannot be applied to the atlanto occipital joint because the vertebral artery takes a redundant course in this area (Fig. 32-8) and can be injured. To insert the electrode in the remaining cervical foramen, except for C2, an oblique view of the cervical spine is helpful. Electrothermocoagulation of the level below C6 and the first four thoracic roots, should be carried out with extreme caution to avoid injuring the important large radicular arteries. The position of the shoulder muscles and scapula may interfere with the needle puncture and make the procedure more difficult. Therefore, open surgical rhizotomy may be a safer approach for this particular region (Figs. 32-9, 32-10, and 32-11).

Thoracic Rhizotomy

The patient is placed on a fluoroscopic operating table, in the prone position, with a pillow under his abdomen and his arms hanging over the table. If the upper thoracic nerves are to be blocked, a pillow should be placed under the upper chest and the patient's head should be hanging off the pillow, downward. By palpation and under the image intensifier, the anatomic relationships of the following bony landmarks are studied: (a) the spinous processes, (b) the costotransverse and facet joints on the anteroposterior view, and (c) the intervertebral foramina on the lateral view. The outline of the structure is traced on the skin with methylene blue to determine the entering point, direction, and angulation of the probe to

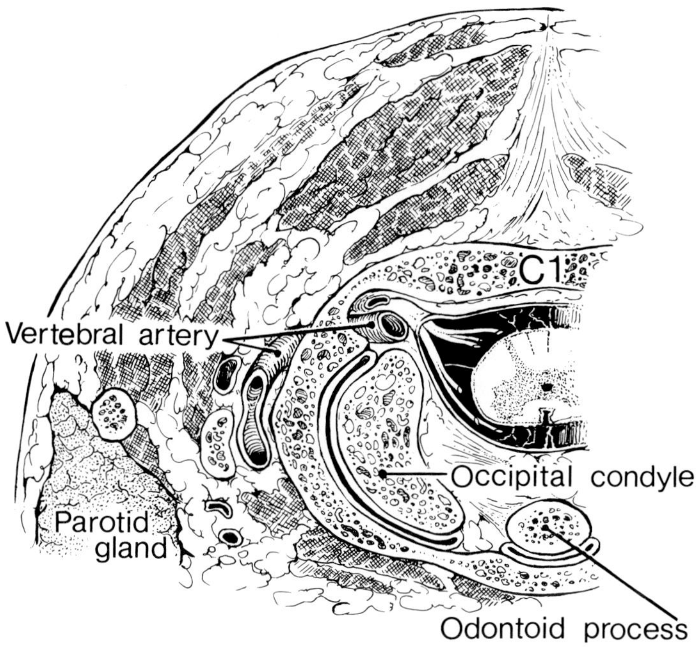

Fig. 32-8. Cross section at the atlanto occipital joint. Note the proximity of the vertebral artery and the C1 nerve root.

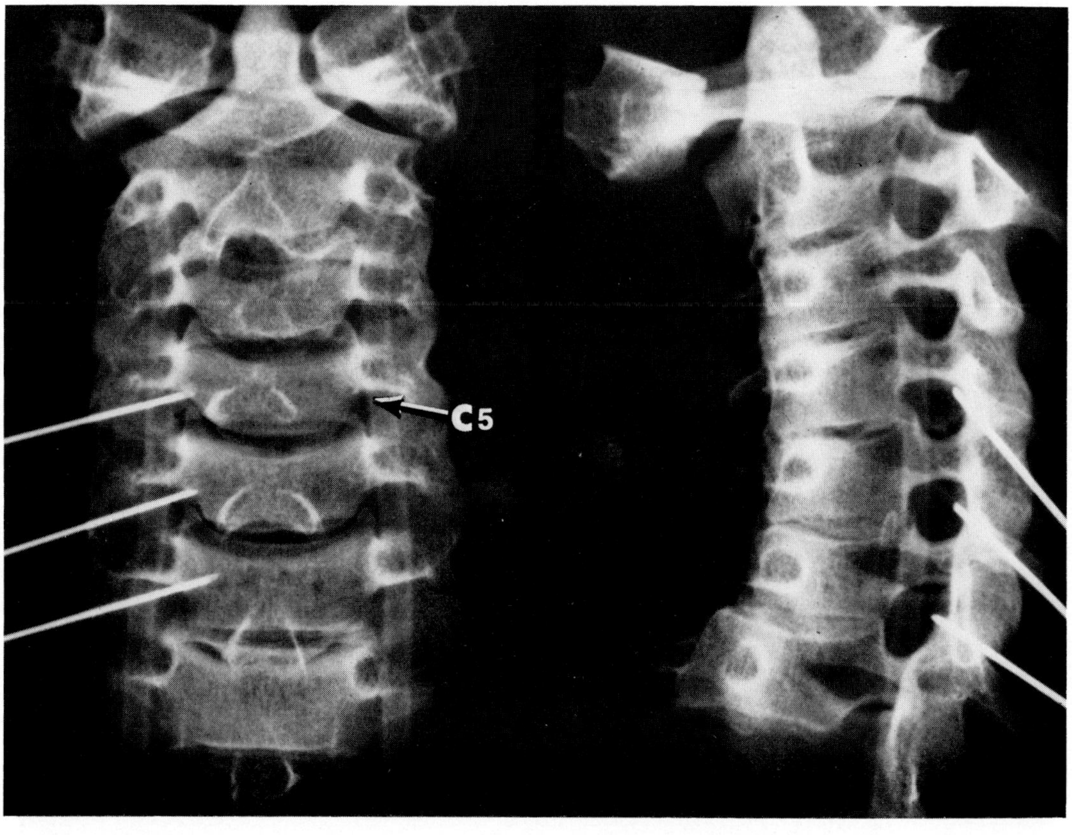

Fig. 32-9. Relationship of the needles to the lower cervical foramens (oblique x-ray view on the left).

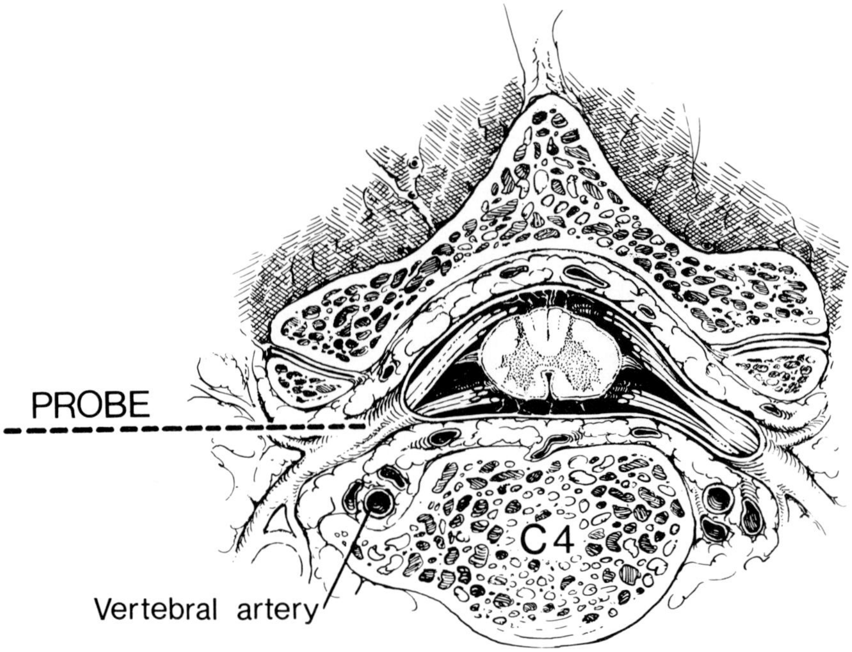

Fig. 32-10. Cross section at the C4 and the direction of the needle.

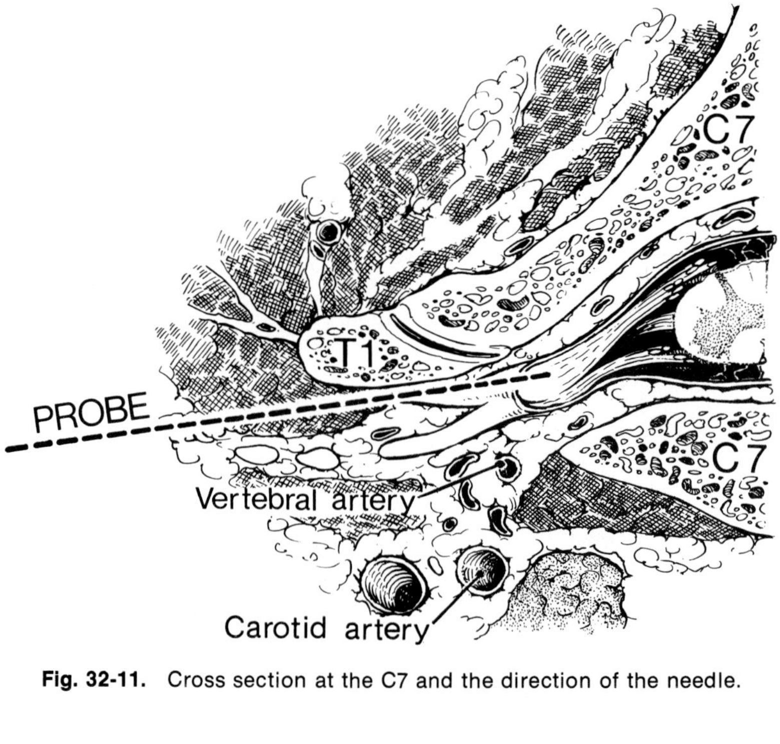

Fig. 32-11. Cross section at the C7 and the direction of the needle.

the target foramen. It is helpful to know that in the thoracic region, the spinous process of one vertebra lie in a line with those of the vertebra immediately below it. For example, the superior edge of the tip of the sixth thoracic vertebra lies in a line with the transverse processes of the seventh thoracic vertebrae (Figs. 32-12 and 32-13).

Under fluoroscopic control in the AP view, a line is traced from the head of the transverse process of the vertebra one level below the target foramen to the neck of the transverse process of the target vertebra. For example, using the sixth thoracic vertebra as the target, a line is drawn from the head of the transverse process of the seventh vertebra to the neck of the transverse process of the sixth thoracic vertebra. The needle entry point is approximately 3.5 to 5 cm from the midline of the vertebral body one level below the target. A local anesthetic is injected and the guiding needle advanced so that it impinges on the head of the transverse process. The needle is then angled toward the neck of the transverse process of the target foramen. Under lateral fluoroscopic control, the target foramen is identified and the needle is then carefully advanced into it. The target, in the AP view, is located 2 to 3 mm caudal to the caudal edge of the facet joint (Fig. 32-14).

After the needle is placed in the target, an attempt should always be made to gently aspirate for spinal fluid and blood. If cerebrospinal fluid is observed, the needle is withdrawn 1 to 2 mm. Often the needle tip impinges on the wall of the foramen (pedicle) before it is advanced deeply enough and multiple attempts to introduce the needle should be avoided. The patient frequently reports radiating pain along the appropriate intercostal nerve to the anterior chest or abdominal wall.

The thermoprobe is introduced after the position of the needle is confirmed. Electrode stimulation is then applied, using the same parameters described for cervical rhizotomy. After the proper location of the needle is confirmed by muscle contraction and by reproducing the pain, trial thermocoagulation is applied at a temperature of 40° to 50°C for 15 seconds, carefully observing flexion and extension movements of all toes, bilaterally, throughout the

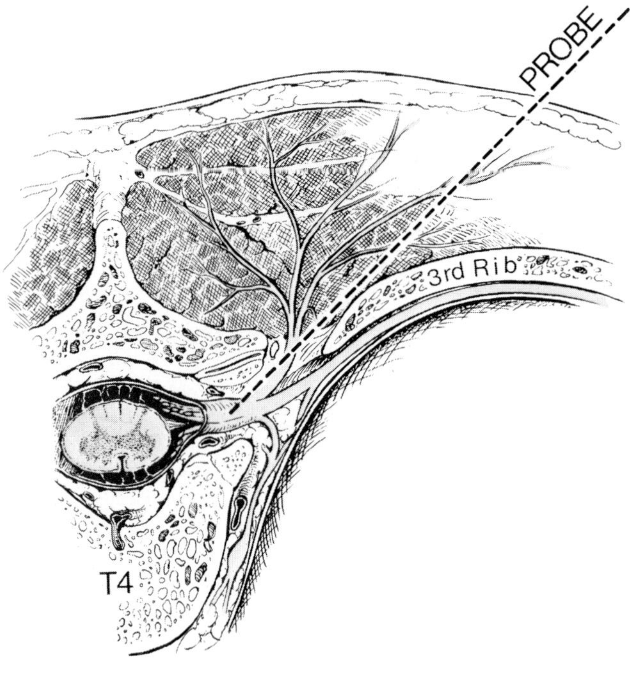

Fig. 32-12. Cross section at the T4 foramen and the direction of the needle.

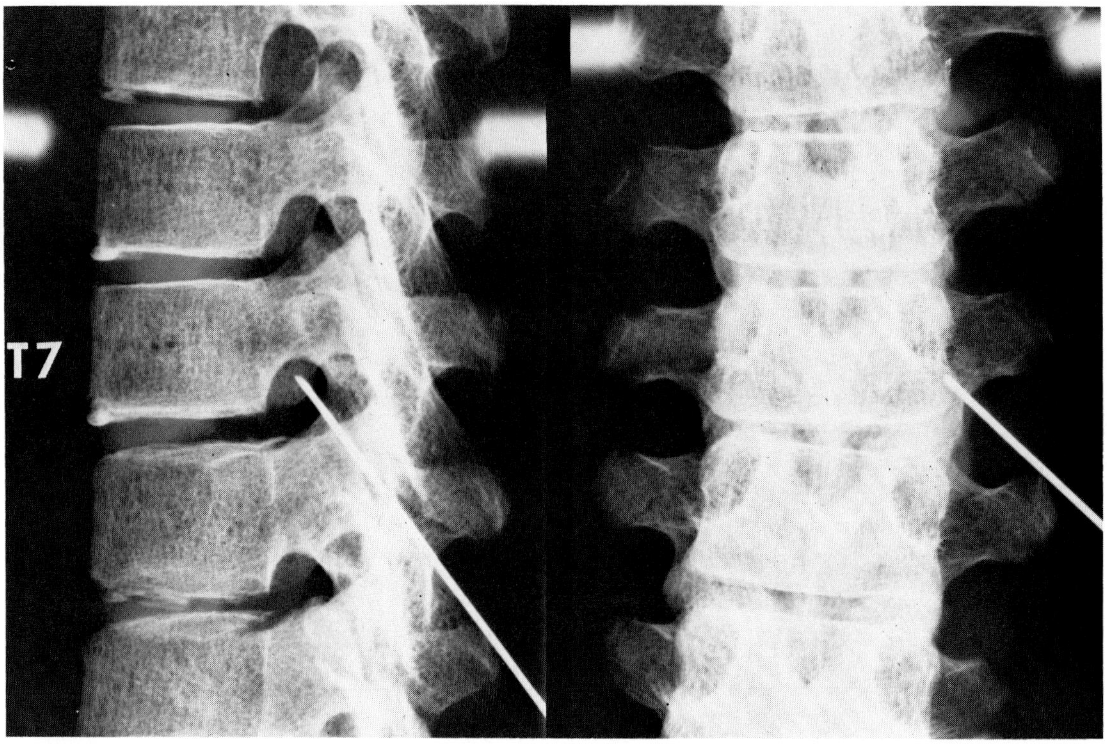

Fig. 32-13. The needle is impinged to the head of the transverse process that is one level below the target foramen, and directed to the target foramen of the thoracic spine.

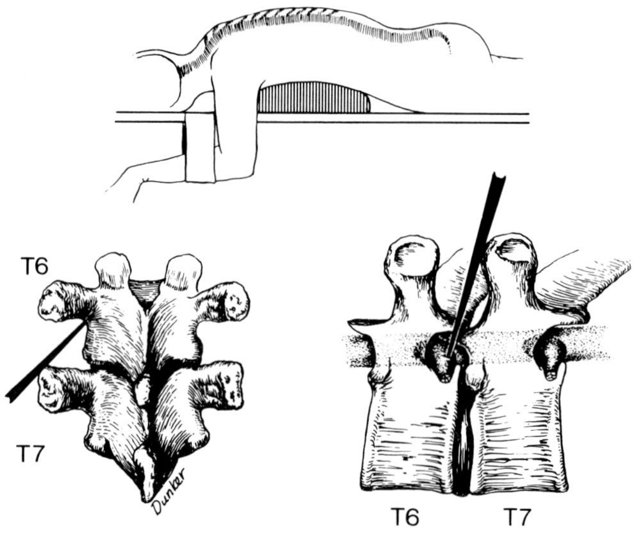

Fig. 32-14. An artist's view of the direction, angulation, and puncture site of the needle for the introduction into the thoracic intervertebral foramen.

treatment period. Treatment is given in increments up to a total of 90 to 120 seconds; a maximum temperature of less than 74°C is applied for denervation of pain fibers.

If the needle enters or touches the pleura, the patient may cough while the needle is being advanced or during heating. The needle should not be inserted lateral to the transverse processes nor ventral to the foramen.

As soon as the procedure is completed chest x-ray films are taken. Two hours after the procedure, follow-up films are taken to be certain that there is no pneumothorax. The patient should be kept under observation, in the recovery room, for a minimum of 2 hours. Since blood pressure may fall, particularly in elderly patients after multiple roots are denervated, blood pressure and pulse are closely monitored.

Intercostal Nerve Denervation

Intercostal nerves and vessels, lie in the intercostal spaces. The nerves lie a little below the blood vessels. The intercostal nerve lies between the pleura and the posterior intercostal membrane, proximal to the angle of the ribs. In the region of the posterior axillary line, the nerves lie between the two muscle layers of the internal and external intercostal muscles. They continue forward in this relationship toward the front of the thorax. The lower six intercostal nerves, at the anterior end of the intercostal space, pass into the abdominal muscles.

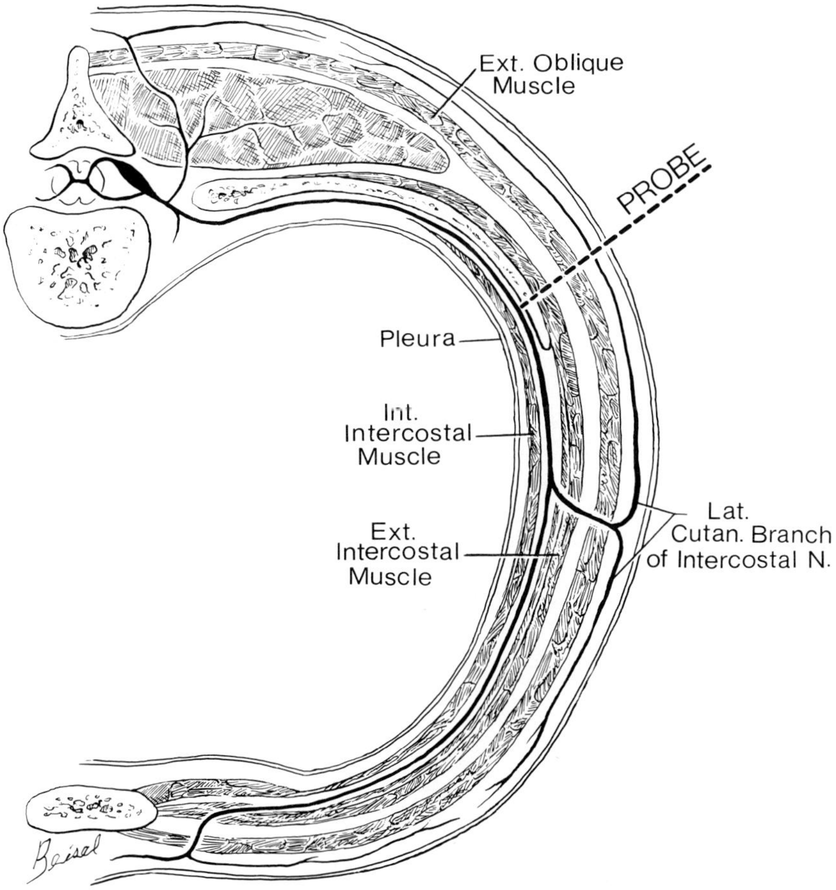

Fig. 32-15. A probe at the posterior axillar line. Note lateral cutaneous branches.

The most important branch of each intercostal nerve, from the standpoint of denervation, is the lateral cutaneous. It arises from the intercostal nerve just anterior to the midaxillary line, pierces the external intercostal and anterior serratus muscles, and then divides into anterior and posterior cutaneous branches. Therefore, if the intercostal nerves are not blocked posteriorly or around the posterior axillary line, it is very easy to miss the lateral cutaneous branch and adequate analgesia will not occur. The rib, at this angle, is approximately 0.6 cm thick (Fig. 32-15).

Under local anesthesia, at the junction of the posterior axillary line and inferior edge of the ribs, a 20-gauge needle, as described for cervical rhizotomy, impinges on the ribs at their inferior margin. Then the tip of the needle slides into the visceral aspect of the ribs, only 2 to 3 mm deep from the inner aspect of the rib. At this point stimulation by 0.2 to 0.5 V, at a rate of 2/sec, is applied to determine the proper location of the needle. After the location is confirmed, incremental heat lesions are made, as described previously. Vital signs should be monitored for 2 hours.[18]

Lumbar Rhizotomy

The patient is placed on the operating table in the lateral recumbent position, with the affected side up. The entry point of the needle is determined by fluoroscopy in the lateral view. The foramina are easily visualized in this view. The needle entry point is usually 4 cm from the midline and the target point of the intervertebral foramen is located in the slightly rostral portion of the intervertebral disc space. The needle is advanced into the dorsal one-third of the foramen. When it is 10 mm away from the target, the x-ray tube is relocated for an anteroposterior examination to advance the needle the remaining depth. The target, in the anteroposterior view, is located 0 to 2 mm medial to the medial edge of the facet joint and 2 to 3 mm caudal to the caudal edge of the joint (Fig. 32-16 and 32-17).

When the needle is placed in the target, an attempt is always made to gently aspirate for spinal fluid or blood. If cerebrospinal fluid is observed, the needle is withdrawn 1 to 2 mm.

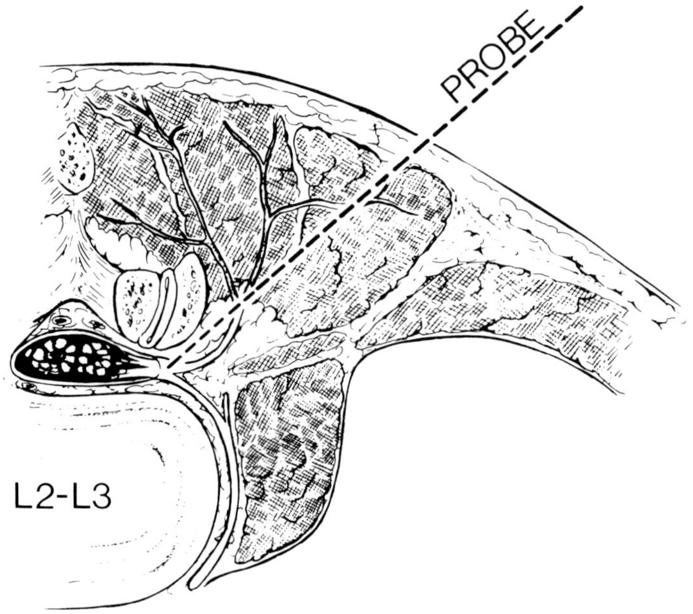

Fig. 32-16. Cross section of the L-2 foramen and the direction of the needle.

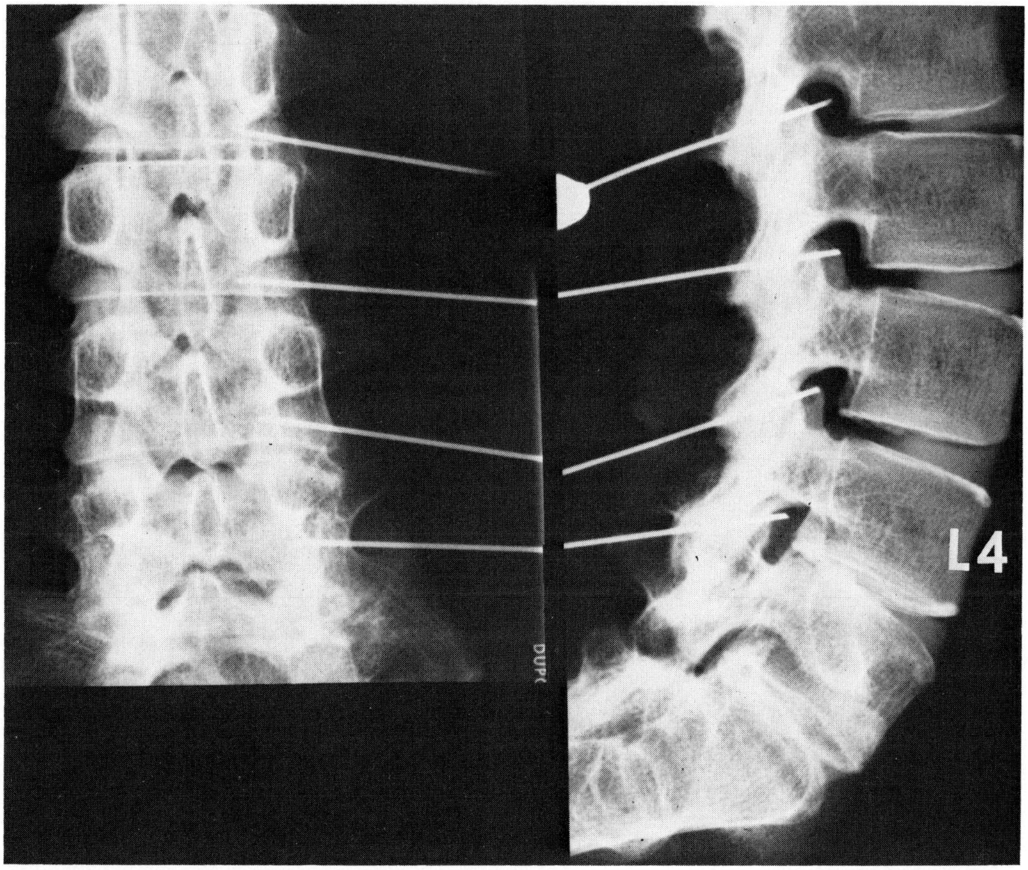

Fig. 32-17. Relationship of the needle to the first, second, third, and fourth lumbar intervertebral foramen as viewed on x-ray film.

A thermoprobe is introduced after the position of the needle is confirmed. Electrode stimulation is then tried, using the same parameters as described for cervical rhizotomy. After proper muscle contraction and reproduction of pain, trial thermocoagulation is performed with a temperature of 40° to 50°C for 15 seconds. Flexion and extension of the toes, bilaterally, are observed during the entire treatment period. This treatment is then given in increments to a total of 90 to 120 seconds, with a maximum temperature of less than 74°C. It is more important to observe muscle contraction in the lower extremity than in the paravertebral muscles, since the latter could result from direct muscle rather than nerve root stimulation. Particular care should be taken to avoid injuring the Adamkiewicz artery, which is in the vicinity of T11 to L1. In my opinion rhizotomy of lumbar or lower cervical nerve roots to alleviate discogenic chronic pain should only be used in patients who already have a sensory or motor impairment, so that the procedure does not increase the degree of disability. It should not be done in patients with chronic pain, who have normal sensory and motor functions of the extremity.

The Fifth Lumbar and Sacral Rhizotomy

The patient is placed in the prone position, with a large pillow under the abdomen, at the level of the iliac crest, to create flexion of the lumbosacral joint. This is particularly important for denervation of the fifth lumbar root. An anteroposterior view by fluoroscopic examination

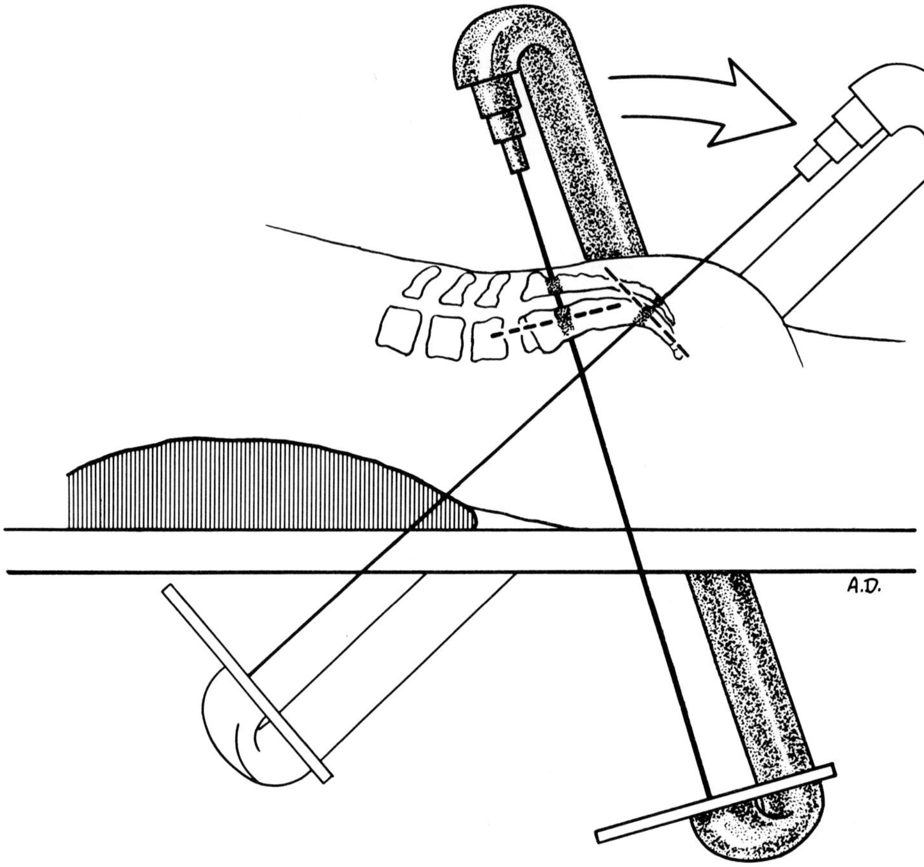

Fig. 32-18. **A.** Artist's view of the position of the patient for a sacral rhizotomy. Note x-ray beam directed at 90° angle toward the longitudinal axis of the sacral spine. This enables fluoroscopic visualization of the sacral foramens.

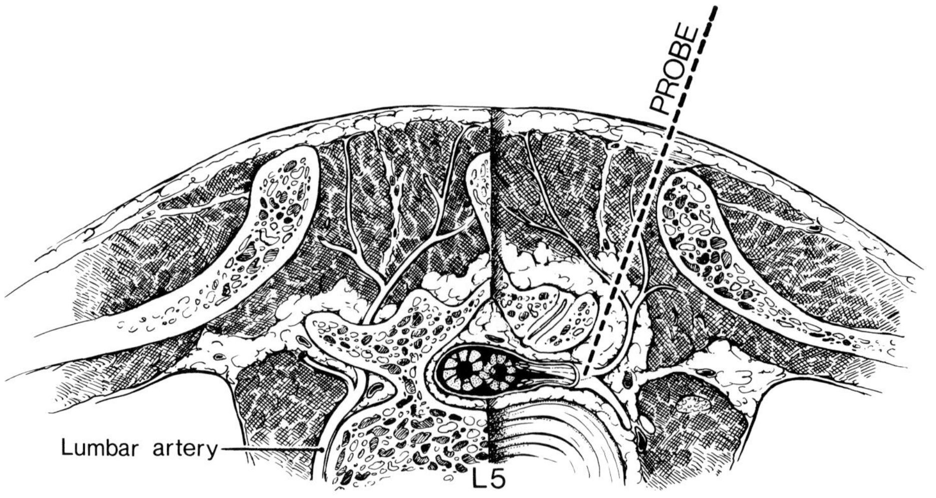

Fig. 32-19. Cross section at the level of the L5-S1 foramen; the direction of the needle; and the relationship of the needle to the L5 root. Note that the posterior superior iliac spine interferes with the needle entry.

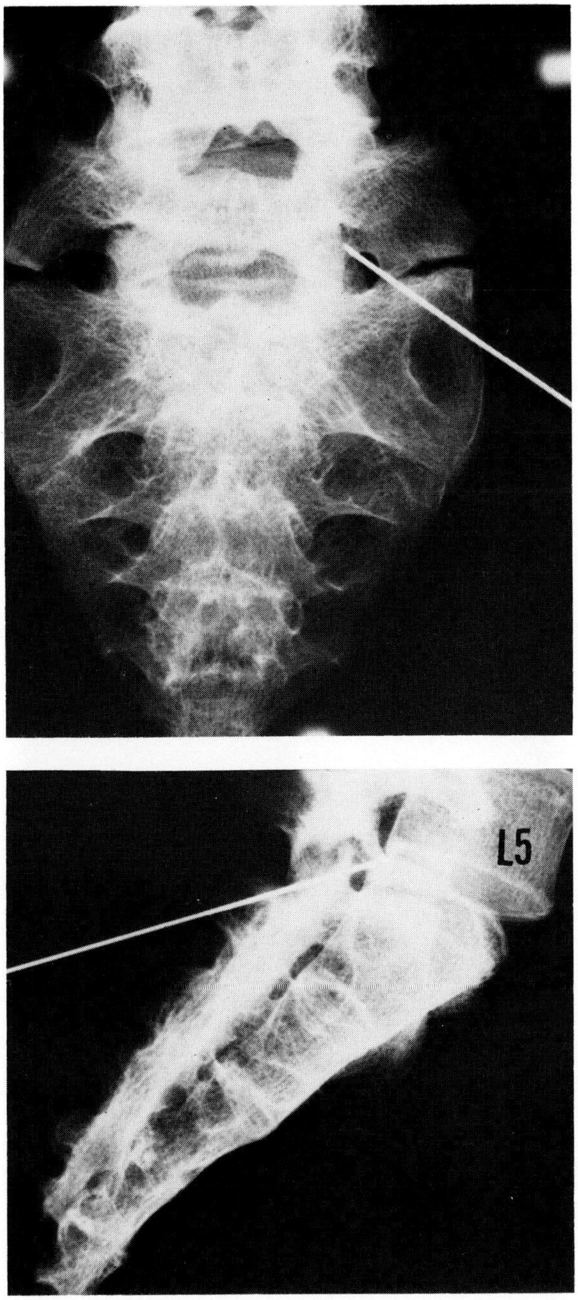

Fig. 32-20. Direction of the needle and its relationship to the 5th lumbar foramen as viewed on x-ray film.

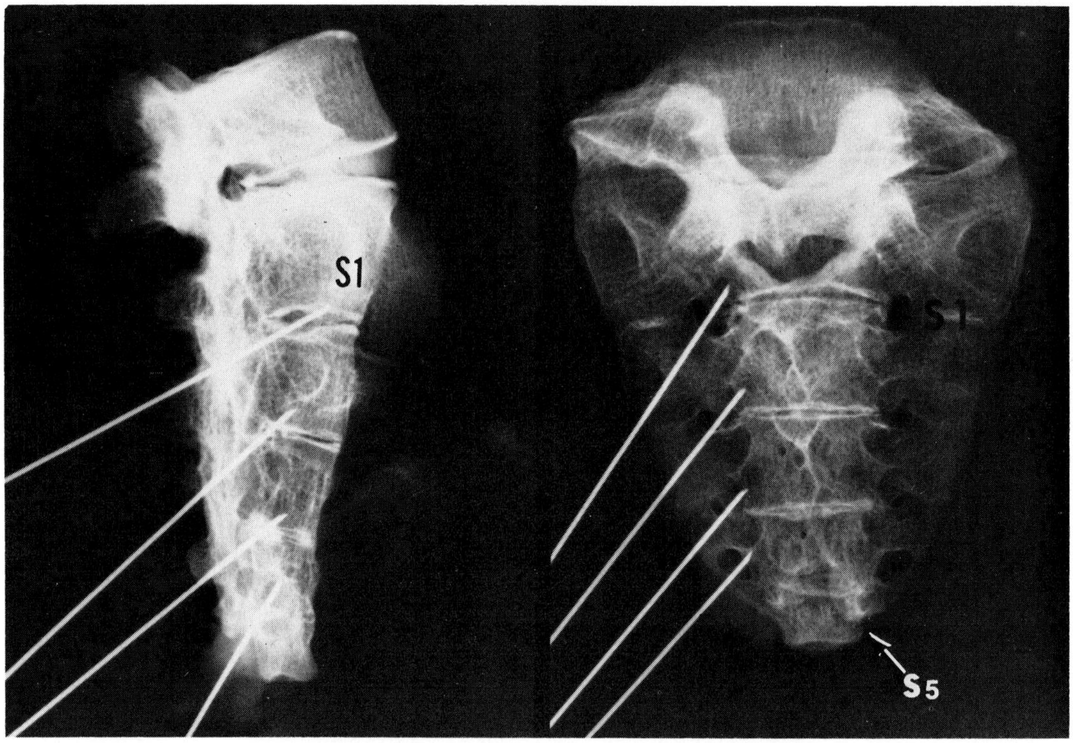

Fig. 32-21. Relationship of the needle to the first, second, third, and fourth sacral foramens as viewed on x-ray film.

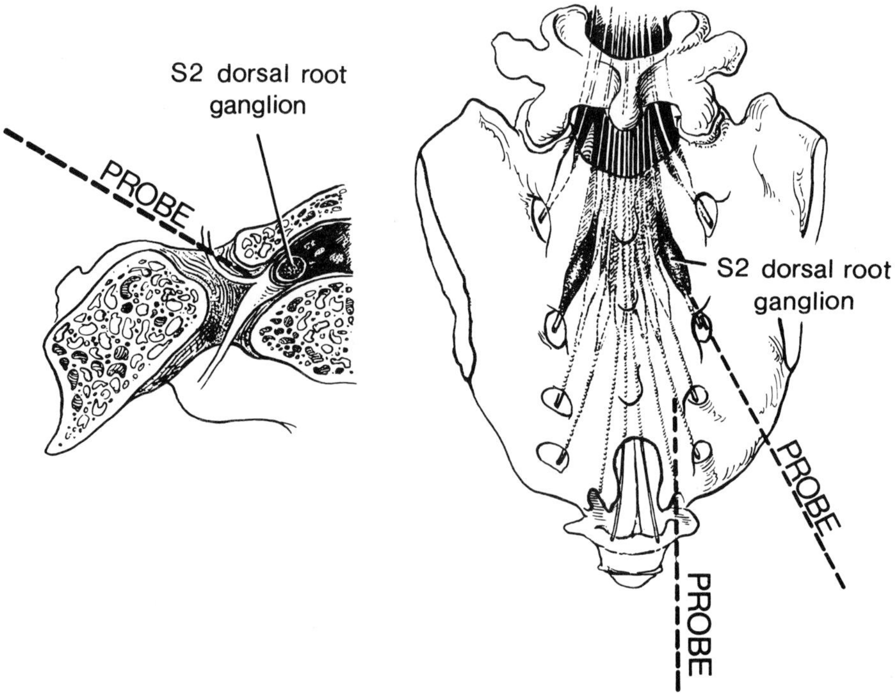

Fig. 32-22. **Left.** Cross section at the level of the second sacral ganglion with probe inserted through the second sacral foramen. **Right.** Superimposed view of sacral spine with ganglia and roots. Note probe inserted through the sacral hiatus, and its tip in contact with fifth and fourth root. A second probe is inserted through the second sacral foramen to the second ganglion.

locates the fifth lumbar and sacral intervertebral foramina. The x-ray beam must be directed at a 90° angle to the longitudinal axis of the sacral spine (Fig. 32-18) to visualize the posterior and anterior sacral foramina. The same type of needle, as described previously, is introduced through the prepped and anesthetized skin into the posterior surface of the sacrum, just next to the target foramen. This procedure permits the operator to estimate needle depth so that it can be advanced further through the foramen. The needle is then relocated, aiming it at the center of the target foramen, under x-ray control. For fifth lumbar denervation, the trunk of the nerve is the target. The rootlets and ganglion cannot be reached due to the iliac crest and posterior superior spine of the pelvis. The needle enters at the medial edge of the posterior superior iliac spine and is aimed toward the neck of the fifth lumbar transverse process. At times, it is difficult to insert the needle because of lumbrosacralization and/or arthritic changes. The depth of the needle is determined by a lateral view fluoroscopic examination. It is always important to aspirate for blood or spinal fluid before local block anesthesia or electrothermocoagulation (Figs. 32-19, 32-20, and 32-21). A sponge is placed between the gluteal folds to prevent the antiseptic solution from spilling over the perineum, which would burn the patient. Pain secondary to carcinoma of the rectum, with colostomy and loss of bladder control, may be treated by denervation of the second, third, and fourth sacral roots. Bladder function should be monitored cystometrically for denervation of the second, third, and fourth sacral roots when bladder and bowel function are intact.[12] The fifth, fourth, and third roots can be reached through the sacral hiatus. Electrical stimulation and fluoroscopic examination are used to guide the probe toward the target root or ganglion (Fig. 32-22).

Summary

A relatively simple technique for interrupting root, ganglion, trunk, and nerve is described as an alternative to open rhizotomy. Clinical observations of trigeminal rhizotomy support the fact that pain can be relieved and proprioception and motor function preserved with this technique. Differential denervation is now possible with the use of radiologic image intensification, means of electrical stimulation, and temperature control. The procedure can be applied to patients who are debilitated due to carcinoma and/or old age, and can be repeated if necessary.

Acknowledgments

Gratitude is due Dr. David Bodian, Department of Anatomy, for his suggestions and for the preparation of the histologic slides used on Figure 32-1.

My thanks go to our secretarial and technical staff, Jean Arnett, Erva Baden, Debbie Gilmer and Richard Kouba, for their careful and conscientious assistance in the completion of the manuscript.

REFERENCES

1. Abbe R: A contribution to the surgery of the spine. *Med Rec 35*:149-152, 1889
2. Bennett WH: A case in which antispasmodic pain in the left lower extremity was completely relieved by subdural division of the posterior roots of certain spinal nerves, all other treatment having proved useless. Death from sudden collapse and cerebral hemorrhage on the twelfth day after the operation, at the commencement of apparent convalescence. *Med Chir Trans (Lond) 72*:329-348, 1889
3. Scoville WB: Extradural spinal sensory rhizotomy. *J Neurosurg 25*:94-95, 1966
4. Dogliotti AM: Traitement des syndromes douloureux de la peripherie par l'alcholisation subarachnoidienne des racines posterieures a leur emergence de la moelle epiniere. *Presse Med 39*:1249-1252, 1931

5. Maher RM: Relief of pain in incurable cancer. *Lancet 1*:18-20, 1955
6. White J, Sweet W: *Pain and the Neurosurgeon, a 40-Year Experience.* Charles C Thomas, Illinois, 1969, p 662
7. Kirschner M: Die Behandlung der Trigeminus Neuralgie (Nach Erfahrungen an 1113 Kranken). *Munchen Med Wochenschr 89*:235-239, 1942
8. Sweet W, Wepsic J: Controlled thermocoagulation of trigeminal ganglion and rootlets for differential destruction of pain fibers. Part 1: Trigeminal neuralgia. *J Neurosurg 40*:143-156, 1974
9. Uematsu S, Udvarhelyi G, Benson DW, et al: Percutaneous radiofrequency rhizotomy. *Surg Neurol 2*:319-325, 1974
10. Hamby WB, Schiffer: Spasmodic torticollis: Results after cervical rhizotomy in 50 cases. *J Neurosurg 31*:323-326, 1969
11. Heimburger R, Slominski O, Griswold P: Cervical posterior rhizotomy for reducing spasticity in cerebral palsy. *J Neurosurg 39*:30-34, 1973
12. Rockwold G, Bradley W, Chou S: Differential sacral rhizotomy in the treatment of neurogenic bladder dysfunction. Preliminary report of six cases. *J Neurosurg 38*:748-754, 1973
13. Vakili H: *The Spinal Cord.* Intercontinental Medical Book Corp., New York, p 20
14. Djindjian R, Hurth M, Houdart R, et al: *Angiography of the Spinal Cord.* University Park Press, Baltimore, 1970, p 3-10
15. Onofrio BM, Campa HK: Evaluation of rhizotomy. Review of 12 years experience. *J Neurosurg 36*:751-755, 1972
16. Pawl P: Percutaneous Radiofrequency Electrocoagulation in the Control of Chronic Pain. *Surg Clin North Am 55*:167-179, 1975
17. Siegfried et al: *Advances and Technical Standard in Neurosurgery.* Vol 2. Edited by H Krayenbühl, et al. Springer-Verlag, New York, 1975
18. Moore DC: *Regional Block, A Handbook for Use in the Clinical Practice of Medicine and Surgery.* Charles C Thomas, Illinois, 1953, pp 113-150
19. White JC: Posterior rhizotomy: A possible substitute for cordotomy in otherwise intractable neuralgias of the trunk and extremities of nonmalignant origin. *Clin Neurosurg 13*:20-41, 1966

CHAPTER 33

Posterior Lumbosacral Facet Coagulation—A Stereotactic Radiofrequency Technique for Treatment of Back Pain

Howard A. Richter

Editorial Note: At the meeting of the American Association of Neurological Surgeons in April, 1973, Shealy, Prieto, Burton and Long described "Radiofrequency Percutaneous Rhizotomy of the Articular Nerve of Luschka." They reported 57 good and 60 excellent results in 180 patients. The categories of patients alleged to be so effectively treated were those with:

1) Chronic back or high leg pain with radiographic evidence of osteoarthritis and degenerative changes in the facets
2) osteoporosis of the spine with severe pain
3) "discogenic" pain
4) compression fracture
5) continuing chronic back pain and/or incapacitating radicular pain after multiple lumbar laminectomies
6) failure of lumbar fusion
7) epidural adhesions
8) adhesive arachnoiditis

Radiofrequency heating of an electrode placed against the posterior or lateral surface of the lumbar articular facets on each side is the objective of the operation. In my hands such heating even to 80°C has never produced any radiation of sensation into a lower limb. With an electrode in trigeminal rootlets, heating to 42° to 50°C suffices to produce severe facial pain. I think we can say with confidence that, whatever is being destroyed by the electrodes against the posterior or lateral aspect of the lumbar articular facets at 80°C, posterior root fibers are not included. The procedure is not a rhizotomy, it is at most a peripheral neurotomy. The allegations of Shealy that RF heating at the site he describes destroys ganglion or posterior root are without any foundation I have been able to detect. (Shealy, C.N. "Facet Rhizotomy," presented at Postgraduate Course—Neurological Surgery, Oct. 22, 1974, Clinical Congress of American College of Surgeons.) This is not an idle point of semantics, since we have an abundance of experience demonstrating frequent prompt recovery of sensation and return of pain following sensory neurotomy or even after a neurectomy with extensive avulsion.

Dr. Donlin Long promptly, and we believe appropriately, withdrew from the positions in the communication cited. The overwhelming majority of the real problem cases are of course those who have already had one or more operations. In a letter to me on June 7, 1973, Dr. Long wrote, "My success rate in the patients with multiple operations has been very poor." He also rapidly changed his terminology for the procedure, describing it in an article in *Spine*, 1976 as "so-called facet denervation." (Reference: Lora, J and Long, DM: So-Called Facet Denervation in the Management of Intractable Back Pain. *Spine 1*:121-126, 1976.) Lora and Long in that article report that no patient who had had two or more operations achieved even 50% pain relief and only ¼ of the 40 patients with one previous operation achieved as much as 50% pain relief. These are all of course relatively short-term followups, varying from 6 months to 2½ years.

I have seen little enough benefit from this procedure done personally so that I am dubious as the existence of any clearcut indications for it, but am scrutinizing with interest the reports of those who are more encouraged.

This chapter is included here with these very strong reservations as to the value of the procedure described.

W. H. Sweet, M.D., D.Sc.

Department of Neurosurgery, Lankenau Hospital and Department of Neurosurgery, Jefferson Medical College, Philadelphia, Pennsylvania 19151

FACET COAGULATION IS A safe, simple percutaneous technique useful in the treatment of back pain and worth having in the neurosurgical armamentarium. Low backaches are ubiquitous and their successful treatment is often elusive. The syndrome of herniated lumbar disc with nerve root compression[1] represents only a modest portion of all patients complaining of low back pain. Even in classic cases of lumbar disc rupture, excellent surgical treatment can result in failure to relieve pain. It has been proposed that patients with low back pain be treated by denervating the facet joints. Rees,[2] in February, 1971, reported using a long scalpel to penetrate the lumbar intertransverse ligament and sever sensory nerve fibers proximal to their entrance into the facet articular capsule. He reported over 2,000 operations with an amazing success rate, greater than 90%. Soon thereafter, Shealy[3] introduced the concept of a transcutaneously placed radiofrquency lesion in the parafacet area, presumably coagulating the nerve to the articular facet. He called this facet *rhizotomy* and later, *denervation of spinal facets*.[4] I call this procedure *paravertebral neurectomy* or *facet coagulation,* since the nerve to the joint of Luschka is postganglionic.[5] The advantage of Shealy's technique is its safety when compared to the use of the scalpel thrust through the skin. The needle allows localization by electrical stimulation and x-ray. Lesions can be limited by controlling the temperature at the radiofrequency electrode tip. I have adopted the procedure described by Shealy and associates.[6] Facet coagulation has been performed by Shealy in the cervical and thoracic regions.[4] The technique is similar to that used in the lumbosacral region.

Selection of Patients

Patients with low back pain, with or without leg pain and lacking sensory loss, muscle weakness, or reflex abnormality are submitted to paravertebral neurectomy without myelography. These patients may have spine tenderness and positive straight-leg raising signs. They all have failed to improve after at least 2 weeks of conservative management, including bedrest, medication with analgesics and sometimes tranquilizers, and occasionally traction. Patients with neurologic signs are evaluated by myelography and preferably not subjected to paravertebral neurectomy, unless the signs are minimal and the myelogram is negative or the patient refuses or won't tolerate laminectomy. Patients who are postlaminectomy and/or postspinal fusion with persistent pain have been treated with this procedure. Patients with spinal arthritis, lumbar strain, and pain radiation into the groin, lower abdomen, and thigh have also been treated with facet coagulation. Patients who fail to improve or have sustained relief after lidocaine paravertebral blocks are not subjected to surgery.

Technique

Prior to the initial radiofrequency coagulation, most patients are subjected to a paravertebral nerve block with 2% lidocaine. This is usually done on the day of admission to the hospital. In the x-ray department, under fluoroscopic control, 18-gauge spinal needles are guided to the appropriate target.

The target point is the same for the nerve block and the facet coagulation. It is at the junction of the transverse process with the facet joint at the appropriate level (Fig. 33-1). The needle is placed at the junction of the transverse process of the lower vertebra, with the facet joint at that level. For example, at L3-4, the needle would be placed at the junction of the upper border of the L4 transverse process with the facet joint of L3-4. The needle is initially placed and aimed somewhat medial so that it can be *walked* down the facet joints to the junction with the transverse process and then placed in the intertransverse ligaments.

For the nerve blocks, the patient is placed on the fluoroscopy table, the skin prepped

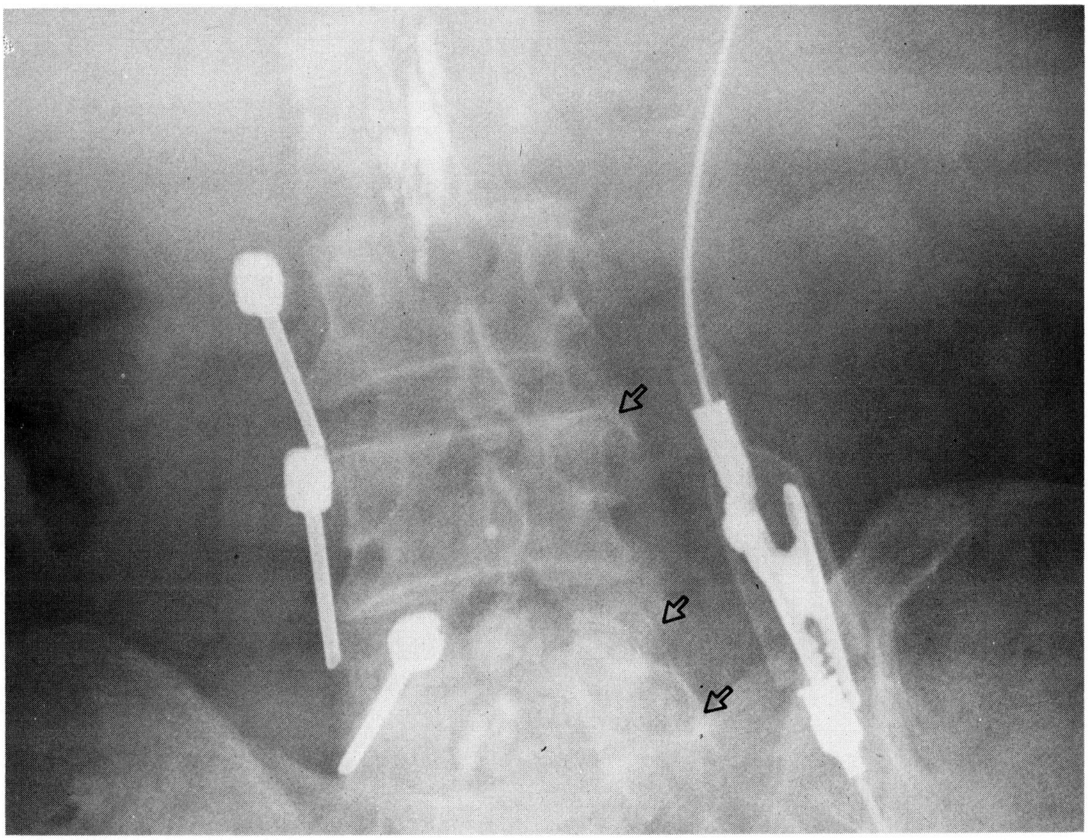

Fig. 33-1. Final PA radiograph for needle position in unilateral facet coagulation L-3, 4, L-4, 5, and L5, S-1 on the left with R-buttock 18-gauge needle ground electrode. Arrows on right indicate target points on unoperated side.

with organic iodine solution and alcohol, and draped. Skin wheals are made with 1% lidocaine at each site and 18-gauge spinal needles passed, without further anesthesia, to the target point, under fluoroscopy. Two milliliters of 2% lidocaine are inserted through each needle and the needles removed. It has not been necessary to obtain lateral films during the nerve blocks. Rarely, lidocaine diffuses into the primary ramus but this has not been a problem. Blocks with lidocaine are usually done at L3-4, L4-5, and L5, S1, bilaterally or unilaterally, as dictated by the patient's pain.

The patient is returned to his room, instructed to stand and walk during the next hour, and then make a judgment as to whether any relief of pain has occurred. The attending surgeon and his resident see the patient independently and compare notes. Based on the effectiveness of the block, a decision is made as to whether it would be worthwhile to proceed with facet coagulation. If there has been a useful degree of pain relief, facet coagulation is attempted the next day.

This procedure may be performed in the operating room or in the x-ray suite. Preoperative medication with meperidine, 100 mg, pentabarbital, 100 mg, and promethazine, 50 mg, intramuscularly, is given 1 hour before the operation. The procedure is done under local anesthesia. The skin is prepped and draped in the same fashion as for lumbar laminectomy. When lidocaine blocks were administered on the previous day, the skin sites for needle puncture are known. If blocks were omitted, a scout PA x-ray film, taken with a sterile metallic marker in place on the lumbar skin, shows the surgeon where to place the needles.

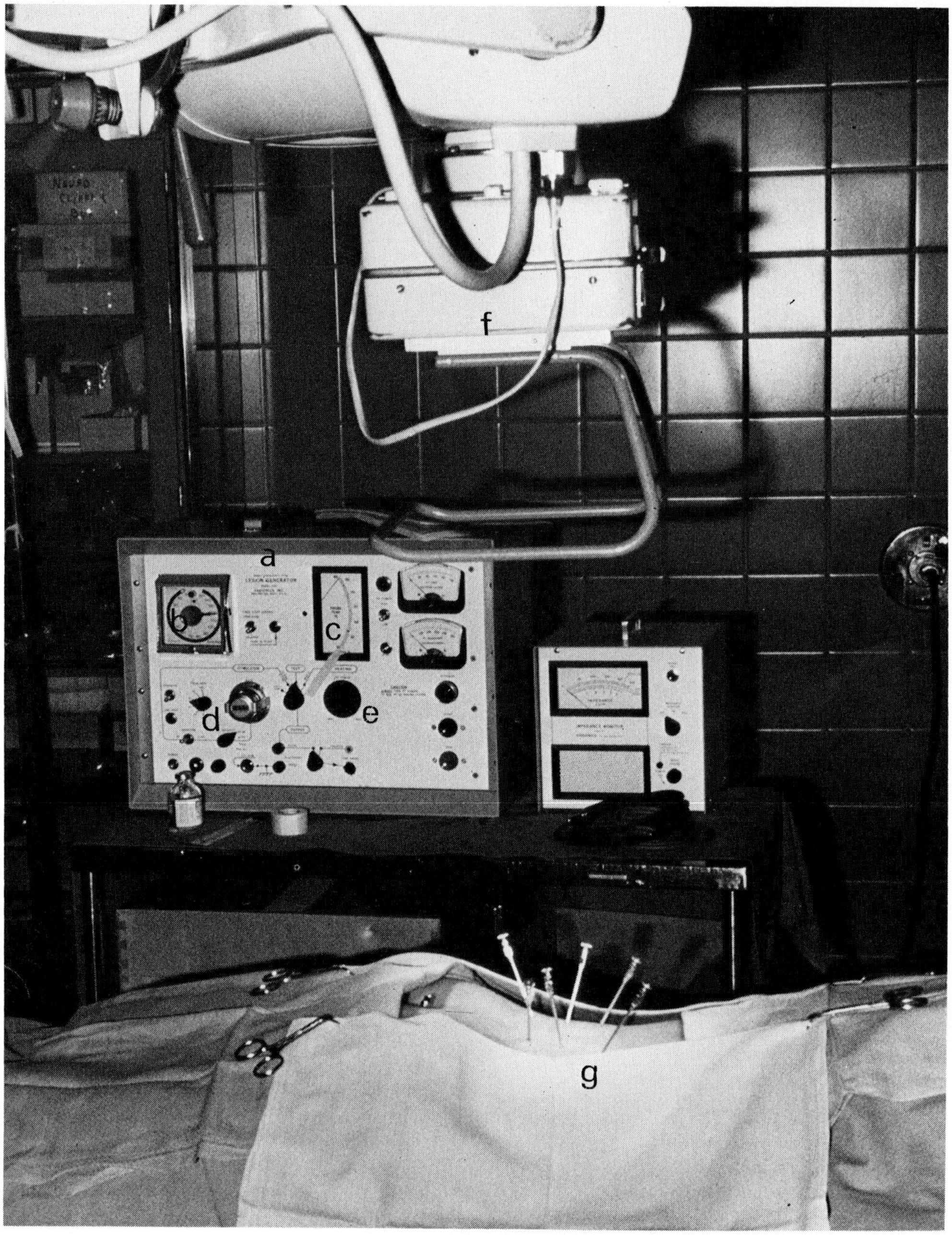

Fig. 33-2. Operative position for facet coagulation. Bilateral guide needles have been inserted. Note: a=lesion generator, b=timer, c=temperature gauge, d=stimulator controls, e=coagulation control, f=portable x-ray machine, g=patient with six 12-gauge needles in lumbar muscles.

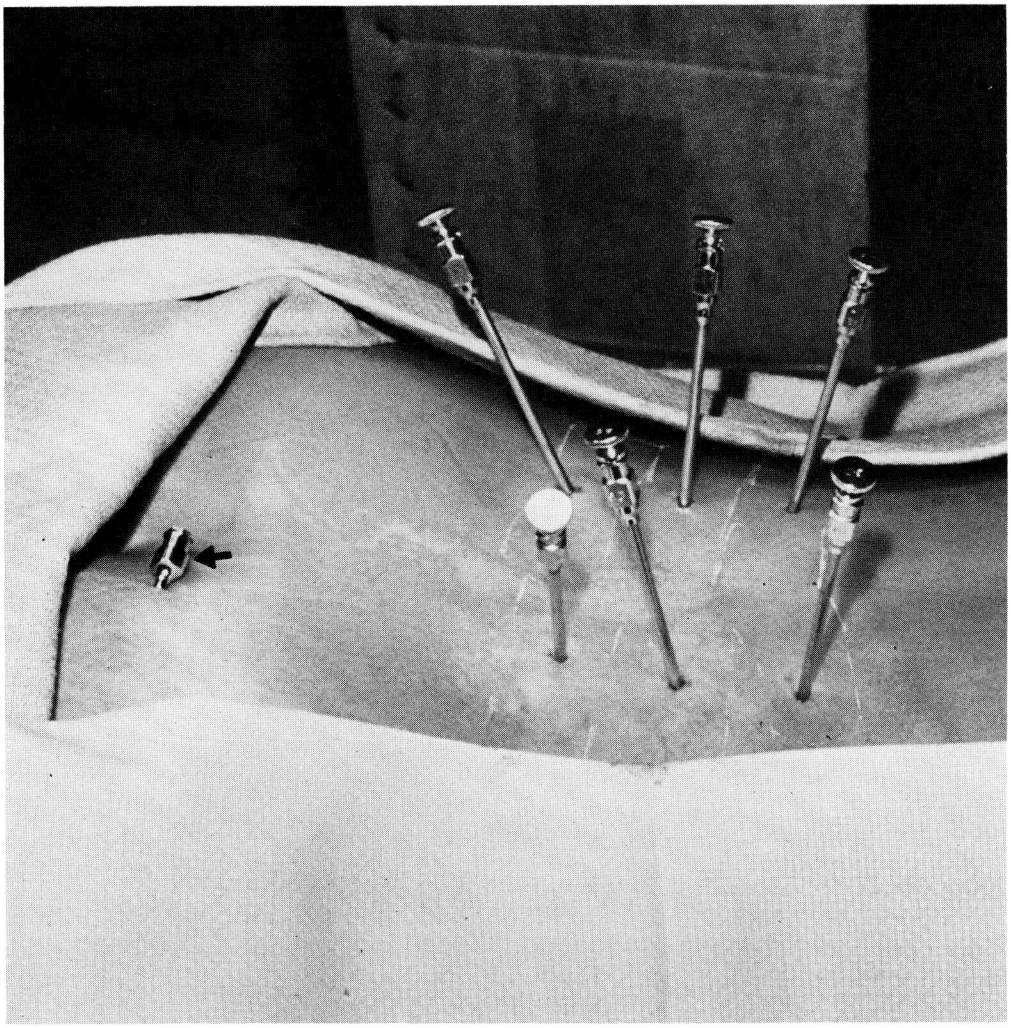

Fig. 33-3. Close-up of 12-gauge needles placed into lumbar muscles but not yet in final position. Arrow denotes 18-gauge spinal-needle ground electrode.

Skin wheals are raised by injecting 1% lidocaine and then an additional 2 ml of 1% lidocaine are placed about 1 inch deep into the lumbar paravertebral muscles at each of the puncture sites. Twelve-gauge, thin-wall needles, such as those supplied by Radionics in their Type SRK Facet Rhizotomy Kit, are used (Figs. 33-2 and 33-3). These are placed through the skin into the muscle and a posteroanterior radiograph taken (Figs. 33-2 and 33-4). Based on this film, the needles are advanced free-hand until they reach the facet joints or bone. Further adjustments of the needles are monitored by x-ray films, until the final target position is shown in the PA view (Figs. 33-1 and 33-4). A lateral radiograph is then taken, using a standard portable x-ray machine. In the correct position, the needle tips, on the lateral film, are not below the dorsum of the lumbosacral spinal canal (Fig. 33-5).

Once the needles are in correct position in both planes, a ground electrode is placed. I use an 18-gauge spinal needle, placed subcutaneously in the buttock, using 8 ml of 1% lidocaine. No complications have occurred from this maneuver. The ground is then attached to the radiofrequency lesion generator and the electrode, measuring 125 mm long, 1.6 mm in

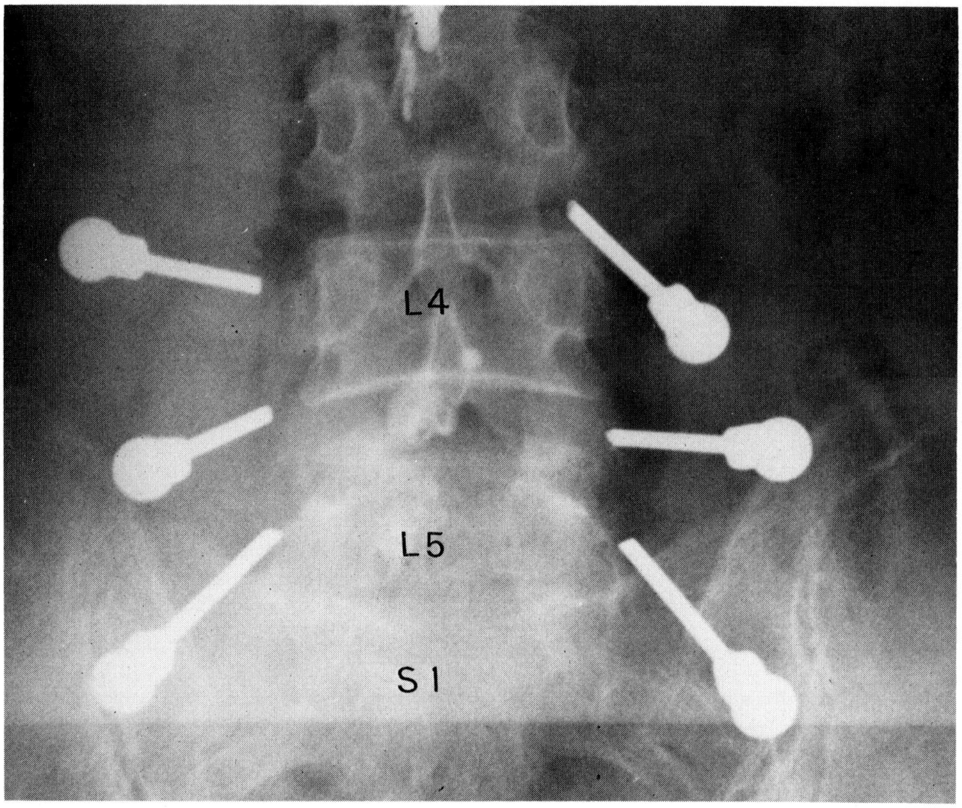

Fig. 33-4. Guide-needle placement for bilateral paravertebral neurectomy. Needles on the right are on target; needles on left require further adjustment medial at L3 and 4 and at L4 and 5 and downward at L5, S1. (Compare to Fig. 33-1.)

diameter, and exposed 7 mm distally, with a thermistor at the tip, is placed through the 12-gauge, thin-wall needle (Fig. 33-6). Provision must be made for temperature measurement, timing, and stimulation.

In bilateral procedures coagulation is completed on one side, beginning at the lowest level, and then performed in a similar fashion on the other side. All guide needles are placed and positioned before coagulation. If the pain is extremely low lumbar or only sacral, the L3-4 lesion is omitted. The electrode is placed through the needle to the intertransverse ligament and the guide needle is then removed 1.5 cm to expose the bared electrode tip at the target site (Fig. 33-6). Electrode stimulation with 50 cps, 1-msec duration current is used to find the threshold voltage. The voltage at which the patient first reports a sensory phenomenon is determined at least twice to be certain of the consistency of the threshold response. Stimulation is then increased slowly to 1 V to see whether or not the patient's pain can be reproduced. The machine is then set to single pulse and the voltage turned to 2.25 V. At least two single-short stimulations at this voltage level are administered as the patient's leg is watched to be sure that movement is not provoked. The patient's response is recorded. If the patient feels any sensation below the knee or there is any leg movement from this stimulation, the electrode is elevated 2 mm, and then the entire cycle of stimulation is repeated. In my experience, this has been totally effective in preventing injury to the root or anterior primary ramus.

Once stimulation is completed, the tip of the needle is heated to 80° for 2 minutes. During

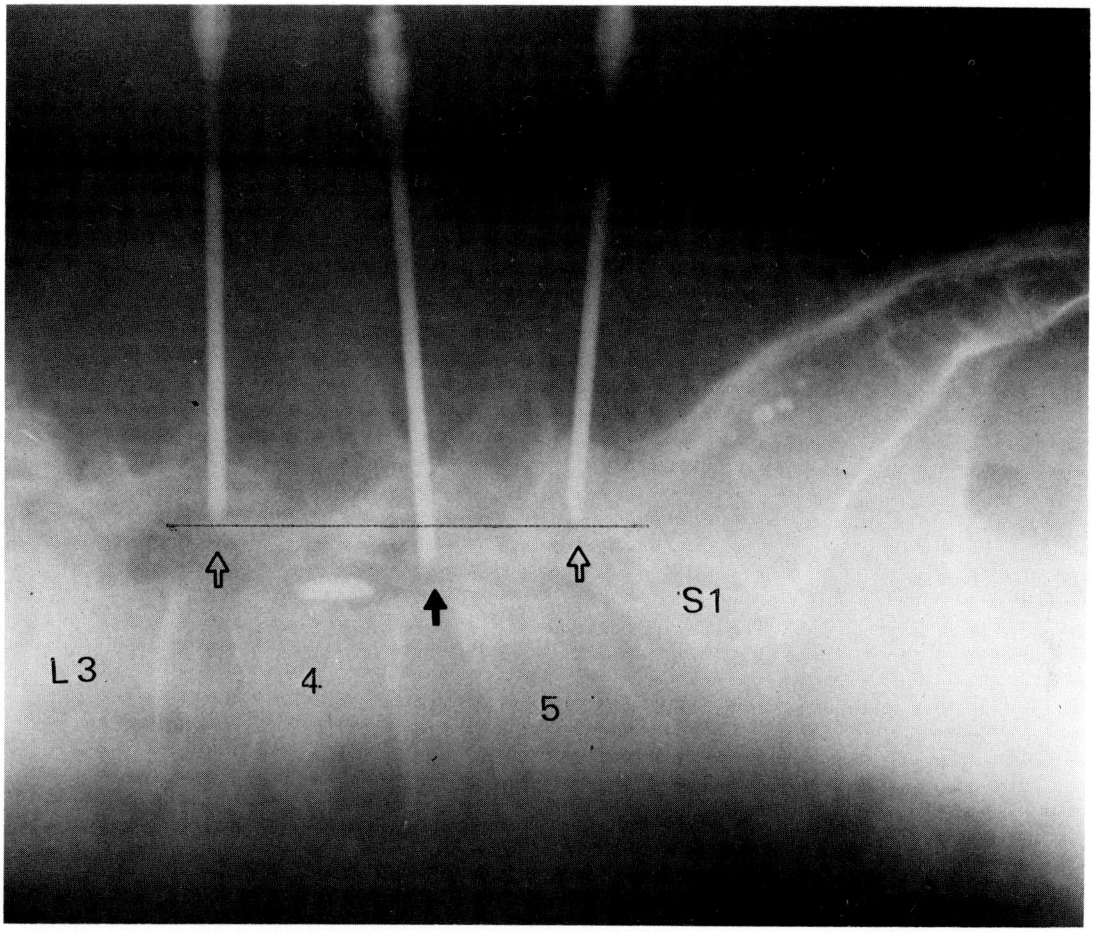

Fig. 33-5. Lateral radiograph illustrating correct depth at L3-4 and L5, S1 (open arrows). At L4-5 the tip is too deep and must be elevated (closed arrows). Solid line indicates dorsum of canal.

the heating, the patient is asked to relate his experience. If he has pain, he is asked to characterize its nature, severity, and location. If the patient's preoperative pain is reproduced during coagulation, it is an encouraging prognostic sign. Stimulation and heating are repeated at each level selected.

Once the coagulations are completed, the needles are removed from the facet joint regions, the ground electrode is removed, slight pressure is held over the needle puncture sites for 3 to 5 minutes, and then small dressings are applied. The patient is returned to his room and is allowed to eat and ambulate that day. By the following day, the patient is usually able to report accurately regarding pain relief, and discharge from the hospital is permitted.

Results and Discussion

Thirty-four facet coagulations have been performed on 27 patients who complained of backache, with or without leg pain. Nineteen females and 8 males, ranging in age from 20 to 81 years (mean of 50 years), comprise this series. Thirteen patients had bilateral and 14 had unilateral procedures. Three patients had repeat procedures.

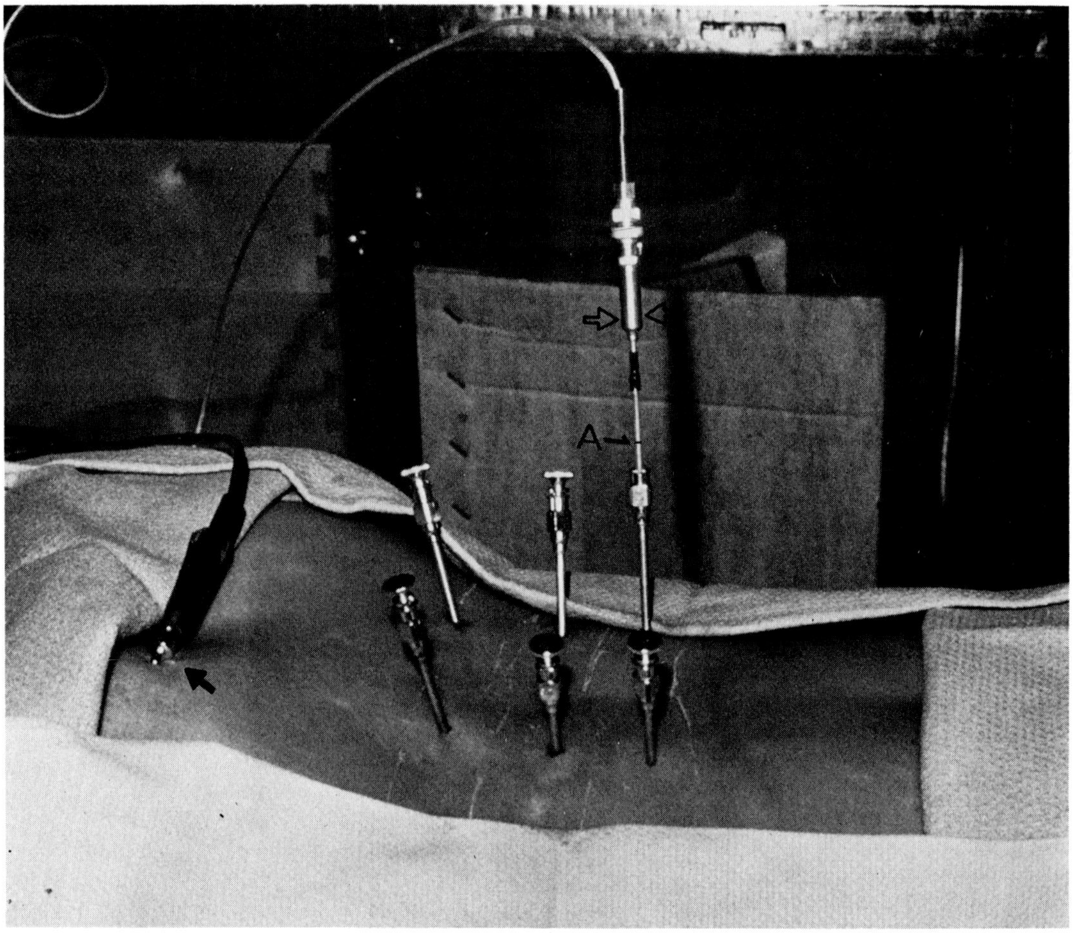

Fig. 33-6. Coagulation electrode in place at L3-4 on the patient's left (open arrows) and the ground wire is connected (closed arrow). Note other needles are now in final position (compare to Fig. 33-3). The guide needle must be elevated to Point A prior to coagulation to expose the electrode tip at the target point.

Table 33-1 lists the results by diagnostic category. The follow-up period was 12 to 36 months (mean equals 30) in 22 patients. The 5 patients who were followed for less than 1 year are marked with an asterisk in the table; of these, pain relief is excellent in 2 and poor in 3. Overall, 38% obtained excellent relief of pain; 18% are fair, with some pain relief; and 43% are poor, with little or no relief. Eliminating patients followed for less than 1 year yields 35% with excellent, 23% with fair, and 41% with poor results. These data may be compared to the results in 182 patients treated by Shealy[4] by lumbar coagulation in which 31% were excellent, 14% good, and 55% failures.

The one patient with a poor result post fusion deserves special mention. She has required six separate bilateral coagulations. Only the most recent procedure failed to relieve her pain, and this was done with fluoroscopy rather than portable radiographs. It is possible the targets were not as accurately located and, therefore, fluoroscopy is not recommended for final x-ray localization during actual coagulation. Stimulation is not as helpful in fusion patients either.

The 5 patients with unoperated lumbar discs all had poor results. Four have had further surgery and are improved. One is incapacitated from cardiac illness and has to live with his pain. It is apparent that facet coagulation should not be recommended as treatment for

Table 33-1. Results of Facet Coagulation for Low Back Pain

Diagnosis	Result: Excellent	Fair	Poor	Total No. of patients
Previous laminectomy–no fusion	3	3	3*	9
Previous laminectomy–with fusion	1*	0	1*	2
Lumbar disc–unoperated	0	0	5*	5
Lumbar spondylosis	3*	0	1	4
Spondylolisthesis	0	0	1	1
"Lumbosacral strain"	3	2	1	6
Totals	10(38%)	5(19%)	12(43%)	27(100%)

*represents one patient less than 1 year postoperative (See text also)

genuine ruptured lumbar disc syndrome. The 1 patient with spondylolisthesis who did poorly had had subsequent open spine surgery with improvement. If these 6 patients are excluded, the overall results would improve to 47% excellent, 23% fair, and 30% poor.

It is clear that facet coagulation is not a panacea. However, a significant number of patients with chronic low back pain have been relieved of their symptoms; none has been made worse, and there have been no complications. On this basis the technique is recommended for use by neurosurgeons in their daily efforts to ease the discomfort of low back pain.

REFERENCES

1. Mixter WJ, Barr JS: Rupture of the intervertebral disc with involvement of the spinal canal. *N Engl J Med 211*:210-215, 1934
2. Rees WES: Multiple bilateral subcutaneous rhizolysis of segmental nerves in the treatment of the intervertebral disc syndrome. *Am Gen Prac 26*:126-127, 1971
3. Shealy CN: Personal communication. Seminar on dorsal column stimulation, Temple University Health Sciences Center, September 23, 1972
4. Shealy CN: Percutaneous radiofrquency denervation of spinal facets. *J Neurosurg 43*:448-451, 1975
5. Fox JL, Rizzoli HV: Identification of radiologic coordinates for the posterior articular nerve of Luschka in the lumbar spine. *Surg Neurol 1*:343-346, 1973
6. Shealy CN, Prieto A, Burton C, et al: Radiofrequency percutaneous rhizotomy of the articular nerve of Luschka: an alternative approach to chronic low back pain and sciatica. Presented at the Annual Meeting of the American Association of Neurological Surgeons, Los Angeles, April 1973

INDEX

Page numbers in *italics* refer to illustrations; page numbers followed by t refer to tables.

a
b
c
d
7 e
8 f
9 g
0 h
1 i
8 2 j